T0226574

Lung Cancer

Guest Editors

LYNN T. TANOUE, MD
RICHARD A. MATTHAY, MD

CLINICS IN CHEST MEDICINE

www.chestmed.theclinics.com

December 2011 • Volume 32 • Number 4

SAUNDERS an imprint of ELSEVIER, Inc.

W.B. SAUNDERS COMPANY
A Division of Elsevier Inc.

1600 John F. Kennedy Boulevard ● Suite 1800 ● Philadelphia, Pennsylvania 19103

http://www.theclinics.com

CLINICS IN CHEST MEDICINE Volume 32, Number 4
December 2011 ISSN 0272-5231, ISBN-13: 978-1-4557-7981-9

Editor: Sarah E. Barth
Developmental Editor: Donald E. Mumford

© **2011 Elsevier Inc. All rights reserved.**

This journal and the individual contributions contained in it are protected under copyright by Elsevier, and the following terms and conditions apply to their use:

Photocopying
Single photocopies of single articles may be made for personal use as allowed by national copyright laws. Permission of the Publisher and payment of a fee is required for all other photocopying, including multiple or systematic copying, copying for advertising or promotional purposes, resale, and all forms of document delivery. Special rates are available for educational institutions that wish to make photocopies for non-profit educational classroom use. For information on how to seek permission visit www.elsevier.com/permissions or call: (+44) 1865 843830 (UK)/(+1) 215 239 3804 (USA).

Derivative Works
Subscribers may reproduce tables of contents or prepare lists of articles including abstracts for internal circulation within their institutions. Permission of the Publisher is required for resale or distribution outside the institution. Permission of the Publisher is required for all other derivative works, including compilations and translations (please consult www.elsevier.com/permissions).

Electronic Storage or Usage
Permission of the Publisher is required to store or use electronically any material contained in this journal, including any article or part of an article (please consult www.elsevier.com/permissions). Except as outlined above, no part of this publication may be reproduced, stored in a retrieval system or transmitted in any form or by any means, electronic, mechanical, photocopying, recording or otherwise, without prior written permission of the Publisher.

Notice
No responsibility is assumed by the Publisher for any injury and/or damage to persons or property as a matter of products liability, negligence or otherwise, or from any use or operation of any methods, products, instructions or ideas contained in the material herein. Because of rapid advances in the medical sciences, in particular, independent verification of diagnoses and drug dosages should be made.

Although all advertising material is expected to conform to ethical (medical) standards, inclusion in this publication does not constitute a guarantee or endorsement of the quality or value of such product or of the claims made of it by its manufacturer.

Clinics in Chest Medicine (ISSN 0272-5231) is published quarterly by Elsevier Inc., 360 Park Avenue South, New York, NY 10010-1710. Months of issue are March, June, September, and December. Periodicals postage paid at New York, NY and additional mailing offices. Subscription prices are $293.00 per year (domestic individuals), $475.00 per year (domestic institutions), $140.00 per year (domestic students/residents), $321.00 per year (Canadian individuals), $583.00 per year (Canadian institutions), $399.00 per year (international individuals), $583.00 per year (international institutions), and $195.00 per year (international and Canadian students/residents). International air speed delivery is included in all Clinics subscription prices. All prices are subject to change without notice. **POSTMASTER:** Send address changes to Clinics in Chest Medicine, Elsevier Health Sciences Division, Subscription Customer Service, 3251 Riverport Lane, Maryland Heights, MO 63043. **Customer Service: Telephone: 1-800-654-2452** (U.S. and Canada); **1-314-447-8871** (outside U.S. and Canada). **Fax: 1-314-447-8029. E-mail: journalscustomerservice-usa@elsevier.com** (for print support); **journalsonlinesupport-usa@elsevier.com** (for online support).

Reprints. For copies of 100 or more of articles in this publication, please contact the Commercial Reprints Department, Elsevier Inc., 360 Park Avenue South, New York, NY 10010-1710. Tel.: 212-633-3812; Fax: 212-462-1935; E-mail: reprints@elsevier.com.

Clinics in Chest Medicine is covered in *MEDLINE/PubMed (Index Medicus), Current Contents/Clinical Medicine, EMBASE/ Excerpta Medica, Science Citation Index,* and *ISI/BIOMED.*

Printed and bound by CPI Group (UK) Ltd, Croydon, CR0 4YY

Transferred to Digital Print 2011

Contributors

GUEST EDITORS

LYNN T. TANOUE, MD
Professor, Pulmonary and Critical Care
Medicine Section, Department of Internal
Medicine, Yale University School of Medicine,
New Haven, Connecticut

RICHARD A. MATTHAY, MD
Boehringer Ingelheim Emeritus Professor
of Medicine and Senior Research Scientist
in Medicine, Pulmonary and Critical Care
Medicine Section, Department of Internal
Medicine, Yale University School of Medicine,
New Haven, Connecticut

AUTHORS

STEVEN M. ALBELDA, MD
Professor of Medicine and Vice-Chief, Division
of Pulmonary, Allergy & Critical Care Medicine,
Department of Medicine, University of
Pennsylvania, Philadelphia, Pennsylvania

DANIEL J. BOFFA, MD
Assistant Professor, Thoracic Surgery, Yale
University School of Medicine, New Haven,
Connecticut

CHRIS T. BOLLIGER, MD, PhD
Division of Pulmonology, Department of
Medicine, University of Stellenbosch,
Tygerberg, Cape Town, South Africa

CHING-FEI CHANG, MD
Department of Medicine, Division of Pulmonary
and Critical Care Medicine, Keck School of
Medicine of University of Southern California,
Los Angeles, California

DAVID T. COOKE, MD
Assistant Professor, Associate Program
Director, Cardiothoracic Surgery Residency,
Division of Cardiothoracic Surgery, The
University of California, Davis Medical Center,
Sacramento, California

CHARLES S. DELA CRUZ, MD, PhD
Assistant Professor, Pulmonary and Critical
Care Medicine Section, Department of Internal
Medicine, Yale University School of Medicine,
New Haven, Connecticut

ROY H. DECKER, MD, PhD
Assistant Professor, Department of
Therapeutic Radiology, Yale University School
of Medicine, New Haven, Connecticut

CHADRICK E. DENLINGER, MD
Assistant Professor of Surgery, Division of
Surgery, Medical University of South Carolina,
Ashley River Tower, Charleston,
South Carolina

FRANK C. DETTERBECK, MD
Professor and Chief, Yale Thoracic Surgery,
Yale School of Medicine, New Haven,
Connecticut

JON O. EBBERT, MD
Professor of Medicine, College of Medicine,
Nicotine Dependence Center, Mayo Clinic,
Rochester, Minnesota

DAVID FELLER-KOPMAN, MD
Assistant Professor of Medicine,
Bronchoscopy and Interventional
Pulmonology, Division of Pulmonary and
Critical Care Medicine, Johns Hopkins
University, Johns Hopkins Hospital,
Baltimore, Maryland

SCOTT GETTINGER, MD
Associate Professor of Medicine, Division
of Medical Oncology, Yale University School
of Medicine, New Haven, Connecticut

MICHAEL K. GOULD, MD, MS
Department of Medicine, Keck School of
Medicine of University of Southern California;
Senior Research Scientist and Assistant
Director, Department of Research and
Evaluation, Kaiser Permanente Southern
California, Pasadena, California

MATTHEW A. GUBENS, MD
Assistant Clinical Professor, Thoracic
Oncology, University of California,
San Francisco, San Francisco, California

ANDREW R. HAAS, MD, PhD
Assistant Professor of Medicine, Division of
Pulmonary, Allergy & Critical Care Medicine,
Department of Medicine, University of
Pennsylvania, Philadelphia, Pennsylvania

J. TAYLOR HAYS, MD
Professor of Medicine, College of Medicine,
Nicotine Dependence Center, Mayo Clinic,
Rochester, Minnesota

ROBERT J. HOMER, MD, PhD
Associate Professor Internal Medicine
Pulmonary, and Professor, Department of
Pathology, Yale School of Medicine,
New Haven, Connecticut

RICHARD D. HURT, MD
Professor of Medicine, College of Medicine,
Nicotine Dependence Center, Mayo Clinic,
Rochester, Minnesota

ANTHONY W. KIM, MD
Assistant Professor, Section of Thoracic
Surgery, Department of Surgery, Yale School
of Medicine, New Haven, Connecticut

COENRAAD F.N. KOEGELENBERG, MD
Division of Pulmonology, Department of
Medicine, University of Stellenbosch,
Tygerberg, Cape Town, South Africa

JILL E. LARSEN, PhD
Hamon Center for Therapeutic Oncology
Research, Simmons Cancer Center, University
of Texas Southwestern Medical Center,
Dallas, Texas

THOMAS LYNCH, MD
Physician-in-Chief, Director, Professor of
Medicine, Division of Medical Oncology,
Yale University School of Medicine, Yale
Cancer Center, Smilow Cancer Hospital at
Yale-New Haven, New Haven, Connecticut

RICHARD A. MATTHAY, MD
Boehringer Ingelheim Emeritus Professor
of Medicine and Senior Research Scientist
in Medicine, Pulmonary and Critical Care
Medicine Section, Department of Internal
Medicine, Yale University School of Medicine,
New Haven, Connecticut

DAVID D. MCFADDEN, MD
Instructor in Medicine, College of Medicine,
Nicotine Dependence Center, Mayo Clinic,
Rochester, Minnesota

HIREN J. MEHTA, MD
Fellow, Division of Pulmonary and Critical Care
Medicine, Medical University of South
Carolina, Charleston, South Carolina

DAVID E. MIDTHUN, MD
Professor of Medicine, Division of Pulmonary
and Critical Care Medicine, Mayo Clinic,
Rochester, Minnesota

JOHN D. MINNA, MD
Hamon Center for Therapeutic Oncology
Research, Simmons Cancer Center, University
of Texas Southwestern Medical Center,
Dallas, Texas

EDMUND MOON, MD
Senior Fellow, Division of Pulmonary, Allergy &
Critical Care Medicine, University of
Pennsylvania, Philadelphia, Pennsylvania

JOEL W. NEAL, MD, PhD
Assistant Professor of Medicine, Stanford
Cancer Institute, Stanford University, Stanford,
California

LUCA PAOLETTI, MD
Pulmonary/Critical Care Fellow, Division
of Pulmonary and Critical Care Medicine,
Medical University of South Carolina,
Charleston, South Carolina

NICHOLAS J. PASTIS, MD
Assistant Professor of Medicine, Division of Pulmonary and Critical Care Medicine, Medical University of South Carolina, Charleston, South Carolina

JONATHAN PUCHALSKI, MD, MEd
Assistant Professor of Medicine, Division of Pulmonary and Critical Care Medicine, Yale University School of Medicine, New Haven, Connecticut

AFSHIN RASHTIAN, MD
Department of Radiation Oncology, Keck School of Medicine of University of Southern California, Los Angeles, California

M. PATRICIA RIVERA, MD, FCCP
Associate Professor of Medicine, Division of Pulmonary and Critical Care Medicine, Department of Medicine, University of North Carolina at Chapel Hill, Chapel Hill, North Carolina

CHRISTOPHER ROSS, MD
Resident, Department of Therapeutic Radiology, Yale University School of Medicine, New Haven, Connecticut

GERARD A. SILVESTRI, MD, MS
Professor of Medicine, Division of Pulmonary and Critical Care Medicine, Medical University of South Carolina, Charleston, South Carolina

DANIEL H. STERMAN, MD
Associate Professor of Medicine, Division of Pulmonary, Allergy & Critical Care Medicine, Department of Medicine, University of Pennsylvania, Philadelphia, Pennsylvania

LYNN T. TANOUE, MD
Professor, Pulmonary and Critical Care Medicine Section, Department of Internal Medicine, Yale University School of Medicine, New Haven, Connecticut

WILLIAM D. TRAVIS, MD
Attending Thoracic Pathologist, Department of Pathology, Memorial Sloan Kettering Cancer Center, New York, New York

ANIL VACHANI, MD
Assistant Professor of Medicine, Division of Pulmonary, Allergy & Critical Care Medicine, Department of Medicine, University of Pennsylvania, Philadelphia, Pennsylvania

FLORIAN VON GROOTE-BIDLINGMAIER, MD
Division of Pulmonology, Department of Medicine, University of Stellenbosch, Tygerberg, Cape Town, South Africa

ELLIOT WAKEAM, MD
Resident in Surgery, Department of Surgery, University of Toronto, Toronto, Ontario, Canada

HEATHER A. WAKELEE, MD
Assistant Professor of Medicine, Stanford Cancer Institute, Stanford University, Stanford, California

NICHOLAS J. PASTIS, MD
Assistant Professor of Medicine, Division of Pulmonary and Critical Care Medicine, Medical University of South Carolina, Charleston, South Carolina

JONATHAN PUCHALSKI, MD, MEd
Assistant Professor of Medicine, Division of Pulmonary and Critical Care Medicine, Yale University School of Medicine, New Haven, Connecticut

ARSHIN PARSHTHAN, MD
Department of Radiation Oncology, Keck School of Medicine of University of Southern California, Los Angeles, California

M. PATRICIA RIVERA, MD, FCCP
Associate Professor of Medicine, Division of Pulmonary and Critical Care Medicine, Department of Medicine, University of North Carolina at Chapel Hill, Chapel Hill, North Carolina

CHRISTOPHER ROSS, MD
Resident, Department of Therapeutic Radiology, Yale University School of Medicine, New Haven, Connecticut

GERARD A. SILVESTRI, MD, MS
Professor of Medicine, Division of Pulmonary and Critical Care Medicine, Medical University of South Carolina, Charleston, South Carolina

DANIEL H. STERMAN, MD
Associate Professor of Medicine, Division of Pulmonary, Allergy, & Critical Care Medicine, Department of Medicine, University of Pennsylvania, Philadelphia, Pennsylvania

LYNN T. TANOUE, MD
Professor, Pulmonary and Critical Care Medicine Section, Department of Internal Medicine, Yale University School of Medicine, New Haven, Connecticut

WILLIAM D. TRAVIS, MD
Attending Thoracic Pathologist, Department of Pathology, Memorial Sloan-Kettering Cancer Center, New York, New York

ANIL VACHANI, MD
Assistant Professor of Medicine, Division of Pulmonary, Allergy & Critical Care Medicine, Department of Medicine, University of Pennsylvania, Philadelphia, Pennsylvania

FLORIAN VON GROOTE-BIDLINGMAIER, MD
Division of Pulmonology, Department of Medicine, University of Stellenbosch, Tygerberg, Cape Town, South Africa

ELLIOT WAKEAM, MD
Resident in Surgery, Department of Surgery, University of Toronto, Toronto, Ontario, Canada

HEATHER A. WAKELEE, MD
Assistant Professor of Medicine, Stanford Cancer Institute, Stanford University, Stanford, California

Contents

> Lung cancer is the leading cause of cancer death in the United States and around the world. A vast majority of lung cancer deaths are attributable to cigarette smoking, and curbing the rates of cigarette smoking is imperative. Understanding the epidemiology and causal factors of lung cancer can provide additional foundation for disease prevention. This article focuses on modifiable risk factors, including tobacco smoking, occupational carcinogens, diet, and ionizing radiation. It also discusses briefly the molecular and genetic aspects of lung carcinogenesis.

> Tobacco use is a chronic medical disorder. Providing evidence-based treatment of tobacco-dependent patients is a challenge, and a team approach provides an efficient treatment model. Tobacco treatment specialists could expand the collective tobacco treatment expertise in the medical setting. Effective tobacco dependence treatment frequently requires tailoring and intensifying of interventions to meet the needs of the individual patient. Stopping smoking reduces the risk of lung cancer and many other cancers, cardiovascular disease, stroke, peripheral vascular disease. Treating tobacco dependence is one of the most cost-effective therapies in medicine and it deserves adequate reimbursement for it to be more widely available.

> The National Lung Screening Study has demonstrated that screening with low-dose spiral computed tomography results in fewer deaths from lung cancer compared with screening with chest radiography (CXR). Previous trials of screening with CXR and sputum cytology failed to exhibit fewer deaths compared with no screening intervention. Early computed tomography (CT) studies showed promise for CT to be a more sensitive test, yet were unable to demonstrate sufficient evidence of efficacy. This review examines the problem of early lung cancer detection, the issues presented by screening, and results of past and recent studies of lung cancer screening.

> This article reviews current concepts in pathologic classification of lung cancer based on the 2004 World Health Organization classification of lung tumors and the 2011 International Association for the Study of Lung Cancer (IASLC)/American Thoracic Society (ATS)/European Respiratory Society (ERS) classification of lung

adenocarcinoma. Preinvasive lesions are discussed. The major changes in lung disease diagnosis affected by the IASLC/ATS/ERS classification are presented. For adenocarcinomas diagnosed in small biopsies, specific terminology and diagnostic criteria are proposed along with recommendations for strategic management of tissue and EGFR mutation testing in patients with advanced adenocarcinoma. Histologic criteria are also presented for other tumors.

It has been proposed that invasive carcinoma of the bronchus develops through a transition from preinvasive lesions to overt malignancy. Newer diagnostic technologies have provided a more sensitive way to diagnose preinvasive lesions and a better understanding of the prevalence of such lesions. The natural history of preinvasive lesions has not been well defined; however, there is evidence that high-grade lesions are at a higher risk of progression to carcinoma. Molecular alterations have been described in preinvasive lesions and may help better predict which lesions will progress. Several noninvasive techniques are available for the treatment of high-grade lesions.

Lung cancer is a heterogeneous disease clinically, biologically, histologically, and molecularly. Understanding the molecular causes of this heterogeneity, which might reflect changes occurring in different classes of epithelial cells or different molecular changes occurring in the same target lung epithelial cells, is the focus of current research. Identifying the genes and pathways involved, determining how they relate to the biological behavior of lung cancer, and their utility as diagnostic and therapeutic targets are important basic and translational research issues. This article reviews current information on the key molecular steps in lung cancer pathogenesis, their timing, and clinical implications.

The revised stage classification system has improved the ability of clinicians to estimate prognosis based on specific staging determinations. Several important questions have been addressed, although many remain and will likely fuel the discussion for subsequent revisions. Perhaps more than previous revisions, the current iteration may cause confusion because of the emphasis on stage-specific treatment recommendations. However, prognosis is only 1 of the factors in a multidisciplinary treatment plan, and clinicians are encouraged to apply randomized trial data whenever possible. This global staging effort is testament to the progress that is possible through international collaboration.

This article discusses the potential benefits and limitations of positron emission tomography (PET) for characterizing lung nodules, staging the mediastinum, identifying occult distant metastasis, determining prognosis and treatment response, guiding plans for radiation therapy, restaging during and after treatment, and selecting targets for tissue sampling. The key findings from the medical literature are presented regarding the capabilities and fallibilities of PET in lung cancer evaluation, including characterization of pulmonary nodules and staging in patients with known or suspected non–small-cell lung cancer. The discussion is limited to PET imaging with fluorodeoxyglucose.

Diagnostic and therapeutic strategies for lung cancer have improved with advancing technology and the acquisition of the necessary skills by bronchoscopists to fully use these advanced techniques. The diagnostic yield for lung cancer has significantly increased with the advent of technologies such as endobronchial ultrasound, navigational systems, and improved imaging modalities. Similarly, the therapeutic benefit of bronchoscopy in advanced lung cancer has begun to be understood for its impact on quality and quantity of life. This article highlights the pulmonologists' diagnostic advances and therapeutic options, with an emphasis on outcomes.

Lung cancer is the leading cause of cancer-related death worldwide, and lung resection remains the only curative approach. In the Western world, lung cancer is one of the main indications for lung resection, despite only 15% to 25% of all lung cancers being operable at the time of presentation. In most cases of operable lung cancer, a substantial part of functional lung tissue has to be resected, leading to a permanent loss of pulmonary function. Resection in patients with insufficient pulmonary reserves can result in permanent respiratory disability. This article reviews the current standards of preoperative assessment.

Standard therapy for early-stage non–small cell lung cancer is lobectomy for patients who are able to tolerate such surgery. However, the risk of postoperative morbidity is not trivial, with a 30% to 40% incidence of postoperative complications and a 1% to 5% incidence of operative mortality. Some patients, though technically resectable, refuse surgery or are considered medically inoperable because of insufficient respiratory reserve, cardiovascular disease, or general frailty. This group is considered either "high risk" or "medically inoperable."

The detection of ground-glass opacity (GGO) is increasingly common. Sufficient data have been accumulated to formulate recommendations for observation, intervention, and treatment modalities. However, an understanding of many nuances and uncertainties in the available data is needed to avoid making management errors. This article discusses the range of possible entities, risk factors and characteristics that help make a presumptive clinical diagnosis, how often and for how long these should be followed when and how a biopsy should be done, how these lesions should be treated, and how multifocal GGOs should be approached.

Both advanced-stage lung cancer and malignant pleural mesothelioma are associated with a poor prognosis. Advances in treatment regimens for both diseases have had only a modest effect on their progressive course. Gene therapy for thoracic malignancies represents a novel therapeutic approach and has been evaluated in several clinical trials. Strategies have included induction of apoptosis, tumor suppressor gene replacement, suicide gene expression, cytokine-based therapy, various vaccination approaches, and adoptive transfer of modified immune cells. This review considers the clinical results, limitations, and future directions of gene therapy trials for thoracic malignancies.

Clinics in Chest Medicine

THE CLINICS ARE NOW AVAILABLE ONLINE!

Access your subscription at:
www.theclinics.com

Preface

Carcinoma of the lung is one of the most prevalent and aggressive types of cancer. It is the leading cause of cancer death in the United States and worldwide. Siegel and colleagues at the American Cancer Society estimated that in 2011 in the United States there would be 221,130 new cases of lung cancer and 156,940 deaths from lung cancer. Fortunately, however, lung cancer death rates in women in the United States decreased for the first time during the years 2003 to 2007, more than a decade after decreasing in men.

Cigarette smoking is the leading cause of lung cancer, with more than 85% of cases being caused by cigarette smoking. Approximately 94 million Americans are current or former smokers. Fifty percent of lung cancer is found in formers smokers. In Europe, Asia, and many undeveloped countries, smoking rates remain high or have even increased. Throughout Asia, cigarette smoking among women, once taboo, is becoming more prevalent.

Three previous issues of *Clinics in Chest Medicine* (1982, 1993, and 2002) were devoted to lung cancer. This issue contains 17 articles by 43 authors from 12 institutions. Nine of the current authors also contributed to the 2002 issue—Drs Albelda, Bolliger, Ebbert, Hurt, Lynch, Matthay, Minna, Tanoue, and Travis. As guest editors, we have selected articles highlighting recent advances in lung cancer epidemiology, etiology, prevention, screening, pathology, molecular biology, staging, diagnosis, and treatment. In the first article, Drs Dela Cruz, Tanoue, and Matthay extensively review the epidemiology, etiology, and prevention of lung cancer. They focus on such etiologic factors as tobacco and other environmental exposures, genetic predisposition, gender, race, ethnicity, and age. In the next article, Dr Hurt and colleagues discuss the neurobiology of nicotine dependence, review pharmacologic therapy for tobacco dependence, and challenge clinicians to learn to recognize and treat nicotine dependence. In the following article, Dr Midthun details the recent positive results of the National Cancer Institute—sponsored trial of screening for lung cancer and discusses the study's implications for clinicians.

In an update on the pathology of lung cancer, Dr Travis highlights the ASLC/ATS/ERS Lung Adenocarcinoma Classification published in 2011 and provides a detailed overview of the current concepts in pathologic classification of lung cancer.

Dr Rivera focuses on preinvasive lesions of the bronchus. She elucidates their prevalence and natural history, their distinctive genetic alterations, and techniques for diagnosing and treating these premalignant lesions. Drs Larsen and Minna extensively review the state of the art in the biology of lung cancer and its clinical implications. They emphasize the clinical, biological, histological, and molecular heterogeneity of lung cancer. Their review brings readers up to date on the current understanding of the molecular causes of this heterogeneity. They outline multiple significant genetic alterations known to be involved in the initiation and/or progression of lung cancer. Continued development of targeted therapies for lung cancer depends on increased understanding of involved molecules and pathways.

Dr Boffa discusses in detail the 7th revised edition of the American Joint Committee on Cancer lung cancer stage classification, the result of a global staging project organized through the International Assocation for the Study of Lung Cancer. This revised staging classification refines clinicians' ability to estimate prognosis based on specific T, N, M staging determination.

Drs Chang, Rashtian, and Gould summarize the capabilities and limitations of positron emission tomography in lung cancer evaluation. Next, the current status of interventional pulmonology in the diagnosis and therapy of lung cancer is detailed by Drs Puchalski and Feller-Kopman. They clarify the role of endobronchial ultrasound, esophageal ultrasound, and electromagnetic navigation, respectively, for diagnosing and staging this disease. In addition, they cover therapeutic modalities, including topical therapies, such as laser, electrocautery, argon plasma coagulation, cryotherapy, brachytherapy, and photodynamic therapy, as well as airway stenting.

Many patients with lung cancer are not candidates for lung resection because of such underlying comorbidities as chronic obstructive pulmonary disease and cardiovascular diseases. Drs Von Groote-Bidlingmaier, Koegelenberg, and Bolliger outline the appropriate functional evaluation of patients before lung resection.

The final seven articles in this symposium address treatment of lung cancer. Dr Mehta and colleagues discuss treatment options for high-risk patients with early-stage lung cancer, focusing primarily on surgical options and

Clin Chest Med 32 (2011) xiii–xiv
doi:10.1016/j.ccm.2011.08.016
0272-5231/11/$ – see front matter © 2011 Elsevier Inc. All rights reserved.

radiation therapy, including stereotactic body radiotherapy (SBRT). Drs Detterbeck and Homer outline a systematic approach to ground glass nodules noted on the chest radiograph and/or chest CT scan. Drs Kim and Cooke elucidate the controversies and challenges in managing additional pulmonary nodules in patients with lung cancer. Dr Paoletti and colleagues summarize advances in treatment of early-stage lung cancer, including video-assisted thoracoscopic surgery, SBRT, and radiofrequency ablation. Drs Gettinger and Lynch discuss impressive advances in treatment of advanced-stage non-small cell lung cancer, including chemotherapy and such molecularly targeted agents as epidermal growth factor receptor and anaplastic lymphoma kinase inhibitors. Drs Neal, Gubens, and Wakelee review advances in the management of small-cell lung cancer (SCLC), pointing out that despite numerous clinical trials and excellent responses to first-line chemotherapy, there have been few substantial clinical advances in the treatment of extensive-stage SCLC over the past 30 years. Dr Vachani and colleagues conclude this symposium with a review of the clinical results, limitations, and future directions of gene therapy trials for thoracic malignancies.

We are deeply grateful to all of the contributors to this symposium, to Chuck Rossi for editorial assistance, and to Sarah Barth at Elsevier for her invaluable guidance and assistance.

This issue is dedicated to the outstanding clinician-academician Dorothy A. White, MD.

Lynn T. Tanoue, MD
Pulmonary and Critical Care Medicine Section
Department of Internal Medicine
Yale University School of Medicine
200 South Frontage Road, LCI 106A
New Haven, CT 06510, USA

Richard A. Matthay, MD
Pulmonary and Critical Care Medicine Section
Department of Internal Medicine
Yale University School of Medicine
200 South Frontage Road, LCI 105E
New Haven, CT 06510, USA

E-mail addresses:
lynn.tanoue@yale.edu (L.T. Tanoue)
Richard.matthay@yale.edu (R.A. Matthay)

Dedication

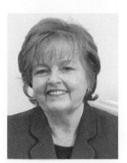

Dorothy A. White, MD

We dedicate this issue of *Clinics in Chest Medicine* to our friend and colleague, the outstanding physician and educator, Dorothy A. White, M.D. (1943–2010). Dr White received her medical degree at SUNY Downstate in 1977, followed by residency in internal medicine at New York Hospital (1977–1980). She was Chief Medical Resident at Memorial Sloan-Kettering Cancer Center in New York City (1980–1981) before training in Pulmonary and Critical Care Medicine at Yale-New Haven Hospital (1982–1984). From 1984 until her death in 2010, Dr White was an attending physician at Memorial Hospital and a faculty member of the Weill Medical College of Cornell University where she was appointed Professor of Medicine in 2001.

Dr White was an international authority on pulmonary disease in the immunocompromised host. Her important contributions in this field spanned pulmonary complications related to cancer, transplantation, and HIV/AIDS. Her work included expertise in drug-induced lung disease and in 1986 she and her colleagues published a sentinel article on this subject in the *American Review of Respiratory Disease*. Dr White was also a leader in education in pulmonary medicine, serving as a member of the Pulmonary Section of the American Board of Internal Medicine (ABIM) from 2000–2006.

Dr White was an outstanding clinician who paid exquisite attention to detail and had extraordinary skills in caring for patients. She was a gifted teacher and mentor for trainees at Memorial Hospital. We will miss her wit, humor, and sharp clinical acumen, and are grateful for her inspiring example as the consummate pulmonary physician.

Lynn T. Tanoue, MD

Richard A. Matthay, MD

Clin Chest Med 32 (2011) xv
doi:10.1016/j.ccm.2011.08.015
0272-5231/11/$ – see front matter © 2011 Elsevier Inc. All rights reserved.

Lung Cancer: Epidemiology, Etiology, and Prevention

Charles S. Dela Cruz, MD, PhD[a],*, Lynn T. Tanoue, MD[b],
Richard A. Matthay, MD[c]

KEYWORDS

• Lung cancer • Tobacco smoking • Epidemiology
• Carcinogens

EPIDEMIOLOGY OF LUNG CANCER

Lung cancer is the leading cause of cancer death in the United States and around the world. Almost as many Americans die of lung cancer every year than die of prostate, breast, and colon cancer combined (**Fig. 1**).[1] Siegel and colleagues[1] reviewed recent cancer data and estimated a total of 239,320 new cases of lung cancer and 161,250 deaths from lung cancer in the United States in 2010.[2] The statistics reflect data from 2007 and, therefore, likely underestimate the current lung cancer burden. Lung cancer has been the most common cancer worldwide since 1985, both in terms of incidence and mortality. Globally, lung cancer is the largest contributor to new cancer diagnoses (1,350,000 new cases and 12.4% of total new cancer cases) and to death from cancer (1,180,000 deaths and 17.6% of total cancer deaths). The 5-year survival rate in the United States for lung cancer is 15.6%, and although there has been some improvement in survival during the past few decades, the survival advances that have been realized in other common malignancies have yet to be achieved in lung cancer. There has been a large relative increase in the numbers of cases of lung cancer in developing countries. Approximately half (49.9%) of the cases now occur in developing countries whereas in 1980, 69% of cases were in developed countries. The estimated numbers of lung cancer cases worldwide has increased by 51% since 1985 (a 44% increase in men and a 76% increase in women). In the United States, cancer of the lung and bronchus ranks second in both genders, with an estimated 115,060 new cases in men (14% of all new cancers) and 106,070 in women (14% of all new cancers).[1,2] The age-adjusted incidence rate of lung cancer is 62 per 100,000 men and women per year in the United States, with the incidence rate higher in men than in women (75.2 vs 52.3 per 100,000).[3] Lung cancer in both genders tops the list on the number of estimated deaths yearly (85,600, or 28% of all cancer deaths for men, and 71,340, or 26% of all cancer deaths for women) (**Fig. 2**).

Lung cancer incidence in men in the United States has been decreasing since the early 1980s. The incidence and mortality rates for lung cancer tend to mirror one another because most patients diagnosed with lung cancer eventually die of it. Siegel and colleagues,[1] in their review of cancer statistics in 2011, noted decreases in death rates from lung cancer in men by 2.0% per year

a Pulmonary and Critical Care Medicine Section, Department of Internal Medicine, Yale University School of Medicine, 300 Cedar Street, TAC S441-C, New Haven, CT 06519, USA
b Pulmonary and Critical Care Medicine Section, Department of Internal Medicine, Yale University School of Medicine, 200 South Frontage Road, LCI 106A, New Haven, CT 06510, USA
c Pulmonary and Critical Care Medicine Section, Department of Internal Medicine, Yale University School of Medicine, 200 South Frontage Road, LCI 105E, New Haven, CT 06510, USA
* Corresponding author.
E-mail address: Charles.delacruz@yale.edu

Clin Chest Med 32 (2011) 605–644
doi:10.1016/j.ccm.2011.09.001
0272-5231/11/$ – see front matter © 2011 Elsevier Inc. All rights reserved.

chestmed.theclinics.com

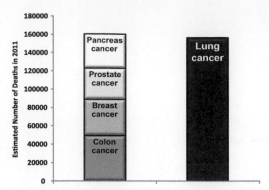

Fig. 1. Estimated deaths from lung cancer compared with colon cancer, breast cancer, prostate cancer, and pancreatic cancer combined. (*Data from* Siegel R, Ward E, Brawley O, et al. Cancer statistics, 2011: the impact of eliminating socioeconomic and racial disparities on premature cancer deaths. CA Cancer J Clin 2011;61(4):212–36.)

from 1994 to 2006 (**Fig. 3**). In women, however, lung cancer death rates continued to increase by 0.3% per year from 1995 to 2005, but more recent data from 2003 to 2006 show a more encouraging trend with a start in decline of 0.9% per year (see **Figs. 3** and **4**). The lung cancer incidence among women has declined over the past decades, from 5.6% between 1975 and 1982, to 3.4% between 1982 and 1990, to 0.4% between 1991 and 2006, and more recently to –2.3% between 2006 and 2008 (see **Fig. 4**). Because of the change in lung cancer incidence in women, recent figures show that lung cancer death rates decreased in women for the first time, more than a decade after decreases in men.[4] The lag in the decline of lung cancer rates in women compared with men has been attributed to the fact that cigarette smoking in women peaked two decades later than in men. Lung cancer mortality rates thus seem to be reaching a plateau, which is an encouraging change from the steep rise in the 1970s (see **Fig. 3**).

The Surveillance, Epidemiology and End Results (SEER) data from 2004 to 2008 reported the median age at diagnosis for cancer of the lung and bronchus as 71 years (**Fig. 5**). No cases were diagnosed in patients younger than 20 years (see **Fig. 5**).[3] Approximately 0.2% of lung cancers was diagnosed in patients between age 20 and 34 years; 1.5% between 35 and 44 years; 8.8% between 45 and 54 years; 20.9% between 55 and 64 years; 31.1% between 65 and 74 years; 29% between 75 and 84 years; and 8.3% at 85 years and older.

Lung cancer arises from the cells of the respiratory epithelium and can be divided into two broad categories. Small cell lung cancer (SCLC) is a highly malignant tumor derived from cells exhibiting neuroendocrine characteristics and accounts for 15% of lung cancer cases. Non–small cell lung cancer (NSCLC), which accounts for the remaining 85% of cases, is further divided into 3 major pathologic subtypes: adenocarcinoma, squamous cell carcinoma, and large cell carcinoma. Adenocarcinoma by itself accounts for 38.5% of all lung cancer cases, with squamous cell carcinoma accounting for 20% and large cell carcinoma accounting for 2.9%.[3,5] In the past several decades, the incidence of adenocarcinoma has increased greatly, and adenocarcinoma has replaced squamous cell carcinoma as the most prevalent type of NSCLC. The 5-year total survival rate for lung cancer in the United States from 2001 to 2007 was 15.6%. Patients with localized disease at diagnosis have a 5-year survival rate of 52%; however, the more than 52% of patients with distant metastasis at diagnosis have a dismal 5-year survival rate of 3.6%, which begs for the need for better screening methods to detect early-stage cancers (**Fig. 6**). (See article elsewhere in this issue by Mithun.)

Lung cancer was the most commonly diagnosed cancer and the leading cause of cancer death in men in 2008 globally.[2] For women, lung cancer was the fourth most commonly diagnosed cancer and the second leading cause of cancer death. Overall, lung cancer accounted for 13% or 1.6 million of total cancer cases and 18% or 1.4 million cancer-related deaths worldwide in 2008. Lung cancer incidence and mortality rates are highest in the United States and the developed countries. In contrast, lung cancer rates in underdeveloped geographic areas, including Central America and most of Africa, are lower, except the rates are slowly increasing (**Fig. 7A**). More developed countries have higher incidence and mortality rates from lung cancers in both genders than less developed countries (see **Fig. 7B, C**). The World Health Organization estimates that lung cancer deaths worldwide will continue to rise, largely as a result of an increase in global tobacco use, especially in Asia. Tobacco use is the principal risk factor for lung cancer, and a large proportion of all pulmonary carcinomas are attributable to the effects of cigarette smoking.[6] Despite efforts to curb tobacco smoking, there are approximately 1.1 billion smokers worldwide, and if the current trends continue, that number would increase to 1.9 billion by 2025.[7] As of 2008, 20.6% (46.0 million) of American adults smoke.[8] Of these, 79.8% (36.7 million) smoke every day and 20.2% (9.3 million) smoke some days. During the past decade, there has been a 3.5% point

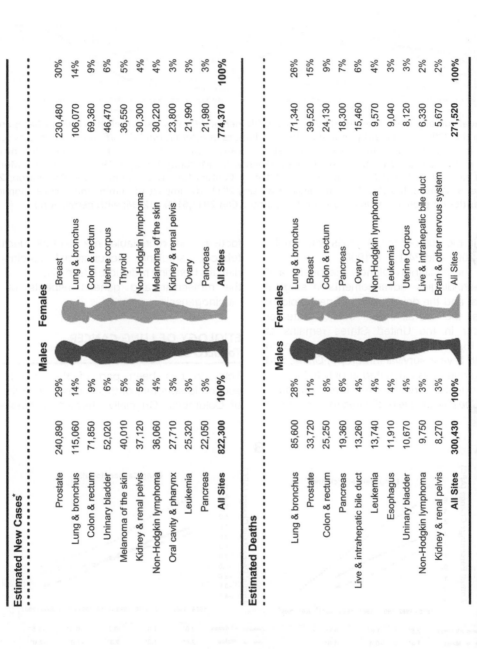

Estimated New Cases*

	Males			Females	
Prostate	240,890	29%	Breast	230,480	30%
Lung & bronchus	115,060	14%	Lung & bronchus	106,070	14%
Colon & rectum	71,850	9%	Colon & rectum	69,360	9%
Urinary bladder	52,020	6%	Uterine corpus	46,470	6%
Melanoma of the skin	40,010	5%	Thyroid	36,550	5%
Kidney & renal pelvis	37,120	5%	Non-Hodgkin lymphoma	30,300	4%
Non-Hodgkin lymphoma	36,060	4%	Melanoma of the skin	30,220	4%
Oral cavity & pharynx	27,710	3%	Kidney & renal pelvis	23,800	3%
Leukemia	25,320	3%	Ovary	21,990	3%
Pancreas	22,050	3%	Pancreas	21,980	3%
All Sites	**822,300**	**100%**	**All Sites**	**774,370**	**100%**

Estimated Deaths

	Males			Females	
Lung & bronchus	85,600	28%	Lung & bronchus	71,340	26%
Prostate	33,720	11%	Breast	39,520	15%
Colon & rectum	25,250	8%	Colon & rectum	24,130	9%
Pancreas	19,360	6%	Pancreas	18,300	7%
Live & intrahepatic bile duct	13,260	4%	Ovary	15,460	6%
Leukemia	13,740	4%	Non-Hodgkin lymphoma	9,570	4%
Esophagus	11,910	4%	Leukemia	9,040	3%
Urinary bladder	10,670	4%	Uterine Corpus	8,120	3%
Non-Hodgkin lymphoma	9,750	3%	Live & intrahepatic bile duct	6,330	2%
Kidney & renal pelvis	8,270	3%	Brain & other nervous system	5,670	2%
All Sites	**300,430**	**100%**	**All Sites**	**271,520**	**100%**

Fig. 2. Ten leading cancer types for the estimated new cancer cases and deaths categorized by gender. (*From* Siegel R, Ward E, Brawley O, et al. Cancer statistics, 2011: the impact of eliminating socioeconomic and racial disparities on premature cancer deaths. CA Cancer J Clin 2011;61(4):212–36; with permission.)

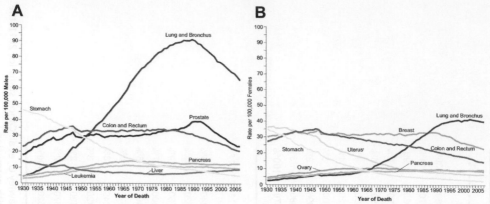

Fig. 3. Annual age-adjusted cancer death rates among (*A*) men and (*B*) women for selected cancers. Rates are age adjusted to the 2000 US standard population. Due to changes in *International Classification of Diseases* coding, numerator information has changed over time. Rates for cancers of the uterus, ovary, lung and bronchus, and colon and rectum are affected by these changes. (*Source*: US Mortality Volumes 1930 to 1959, US Mortality Data, 1960 to 2007. National Center for Health Statistics, Centers for Disease Control and Prevention; 2006.) (*From* Siegel R, Ward E, Brawley O, et al. Cancer statistics, 2011: the impact of eliminating socioeconomic and racial disparities on premature cancer deaths. CA Cancer J Clin 2011;61(4):212–36; with permission.)

decrease in the number of US adults who smoke (20.6% in 2008 and 24.1% in 1998).

Despite the availability of new diagnostic and genetic technologies, advancements in surgical techniques, and the development of new biologic treatments, the overall 5-year survival rate for lung cancer in the United States remains at a dismal 15.6%.[9] The situation globally is even worse, with 5-year survival in Europe, China, and developing countries estimated at only 8.9%.

This introductory article to the current edition of *Clinics in Chest Medicine* dedicated to lung cancer

focuses on modifiable risk factors, including tobacco smoking, occupational carcinogens, diet, and ionizing radiation. It also discusses briefly the molecular and genetic aspects of lung carcinogenesis.

ETIOLOGY OF LUNG CANCER
Tobacco Smoking

Tobacco has been part of the cultural and economic structure of this country since the time of Columbus. Originally chewed or smoked in

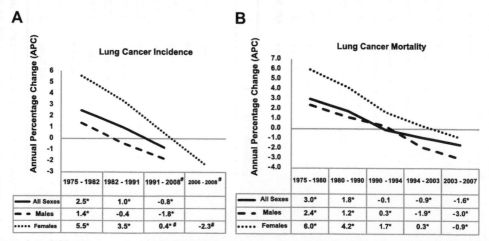

Fig. 4. Trends in (*A*) lung cancer incidence and (*B*) lung cancer mortality rates in the United States as evaluated by the annual percentage change (APC). A negative APC value means that the trend is a decrease; a positive APC value refers to an increase trend. Asterisk refers to statistically significant APC value; # refers to the APC value of 0.5 for women for the period 1991–2006; and the APC trend value of −2.3 refers to the period 2006–2008. (*Data from* Howlander N, Noone A, Krapcho M, et al. Cancer of the lung and bronchus [invasive]. In: Institute NC, editor. SEER Cancer Statistics Review 1975–2008; 2011.)

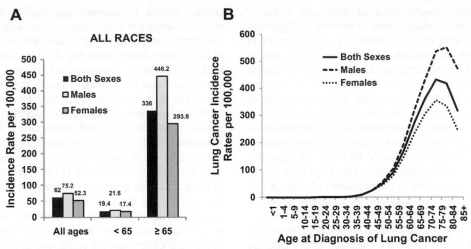

Fig. 5. US age-adjusted lung cancer incidence by gender, age, and race. (*A*) Separated by age <65 years and age ≥65 years. (*B*) Separated by age from <1 to 85+ years. Rates are per 100,000 and are age-adjusted to the 2000 US standard population. (*Data from* Howlader N, Noone AM, Krapcho M, et al, editors. SEER Cancer Statistics Review, 1975–2008. Bethesda (MD): National Cancer Institute; 2010. Available at: http://seer.cancer.gov/csr/1975_2008/, based on November 2010 SEER data submission, posted to the SEER web site, 2011.)

pipes, tobacco became widely available in cigarette form after the development of cigarette wrapping machinery in the mid-1800s. Before World War I, cigarette use in the United States was modest. Wynder and Graham estimated that the average adult smoked fewer than 100 cigarettes per year in 1900.[10] Fifty years later, this number rose to approximately 3500 cigarettes per person per year and reached a maximum of approximately 4400 cigarettes per person per year in the mid-1960s (**Fig. 8**).[11] In 1964, the US Public Health Service published a landmark report from the Surgeon General on smoking and its effects on health.[12] That seminal report stated the following important principal findings. (1) Cigarette smoking was associated with a 70% increase in the

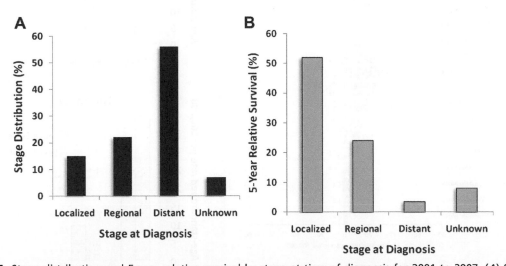

Fig. 6. Stage distribution and 5-year relative survival by stage at time of diagnosis for 2001 to 2007. (*A*) Stage distribution and (*B*) 5-year relative survival based on stage at diagnosis of lung cancer. Localized disease defined by confinement to primary site. Regional refers to spread to regional lymph nodes. Distant refers to when cancer has metastasized. Unknown includes unstaged cancers. Stage distribution is based on summary stage 2000 documentations. (*Data from* Howlader N, Noone AM, Krapcho M, et al, editors. SEER Cancer Statistics Review, 1975–2008. Bethesda (MD): National Cancer Institute; 2010. Available at: http://seer.cancer.gov/csr/1975_2008/, based on November 2010 SEER data submission, posted to the SEER web site, 2011.)

age-specific death rates of men and a lesser increase in the death rates of women. (2) Cigarette smoking was causally related to lung cancer in men. The magnitude of the effect of cigarette smoking far outweighed all other factors leading to lung cancer. The risk for lung cancer increased with the duration of smoking and the number of cigarettes smoked per day. The report estimated that the average male smoker had an approximately 9-fold to 10-fold risk for lung cancer, whereas heavy smokers had at least a 20-fold risk. (3) Cigarette smoking was believed more important than occupational exposures in the causation of lung cancer in the general population. (4) Cigarette smoking was the most important cause of chronic bronchitis in the United States. (5) Male cigarette smokers had a higher death rate from coronary artery disease than male nonsmokers.

The report concluded, "Cigarette smoking is a health hazard of sufficient importance in the United States to warrant appropriate remedial action." Since the publication of the report, yearly per capita consumption of cigarettes has declined in the United States (see **Fig. 8**).[11] It is estimated that 20.6% of all American adults over age 18 years continue to smoke, a figure that has only minimally decreased since approximately 1997, based on a recent *Morbidity and Mortality Weekly Report* report by Dube and colleagues.[13] Of these smokers, 80.1% (36.3 million people) smoke every day and 19.9% (9 million) smoke some days. More men (23.5%) than women (17.9%) smoke. The decline in smoking rates is steeper for black men and white men than for white women and black women. The prevalence of smoking is 31.1% among persons below the federal poverty level. For adults older than 25 years, the prevalence of smoking was 28.5% among persons with less than a high school diploma compared with 5.6% among persons with a graduate degree.[13] There

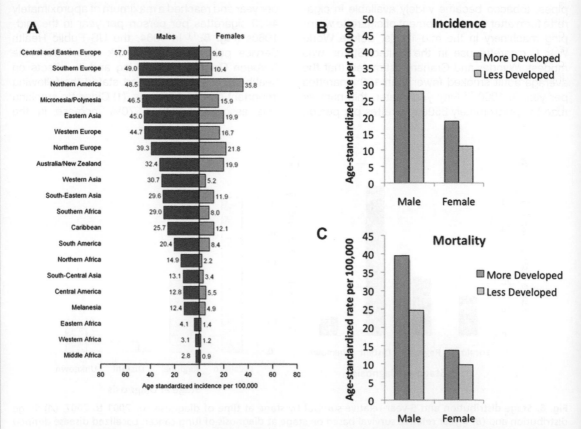

Fig. 7. Age-standardized lung cancer incidence and mortality rates by gender and world area. Lung cancer incidence by gender and world area (A). Incidence (B) and mortality rates (C) of lung cancer by gender for more developed and less developed areas in the world, 2008. Rates are standardized to the world standard population. (*Adapted from* Jemal A, Bray F, Center MM, et al. Global cancer statistics. CA Cancer J Clin 2011;61(2):69–90; with permission.)

were also regional differences in the United States, with the West having the lowest prevalence (16.4%) and higher prevalence observed in the South (21.8%) and the Midwest States (23.1%).[8] More than 80% of adult smokers begin before the age 18 years. In 2009, 1 in 5 American high school students reported smoking cigarettes in the preceding 30 days.[14] The smoking rate has declined but has slowed of late; the smoking prevalence increased from 27.5% in 1991 to 36.4% in1997, declined to 21.9% in 2003, and then declined less to 19.5% in 2009.[15]

One of the first descriptions of lung cancer was in 1912 by Adler[16] in an extensive review of autopsy reports from hospitals in the United States and western Europe, which found 374 cases of primary lung cancer. This represented less than 0.5% of all cancer cases. He concluded, "primary malignant neoplasms of the lung are among the rarest forms of disease." In 1920, lung cancer constituted only 1% of all malignancies in the United States. During the next several decades, researchers in the United States and abroad noted a significant increase in the incidence of carcinoma of the lung. In a series of 185,434 autopsy cases collected between 1897 and 1930, Hruby and Sweany[17] noted that the incidence of lung cancer had increased disproportionately to the incidence of cancer in general.

The first scientific report that associated cigarette smoking with an increased risk of premature death was in 1938, when Pear[18] showed the degree of adverse effect on longevity increased with the amount of smoking (Fig. 9). The finding that tar applied to the skin of animals produced lung carcinoma raised concern that inhalation of tar products could be an important factor in the increase in lung cancer incidence. Observations in patients and experimental studies in animals have shown that tobacco tar liberated from the burning of tobacco was a carcinogenic agent.[19] Other uncontrolled patient series highlighted the potential role of cigarette smoking in the increase in lung cancer incidence.[20–23] In 1941, Ochsner and DeBakey stated in their review of lung carcinoma, "it is our definite conviction that the increase in the incidence of pulmonary carcinoma is due largely to the increase in smoking."[21]

In 1950, two large landmark epidemiologic studies established the role of tobacco smoking as a causal factor in bronchogenic carcinoma.[24,25] In a case-control study in United Kingdom, Doll and Hill[24] described an association between carcinoma of the lung and cigarette smoking and the effect of the amount of cigarette use on the development of lung cancer.[18,24,26] In another case-control study in the United States, Wynder and Graham[25] examined 605 cases of lung cancer in men compared with a general male hospital population without cancer. The American investigators found that 96.5% of lung cancers were in men who were moderate to heavy smokers for many

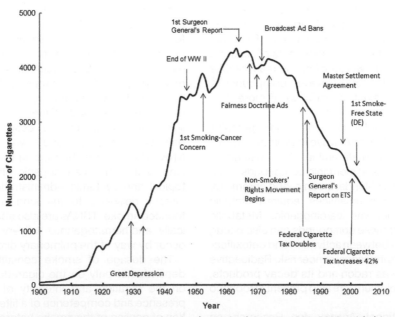

Fig. 8. The adult per capita cigarette consumption in the United States, 1900–2006, with historical highlights. (*Adapted from* Warner KE, Mendez D. Tobacco control policy in developed countries: yesterday, today, and tomorrow. Nicotine Tob Res 2010;12(9):876–87; with permission.)

years. The authors concluded, (1) the excessive and prolonged use of tobacco was an important factor in the induction of lung cancer; (2) lung cancer in a nonsmoker was rare (however, this is currently not the case [discussed later in section on never smokers]); and (3) there could be a lag period of 10 years or more between cessation of smoking and the clinical onset of carcinoma. Subsequently, the Surgeon General of the United States re-emphasized in 2004 the conclusions of the 1964 report that "cigarette smoking is the major cause of lung cancer."[27]

Cigarette smoke is a complex aerosol composed of gaseous and particulate compounds. The smoke consists of mainstream smoke and sidestream smoke components. Mainstream smoke is produced by inhalation of air through the cigarette and is the primary source of smoke exposure for the smoker. Sidestream smoke is produced from smoldering of the cigarette between puffs and is the major source of environmental tobacco smoke (ETS). The primary determinant of tobacco addiction is nicotine, and tar is the total particulate matter of cigarette smoke after nicotine and water have been removed. Exposure to tar seems to be a major component of lung cancer risk. The Federal Trade Commission determines the nicotine and tar content of cigarettes by measurements made on standardized smoking machines. The composition of mainstream smoke, however, can vary greatly depending on the intensity of inhalation by a smoker. Although the use of filter tips decreases the amount of nicotine and tar in mainstream smoke, the effect of filter tips also varies because the compression of the tips by lips or fingers and the depth of inhalation of the smoker. There are more than 4000 chemical constituents of cigarette smoke: 95% of the weight of mainstream smoke comes from 400 to 500 gaseous compounds[28]; the rest of the weight is made up of more than 3500 particulate components.

Mainstream smoke contains many potential carcinogens, including polycyclic aromatic hydrocarbons (PAHs), aromatic amines, N-nitrosamines, and other organic and inorganic compounds, such as benzene, vinyl chloride, arsenic, and chromium. The PAHs and N-nitrosamines require metabolic activation to become carcinogenic. Metabolic detoxification of these compounds can also occur, and the balance between activation and detoxification likely affects individual cancer risk. Radioactive materials, such as radon and its decay products, bismuth, and polonium, are also present in tobacco smoke.

The International Agency for Research on Cancer (IARC) has identified at least 50 carcinogens in tobacco smoke.[29,30] The agents that

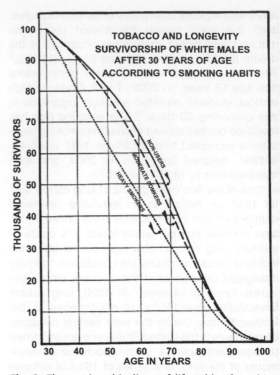

Fig. 9. The survivorship lines of life tables for white men falling into 3 categories relative to the usage of tobacco. (A) Nonusers (*solid line*); (B) moderate smokers (*dashed line*); (C) heavy smokers (*dotted line*). (*Adapted from* Pear R. Tobacco smoking and longevity. Science 1938;87:216; with permission.)

seem of particular concern in lung carcinoma are the tobacco-specific N-nitrosamines (TSNAs) formed by nitrosation of nicotine during tobacco processing and during smoking. Eight TSNAs have been described, including 4-(methylnitrosamino)-1(3-pyridyl)-1-butanone (NNK), which is known to induce adenocarcinoma of the lung in experimental animals. Other TSNAs have been linked to cancer of the esophagus, bladder, pancreas, oral cavity, and larynx. Of the TSNAs, NNK, which seems the most important inducer of lung cancer, has carcinogenic effects with both topical and systemic administration. TSNAs are directly delivered to the lung by inhalation of tobacco smoke. TSNAs are also absorbed systemically, and hematogenous delivery to the lung can occur by way of the pulmonary circulation.

The dosage of smoke constituents received depends not only on the cigarette itself but also on the duration and intensity of inhalation, the presence and competence of a filter, and the duration of cooling of the smoke before inhalation. The primary factor determining intensity of cigarette use is the nicotine dependence of the smoker, and although cigarettes now contain less nicotine and tar than in the past, smokers tend to smoke more intensively with higher puffs per minute and deeper inhalations to satisfy their nicotine need. Therefore, the measurements of tar and nicotine content made by smoking machines may significantly underestimate individual exposure. Low-yield filtered cigarettes might be a contributing factor to the increase in the incidence of adenocarcinoma of the lung.[31] The nicotine-addicted smoker smokes low-yield cigarettes far more intensively than nonfiltered higher-yield cigarettes, and with deeper inhalation, higher-order bronchi in the peripheral lung are exposed to carcinogen-containing smoke as opposed to the major bronchi alone. These peripheral bronchi lack protective epithelium and are exposed to carcinogens, including TSNAs, which have been linked to the induction of adenocarcinoma.

Tobacco carcinogens, such as NNK, can bind to DNA and create DNA adducts, which are pieces of DNA covalently bonded to a cancer-causing chemical, such as PAH in cigarette smoke. Repair processes may remove these DNA adducts and restore normal DNA, or cells with damaged DNA may undergo apoptosis. Failure of the normal DNA repair mechanisms to remove DNA adducts, however, can lead to permanent mutations. NNKs can mediate an array of signaling pathway activation that includes modulation of critical oncogenes and tumor suppressor genes that ultimately can result in uncontrolled cellular proliferation and tumorigenesis.[32]

NNK is associated with DNA mutations resulting in the activation of K-*ras* oncogenes.[33,34] K-*ras* oncogene activation has been detected in 24% of human lung adenocarcinomas[35] and is present in adenocarcinoma of the lung in ex-smokers, suggesting that such mutations do not revert necessarily with the cessation of tobacco smoking.[36] This may in part explain the persistent elevation in lung cancer risk in exsmokers even years after discontinuing cigarette use. In addition, a specific chemical constituent of tobacco smoke, benzo[a]pyrene metabolite, can damage various p53 tumor-suppressor gene loci that are known to be abnormal in approximately 60% of primary lung cancer cases.[37] Related PAHs found in tobacco smoke are also capable of targeting other lung cancer mutational hotspots.[38]

One in 9 smokers eventually develops lung cancer.[39] The relative risk of lung cancer in long-term smokers has been estimated as 10-fold to 30-fold compared with lifetime nonsmokers.[40] The cumulative lung cancer risk among heavy smokers can be as high as 30% compared with a lifetime risk of less than 1% in nonsmokers.

The lung cancer risk is proportional to the quantity of cigarette consumption, because factors, such as the number of packs per day smoked, the age of onset of smoking, the degree of inhalation, the tar and nicotine content of cigarettes, and use of unfiltered cigarettes, become important.[41,42] There is no question that tobacco smoking remains the most important modifiable risk factor for lung cancer. It has been estimated that up to 20% of all cancer deaths worldwide could be prevented by the elimination of tobacco smoking.[43] It is also clear that individual susceptibility is a factor in carcinogenesis. Although more than 80% of lung cancers occur in persons with tobacco exposure, fewer than 20% of smokers develop lung cancer. This variability in cancer susceptibility is likely affected by other environmental factors or by genetic predisposition.

Other Types of Smoking

Other forms of tobacco use, such as cigar smoking and pipe smoking, have been associated with increased risk for lung cancer. The risk seems weaker, however, than with cigarette smoking. Most cigars are composed of primarily of a single type of tobacco that is air cured and fermented but can vary in their size and shape to contain from 1 g to 20 g of tobacco. Smoking 5 cigars a day on average is equivalent to smoking 1 pack a day of cigarettes. A large prospective study of more than 130,000 men over 12 years showed that cigar smokers have a relative risk of lung cancer of 5.1 compared with non–cigar smokers.[44] Another study showed a relative risk of 2.1 for lung cancer compared with nonsmokers, with men who smoked 5 or more cigars a day having the greatest risk.[45] The increased risk for lung cancer as a result of pipe smoking is comparable to cigar smoking.[46,47] A large cohort study showed that active pipe smoking was associated with a relative risk for lung cancer of 5.0.[48] Cigar and pipe smokers have a greater risk for lung cancer than lifelong nonsmokers or former smokers.[49]

The effects of inhaling smoke from recreational drugs, such as marijuana and cocaine, are less studied than the effects of tobacco smoke. Metaplastic histologic and molecular changes similar to premalignant alterations have been described in the bronchial epithelium in habitual smokers of marijuana or cocaine.[50,51] A clear association has not been fully established, however, between such inhalant drug use and lung cancer. A case-control study showed that there is an 8% increased risk for lung cancer for each joint-year of marijuana smoking after adjusting for tobacco cigarette smoking.[52] Similarly, there is a 7%

increased risk for lung cancer for each pack-year of cigarette smoking after adjusting for marijuana smoking. The relationship between cocaine smoking and lung cancer is not well studied.

Never Smokers

The term, *never smokers*, refers to persons who have smoked fewer than 100 cigarettes in their lifetime, including lifetime nonsmokers. Most studies that track the trend of lung cancer rates often include both smokers and never smokers, and few studies independently study the trends over time for never smokers because of the limited longitudinal collection and the limited reliability of smoking information in population-based registries. From what is available, however, the overall global statistics estimate that 15% of lung cancers in men and up to 53% in women are not attributable to smoking, with never smokers accounting for 25% of all lung cancer cases worldwide.[53] If lung cancer in never smokers were considered separately, it would rank as the seventh most

common cause of cancer death worldwide before cervical, pancreatic, and prostate cancer (**Fig. 10**).[54] In countries in South Asia, up to 80% of women with lung cancer are never smokers (**Fig. 11**).[55] In the United States, one study estimated that 19% of lung cancer in women and 9% of lung cancer in men occurs in never smokers.[56] The age-adjusted rate for lung cancer in never smokers (ages 40–79 years) ranged from 11.2 to 13.7 per 100,000 person-years for men and from 15.2 to 20.8 per 100,000 person-years for women. The rates are 12 to 30 times higher in current smokers of the same age group.

The incidence of lung cancer in never smokers seems to have a geographic variation. For example, a series following 12,000 patients with lung cancer in California found a dramatic increase in bronchoalveolar carcinoma in never smokers from 19% during 1995 to 1999 to 26% during 1999 to 2003.[57] The percentage of other types of lung cancer in never smokers also increased from 8.6% to 9.4%. Another study in the United States found a small but statistically significant

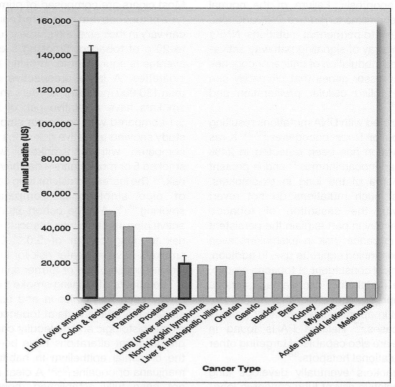

Fig. 10. Common causes of cancer deaths in the United States with focus on never smokers. Total lung cancer deaths, estimated at 161,840 in 2008, have been split into ever smokers and never smokers. Error bars reflect that the number of lung cancer deaths in never smokers, including cases attributable to secondhand smoke exposure and cases not attributable to tobacco, are estimated to total 16,000 to 24,000 per year. (*Adapted from* Rudin CM, Avila-Tang E, Samet JM. Lung cancer in never smokers: a call to action. Clin Cancer Res 2009;15(18):5622–5; with permission.)

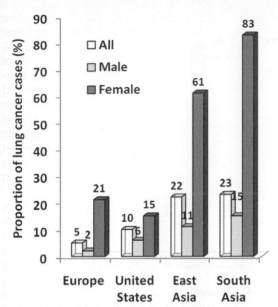

Fig. 11. Geographic and gender variations of lung cancers in never smokers. Systematic compilation of published study involving 18 reports with 82,0237 cases. A marked gender bias was observed whereby lung cancer in never smokers seems to affect women more frequently than men, irrespective of geography. The proportion of female lung cancer cases in never smokers is particularly high in East Asia and South Asia. (*Adapted from* Sun S, Schiller JH, Gazdar AF. Lung cancer in never smokers—a different disease. Nat Rev Cancer 2007;7(10):778–90; with permission.)

increase in the mortality rate in women with non–smoking-associated lung cancers from 12.3% in the years 1959 to 1972 to 14.7% in the years 1982 to 2000.[41] A corresponding increase did not occur in men. In Japan, the percentage of never smoker NSCLC increased from 16% to 33% over a 30-year period ending in 2004.[58] A European case-control study, however, comparing data from 1950 and 1990, showed no significant change in the percentage of never smokers in male lung cancer patients and a decrease in the percentage of never smokers among female lung cancer patients.[59] Similarly, an analysis of 13 American cohorts and 22 cancer registry studies found no substantial change in the rate of lung cancer in women never smokers.[60] Two major epidemiologic trends seem to be emerging in lung cancer in never smokers: (1) women are more frequently affected than men and (2) it is more prevalent in certain parts of the world, such as Asia.

Although all histologic types of lung cancer are associated with cigarette smoking, in smokers the association is stronger for SCLC and for squamous cell carcinoma. In contrast, adenocarcinoma of the lung is more common in never smokers (62% vs 18%, based on 5144 cases[55]) compared with smokers (19% vs 53% based on 21,853 cases[61]) (**Fig. 12**). Adenocarcinoma, however, is becoming more common even among smokers.[62,63] This finding may be attributable to the deeper inhalation of lowered tar-containing and nicotine-containing cigarettes, leading to a more peripheral distribution of cigarette smoke in the lung.[64] Adenocarcinoma is becoming a common lung cancer type in young patients, however, especially never smokers.[65] Other series have also shown the common prevalence of adenocarcinoma in never smokers.[56,66] Although there has been no predominant causal factor that can fully explain lung cancer in never smokers, the risk factors considered important for never smokers include secondhand smoke; radon exposure; environmental exposures, such as indoor air pollution, asbestos, and arsenic; history of lung disease; and genetic factors.[67] A population-based case-control study in Canada found that occupational exposures, history of lung disease, and family history of early-onset cancer were important risk factors for lung cancer among never smokers.[68] In this study, potential environmental sources of increased risk included exposure to solvents, paints, or thinners; welding equipment; and smoke, soot, or exhaust. This finding is particularly important because there are few data on occupational exposures and lung cancer among never smokers. Other studies have also shown an association between lung cancer in never smokers and a family history of lung cancer, a finding that suggests a role for genetic factors.[69–71] For example, a case-control study following 2400 relatives of 316 never smokers with lung cancer cases showed a 25% excess risk for cancer in first-degree relatives of lung cancer cases.[70] Specific genetic factors in these studies have not been identified. Some studies, however, suggest the role of the epidermal growth factor receptor gene (*EGFR*) pathway, the human repair gene (*hMSH2*), and various cytochrome P450 and glutathione-*S*-transferase enzymes.[72–75] No unique susceptibility gene has been identified that distinguishes lung cancers in never smokers from smokers. Recent data have shown, however, an increased frequency of *EGFR* mutations in lung adenocarcinomas of never smokers, especially in Asian cohorts (**Fig. 13**).[76–79]

Lung cancers among never smokers in Asia (Hong Kong, Singapore, and Japan) are diagnosed at an earlier age than in smokers.[66,80] These findings have not been reproduced in the United States or Europe.[56,81] It has been suggested that the investigation threshold in symptomatic never smokers is higher, leading to diagnosis at later

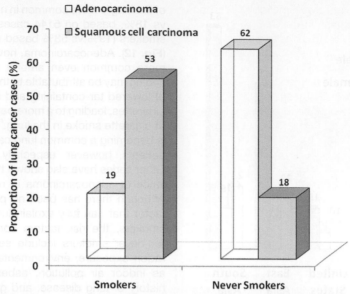

Fig. 12. Different histologic features of lung cancer in never smokers. Histologic distribution of lung cancers in never smokers compared with smokers. Cases of bronchioloalveolar carcinoma included with adenocarcinoma. Histologic subtypes were classified as adenocarcinoma, squamous cell carcinoma, or others. Ratio of the number of adenocarcinoma to squamous cell carcinoma was 0.4:1 in smokers, whereas it was 3.4:1 in never smokers. (*Adapted from* Sun S, Schiller JH, Gazdar AF. Lung cancer in never smokers—a different disease. Nat Rev Cancer 2007;7(10):778–90; with permission.)

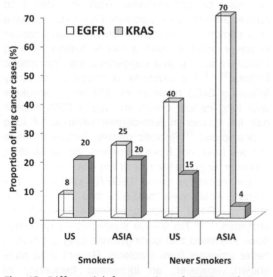

Fig. 13. Differential frequencies of EGFR and K-ras mutations reported in lung adenocarcinomas in East Asia compared with the United States in never smokers and ever smokers. Activating mutations in both genes are found predominantly in adenocarcinomas, and occur in nonoverlapping cohorts. (*Adapted from* Rudin CM, Avila-Tang E, Harris CC, et al. Lung cancer in never smokers: molecular profiles and therapeutic implications. Clin Cancer Res 2009;15(18): 5646–61; with permission.)

stages in never smokers.[66] Despite this potential delayed diagnosis and later presentation of lung cancer in never smokers, the survival rate for never smokers is better than for smokers, independent of stage of disease, treatment received, and presence of comorbidities.[57,81,82] A multivariate analyses of lung adenocarcioma found that the never smoking status was an independent predictor of improved survival (23% 5-year survival rate for never smokers and 16% for current smokers).[81] Such findings have suggested that the cancer in never smokers may display a distinct biologic and natural history. There are also epidemiologic, clinicopathologic, and molecular differences between lung cancers in never smokers and smokers, differences that have led some investigators to suggest that lung cancer in never smokers may be a different disease. Microarray gene-profiling studies have found that lung adenocarcinomas are heterogeneous, and the profiles of cancer in smokers and never smokers are different.[83,84] In 2010, the first genome-wide association study (GWAS) reported genetic variations in chromosome 13q31.3 that altered the expression of glypican 5 (*GPC5*), a heparin sulfate proteoglycan with many known functions involving cell growth and differentiation and tissue responses.[85] Another GWAS focusing on lung adenocarcinomas in female Han Chinese never smokers in Taiwan identified genetic variation in the *CLPTM1L-TERT* locus of chromosome 5p15.33 as associated with risk for lung cancer in this population.[86] This 5p15.33 chromosome contains two well-known genes, telomerase reverse transcriptase (*TERT*) and cleft lip and palate transmembrane 1-like (*CLPTM1L*), both of which have been implicated in carcinogenesis.

Genetic Factors

There is a genetic component to the pathogenesis of lung cancer, whether it relates to host susceptibility to lung cancer, with or without exposure to cigarette smoke to the development of certain types of lung cancer, or to an individual's responsiveness to biologic therapies. A lung cancer risk prediction analysis developed by Spitz and

colleagues[87,88] incorporated multiple variables, such as smoking history, exposure to environmental tobacco smoke, occupational exposures to dusts and to asbestos, and family history of cancer. They showed the influence of a family history of cancer on the risk for lung cancer in never smokers, former smokers, and current smokers (**Table 1**). Cassidy and colleagues[89] also highlighted the significantly increased risk for lung cancer specifically for persons with a family history of early-onset lung cancer (<60 years of age) (**Table 2**).

Recently, Schwartz and colleagues[90] reviewed the molecular epidemiology of lung cancer, focusing on host susceptibility genetic markers to lung carcinogens. (See the article by Larsen and Minna elsewhere in this issue.) The susceptibility genetic factors include high-penetrance, low-frequency genes; low-penetrance, high-frequency genes;

Table 1
Multivariable logistic model for lung cancer by smoking status

Risk Factor	P Value	OR (95% CI)
Never smoker		
ETS (yes vs no)	.0042	1.80 (1.20–2.89)
Family history (≥2 vs <2)[a]	<.001	2.00 (1.39–2.90)
Former smoker		
Emphysema (yes vs no)	<.001	2.65 (1.95–3.60)
Dust exposure (yes vs no)	<.001	1.59 (1.29–1.97)
Family History (≥2 vs <2)[a]	<.001	1.59 (1.28–1.98)
Age stopped smoking		
<42 years	Reference	
42–54 years	.1110	1.24 (0.95–1.61)
≥54 years	.0018 (P for trend = .017)	1.50 (1.16–1.94)
Current smoker		
Emphysema (yes)	<.001	2.13 (1.58–2.88)
Pack-years		
<28	Reference	
28–41.9	.1932	1.25 (0.89–1.74)
42–57.4	.0241	1.45 (1.05–2.01)
≥57.5	<.001 (P for trend <.001)	1.85 (1.35–2.53)
Dust exposure (yes vs no)	.0075	1.36 (1.09–1.70)
Asbestos exposure (yes vs no)	.0127	1.51 (1.09–2.08)
Family history[b]		
0	Reference	
≥1	.0021	1.47 (1.15–1.88)

[a] Number of first-degree relatives with any cancer.
[b] Number of first-degree relatives with a smoking-related cancers, such as lung cancers, cancers, renal cancer, cancers of upper digestive tract, esophagus, pancreas, bladder, and cervix.
Data from Spitz MR, Hong WK, Amos CI, et al. A risk model for prediction of lung cancer. J Natl Cancer Inst 2007; 99(9):715–26.

Table 2
Liverpool lung project—multivariable risk model lung cancer

Risk Factor	P Value	OR (95% CI)
Smoking duration	<.001	
Never		1.00 Reference
1–20 years		2.16 (1.21–3.85)
21–40 years		4.27 (2.62–6.94)
41–60 years		12.27 (7.41–20.30)
>60 years		15.25 (5.71–40.65)
Prior diagnosis of pneumonia	.002	
No		1.00 Reference
Yes		1.83 (1.26–2.64)
Occupational exposure to asbestos	<.001	
No		1.00 Reference
Yes		1.89 (1.35–2.62)
Prior diagnosis of malignant tumor	.005	
No		1.00 Reference
Yes		1.96 (1.22–3.14)
Family history of lung cancer	.01	
No		1.00 Reference
Early onset (<60 years)		2.02 (1.18–3.45)
Late onset (≥60 years)		1.18 (0.79–1.76)

Data from Cassidy A, Myles JP, van Tongeren M, et al. The LLP risk model: an individual risk prediction model for lung cancer. Br J Cancer 2008;98(2):270–6.

and acquired epigenetic polymorphisms. Takemiya and colleagues[91] and Yamanaka and colleagues[92] showed the association of lung cancer with rare mendelian cancer syndromes, such as Bloom and Werner syndromes. Studies on familial aggregation have supported the hypothesis that there is a hereditary component to the risk for lung cancer. These familial association approaches have been used to discover high-penetrance, low-frequency genes. A meta-analysis involving 32 studies showed a 2-fold increased risk for lung cancer in persons with a family history of lung cancer with an increased risk also present in nonsmokers.[93] Bailey-Wilson and colleagues,[94] using family linkage approaches, reported the first association of familial lung cancer to the region on chromosome 6q23–25 (146cM–164cM). The addition of smoking history to the effect of this inheritance was associated with a 3-fold increase risk for lung cancer.

There have also been many studies on candidate susceptibility genes that are of low penetrance and high frequency. The approach has been to target genes known to be involved in the absorption, metabolism, and accumulation of tobacco or other carcinogens in lung tissue.

For example, genetic polymorphisms encoding enzymes involved in the activation and conjugation of tobacco smoke compounds, such as PAHs, nitrosamines, and aromatic amines, have been widely studied. Metabolism of these compounds occurs through either phase I enzymes (oxidation, reduction, and hydrolysis) or phase II (conjugation) enzymes. Some of the frequently studied enzymes in this system include CYP1A1, the glutathione S-transferases (GST), microsomal epoxide hydrolase 1 (mEH/EPHX1), myeloperoxidase (MPO), and reduced form of nicotinamide adenine dinucleotide phosphate quinine oxidoreductase 1 (NQO1). Polymorphisms in CYP1A1 and their association with lung cancer risks have been conflicting. A meta-analysis involving 16 studies by Le Marchand and colleagues[95] showed no significant risk associated with the CYP1A1 Ile462Val allele; however, in pooled analysis, a significant 55% increased risk for squamous cell carcinoma in whites was observed, especially in women and nonsmokers. GST gene products help conjugate electrophilic compounds to the antioxidant glutathione. GSTM1 in its null form occurs in 50% of the population, and studies by Benhamou and colleagues[96] showed a 17% increased lung cancer risk in persons who were GSTM1 null. A more recent and larger meta-analysis involving more than 53,000 case-controls by Ye and colleagues[97] showed an 18% increase risk for lung cancer among persons who were GSTMI null, but this significant association was not present when the analysis was limited to larger studies only. Amos and colleagues[98] performed a GWAS scan of tagged single nucleotide polymorphisms in histologically confirmed NSCLC in an effort to identify common low-penetrance alleles that influence lung cancer risk. They identified a susceptibility locus for lung cancer at chromosome 15q25.1, a region that contains the nicotinic acetylcholine receptor genes.

Results from the many candidate gene polymorphism studies focusing on a single polymorphism in one gene have been mixed. This has led to studies to look at gene-gene interactions, which require even a larger study population. For example, Zhou and colleagues[99] studied the interaction between variants in genes coding for NAT2 (which activates arylamine cigarette smoke metabolites and deactivates aromatic amines) and mEH (which activates PAHs and deactivates various epoxides). They found significant interactions between NAT2 variants associated with certain acetylation pheynotype and mEH variants associated with certain activity level with the risk of lung cancer. For example, a 2-fold increase risk for lung cancer was observed in 120 pack-year smokers who had the NAT2 slow-acetylation and mEH high-activity genotype. Alternatively, in nonsmokers, a 50% decrease risk for lung cancer was observed among persons with the combined NAT2 slow-acetylation and mEH high-activity genotype. Susceptibility to carcinogenic agents may also be affected by individual differences in mutagen sensitivity. Spitz and colleagues[100] reviewed the phenotypic studies of DNA repair capacity and lung cancer risks.

Polymorphisms in genes involved in DNA repair enzymes active in base excision repair (XRCC1 and OGG1), nucleotide excision repair (ERCC1, XPD, and XPA), and double-strand break repair (XRCC3), and different mismatch repair pathways have also been studied as they relate to lung cancer risks. Chronic inflammation in response to repetitive tobacco exposure has been theorized as involved in lung tumorigenesis. Genes encoding for the interleukins (IL-1, IL-6, and IL-8). The cyclooxygenase enzymes (eg, COX-2) involved in inflammation, or the metalloproteases (MMP-1, MMP-2, MMP-3, and MMP-12) involved in repair during inflammation have been associated with lung cancer risk. Several cell cycle–related genes have been implicated in lung

cancer susceptibility, including the tumor suppressor genes p53 and p73, mouse double minute 2 (MDM2), and the apoptosis genes encoding FAS and FASL.

Wu and colleagues[101] showed that the presence of mutagen sensitivity is associated with an increased risk for lung cancer. Spitz and colleagues[100] noted that the combined risk for lung cancer was greater in individuals with mutagen sensitivity who smoked than in persons with either smoking or mutagen sensitivity characteristics alone. DNA adducts can be measured as biomarkers to represent the degree of carcinogenesis. Several of the lung cancer susceptibility genes (discussed previously) have been associated with increased levels of DNA adducts. Acquired or epigenetic changes to DNA chromosome can also lead to increased lung cancer susceptibility. These events include changes, such as DNA methylation, histone deacetylation, and phosphorylation, all of which can affect gene expression. Despite many genetic association studies, the specific genes responsible for the enhanced risk for lung cancer remain poorly understood. Work is under way to pool findings to achieve greater study sample sizes in collaborative efforts, such as the Genetic Susceptibility to Environmental Carcinogens and the International Lung Cancer Consortium.

Lung cancer susceptibility is determined at least in part by host genetic factors. Persons with genetic susceptibility might therefore be at higher risk if they smoke tobacco. As technology advances, it may be possible to target subgroups identified as genetically high risk for lung cancer for specific interventions, including intensive efforts at smoking cessation, screening, and prevention programs.

Gender

Lung cancer surpassed breast cancer as the leading cause of cancer deaths in women in the late 1980s, and now almost twice as many women die of lung cancer than breast cancer.[1] Since 1950 there has been more than a 600% increase in the lung cancer mortality rate in women. In the United States, the cigarette smoking rate for women increased during the period from 1930 to 1960, and this increase was followed two decades later by an increase in lung cancer in women starting in 1960.[102,103] Cigarette smoking peaked during World War II among men born in the 1920s. The smoking rate in women peaked approximately a decade later among those who were born in the 1930s. Lung cancer deaths are expected to keep falling in both genders because older men and women and their younger counterparts smoke less. Smoking prevalence is higher among men (23.1%) than women (18.3%); however, this difference is narrowing.[9] Fortunately, the lung cancer death rate in women is beginning to plateau, with an annual increase of 0.2% in 2005.[104] Lung cancer death rates for women fell for the first time in four decades amid continued declines in the overall cancer death rate (see **Fig. 4**).[4] There has been a drop of 2.5% in lung cancer deaths among men and a 0.9% decline in lung cancer deaths in women. Even though the overall age-adjusted lung cancer incidence is still higher in men than women, this difference is decreasing due to a continued decrease in the male incidence of lung cancer. Cigarette smoking remains the most important factor for the development of lung cancer in women with some suggesting up to 80% of cases in women are related to smoking.[105] Alternatively, for never smokers (discussed previously), the age-adjusted incidence rate of lung cancer is higher for women than men based on the compilation of several prospective cohort studies (14.4–20.8 per 100,000 person-years for women compared with 4.8–13.7 per 100,000 person-years for men).[56]

Whether women are more or less susceptible than men to the carcinogenic effects of cigarette smoke is controversial. The American Cancer Society Cancer Prevention Study II, which followed 1 to 2 million subjects between 1982 and 1988, reported an overall risk for lung cancer in women smokers of 11.94, compared with an overall risk of 22.36 in male smokers, after taking into account the intensity of smoking.[106] Recent analysis of the SEER data from 1997 to 2006 showed that the lung cancer mortality rate is 74.08 per 100,000 man-years compared with 40.81 per 100,000 woman-years.[107] Other studies have suggested, however, that women may be actually more vulnerable to carcinogens in tobacco smoke than men.[108–111] A study using the American Health Foundation data found that the odds ratio (OR) for the major lung cancer types has been consistently higher for women than for men at every level of exposure to cigarette smoke.[111] The dose-response ORs for lung cancer in women were 1.2-fold to 1.7-fold higher than in men. A Canadian case-control study of male–female differences in lung cancer covering the period 1981 to 1985 showed that with a history of 40 pack-years of cigarette smoking relative to lifelong nonsmoking, the OR for women developing lung cancer was 27.9 versus 9.6 in men.[110] In both these studies, the increase in lung cancer risk held for all major histologic types.

The observed gender differences in susceptibility may be related to gender-related differences in nicotine metabolism and in metabolic activation or detoxification of lung carcinogens. Such gender differences in clearance of plasma nicotine by cytochrome P450 enzymes have been reported. For example, several reports have commented on gender differences in lung cancer observed at the molecular level. Ryberg and colleagues[112] noted that women with lung cancer have higher levels of DNA adducts than men. Such patients might be anticipated more susceptible to carcinogens, which might explain why women seem to develop lung cancer with lower-intensity cigarette exposure. Furthermore, hormonal factors may also play a role in susceptibility. A case-control study showed that estrogen replacement therapy was significantly associated with an increased risk for adenocarcinoma (OR 1.7), whereas the combination of cigarette smoking and estrogen replacement increased that risk substantially (OR 32.4).[113] Conversely, early menopause (age 40 years or younger) was associated with a decreased risk for adenocarcinoma (OR 0.3). More recent large randomized studies suggest that the use of hormonal therapies, such as estrogen and progestin, is associated with an increased risk for lung cancer in women.[114] For example, the Vitamins and Lifestyle study followed perimenopausal women for 6 years and found the risk for lung cancer was increased in those who used estrogen and progestin.[114] The observed risk was proportional to the duration of hormone exposure, with approximately 50% increased risk for those who used hormone replacement therapy for 10 years or longer. Two studies as part of the Women's Health Initiative found a statistically nonsignificant trend toward increased incidence of NSCLC and an increased number of deaths from lung cancer in women taking hormone therapy compared with those taking placebo.[115,116]

A second issue is whether cigarette smoking may be associated with a higher risk for nonmalignant lung disease in women than in men. Neither of two large population studies, the British Doctors Study in the United Kingdom[117,118] or the Lung Health Study in the United States,[119] found gender differences in mortality from smoking-related chronic obstructive pulmonary disease (COPD). Other studies, however, including a study by Chen and colleagues,[120] suggest that cigarette smoking may be more harmful to the pulmonary function in women than in men. In this study, changes in forced expiratory volume in the first second of expiration (FEV_1) and maximal midexpiratory flow rate increased with increasing pack-years more rapidly in women smokers than in their male counterparts. These changes were independent of age, height, and weight. Beck and colleagues[121] in a study of

4690 white subjects found that for a given level of smoking, women had more changes in FEV_1 and maximal expiratory flow at 25% and 50% of vital capacity at a younger age (15–24 years) than men (40–45 years). Because smokers with spirometric evidence of airway obstruction are at higher risk for lung cancer, the suggestion that women have increased susceptibility to smoking-induced airway disease may be important in the consideration of their risk for lung cancer.[121]

Finally, it also seems that lung cancer is more common in nonsmoking women than in nonsmoking men. In an early study of tobacco smoking, Wynder and Graham[10] noted that a greater percentage of cancers in nonsmokers occurred in women than men. The number of women in that study was relatively small, however, and few women had at that time smoked for the duration of decades. Since then, it has become clear that women never smokers are more likely than male never smokers to develop lung cancer. In a case-control study by Zang and Wynder[111] of 1889 lung cancer subjects and 2070 control subjects, the proportion of never smoking lung cancer patients was more than twice as high for women than for men. The reasons for this finding are not clear, but speculation has been raised regarding the potential of women having greater susceptibility to nontobacco environmental carcinogens or increased exposure to ETS or the existence of gender-linked differences in the metabolism of nontobacco environmental carcinogens.

Race and Ethnicity

Race is a complex variable that often has a strong socioeconomic association. Racial differences in disease states can shed light, however, on the specific issues of a particular subpopulation. Menck[122] showed that the incidence of lung cancer is substantially higher among blacks and Native Hawaiians and other Polynesians and lower among Japanese Americans and Hispanics than among whites in the United States. These differences initially have been attributed to the variations in cigarette smoking pattern among the different ethnic and racial groups. Recent smoking data show that among the different groups, Asians (9.9%) had the lowest smoking prevalence in the United States, whereas American Indians and Alaska Natives (32.4%) had significantly higher prevalence than the other groups.[8] Smoking prevalence among whites (22%) and blacks (21.3%) were significantly higher than among Hispanics (15.8%). The Department of Health and Human Services reported, however, that the age-adjusted prevalence of cigarette smoking was similar among blacks and whites (30.1% and

27.3%, respectively). In addition, only 8% of black smokers smoked at least 25 cigarettes per day compared with 28% of white smokers. Native Hawaiians also had higher rates of lung cancer than whites and Asians despite having similar smoking habits. Haiman and colleagues[123] reported in their Multiethnic Cohort Study that among participants who smoked no more than 30 cigarettes per day, black Americans and Native Hawaiians had significantly greater risk for lung cancer than did whites. The relative risk for lung cancer among subjects smoking less than 20 cigarettes per day were 0.21 to 0.39 for Japanese Americans and Latinos, and 0.45 to 0.57 for whites as compared with black Americans. The differences in lung cancer risks were not significant, however, among all racial groups who exceeded 30 cigarettes per day of smoking. Recent SEER report based on data from 2004 to 2008 showed that black men, but not black women, in the United States had a higher age-adjusted incidence of lung cancer than their white counterparts at all age groups (**Fig. 14**).

Smokers with a history of early-onset lung cancer in a first-degree relative have a higher risk for lung cancer with increasing age than smokers without such a family history. Coté and colleagues[124] showed in a case-control study that first-degree relatives of black persons with early-onset lung cancer have a greater risk for lung cancer than their white counterparts (25.1% vs 17.1%, respectively). These cumulative differences in risk for lung cancer among blacks and whites are further amplified by increasing cigarette smoking exposure. The explanation for these observed racial or ethnic variations in risk for lung cancer is not known. Black Americans also have higher mortality rates from lung cancer than white Americans.[8] This difference in mortality rates has been attributed not only to the higher incidence rates but also to the poorer survival of black patients with lung cancer than white patients. For example, from 1995 to 2000, the 5-year survival rate was 14.3% lower in black Americans compared with white Americans. The reasons for these racial differences are not known. Brooks and colleagues[125] hypothesized a potential role for greater use of menthol cigarettes among black Americans than among white Americans (69% vs 22%) or the deeper inhalation of menthol cigarettes compared with nonmenthol cigarettes. No evidence, however, supports this hypothesis.

Age

The average age of most populations in developed nations is increasing, and cancer is a disease of

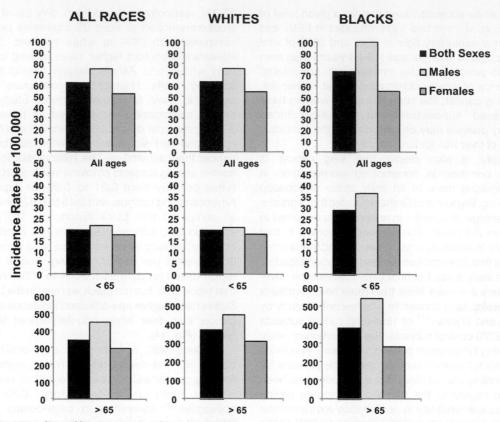

Fig. 14. Age-adjusted lung cancer incidence by gender, age, and race. Rates are per 100,000 and are age adjusted to the 2000 US standard population. Note the different scale, which highlights the predominant incidence of lung cancer in the population age >65 years for both genders and races. (*Data from* Siegel R, Ward E, Brawley O, et al. Cancer statistics, 2011: the impact of eliminating socioeconomic and racial disparities on premature cancer deaths. CA Cancer J Clin 2011;61(4):212–36; and Howlader N, Noone AM, Krapcho M, et al, editors. SEER Cancer Statistics Review, 1975–2008. Bethesda (MD): National Cancer Institute; 2010. Available at: http://seer.cancer.gov/csr/1975_2008/, based on November 2010 SEER data submission, posted to the SEER web site, 2011.)

the elderly. Although smoking prevalence is lowest among persons aged 65 years and older (9.3%) compared with persons aged 18 to 24 years (21.4%), 25 to 44 years (23.7%) and 45 to 64 years (22.6%),[8] (see **Fig. 14**), more than 65% of patients with lung cancer are older than 65. Specifically, 31.1% of patients with lung cancer are between 65 and 74 years, 29% between 75 and 84 years, and 8.3% are 85 years old and older.[3] The mean age at the time of diagnosis is over 70. This difference between lower current smoking prevalence and the higher cancer rate in the elderly population likely reflects heavy smoking history in current elderly population. In the past decade, the incidence and mortality from lung cancer have decreased among persons aged 50 years and younger but have increased among persons aged 70 years and older.[126] The 5-year survival rate for lung cancer decreases incrementally with age for both genders (**Fig. 15**). "Older patients"

are usually considered those older than 70 years with the "very elderly" those 80 years or older. Patients older than 80 years constitute 14% of all patients with lung cancer in the United States but account for almost a quarter of all lung cancer deaths. It has been estimated that the number of lung cancer patients aged 85 years and older will quadruple by 2050. Few studies have examined management of the elderly population with lung cancer. Recent reviews concluded that elderly patients, specially the functionally fit elderly, with lung cancer can benefit from many of the treatments used for younger patients, including surgery for early-stage disease and single-agent chemotherapy for advanced disease.[127,128]

Diet and Obesity

It has been suggested that diet is responsible for approximately 30% of all cancers.[129] Many

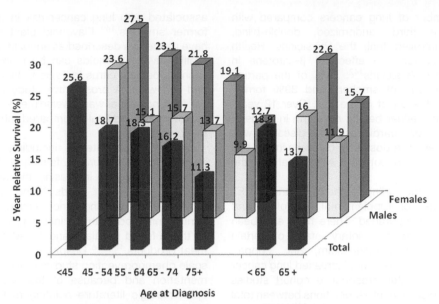

Fig. 15. Five-year relative survival (%) from lung cancer based on age at diagnosis. Based on data from 2001 to 2008 covering SEER 17 areas. (*Data from* Howlader N, Noone AM, Krapcho M, et al, editors. SEER Cancer Statistics Review, 1975–2008. Bethesda (MD): National Cancer Institute; 2010. Available at: http://seer.cancer.gov/csr/1975_2008/, based on November 2010 SEER data submission, posted to the SEER web site, 2011.

reports suggest that dietary factors contribute to the risk for lung cancers.[130] For example, low serum concentrations of antioxidants, such as vitamins A, C, and E, have been associated with the development of lung cancer.[131,132] Vitamin A has both an animal (retinol) and a vegetable (carotenoid) source; the vegetable component only has been shown to have protective effects against lung cancer. In particular, β-carotene, a prominent carotenoid, has been shown to have the greatest protective effect against lung cancer.[133] Vitamins C and E (α-tocopherol) have also been shown to have some protective effect.[134,135]

One of the most widely cited reports of the effect of diet on the development of cancer was a prospective survey of approximately 2000 men aged 40 to 55 years employed by the Western Electric Company where detailed dietary histories were recorded in 1957 and followed for more than 19 years.[136] In this study, β-carotene intake was inversely related to lung cancer incidence, suggesting that vitamin A and β-carotene may have a protective effect against lung cancer. Byers and colleagues[137] evaluated 27 such studies published before 1994 and concluded that persons in the lowest quartile of carotene intake had an approximately 50% to 100% increase in lung cancer risk compared with persons in the highest quartile of carotene intake. In response to these positive observations, three large-scale intervention trials have been conducted to try to determine

the relationship between vitamin supplementations and lung cancer. Unfortunately, these studies showed that vitamin supplementation did not reduce lung cancer risk and in some circumstances increased the incidence of lung cancer. The Alpha-Tocopherol, Beta Carotene Cancer Prevention (ATBC) Study was a randomized, double-blind, placebo-controlled trial designed to determine whether daily supplementation of α-tocopherol, β-carotene, or both could reduce the incidence of cancers, including lung cancer.[138] The study enrolled 29,133 male smokers aged 50 to 60 years in Finland. Unexpectedly, a higher than expected mortality, primarily due to lung cancer and heart disease, was observed in the group receiving β-carotene. Omenn and colleagues[139,140] then reported results of the Beta-Carotene and Retinol Efficacy Trial (CARET), also a randomized, double-blind, placebo-controlled study. The study was intended to determine whether dietary supplementation with β-carotene, vitamin A, or both would decrease the incidence of lung cancer. It enrolled 18,314 men and women considered at increased risk for lung cancer. The CARET study was stopped 21 months early because of "clear evidence of no benefit and substantial evidence of harm" in the group that received β-carotene and retinol palmitate, especially women.[139,141] The group that received both vitamin A and β-carotene had a 17% increase in mortality and a 28% increase in the number of lung cancers compared with placebo. A third randomized, double-blind, placebo-controlled trial, the Physicians' Health Study, evaluated the effect of β-carotene in 22,071 male physicians[142]; 11% of the participants were current smokers and 39% former smokers at the onset of the trial. Over 12 years of follow-up, neither benefit nor harm in terms of malignancy or cardiovascular disease was demonstrated. The dose of β-carotene in this trial was lower than in both the ATBC trial and the CARET study.

Because of the findings of the ATBC and CARET trials, the use of supplemental β-carotene and vitamin A is discouraged. There have also been suggestions that low dietary intake of certain minerals, including magnesium, zinc, copper, and iron, is associated with increased lung cancer risk; however, later prospective cohort studies observed no significant associations between total mineral intake and lung cancer risk.[143,144] The role of dietary supplementation in cancer chemoprevention is currently unsettled. These studies should serve as a reminder, however, that indiscreet and excessive intake of vitamins or other chemicals can be potentially harmful.

A diet rich in fruits and vegetables has been linked to decreased cancer incidence as suggested by a large cohort study in the Netherlands, with the protective effects stronger in current than in former smokers.[145] In this study, no specific type of vegetable or fruit was identified as particularly responsible for the effect. Consumption of vegetables described as cruciferous, such as broccoli and cabbage, which are rich in isothiocyanates, has some protective effect against lung cancer.[146] When study participants were stratified according to their GSTM1 and GSTT1 gene status, which are genes important at eliminating isothiocanates, the protective effect of the cruciferous vegetable consumption was best seen in subjects with the null gene.[146] Overall, it has been shown that low or no intake of fruits or vegetables has been associated with up to 3-fold risk for lung cancer.[147] It has been also further suggested that consuming fruits or vegetables raw rather than cooked is associated with a further reduction in risk for lung cancer because important carotenoids can be destroyed with cooking.[148] A large prospective study (the NIH-AARP Diet and Health Study) showed no relation between total intake of fruit and vegetables with lung cancer risk.[149] The study did show, however, that higher consumption of several botanic groups, such as rosaceae (apples, peaches, and strawberries), convolvulaceas (sweet potatoes and yams), and umbelliferae (carrots), was significantly inversely associated with lung cancer risk in men and in former smokers.[149] Flavonoid plant metabolites have properties described as antioxidant and antiproliferative. Flavonoids can be found in foods, such as berries, citrus fruits, tea, dark chocolate, and red wine. A prospective study showed the risk for lung cancer was lower in men with the highest total flavonoid intake compared with those with the lowest intake.[150]

Certain dietary items, including red meat, dairy products, saturated fats, and lipids, have been suggested as increasing the risk for lung cancer.[151–154] Other foods found to have an adverse effect on lung cancer include items that contain nitrosodimethylamines and nitrites, such as those found in salami and salted and smoked meat products.[155,156] Despite the negative large-scale chemoprevention studies of vitamin supplementation and because of the large body of epidemiologic literature pointing to the benefits of fruits and vegetables, health authorities continue to recommend a balanced dietary intake of fruits and vegetables, including those containing β-carotene.

Because of the current obesity epidemic, discussion of dietary factors cannot be complete without mention of the role of excessive weight in lung cancer. In 2005, 23.25% of the world's adult population (937 million people) was overweight and 9.8% (396 million) was obese with a body mass index (BMI) of greater than 30 kg/m^2.[157] These numbers are greater in industrialized countries where more than one-fifth of the adult population is obese. In the United States, 35.1% of adults aer classified as obese.[158] Excessive body weight has been associated with increased risk for endometrial, breast, and colorectal cancer but not for lung cancer. A meta-analysis by Renehan and colleagues[159] reported that there was an inverse association between BMI and lung cancer risk and obesity may even have a protective role. In the absence of cigarette smoking, however, the association between BMI and lung cancer was not significant. It has been proposed that the observed BMI and cancer association may be related to residual strong confounding effects of smoking itself.[160] For example, smokers tend to have lower mean BMI than age-matched and gender-matched nonsmokers.[161] Smokers have a lower BMI than nonsmokers, and they gain weight when they quit smoking. It has been suggested also that leanness was associated with increased lung cancer risk, but the studies were small and did not clearly exclude the confounding effects of smoking or pre-existing diseases.[162] More recent studies by Kabat and colleagues,[163] after adjusting for pack-years of smoking and other relevant covariates in a female cohort, showed that there was evidence for inverse associations of BMI and lung cancer risk in current and former smokers; whereas in never smokers, BMI was positively associated with lung cancer. A different study showed that waist circumference was positively associated with lung cancer risk in the smokers.[164] Recent prospective studies in Chinese men showed an inverse relationship between BMI and lung cancer mortality after adjustment for potential obvious confounders, such as smoking.[165,166] These studies did not have information on exposure to cooking fumes that have been reported to play a role in lung cancer in the Chinese population.[167]

Other Lung Diseases and Airways Obstruction

Some nonmalignant diseases have been associated with an increased risk for lung cancer, the strongest association being with COPD. Tobacco smoking is the primary cause of both lung cancer and COPD. A study of women never smokers with lung cancer showed a statistically significant association between the presence of airflow obstruction and the development of lung cancer.[168] There is other evidence that airflow obstruction is a risk for lung cancer.[169,170] This conclusion is supported by the Lung Health Study in which 5887 male and female smokers with spirometric evidence of mild to moderate COPD were monitored over a 5-year period with or without smoking cessation counseling or bronchodilator therapy.[171] Lung cancer was the most common cause of death, accounting for 38% of all deaths and lung cancer deaths exceeded deaths from cardiovascular disease by nearly 50%. More recent studies in large cohorts have shown that COPD is significantly associated with an increased risk for lung cancer, especially in men.[172,173] Because COPD affects an estimated 40% to 70% of patients with lung cancer, a coexisting disease of lung cancer and COPD likely reflects a common smoking exposure. Potential confounders by age, gender, and smoking history or the effects of lung cancer on spirometry could have resulted in the overdiagnosis of COPD in patients with lung cancer. A recent study evaluated 602 patients with lung cancer and found that 50% of them had prebronchodilator pulmonary function test results consistent with a diagnosis of COPD with Global Initiative for Chronic Obstructive Lung Disease stage 2 and higher, independent of age, gender, and smoking history, with an OR of 11.6.[174] The prevalence of COPD in newly diagnosed lung cancer was 6-fold greater than matched smokers, suggesting that COPD itself is an important independent risk factor with potential relationship to the pathogenesis of lung cancer.

COPD is characterized by chronic inflammation that responds to corticosteroids, and chronic inflammation itself has been suggested as associated with lung cancer. A Dutch study found that the likelihood of developing lung cancer was increased if C-reactive protein, a measure of generalized inflammation, was greater than 3 mg/L compared with patients with lower levels (<1 mg/L).[175] A large retrospective study of patients with COPD patients found that the risk for lung cancer was lower among patients who took high-dose inhaled corticosteroids compared with patients taking lower doses or none at all.[176] These results suggest that inhaled corticosteroids may have a chemoproventive role in lung cancer among patients with COPD. A study by Yang and colleagues[177] tested whether α_1-antitrypsin deficiency carriers have a higher risk for lung cancer, after adjusting for the effects of tobacco smoke exposure and COPD. Using a multiple logistic regression analysis, they found a significantly increased lung cancer risk (approximately 2-fold increased risk) among α_1-antitrypsin deficiency carriers from two parallel case-control cohorts.

Interstitial fibrosis has also been associated with an increase in lung cancer risk. Hubbard and colleagues[178] evaluated 890 patients with cryptogenic fibrosing alveolitis (idiopathic pulmonary fibrosis) and 5884 control subjects and found that the incidence of lung cancer in patients with fibrosis was markedly increased, even after adjustment for smoking. Patients with such fibrosis had an OR for lung cancer of 8.25 compared with control subjects. Other fibrosing diseases, including asbestosis and scleroderma-related lung disease, also seem to have an increased association with lung cancer (asbestos-related disease is discussed later). The association of scleroderma with lung cancer, however, is weaker. A British study followed patients with idiopathic pulmonary fibrosis and found the incidence of lung cancer markedly increased compared with the general population.[179] Although the mechanisms by which pulmonary interstitial disease may predispose to malignancy are not clear, various hypotheses have been raised, including malignant transformation related to chronic inflammation, epithelial hyperplasia, impaired clearance of carcinogens, and infections.

Infections

Infection as a causative factor in lung cancer has been evoked but remains debatable. For example, oncogenic viruses have been proposed as a cause of lung cancer. Early studies on sheep pulmonary adenomatosis caused by the Jaagsiekte sheep retrovirus show pathologic similarities to human bronchioloalveolar carcinoma; however, there is not enough evidence to link these two diseases and prove the involvement of viruses in the development of human bronchioloalveolar carcinoma.[180] More recent findings have suggested a potential role for human papillomavirus (HPV), known to cause carcinoma in other tissues. The possible involvement of HPV in bronchial squamous cell lesions was first suggested by Syrjänen,[181] who described epithelial changes in bronchial carcinomas that closely resemble those of established HPV condylomatous lesions in the female genital tract.[181] HPV DNA within squamous cell carcinoma lung cancer tissues has been detected. There is inconsistency, however, in the reported prevalence of infection by HPV in patients with lung cancer in different countries with racial and geographic variations. High incidence of HPV DNA in lung cancer has been reported in Asian cohorts, especially in nonsmokers; alternatively, studies in Western Europe failed to show an etiologic role of HPV in lung cancer.[182–184] HPV serotypes 16 and 18 are associated with lung cancer more than any other serotypes. E6 and E7 oncogenes from these HPV serotypes have been shown to immortalize human tracheal epithelial cells, which themselves are highly prone to genetic damage.[185] Currently, studies testing lung cancer specimens for HPV have yielded mixed results, and such variability of the frequency of HPV-positive lung cancer may be due to genetic susceptibility; methodologic approaches to detect HPV, such as those that involve the use of polymerase chain reaction (PCR); in situ hybridization and immunohistochemistry; and environmental and high-risk behavior variables. It would be interesting to see if HPV-directed vaccine for cervical cancer has any impact on the incidence of lung cancer.

Epstein-Barr virus, associated with Burkitt lymphoma and nasopharyngeal carcinoma, has been strongly associated with lymphoepithelioma-like carcinoma, a rare form of lung cancer, in Asian patients, but this association has not been observed in the Western population.[186] Other viruses suggested as etiologic for lung cancer include BK virus, JC virus, the human cytomegalovirus, simian virus 40, and measles virus; however, the results have remained inconclusive.[187–190] More recently, DNA from Torque teno virus, a new virus, has been detected at high levels in idiopathic pulmonary fibrosis patients with lung cancer, and although suggestive that Torque teno virus infection might be associated with the development of lung cancer in idiopathic pulmonary fibrosis, more studies are needed to confirm these findings and determine their clinical significance.[191]

It has also been suggested that Chlamydia pneumonia, a common cause of acute respiratory infection, especially in cigarette smoke –exposed individuals, might be involved in lung cancer carcinogenesis.[192] Identification of C pneumoniae as etiologically related to lung cancer, whether independent of tobacco smoking or as a cofactor, could have profound implications, particularly in the area of lung cancer prevention. Using serology to define Chlamydia infection, multiple epidemiologic studies have reported higher lung cancer risk associated with positive serology compared with those without such evidence of infection.[192] Although there were concerns about measurement differences, the results were consistent and suggested a potentially novel association of this organism with lung cancer. Although Chlamydia is not a known oncogenic pathogen, some investigators have hypothesized that the inflammation resulting from the infection can lead to reactive oxygen species that can cause DNA damage, cell injury, and repair, increasing the risk of mutations, which can confer selective advantages that lead to cancer. Such infection can also act synergistically with cigarette smoking to increase the risk of lung cancer. Similar to the concerns related to the evidence for various viruses as causes of lung cancer, however, further investigations are needed to solidify the evidence for a causal role of Chlamydia in lung cancer.

Some studies have reported association of pulmonary tuberculosis with lung cancer.[193,194] A cohort study from Taiwan showed an increased risk for lung cancer in tuberculosis patients with hazard ratio of 3.3 after adjusting for confounding factors, such as COPD and smoking-related cancers other than lung cancer. The effect of tuberculosis was even greater when combined with COPD or with other smoking-related cancers.[194] Other investigators speculate that the tuberculosis-related inflammation and scarring contribute to lung cancer pathogenesis.[193]

Lung cancer has become a new challenge in HIV-infected individuals. AIDS-related mortality has dramatically fallen since the advent of highly active antiretroviral treatments; however, this has been accompanied by an increase in the proportion of deaths attributable to non–AIDS-defining tumors, especially lung cancer.[195,196] The increased risk of lung cancer relative to the general population of the same age seems due in part to the higher prevalence of smoking among HIV-infected patients. In a study of 2840 HIV-infected patients, HIV was associated with a hazard ratio of 3.6 for lung cancer after controlling for smoking status.[197] Although smoking is a key risk factor for lung cancer in HIV-infected patients, several other factors may contribute to the higher incidence of lung cancer. These include greater prevalence of co-infection with oncogenic viruses, such as human herpesvirus 8, HPV, and Epstein-Barr virus, and the potential direct effects of the HIV virus and the consequences of long-term immunosuppression.[198] For example, the HIV tat protein can transactivate cellular genes or proto-oncogenes, whereas other HIV genes inhibit tumor suppressor genes.[199] HIV-infected cancer patients have a worse prognosis than similarly staged non–HIV-infected patients with the same cancer.[200] They are also more likely to have more advanced disease at diagnosis.[201] Studies have reported that HIV-infected patients were younger, were more likely to be smokers, and had significantly reduced median survival.[201,202] Taken together, evidence suggests that infection may play a role in lung cancer; however, definite proof of a causal relationship is currently lacking.

Environmental Tobacco Smoke

Secondhand smoke, also referred to as ETS, can contribute to an increased risk for lung cancer with a dose-dependent relationship between the degree of exposure and the relative risk. One study showed that household exposure of 25 or more smoker-years before adulthood doubled the risk for lung cancer; exposure of less than 25 smoker-years did not increase risk. The investigators estimated that at least 17% of lung cancers in nonsmokers are attributable to exposure to high levels of ETS during childhood and adolescence.[203] The Surgeon General reported in the early 1970s on the health consequences of smoking and raised concerns about hazards relating to such environmental smoke exposure.[12] Because nonsmokers exposed to ETS have an increased rate of smoke-related problems, including upper respiratory symptoms and eye irritation, and because there is an increased frequency of respiratory illnesses in children, it was suggested that the acknowledged carcinogenic effect of active tobacco smoking might also be present in those involuntarily exposed. Other reports showed an increased risk for lung cancer in nonsmoking women married to men who smoke.[204,205] A summary analysis of a large number of epidemiologic studies on the risk for lung cancer in nonsmokers found an excess risk for lung cancer of 24% in nonsmokers who lived

with a smoker.[206] This should be interpreted from the perspective that the background risk for lung cancer in a nonsmoker is low and contrasted with the 1000-fold increase of lung cancer risk in lifelong active smokers. Another study in nonsmoking women found that tobacco use by the spouse was associated with a 30% excess risk for all types of lung cancer.[207] These studies showed a dose-response relationship of the risk for lung cancer with both the number of cigarettes smoked by the spouse and the duration of exposure.[206,207]

In 1986, the National Research Council commissioned a review of the effects of ETS as a potential causal agent of lung cancer in nonsmokers exposed to household cigarette smoke.[208] Review of all the available evidence yielded an overall OR of 1.34 in lung cancer risk associated with ETS. In nonsmokers this translates into an approximately 30% increase of risk for lung cancer. At the same time, the US Department of Health and Human Services in a report on the health consequences of involuntary tobacco smoke exposure concluded that involuntary smoking is a cause of disease, including lung cancer, in healthy nonsmokers.[209] The US Environmental Protection Agency[210] and the IARC[211] both currently classify ETS as containing lung carcinogens. Cardenas and colleagues[212] examined lung cancer mortality and ETS within the context of the American Cancer Society Cancer Prevention Study. These investigators performed a prospective comparative evaluation of 133,835 never smokers with smoking spouses versus 154,000 never smokers with nonsmoking spouses. They concluded that the relative risk for lung cancer in women with smoking husbands was 1.2, which represented an increase in lung cancer incidence of 20%. The relative risk in nonsmoking men with smoking wives was somewhat less but still elevated at 1.1. These figures are consistent with data from prior studies evaluating lung cancer risk from ETS. Pooled data from 8 such studies in the United States from 1981 to 1991 found the relative risk for lung cancer in nonsmokers living with smokers to be 1.23.[213]

ETS consists of both mainstream (exhaled) smoke and sidestream smoke. Various carcinogens have been identified in ETS, including benzene, benzo[a]pyrene, and NNK. Hecht and colleagues[214] reported that male nonsmokers exposed to sidestream smoke generated by machine smoking of cigarettes had measurable carcinogenic metabolites in their urine. In the third National Health and Nutrition Examination Survey conducted between 1988 and 1991, Pirkle and colleagues[215] reported that a surprising 88% of nontobacco users had detectable levels of serum cotinine, a metabolite of nicotine, presumably from exposure to ETS. The presence of ETS is pervasive and harmful. Therefore, efforts on public smoking limitations will be of great benefit in this regard. With 19.8% of the American adult population still smoking, however, ETS will continue to be a major public health issue until cigarette smoking altogether is eliminated.[216] The exact number of cases of lung cancer due to involuntary smoking is difficult to calculate. Beckett, however, estimates that the number of lung cancer deaths in the United States attributable to ETS is comparable to the annual number caused by asbestos or radon.[217]

Biomass and Wood-smoke Exposure

In many parts of the world, wood is burned for cooking and heating purposes. Approximately 3 billion people worldwide rely on solid fuels as their primary source of domestic energy for cooking and heating. In China, for example, incomplete combustion of coal in homes has been linked with lung cancer.[218] A case-control study followed a group of residents living in underground dwellings who burn coal and unprocessed biomass, such as crop residues, wood, sticks, and twigs, for heating and cooking. They found that the OR for lung cancer associated with such coal use compared with that for biomass in the house was 1.29, after adjusting for smoking.[219] The IARC has recently classified indoor emissions from household coal combustion as a human carcinogen and emissions from biomass fuel primarily from wood as probable human carcinogen. A study using data from this consortium found that compared with nonsolid fuel users, predominant coal users (OR 1.64; in particular, coal users in Asia with OR 4.93), and predominant wood users in North American and European countries (OR of 1.21) exhibited higher risk for lung cancer.[220] A European cohort showed similar association of solid fuel use for heating and cooking with lung cancer risk; OR of lung cancer in lifetime users of solid fuel was 1.80; switching to nonsolid fuels resulted in lowered risk.[221] It has been suggested that the lung cancer that arise from wood smoke may behave differently from lung cancer due to tobacco smoke. Wood smoke exposure was found an important factor in predicting favorable response of NSCLC to tyrosine kinase inhibitor therapy.

Environmental Air Pollution

Air pollution has become a worldwide problem given the current staggering rate of globalization and industrialization. Wilkins[222] chronicled the most impressive example of the severe adverse effect of air pollution: the 1952 "great smog" of London, during which thousands of persons died

in a week from heavy pollution. This led to the implementation of the Clean Air Act 4 years later. The effects of low levels of air pollution exposure over a longer period of time are harder to measure, especially the long-term and accumulative effects on lung cancer risks. Air pollution is worsening in developing countries; the highest concentrations of suspected particulates, sulfur dioxide, and smoke have been recorded in large cities of these countries. Outdoor air pollution has long been thought to increase the risk for lung cancers. Advances in analytic methods used to detect specific pollutants have helped investigators study the effects of such airborne particulates. Early studies by Pershagen[223] involving urban-rural comparisons have shown that an "urban factor" is associated with a 10% to 40% increase in lung cancer deaths. A case-control study in Sweden by Nyberg and colleagues[224] showed a relative risk for lung cancer of 1.44 for persons exposed to more than 29.3 $\mu g/m^3$ of nitric oxide (as a measure of traffic air pollutant) over 21 to 30 years compared with exposures to lower than 12.8 $\mu g/m^3$ of nitric oxide. Two large United States cohort studies by Dockery[225] and Pope and colleagues[226] suggest that there is an excess risk for lung cancer of approximately 19% per 10 $\mu g/m^3$ increment in the long-term average exposure to fine particulates after adjustments for multiple confounding factors. Pope and coworkers[226] found as part of the Cancer Prevention Study II that fine particulate and sulfur oxide-related pollution were associated with 8% increased risk for lung cancer mortality for each 10 $\mu g/m^3$ elevation in long-term average ambient concentration of fine particles less than 2.5 μm in diameter. Despite these studies, it is still difficult to pinpoint the carcinogenic role played by single constituents of air pollution.

Various potential carcinogenic components are thought to be emitted from different sources of fossil fuel combustion products. Cohen[227] and Pope and coworkers[226] suggested that there is a range gradient of relative risk for lung cancer associated with exposure to combustion products, from 7.0 to 22.0 in cigarette smokers, to 2.5 to 10.0 in coke oven workers, to 1.0 to 1.6 in residents of areas with high levels of air pollution, to 1.0 to 1.5 in nonsmokers exposed to environmental tobacco smoke. Diesel exhaust composed of a complex mixture of gases and fine particles represents an important component of air pollution. Some of these gaseous components, such as benzene, formaldehyde, and 1,3-butadiene, are suspected of causing or known to cause cancer in humans. Studies in the late 1980s concluded that there was a weak association between diesel engine exhaust exposure and cancer. Later work, however, that included two large independent meta-analyses by Lipsett and Campleman[228] and Bhatia and colleagues,[229] provided strong support that occupational exposures to diesel exhaust, especially in persons in the trucking industry, is associated with an approximately 30% to 50% increase in the relative risk for lung cancer. Data linking gasoline engine exhaust and lung cancer are less compelling.

Occupational Carcinogens

Several workplace substances have been suggested to be or have been proved carcinogens in the lung. The IARC has identified arsenic, asbestos, beryllium, cadmium, chloromethyl ethers, chromium, nickel, radon, silica, and vinyl chloride as carcinogens. The occupations associated with exposure to these agents are shown in **Tables 3** and **4**. In 2000, it was estimated that 10% of lung cancer deaths among men (88,000 deaths) and 5% among women (14,300 deaths) worldwide could be attributable to exposure to 8 occupational lung carcinogens, namely asbestos, arsenic, beryllium, cadmium, chromium, nickel, silica, and diesel fumes.[230,231] Steeland and colleagues[232,233] estimated that approximately 6800 to 17,000 lung cancers were a result of exposure to chemicals in the workplace.

Asbestos

Asbestos is the most widely known and most common occupational cause of lung cancer. Asbestos is a class of naturally occurring fibrous minerals consisting primarily of 2 types: (1) serpentine (chrysotile) and (2) amphibole (amosite, crocidolite, and tremolites). Asbestos has been used commercially since the late 1800s, and its fire-retardant qualities and strength have made it useful in construction and insulating materials. As early as the 1940s in Germany, asbestos was noted as a lung carcinogen.[234] The wide recognition of its carcinogenicity, however, dates to reports in the United Kingdom in the 1950s, including that by Doll.[235] Asbestos exposure can also result in pleural and pulmonary manifestations. Asbestos-related pleural disease can present as effusion, pleurisy, or both. Chronic pleural involvement is seen as areas of pleural thickening (pleural plaques) that usually involve the parietal pleura and that are often calcified. The presence of pleural plaques does not herald the development of mesothelioma and has not been proved a marker of increased risk for lung cancer. Inhalation of asbestos fibers can result in parenchymal lung disease, specifically interstitial lung disease, known as *asbestosis*. All the major types of asbestos can cause interstitial lung disease, although amphibole fibers may be more fibrogenic than chrysotile fibers. The presentation of asbestosis is essentially identical to that of nonspecific interstitial lung disease as well as idiopathic pulmonary fibrosis. Asbestosis develops above a threshold fiber dose of approximately 25 to 105 fibers per mL per year, where the threshold dose is usually reached only in workers, including asbestos insulators, miners, millers, and textile workers, who have heavy occupational exposure.[236] The development of interstitial fibrosis usually requires prolonged exposure over months to years. Such fibrotic disease can follow shorter, more intense exposure, as occurs in shipyard workers. The latency period from exposure to presentation of disease is inversely proportional to exposure level. In the United States, the national rate of lung cancer in the form of mesothelioma is 13.8 per million population per year, with higher rates, exceeding 20 per million per year, in Maine, New Jersey, Pennsylvania, Washington, Wyoming, and West Virginia (**Fig. 16**).[237]

The distinction between asbestos exposure and asbestosis is important because of the controversy as to which represents the actual risk factor for lung cancer. Two reviews discussing the extensive available epidemiologic data illustrate this controversy. Jones and colleagues[238] in their extensive literature review highlight several important points. First, it is widely recognized that lung fibrosis of many causes, including idiopathic pulmonary fibrosis and interstitial disease associated with connective tissue disease, is associated with an increased risk for lung cancer. Second, in animal experiments asbestos-exposed animals that developed lung cancer only when they also developed pulmonary fibrosis. Third, pleural plaques, a marker for asbestos exposure, have not proved a reliable marker for increased risk for lung cancer. These investigators conclude that the issue of whether asbestosis is a necessary precursor to asbestos-attributable lung cancer cannot be definitively settled. Their assessment, however, was that the available data strongly support that hypothesis. In contrast, in an extensive assessment of the medical literature Egilman and Reinert conclude, "asbestos meets accepted criteria for causation of lung cancer in the absence of clinical or histologic parenchymal asbestosis."[239] Their evaluation of pathologic and epidemiologic studies resulted in the conclusion that asbestos can act as a carcinogen independent of the presence of asbestosis.

The question of whether asbestos exposure alone or asbestosis per se represents the risk factor for lung cancer remains an area of debate. A review of 9 epidemiologic studies by Hessel and colleagues[240] in 2005 concluded that because

Table 3
Occupational carcinogens and associated occupational exposures

Known Carcinogen	Occupational Exposure
Arsenic	Copper, lead, or zinc ore smelting Manufacture of insecticides Mining
Asbestos	Asbestos mining Asbestos textile production Brake lining work Cement production Construction work Insulation work Shipyard work
Beryllium	Ceramic manufacture Electronic and aerospace equipment manufacture Mining
Chloromethyl ethers	Chemical manufacturing
Chromium	Chromate production Chromium electroplating Leather tanning Pigment production
Nickel	Nickel mining, refining, electroplating Production of stainless and heat-resistant steel Polycyclic aromatics Aluminum production Hydrocarbon compounds Coke production Ferrochromium alloy production Nickel-containing ore smelting Roofing
Radon	Mining
Silica	Ceramics and glass industry Foundry industry Granite industry Metal ore smelting Mining and quarrying

Table 4
Suspected occupational carcinogens and associated occupational exposures

Suspected Carcinogen	Occupational Exposures
Acrylonitrile	Textile manufacture Plastics, petrochemical manufacture
Cadmium	Electroplating Pigment production Plastics industry
Formaldehyde	Formaldehyde resin production Synthetic fibers Insulation work Insulation production
Vinyl chloride	Plastic production Polyvinyl chloride production

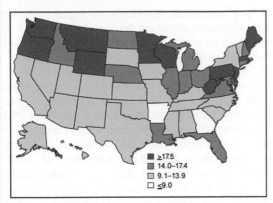

Fig. 16. Malignant mesothelioma death rate per 1 million population by state in the United States from 1999 to 2005. Map of the United States indicates the malignant mesothelioma death rate per 1 million population for each state during 1999–2005. The state death rate was greater than the national rate of 13.8 per million population per year in 26 states; in 6 states (Maine, New Jersey, Pennsylvania, Washington, Wyoming, and West Virginia), the rate exceeded 20 per million per year. (*Adapted from* Bang KM, Mazurek JM, Storey E, et al. Malignant mesothelioma mortality—United States, 1999–2005. MMWR 2009;58(15):393–6.)

of the relative insensitivity of chest radiographs and the uncertain specificity of histologic findings or CT, it is unlikely that epidemiologic studies alone can determine whether asbestos-related lung cancer arises only in the presence of pulmonary fibrosis. Recent studies have found that asbestos exposure was associated with a relative risk for lung cancer of 3.5 after adjusting for age, smoking, and vitamin intake.[241] This risk for lung cancer associated with asbestos exposure is dose-dependent but varied with the type of asbestos fiber exposure. The risk for lung cancer seems higher for workers exposed to amphibole fibers than for those exposed to chrysotile fibers, after adjusting for similar exposure level. The presence of interstitial fibrosis, such as in the form of asbestosis in persons exposed to asbestos, is associated with increased likelihood for lung cancer than patients with asbestos exposure without the associated fibrosis.[241] The study concluded that asbestosis was a better predictor of excess lung cancer risk than measures of asbestos exposure. Another study found excess risk for lung cancer was restricted to asbestos workers with radiographic evidence of asbestosis even though exposures to asbestos were similar to workers without such evidence.[242]

From a public health perspective, however, the issue is important because of concerns about lung cancer risk related to asbestos in the general environment. Jones and colleagues[238] noted that all persons living in industrialized countries have accumulated asbestos fibers in their lungs; in adults, the number of fibers is estimated in the millions. Asbestosis, however, requires prolonged and intense exposure to asbestos and does not occur at the level of everyday asbestos exposure. The risk for lung cancer from nonoccupational asbestos exposure in the general environment is extremely low. Moreover, Hughes and Weill[242] point out that if, as postulated, asbestosis is a necessary prerequisite to the development of cancer, the extrapolation of risk for lung cancer related to occupational asbestos exposure to the risk from exposure to asbestos in the general environment would substantially overestimate that risk. Another controversy in the area of asbestos and lung cancer is whether all types of fibers are carcinogenic. Epidemiologic and experimental data suggest that amphibole fibers are more carcinogenic than chrysotile.[243] In the United States, chrysotile has been by far the most commonly used type of asbestos. Thus, although all fibers may be carcinogenic, public concern about low-level asbestos exposure and lung cancer should be appropriately tempered.

Tobacco smoking clearly potentiates the observed carcinogenic effect of asbestos; however, the magnitude of the combined effect is not clear. It is also unclear whether the interaction of these two agents results in an additive or synergistic increase in the risk for lung cancer. When considering the addition of cigarette smoke exposure to asbestos, the risk for lung cancer is further increased. One report found that the risk for death from lung cancer in asbestos workers increased by 16-fold if the asbestos workers smoked more than 1 pack per day and by 9-fold if they smoked less than 1 pack per day compared with asbestos workers without significant smoking history.[244] The relative risk for lung cancer with asbestos exposure alone is 6-fold, with cigarette smoking alone 11-fold, but with exposure to both asbestos and cigarette smoke, the increase may be as high as 59-fold. The nature of the interaction in terms of relative risk, however, is again not clear. What is clear is that most lung cancers occur in asbestos-exposed workers who smoke. Smoking cessation should, therefore, be the most important goal of cancer prevention programs in this population, with particular targeting of the subgroup of workers with asbestosis. It is unclear if asbestosis is a marker for heavier exposure to asbestos or if the inflammation and fibrotic changes in the pathogenesis of asbestosis itself is mediating the cancer process. With recognition of the many health risks related to asbestos, its use has precipitously declined in the United States since the 1970s (**Fig. 17**).[237]

Radon

Mining is the oldest occupation associated with lung cancer. An illness described as a wasting pulmonary disease of miners and metal smelters has been associated with early mortality. The cause of this illness at the time, known as *miners' phthisis*, was variably attributed to dust or metal exposure, tuberculosis, or even inbreeding among mining communities. Early autopsy study performed on miners exposed to ores in the Central European mines documented that the process was actually neoplastic. Frank[245] points out that these same mines produced the material from which Marie Curie later isolated radium. Although the etiologic factors causing the increased lung cancer risk were originally speculated as dust-related pneumoconioses, arsenic, or cobalt, the actual carcinogens have been identified as radioactive materials, primarily radon and its decay products.

Radon (radon 222) is a naturally occurring decay product of radium 226, itself a decay product of uranium 238. Uranium and radium are ubiquitous

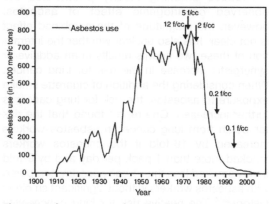

Fig. 17. Asbestos use and permissible exposure limits in the United States from 1900 to 2007. The amount of asbestos use, in thousands of metric tons, and the Occupational Safety and Health Administration permissible asbestos exposure limits in the United States during 1900–2007 are shown. Asbestos use increased from 1000 metric tons in 1900 to a peak of 803,000 metric tons in 1973, then decreased to approximately 1700 metric tons in 2007. Permissible asbestos exposure limits were 12 fibers per cubic centimeter (f/cc) in 1971, 5 f/cc in 1972, 2 f/cc in 1976, 0.2 f/cc in 1986, and 0.1 f/cc in 1994. Arrows indicate year when the Occupational Safety and Health Administration permissible exposure limits were put in place. (*Adapted from* Bang KM, Mazurek JM, Storey E, et al. Malignant mesothelioma mortality—United States, 1999–2005. MMWR 2009;58(15):393–6.)

in soil and rock, although in highly variable concentration. At usual temperatures, radon is released as a radium decay product as an inert radioactive gas. Radon itself decays with a half-life of 3.82 days into a series of radioisotopes, known as *radon decay products (or radon daughters)*, that have half-lives measured in seconds to minutes. These products include polonium 218 and polonium 214, which emit alpha particles. α-Radiation is highly damaging to tissues including the respiratory epithelium. Inhalation of these radon decay products and subsequent alpha particle emission in the lung may cause damage to cells and genetic material. Ultimately, radon decay produces lead 210, which has a half-life of 22 years. Radon is a well-established carcinogen with extensive data available both as an occupational hazards as well as exposures experienced by the general population. Evidence from epidemiologic studies of underground miners shows a linear relationship between radon exposure and lung cancer risk.[246,247] It has been found that uranium miners in Germany exposed to radon and the decay products have an increased risk for lung cancer, especially 15 to 24 years after exposure and in miners younger than 55 years.[248] Pooled original data from 11 cohort studies of radon-exposed underground miners showed that almost 40% of all lung cancer deaths may be due to radon progeny exposure, with 70% of lung cancer deaths in never-smokers and 39% in smokers. Moreover, this report concludes that 10% of all lung cancer deaths might be due to indoor radon, with 11% of lung cancer deaths in smokers and 30% of lung cancers in never smokers.[249]

There is an increased risk for lung cancer in smoking miners compared with nonsmoking miners, with both potentially acting in an additive and potentially a synergistic and multiplicative fashion.[250,251] Smokers and nonsmoking residents of smoking households are at increased risk for lung cancer even when radon levels are low. The combination of exposure to the two carcinogens is worse than exposure to either alone. The numbers of lung cancer cases reported in nonsmoking miners is small because miners have a high prevalence of cigarette smoking. In a study of underground uranium miners from Colorado, however, nonsmoking miners had a higher relative risk for lung cancer compared with all miners.[252] Such work emphasizes the potential importance of radon as a carcinogen in the nonsmoking population at large. Uranium mining has now ceased in the United States. Radon exposure, however, continues to be an occupational concern in nonuranium mining and underground work as well as in uranium and nonuranium mines around the world. In the United States, occupational exposure to radon is legislatively controlled. Individual exposure records are mandated for all workers in areas where the concentration of radon exceeds 0.3 work level, with an annual cumulative exposure limit of 4 work-level month. The Biological Effects of Ionizing Radiation IV study estimated that a 40-year exposure at this level would increase a person's lifetime risk for lung cancer 2-fold.[253] This is at best an approximate estimate, however. Continued longitudinal evaluation of occupationally exposed persons is needed to improve understanding of the carcinogenic effects of radon.

In recent years, the possible risk for lung cancer in the general population associated with radon exposure has been a concern. The National Council on Radiation Protection and Measurements has identified radon and its decay products as the largest component of environmental radiation to persons living in the United States. These findings in conjunction with extrapolation of data collected in groups with high occupational radon exposure have escalated concern about the risks of lung cancer related to domestic radon. Radon is a ubiquitous indoor air pollutant in homes, and it has been projected that radon is the second leading cause of lung cancer after smoking. The concentration of radon gas in an environment varies depending on two factors: the richness of the source of radium and the degree to which the air around that source is ventilated. Therefore, certain sites may be more likely to have a high radon concentration, with the prototypical situation being underground mines with poorly ventilated passageways. In a 1991 survey of homes in the United States, Samet and colleagues[254] reported a mean indoor radon level of approximately 1.25 pCi/L. In this survey, the range of indoor radon levels was broad. Most homes had levels only slightly higher than outdoor environmental levels, but a few had levels ranging in excess of 100 pCi/L. The primary factor determining radon gas concentration in homes is the concentration of radium in the soil and rock beneath those structures. Building materials, well water, and natural gas are less common sources, usually contributing only minimally to indoor radon concentrations. Indoor-to-outdoor air exchange may also affect radon concentration within the home.

Broad concern for the public health implications of domestic radon exposure has been heightened by the documented carcinogenic effect of radon in miners as described. The potential for mutagenic and carcinogenic effects of low-level α radiation, however, has been an area of controversy. Several studies examining lung cancer risks from domestic exposure have been performed. In a meta-analysis of 8 such studies that included 4263 patients with lung cancer and 6612 controls, Lubin and Boice[255] concluded that greater residential exposure levels were associated with an increased overall relative risk for lung cancer of 1.14. This conclusion is consistent with extrapolation of risk from studies performed in miners as well as with actual calculated risks in miners with low cumulative radon exposure. This meta-analysis did not demonstrate any greater increase in lung cancer risk than what would be extrapolated from radon exposure in miners. Using miner-based risk models, it is now estimated that domestic radon may account for 7000 to 36,000 lung cancer deaths in the United States per year. There are studies that dispute this projection, however, or demonstrate no increased risk even with high indoor domestic radon levels.[256-258] Cohen[227,259] concluded that use of a theoretic linear no-threshold relationship to extrapolate known risks in miners with high radon exposure levels to risk in persons with residential radon exposure grossly overestimates lung cancer risk. Cohen pointed out that the effects of low-dose, low-rate radiation have never been adequately evaluated, and he contested the assumptions inherent in extrapolation of high radon exposure in miners to domestic situations. Hei and colleagues[260] shed some insight into the effects of a single alpha particle hit to a cell as this is most relevant to radon exposure in the general population where the probability of multiple hits on a single cell is low given the level of environmental radon. They found that a majority of cells transversed by a single alpha particle survive such radon exposure. Up to 10% of cells can survive even up to 8 alpha particles traversals. Moreover, in the cells that survive such alpha particle exposure, the frequency of gene mutation after a single traversal was enhanced 2-fold, more with additional traversals by alpha particles. Therefore, small numbers of bronchial epithelial cells can be at significant risk for radiation-induced mutation in the setting of environmental radon levels. Assuming that genetic mutation may be an early step in induction of cancer, these data suggest that environmental and indoor radon exposure does indeed constitute a significant public health problem in its potential contribution to the development of lung cancer.

Other occupational carcinogens

Other lung carcinogens have been identified, relating to a wide array of occupations (see **Tables 3** and **4**). Worldwide, there are estimated 152,000 deaths from lung cancer and approximately 1.6

million disability-adjusted life years from lung cancer due to exposure to occupational exposures to carcinogens.[230] Steenland and colleagues[233] from the National Institute for Occupational Safety and Health estimated that approximately 9000 to 10,000 men and 900 to 1900 women per year in the United States develop lung cancer from exposure to occupational carcinogens. Although more than half of these are related to asbestos, a substantial number is attributable to other exposures. Furthermore, because these figures apply only to known carcinogens, they likely underestimate the actual number of lung cancer cases related to occupational exposures and represent another area in which prevention may play an important role.

PREVENTION OF LUNG CANCER

Multiple genetic, cellular, and local tissue alterations are involved in a chronic process that leads to lung carcinogenesis. The transformation of normal cells to preneoplastic cells to actual malignant cells involves changes that include DNA damages, genetic and epigenetic changes and the progression to unyielded proliferation of cells and invasion outside the boundaries of local tissues that is characterized as metastases. Exposure to various carcinogens alters normal cells long before clinically detectable invasive malignant tumors occur. Overwhelmingly, the major risk factor for lung cancer is cigarette smoking with a relative risk of 20 to 25 and an attributable risk of 85% to 90%.[261] The remaining risk factors contributing to lung cancer include environmental tobacco smoke, occupational exposure to asbestos and radon progenies, and diet. The incidence of lung cancer and therefore its related mortality can be reduced by early detection, treatment of disease, chemoprevention, and smoking avoidance and cessation.[261] Of these, only smoking prevention and cessation programs aimed at reducing smoking rates have been shown to reduce lung cancer risk.

Prevention of smoking initiation prevents the sequence of events leading to cancer. Despite intensive antismoking campaigns and widespread public awareness of the risks associated with smoking, there seems to be a committed smoking cohort that includes a 19.8% of the population of the United States.[216] There is no question that smoking cessation can decrease the risk for lung cancer. Peto and colleagues[59] reported two large case-control studies from approximately 1950 and from 1990 in the United Kingdom. In 1990, cessation of smoking had nearly halved what would have been the anticipated number of lung cancer cases. Lung cancer risk also seemed related to age at smoking cessation. For men who had stopped smoking at ages 60, 50, 40, and 30 years, the cumulative risks of lung cancer by age 70 years were 10%, 6%, 3%, and 2%, respectively. Jemal and colleagues,[262] in an evaluation of data collected by the National Center for Health Statistics in the United States, however, identified a slowing in the rate of decrease of the birth cohort trend in lung cancer mortality for whites born after 1950, which they interpreted as a reflection of the impact of increasing teenage smoking. Although there has been debate as to whether age at initiation of smoking is an independent risk factor for lung cancer, their report supports data reported by Wiencke[263] that patients in the youngest quartile of age at smoking initiation (7–15 years of age) have the highest levels of DNA adducts. Therefore, because a large percentage of persons in the United States and an increasing number of persons worldwide continue to smoke, efforts to prevent smoking initiation, particularly in children and teenagers, are of paramount importance. Furthermore, smoking cessation as the other method of primary prevention needs to be continually reinforced.

Smokers who quit for more than 15 years have an 80% to 90% reduction in their risk for lung cancer compared with persons who continue to smoke. Smokers who stop smoking even well into middle age avoid most of their subsequent risk for lung cancer, and stopping before middle age avoids more than 90% of the risk attributable to tobacco.[59] It is this primary prevention that should be the main focus of every society to reduce the risks for lung cancer. (See discussion of the prevention of lung cancer by smoking cessation by Hurt and colleagues elsewhere in this issue.) Lung cancer risk among former smokers has been shown to decrease with increasing duration of smoking abstinence.[264] Studies have observed a 50% or greater lung cancer risk reduction in the first decade of smoking abstinence for former smokers compared with current smokers.[265,266] In the Women's Health Study of women ages 55 to 69 years, there was a beneficial effect of smoking cessation among recent and distant former smokers. There are some investigators who argue that lung cancers may be triggered by smoking cessation.[267,268] The process of lung cancer development, however, takes place over many years. With the median interval of cessation to diagnosis of 2.7 years, the majority of former smokers with lung cancer likely harbored cancer at the time of smoking cessation.[269] A study described spontaneous smoking cessation before lung cancer diagnosis and challenged the widely believed notion that cessation was due to disease symptoms[26] but instead spontaneous smoking cessation represent a presenting symptom of lung cancer itself. They speculate that lung cancers may produce factors that block or emulate the effects of nicotine.[269]

The risk for lung adenocarcinoma, however, remained elevated for up to 30 years for both former heavier and former lighter smokers, highlighting the importance of emphasis on smoking prevention for all smokers.[270] Chemoprevention has been advocated as an approach to reduce lung cancers with the idea of treating in the early steps in lung carcinogenesis. Chemoprevention, a termed coined initially by Sporn and colleagues[271] in 1976, consists of the use of specific natural or non-natural agents, dietary or pharmacologic, to interfere with the development of cancer cells by preventing the DNA damage that initiates carcinogenesis or by halting the progression of premalignant cells.[272] Kelley and McCrory[261] and Dragnev and colleageus[273] extensively reviewed the studies related to lung cancer chemoprevention strategies. Chemoprevention strategies can be used for primary prevention of lung cancer in persons with known high-risk factors, for secondary prevention in persons with disease precursors, or for tertiary prevention in persons with a prior cancer that had been treated with curative intent. Chemoprevention has been used with some success in breast cancer (tamoxifen), prostate cancer (finasteride), and colon cancer (celocoxib); however, no agents have been validated as effective chemoprevention for lung cancer.[274,275] There have been various large chemoprevention of lung cancer trials testing for various agents, such as retinol (vitamin A), β-carotene, N-acetylcysteine, and selenium; however, none of these trials has shown evidence for efficacy.[261] As discussed previously, there is evidence to suggest that the use of β-carotene and isotretinoin for lung cancer chemoprevention in high-risk persons may increase their risk for lung cancer, especially in those who continue to smoke.[273] Currently there are chemoprevention trials being conducted involving agents, such as COX inhibitors, prostacyclin analogues, leukotriene modifiers, green tea, and broccoli sprout extracts, with future trials planned using peroxisome proliferator-activated receptor gamma (PPAR-γ) agonists or mammalian target of rapamycin inhibitors. For a successful lung cancer chemoprevention trial, incorporation of a highly defined risk population based on known lung cancer epidemiology and reliable biomarkers is needed. Until these chemopreventative agents are shown to be efficacious, smoking cessation and tobacco control are the main forms of prevention.

SUMMARY

A vast majority of lung cancer deaths are attributable to cigarette smoking, and curbing the rates of cigarette smoking is imperative. Understanding the epidemiology and causal factors of lung cancer can provide additional foundation for disease prevention. The role of tobacco as an etiologic factor in lung cancer has been convincingly established. Likewise, ionizing radiation and certain occupational exposures have been recognized as carcinogenic. At present, the 5-year survival rate for lung cancer is only 15.6%. This is in stark contrast to the 5-year survival rates for the other leading causes of cancer death in the United States, including cancers of the colon (66%), skin (melanoma 93%), breast (90%), and prostate (100%).[1] The absolute number of lung cancer cases continues to be alarming, with the continued rise of lung cancer in women a particularly disturbing feature. The challenge in the future will be to modify the impact of these identified external sources of risk while continuing to expand knowledge of the genetic and molecular basis of carcinogenesis. Early diagnosis of lung cancer is imperative because the 5-year survival rate for treated stage I lung cancer is substantially better than for stages II to IV. The issue of benefit related to lung cancer screening is being actively revisited. The American Cancer Society does not currently recommend routine screening for lung cancer. The American College of Chest Physicians guidelines for lung cancer screening only recommend it for persons who are part of a clinical trial. Prior trials from the 1970s and 1980s demonstrating no reduction in cancer mortality despite screening by chest radiograph effectively eliminated such testing. Petty[276] points out that groups at high risk, specifically heavy smokers with spirometric and clinical evidence of airflow obstruction, can be easily identified. Many clinicians think that screening with chest radiography and sputum cytology in such groups might be justifiable. Recent National Lung Screening Trial study shows that using low-dose CT scans to screen for lung cancer resulted in a 20% reduction in deaths from the disease.[277] As promising as the National Lung Screening Trial results are, official guidelines on CT scan for lung cancer screening are not available pending careful evaluation of the new data to determine who should or should not consider undergo screen for early lung cancer detection. It is hoped that ongoing trials evaluating chest radiography, chest CT scanning, and sputum cytology will clarify this important controversial issue.

At present, with approximately a quarter of the American population still smoking cigarettes, continued efforts must be directed at smoking cessation and at preventing persons from becoming addicted to smoking. Although work in the field of lung cancer treatment continues to be and remains important, the dismal survival rate associated with this disease demands that the medical profession contribute to efforts aimed at limiting its primary cause. If tobacco smoking could be eliminated, or at least severely curtailed, and if some of the other known exposure risks of lung cancer are addressed, only then may lung cancer be able to be returned to its designation by Adler[16] at the turn of the twentieth century as "among the rarest forms of disease."

REFERENCES

1. Siegel R, Ward E, Brawley O, et al. Cancer statistics, 2011: the impact of eliminating socioeconomic and racial disparities on premature cancer deaths. CA Cancer J Clin 2011;61(4):212–36.
2. Jemal A, Bray F, Center MM, et al. Global cancer statistics. CA Cancer J Clin 2011;61(2):69–90.
3. Howlader N, Noone AM, Krapcho M, et al, editors. SEER Cancer Statistics Review, 1975–2008. Bethesda (MD): National Cancer Institute; 2010. Available at: http://seer.cancer.gov/csr/1975_2008/, based on November 2010 SEER data submission, posted to the SEER web site, 2011.
4. Kohler B, Ward E, McCarthy B, et al. Annual report to the nation on the status of cancer, 1975-2007, featuring tumors of the brain and other nervous system. J Natl Cancer Inst 2011;103:1–23.
5. Herbst RS, Heymach JV, Lippman SM. Lung cancer. N Engl J Med 2008;359(13):1367–80.
6. Parkin DM, Pisani P, Lopez AD, et al. At least one in seven cases of cancer is caused by smoking. Global estimates for 1985. Int J Cancer 1994; 59(4):494–504.
7. Guindon GE, Boisclair D. Past, current and future trend in tobacco. Washington, DC: International Bank for Reconstruction and Development. The World Bank; 2009. p. 13–6.
8. Dube S, McClave A, James C, et al. Vital signs: current cigarette smoking among adults aged ≥18 years—United States, 2009. MMWR 2010;59: 1135–40.
9. Minna J, Schiller J. Harrison's principles of internal medicine. 17th edition. New York: McGraw-Hill; 2008.
10. Wynder EL, Graham EA. Tobacco smoking as a possible etiologic factor in bronchiogenic carcinoma; a study of 684 proved cases. J Am Med Assoc 1950;143(4):329–36.
11. Warner KE, Mendez D. Tobacco control policy in developed countries: yesterday, today, and tomorrow. Nicotine Tob Res 2010;12(9):876–87.
12. U.S. Public Health Service, office of the Surgeon General: The health consequences of smoking. National Clearinghouse for Smoking Health; 1972.
13. Dube S, Asman K, Malarcher A, et al. Cigarette smoking among adults and trends in smoking cessation—United States 2008. Office on Smoking and Health, National Center for Chronic Disease Prevention and Health Promotion, CDC; 2009.
14. Eaton D, Kann L, Kinchen S, et al. Youth Risk Behavior Surveillance – United States, 2009. In: Department of Health and Human Services. MMWR. 2010;59:1–36.
15. Office on Smoking and Health DoAaSH, National Center for Chronic Disease Prevention and Health Promotion, CDC. Cigarette use among high school students—United States, 1991-2007. MMWR Morb Mortal Wkly Rep 2008;57:689–91.
16. Adler I. Primary malignant growth of the lung and bronchi. New York: Longman, Green, Company; 1912.
17. Hruby A, Sweany H. Primary carcinoma of the lung. Arch Intern Med 1933;52:497.
18. Pear R. Tobacco smoking and longevity. Science 1938;87(2253):216–7.
19. Robert PN. Angel H Roffo: The forgotten father of experimental tobacco carcinogenesis. Bulletin of the World Health Organization 2006;84:494–6.
20. Tylecote F. Cancer of the lung. Lancet 1927;2:256.
21. Ochsner A, DeBakey M. Primary pulmonary malignancy: treatment of total pneumonectomy. Analysis of seventy-nine collected cases and presentation of seven personal cases. Surg Gynecol Obstet 1939;68:435.
22. Levin ML, Goldstein H, Gerhardt PR. Cancer and tobacco smoking; a preliminary report. J Am Med Assoc 1950;143(4):336–8.
23. McNally W. The tar in cigarette smoke and its possible effects. Am J Cancer 1932;16:1502.
24. Doll R, Hill AB. Smoking and carcinoma of the lung; preliminary report. Br Med J 1950;2(4682):739–48.
25. Wynder EL, Graham EA. Etiologic factors in bronchiogenic carcinoma with special reference to industrial exposures; report of eight hundred fifty-seven proved cases. A M A Arch Ind Hyg Occup Med 1951;4(3):221–35.
26. Doll R, Peto R, Boreham J, et al. Mortality in relation to smoking: 50 years' observations on male British doctors. BMJ 2004;328(7455):1519.
27. U.S. Department of Health and Human Services PHS, Centers for Dsiease Control and Prevention. The health consequences of smoking: a report of the Surgeon General, vol. 7829. Washington, DC: CDC Publication; 2004.

28. Hoffmann D, Hoffmann I. The changing cigarette, 1950-1995. J Toxicol Environ Health 1997;50(4): 307–64.

29. Smith CJ, Perfetti TA, Rumple MA, et al. "IARC group 2A Carcinogens" reported in cigarette mainstream smoke. Food Chem Toxicol 2000;38(4): 371–83.

30. Smith CJ, Perfetti TA, Mullens MA, et al. "IARC group 2B Carcinogens" reported in cigarette mainstream smoke. Food Chem Toxicol 2000;38(9): 825–48.

31. Wynder EL, Hoffmann D. Smoking and lung cancer: scientific challenges and opportunities. Cancer Res 1994;54(20):5284–95.

32. Akopyan G, Bonavida B. Understanding tobacco smoke carcinogen NNK and lung tumorigenesis. Int J Oncol 2006;29(4):745–52.

33. Hoffmann D, Djordjevic MV, Rivenson A, et al. A study of tobacco carcinogenesis. LI. Relative potencies of tobacco-specific N-nitrosamines as inducers of lung tumours in A/J mice. Cancer Lett 1993;71(1–3):25–30.

34. Belinsky SA, Devereux TR, Maronpot RR, et al. Relationship between the formation of promutagenic adducts and the activation of the K-ras protooncogene in lung tumors from A/J mice treated with nitrosamines. Cancer Res 1989;49(19):5305–11.

35. Rodenhuis S, Slebos RJ. Clinical significance of ras oncogene activation in human lung cancer. Cancer Res 1992;52(Suppl 9):2665s–9s.

36. Westra WH, Slebos RJ, Offerhaus GJ, et al. K-ras oncogene activation in lung adenocarcinomas from former smokers. Evidence that K-ras mutations are an early and irreversible event in the development of adenocarcinoma of the lung. Cancer 1993;72(2):432–8.

37. Denissenko MF, Pao A, Tang M, et al. Preferential formation of benzo[a]pyrene adducts at lung cancer mutational hotspots in P53. Science 1996; 274(5286):430–2.

38. Smith LE, Denissenko MF, Bennett WP, et al. Targeting of lung cancer mutational hotspots by polycyclic aromatic hydrocarbons. J Natl Cancer Inst 2000;92(10):803–11.

39. Jemal A, Ward E, Hao Y, et al. Trends in the leading causes of death in the United States, 1970-2002. JAMA 2005;294(10):1255–9.

40. Mattson ME, Pollack ES, Cullen JW. What are the odds that smoking will kill you? Am J Public Health 1987;77(4):425–31.

41. Harris JE, Thun MJ, Mondul AM, et al. Cigarette tar yields in relation to mortality from lung cancer in the cancer prevention study II prospective cohort, 1982-8. BMJ 2004;328(7431):72.

42. Loeb LA, Ernster VL, Warner KE, et al. Smoking and lung cancer: an overview. Cancer Res 1984; 44(12 Pt 1):5940–58.

43. Pisani P, Bray F, Parkin DM. Estimates of the world-wide prevalence of cancer for 25 sites in the adult population. Int J Cancer 2002;97(1): 72–81.

44. Shapiro JA, Jacobs EJ, Thun MJ. Cigar smoking in men and risk of death from tobacco-related cancers. J Natl Cancer Inst 2000;92(4):333–7.

45. Iribarren C, Tekawa IS, Sidney S, et al. Effect of cigar smoking on the risk of cardiovascular disease, chronic obstructive pulmonary disease, and cancer in men. N Engl J Med 1999;340(23): 1773–80.

46. Boffetta P, Pershagen G, Jöckel KH, et al. Cigar and pipe smoking and lung cancer risk: a multicenter study from Europe. J Natl Cancer Inst 1999;91(8):697–701.

47. Boffetta P, Nyberg F, Agudo A, et al. Risk of lung cancer from exposure to environmental tobacco smoke from cigars, cigarillos and pipes. Int J Cancer 1999;83(6):805–6.

48. Henley SJ, Thun MJ, Chao A, et al. Association between exclusive pipe smoking and mortality from cancer and other diseases. J Natl Cancer Inst 2004;96(11):853–61.

49. Wald NJ, Watt HC. Prospective study of effect of switching from cigarettes to pipes or cigars on mortality from three smoking related diseases. BMJ 1997;314(7098):1860–3.

50. Fligiel SE, Roth MD, Kleerup EC, et al. Tracheobronchial histopathology in habitual smokers of cocaine, marijuana, and/or tobacco. Chest 1997; 112(2):319–26.

51. Barsky SH, Roth MD, Kleerup EC, et al. Histopathologic and molecular alterations in bronchial epithelium in habitual smokers of marijuana, cocaine, and/or tobacco. J Natl Cancer Inst 1998; 90(16):1198–205.

52. Aldington S, Harwood M, Cox B, et al. Cannabis use and risk of lung cancer: a case-control study. Eur Respir J 2008;31(2):280–6.

53. Parkin DM, Bray F, Ferlay J, et al. Global cancer statistics, 2002. CA Cancer J Clin 2005;55(2): 74–108.

54. Rudin CM, Avila-Tang E, Samet JM. Lung cancer in never smokers: a call to action. Clin Cancer Res 2009;15(18):5622–5.

55. Sun S, Schiller JH, Gazdar AF. Lung cancer in never smokers—a different disease. Nat Rev Cancer 2007;7(10):778–90.

56. Wakelee HA, Chang ET, Gomez SL, et al. Lung cancer incidence in never smokers. J Clin Oncol 2007;25(5):472–8.

57. Zell JA, Ou SH, Ziogas A, et al. Epidemiology of bronchioloalveolar carcinoma: improvement in survival after release of the 1999 WHO classification of lung tumors. J Clin Oncol 2005;23(33): 8396–405.

58. Yano T, Miura N, Takenaka T, et al. Never-smoking nonsmall cell lung cancer as a separate entity: clinicopathologic features and survival. Cancer 2008; 113(5):1012–8.

59. Peto R, Darby S, Deo H, et al. Smoking, smoking cessation, and lung cancer in the UK since 1950: combination of national statistics with two case-control studies. BMJ 2000;321(7257):323–9.

60. Thun MJ, Hannan LM, Adams-Campbell LL, et al. Lung cancer occurrence in never-smokers: an analysis of 13 cohorts and 22 cancer registry studies. PLoS Med 2008;5(9):e185.

61. Gabrielson E. Worldwide trends in lung cancer pathology. Respirology 2006;11(5):533–8.

62. Kenfield SA, Wei EK, Stampfer MJ, et al. Comparison of aspects of smoking among the four histological types of lung cancer. Tob Control 2008; 17(3):198–204.

63. Bryant A, Cerfolio RJ. Differences in epidemiology, histology, and survival between cigarette smokers and never-smokers who develop non-small cell lung cancer. Chest 2007;132(1):185–92.

64. Gray N. The consequences of the unregulated cigarette. Tob Control 2006;15(5):405–8.

65. Liu NS, Spitz MR, Kemp BL, et al. Adenocarcinoma of the lung in young patients: the M. D. Anderson experience. Cancer 2000;88(8):1837–41.

66. Toh CK, Gao F, Lim WT, et al. Never-smokers with lung cancer: epidemiologic evidence of a distinct disease entity. J Clin Oncol 2006;24(15):2245–51.

67. Yang P. Lung cancer in never smokers. Semin Respir Crit Care Med 2011;32(1):10–21.

68. Brenner DR, Hung RJ, Tsao MS, et al. Lung cancer risk in never-smokers: a population-based case-control study of epidemiologic risk factors. BMC Cancer 2010;10:285.

69. Gorlova OY, Zhang Y, Schabath MB, et al. Never smokers and lung cancer risk: a case-control study of epidemiological factors. Int J Cancer 2006; 118(7):1798–804.

70. Gorlova OY, Weng SF, Zhang Y, et al. Aggregation of cancer among relatives of never-smoking lung cancer patients. Int J Cancer 2007;121(1):111–8.

71. Wu PF, Lee CH, Wang MJ, et al. Cancer aggregation and complex segregation analysis of families with female non-smoking lung cancer probands in Taiwan. Eur J Cancer 2004;40(2):260–6.

72. Bell DW, Gore I, Okimoto RA, et al. Inherited susceptibility to lung cancer may be associated with the T790M drug resistance mutation in EGFR. Nat Genet 2005;37(12):1315–6.

73. Wenzlaff AS, Cote ML, Bock CH, et al. CYP1A1 and CYP1B1 polymorphisms and risk of lung cancer among never smokers: a population-based study. Carcinogenesis 2005;26(12):2207–12.

74. Wenzlaff AS, Cote ML, Bock CH, et al. GSTM1, GSTT1 and GSTP1 polymorphisms, environmental tobacco smoke exposure and risk of lung cancer among never smokers: a population-based study. Carcinogenesis 2005;26(2):395–401.

75. Jung CY, Choi JE, Park JM, et al. Polymorphisms in the hMSH2 gene and the risk of primary lung cancer. Cancer Epidemiol Biomarkers Prev 2006; 15(4):762–8.

76. Pao W, Miller V, Zakowski M, et al. EGF receptor gene mutations are common in lung cancers from "never smokers" and are associated with sensitivity of tumors to gefitinib and erlotinib. Proc Natl Acad Sci U S A 2004;101(36):13306–11.

77. Shigematsu H, Lin L, Takahashi T, et al. Clinical and biological features associated with epidermal growth factor receptor gene mutations in lung cancers. J Natl Cancer Inst 2005;97(5):339–46.

78. Kosaka T, Yatabe Y, Endoh H, et al. Mutations of the epidermal growth factor receptor gene in lung cancer: biological and clinical implications. Cancer Res 2004;64(24):8919–23.

79. Rudin CM, Avila-Tang E, Harris CC, et al. Lung cancer in never smokers: molecular profiles and therapeutic implications. Clin Cancer Res 2009; 15(18):5646–61.

80. Shimizu H, Tominaga S, Nishimura M, et al. Comparison of clinico-epidemiological features of lung cancer patients with and without a history of smoking. Jpn J Clin Oncol 1984;14(4):595–600.

81. Nordquist LT, Simon GR, Cantor A, et al. Improved survival in never-smokers vs current smokers with primary adenocarcinoma of the lung. Chest 2004; 126(2):347–51.

82. Tammemagi CM, Neslund-Dudas C, Simoff M, et al. Smoking and lung cancer survival: the role of comorbidity and treatment. Chest 2004;125(1):27–37.

83. Takeuchi T, Tomida S, Yatabe Y, et al. Expression profile-defined classification of lung adenocarcinoma shows close relationship with underlying major genetic changes and clinicopathologic behaviors. J Clin Oncol 2006;24(11):1679–88.

84. Lam DC, Girard L, Suen WS, et al. Establishment and expression profiling of new lung cancer cell lines from Chinese smokers and lifetime never-smokers. J Thorac Oncol 2006;1(9):932–42.

85. Li Y, Sheu CC, Ye Y, et al. Genetic variants and risk of lung cancer in never smokers: a genome-wide association study. Lancet Oncol 2010;11(4):321–30.

86. Hsiung CA, Lan Q, Hong YC, et al. The 5p15.33 locus is associated with risk of lung adenocarcinoma in never-smoking females in Asia. PLoS Genet 2010;6(8):1–9.

87. Spitz MR, Hong WK, Amos CI, et al. A risk model for prediction of lung cancer. J Natl Cancer Inst 2007;99(9):715–26.

88. Spitz MR, Etzel CJ, Dong Q, et al. An expanded risk prediction model for lung cancer. Cancer Prev Res (Phila) 2008;1(4):250–4.

89. Cassidy A, Myles JP, van Tongeren M, et al. The LLP risk model: an individual risk prediction model for lung cancer. Br J Cancer 2008;98(2):270–6.

90. Schwartz AG, Prysak GM, Bock CH, et al. The molecular epidemiology of lung cancer. Carcinogenesis 2007;28(3):507–18.

91. Takemiya M, Shiraishi S, Teramoto T, et al. Bloom's syndrome with porokeratosis of Mibelli and multiple cancers of the skin, lung and colon. Clin Genet 1987;31(1):35–44.

92. Yamanaka A, Hirai T, Ohtake Y, et al. Lung cancer associated with Werner's syndrome: a case report and review of the literature. Jpn J Clin Oncol 1997;27(6):415–8.

93. Matakidou A, Eisen T, Houlston RS. Systematic review of the relationship between family history and lung cancer risk. Br J Cancer 2005;93(7):825–33.

94. Bailey-Wilson JE, Amos CI, Pinney SM, et al. A major lung cancer susceptibility locus maps to chromosome 6q23-25. Am J Hum Genet 2004;75(3):460–74.

95. Le Marchand L, Guo C, Benhamou S, et al. Pooled analysis of the CYP1A1 exon 7 polymorphism and lung cancer (United States). Cancer Causes Control 2003;14(4):339–46.

96. Benhamou S, Lee WJ, Alexandrie AK, et al. Meta- and pooled analyses of the effects of glutathione S-transferase M1 polymorphisms and smoking on lung cancer risk. Carcinogenesis 2002;23(8):1343–50.

97. Ye Z, Song H, Higgins JP, et al. Five glutathione s-transferase gene variants in 23,452 cases of lung cancer and 30,397 controls: meta-analysis of 130 studies. PLoS Med 2006;3(4):e91.

98. Amos CI, Wu X, Broderick P, et al. Genome-wide association scan of tag SNPs identifies a susceptibility locus for lung cancer at 15q25.1. Nat Genet 2008;40(5):616–22.

99. Zhou W, Liu G, Thurston SW, et al. Genetic polymorphisms in N-acetyltransferase-2 and microsomal epoxide hydrolase, cumulative cigarette smoking, and lung cancer. Cancer Epidemiol Biomarkers Prev 2002;11(1):15–21.

100. Spitz MR, Wei Q, Dong Q, et al. Genetic susceptibility to lung cancer: the role of DNA damage and repair. Cancer Epidemiol Biomarkers Prev 2003;12(8):689–98.

101. Wu X, Delclos GL, Annegers JF, et al. A case-control study of wood dust exposure, mutagen sensitivity, and lung cancer risk. Cancer Epidemiol Biomarkers Prev 1995;4(6):583–8.

102. Weir HK, Thun MJ, Hankey BF, et al. Annual report to the nation on the status of cancer, 1975-2000, featuring the uses of surveillance data for cancer prevention and control. J Natl Cancer Inst 2003;95(17):1276–99.

103. Thomas L, Doyle LA, Edelman MJ. Lung cancer in women: emerging differences in epidemiology, biology, and therapy. Chest 2005;128(1):370–81.

104. Jemal A, Thun MJ, Ries LA, et al. Annual report to the nation on the status of cancer, 1975-2005, featuring trends in lung cancer, tobacco use, and tobacco control. J Natl Cancer Inst 2008;100(23):1672–94.

105. Wingo PA, Ries LA, Giovino GA, et al. Annual report to the nation on the status of cancer, 1973-1996, with a special section on lung cancer and tobacco smoking. J Natl Cancer Inst 1999;91(8):675–90.

106. Halpern MT, Gillespie BW, Warner KE. Patterns of absolute risk of lung cancer mortality in former smokers. J Natl Cancer Inst 1993;85(6):457–64.

107. Cook MB, McGlynn KA, Devesa SS, et al. Sex disparities in cancer mortality and survival. Cancer Epidemiol Biomarkers Prev 2011;20(8):1629–37.

108. Brownson RC, Chang JC, Davis JR. Gender and histologic type variations in smoking-related risk of lung cancer. Epidemiology 1992;3(1):61–4.

109. McDuffie HH, Klaassen DJ, Dosman JA. Female-male differences in patients with primary lung cancer. Cancer 1987;59(10):1825–30.

110. Risch HA, Howe GR, Jain M, et al. Are female smokers at higher risk for lung cancer than male smokers? A case-control analysis by histologic type. Am J Epidemiol 1993;138(5):281–93.

111. Zang EA, Wynder EL. Differences in lung cancer risk between men and women: examination of the evidence. J Natl Cancer Inst 1996;88(3–4):183–92.

112. Ryberg D, Hewer A, Phillips DH, et al. Different susceptibility to smoking-induced DNA damage among male and female lung cancer patients. Cancer Res 1994;54(22):5801–3.

113. Taioli E, Wynder EL. Re: Endocrine factors and adenocarcinoma of the lung in women. J Natl Cancer Inst 1994;86(11):869–70.

114. Slatore CG, Chien JW, Au DH, et al. Lung cancer and hormone replacement therapy: association in the vitamins and lifestyle study. J Clin Oncol 2010;28(9):1540–6.

115. Heiss G, Wallace R, Anderson GL, et al. Health risks and benefits 3 years after stopping randomized treatment with estrogen and progestin. JAMA 2008;299(9):1036–45.

116. Chlebowski RT, Schwartz AG, Wakelee H, et al. Oestrogen plus progestin and lung cancer in postmenopausal women (Women's Health Initiative trial): a post-hoc analysis of a randomised controlled trial. Lancet 2009;374(9697):1243–51.

117. Doll R, Peto R. Mortality in relation to smoking: 20 years' observations on male British doctors. Br Med J 1976;2(6051):1525–36.

118. Doll R, Gray R, Hafner B, et al. Mortality in relation to smoking: 22 years' observations on female British doctors. Br Med J 1980;280(6219):967–71.

119. Tashkin DP, Altose MD, Bleecker ER, et al. The lung health study: airway responsiveness to inhaled methacholine in smokers with mild to moderate airflow limitation. The Lung Health Study Research Group. Am Rev Respir Dis 1992;145(2 Pt 1):301–10.

120. Chen Y, Horne SL, Dosman JA. Increased susceptibility to lung dysfunction in female smokers. Am Rev Respir Dis 1991;143(6):1224–30.

121. Beck GJ, Doyle CA, Schachter EN. Smoking and lung function. Am Rev Respir Dis 1981;123(2):149–55.

122. Menck H, Hnederson BE. Cancer incidence patterns in the Pacific Basin. Natl Cancer Mongr 1982;62:101–9.

123. Haiman CA, Stram DO, Wilkens LR, et al. Ethnic and racial differences in the smoking-related risk of lung cancer. N Engl J Med 2006;354(4):333–42.

124. Coté ML, Kardia SL, Wenzlaff AS, et al. Risk of lung cancer among white and black relatives of individuals with early-onset lung cancer. JAMA 2005;293(24):3036–42.

125. Brooks DR, Palmer JR, Strom BL, et al. Menthol cigarettes and risk of lung cancer. Am J Epidemiol 2003;158(7):609–16 [discussion: 617–20].

126. Wingo PA, Cardinez CJ, Landis SH, et al. Long-term trends in cancer mortality in the United States, 1930-1998. Cancer 2003;97(Suppl 12):3133–275.

127. Blanchard EM, Arnaoutakis K, Hesketh PJ. Lung cancer in octogenarians. J Thorac Oncol 2010;5(6):909–16.

128. Gridelli C, Langer C, Maione P, et al. Lung cancer in the elderly. J Clin Oncol 2007;25(14):1898–907.

129. Willett WC, Trichopoulos D. Nutrition and cancer: a summary of the evidence. Cancer Causes Control 1996;7(1):178–80.

130. Ruano-Ravina A, Figueiras A, Barros-Dios JM. Diet and lung cancer: a new approach. Eur J Cancer Prev 2000;9(6):395–400.

131. Boone CW, Kelloff GJ, Malone WE. Identification of candidate cancer chemopreventive agents and their evaluation in animal models and human clinical trials: a review. Cancer Res 1990;50(1):2–9.

132. Woodson K, Tangrea JA, Barrett MJ, et al. Serum alpha-tocopherol and subsequent risk of lung cancer among male smokers. J Natl Cancer Inst 1999;91(20):1738–43.

133. Buring JE, Hennekens CH. Beta-carotene and cancer chemoprevention. J Cell Biochem Suppl 1995;22:226–30.

134. Stefani ED, Boffetta P, Deneo-Pellegrini H, et al. Dietary antioxidants and lung cancer risk: a case-control study in Uruguay. Nutr Cancer 1999;34(1):100–10.

135. Yong LC, Brown CC, Schatzkin A, et al. Intake of vitamins E, C, and A and risk of lung cancer. The NHANES I epidemiologic followup study. First National Health and Nutrition Examination Survey. Am J Epidemiol 1997;146(3):231–43.

136. Shekelle RB, Lepper M, Liu S, et al. Dietary vitamin A and risk of cancer in the Western Electric study. Lancet 1981;2(8257):1185–90.

137. Byers TE, Graham S, Haughey BP, et al. Diet and lung cancer risk: findings from the Western New York Diet Study. Am J Epidemiol 1987;125(3):351–63.

138. The effect of vitamin E and beta carotene on the incidence of lung cancer and other cancers in male smokers. The Alpha-Tocopherol, Beta Carotene Cancer Prevention Study Group. N Engl J Med 1994;330(15):1029–35.

139. Omenn GS, Goodman GE, Thornquist MD, et al. Effects of a combination of beta carotene and vitamin A on lung cancer and cardiovascular disease. N Engl J Med 1996;334(18):1150–5.

140. Omenn GS, Goodman GE, Thornquist MD, et al. Risk factors for lung cancer and for intervention effects in CARET, the Beta-Carotene and Retinol Efficacy Trial. J Natl Cancer Inst 1996;88(21):1550–9.

141. Goodman GE, Thornquist MD, Balmes J, et al. The Beta-Carotene and Retinol Efficacy Trial: incidence of lung cancer and cardiovascular disease mortality during 6-year follow-up after stopping beta-carotene and retinol supplements. J Natl Cancer Inst 2004;96(23):1743–50.

142. Hennekens CH, Buring JE, Manson JE, et al. Lack of effect of long-term supplementation with beta carotene on the incidence of malignant neoplasms and cardiovascular disease. N Engl J Med 1996;334(18):1145–9.

143. Mahabir S, Spitz MR, Barrera SL, et al. Dietary zinc, copper and selenium, and risk of lung cancer. Int J Cancer 2007;120(5):1108–15.

144. Mahabir S, Forman MR, Dong YQ, et al. Mineral intake and lung cancer risk in the NIH-American Association of Retired Persons Diet and Health study. Cancer Epidemiol Biomarkers Prev 2010;19(8):1976–83.

145. Voorrips LE, Goldbohm RA, Verhoeven DT, et al. Vegetable and fruit consumption and lung cancer risk in the Netherlands Cohort Study on diet and cancer. Cancer Causes Control 2000;11(2):101–15.

146. Brennan P, Hsu CC, Moullan N, et al. Effect of cruciferous vegetables on lung cancer in patients stratified by genetic status: a mendelian randomisation approach. Lancet 2005;366(9496):1558–60.

147. Fontham ET. Protective dietary factors and lung cancer. Int J Epidemiol 1990;19(Suppl 1):S32–42.

148. Cooper DA, Eldridge AL, Peters JC. Dietary carotenoids and lung cancer: a review of recent research. Nutr Rev 1999;57(5 Pt 1):133–45.

149. Wright ME, Park Y, Subar AF, et al. Intakes of fruit, vegetables, and specific botanical groups in relation to lung cancer risk in the NIH-AARP Diet and Health Study. Am J Epidemiol 2008;168(9):1024–34.

150. Mursu J, Nurmi T, Tuomainen TP, et al. Intake of flavonoids and risk of cancer in Finnish men: The Kuopio Ischaemic Heart Disease Risk Factor Study. Int J Cancer 2008;123(3):660–3.

151. Swanson CA, Brown CC, Sinha R, et al. Dietary fats and lung cancer risk among women: the Missouri Women's Health Study (United States). Cancer Causes Control 1997;8(6):883–93.

152. Alavanja MC, Brownson RC, Benichou J. Estimating the effect of dietary fat on the risk of lung cancer in nonsmoking women. Lung Cancer 1996;14(Suppl 1):S63–74.

153. De Stefani E, Fontham ET, Chen V, et al. Fatty foods and the risk of lung cancer: a case-control study from Uruguay. Int J Cancer 1997; 71(5):760–6.

154. Goodman MT, Kolonel LN, Yoshizawa CN, et al. The effect of dietary cholesterol and fat on the risk of lung cancer in Hawaii. Am J Epidemiol 1988;128(6):1241–55.

155. Hecht SS. Approaches to cancer prevention based on an understanding of N-nitrosamine carcinogenesis. Proc Soc Exp Biol Med 1997; 216(2):181–91.

156. De Stefani E, Deneo-Pellegrini H, Carzoglio JC, et al. Dietary nitrosodimethylamine and the risk of lung cancer: a case-control study from Uruguay. Cancer Epidemiol Biomarkers Prev 1996;5(9): 679–82.

157. Kelly T, Yang W, Chen CS, et al. Global burden of obesity in 2005 and projections to 2030. Int J Obes (Lond) 2008;32(9):1431–7.

158. Catenacci VA, Hill JO, Wyatt HR. The obesity epidemic. Clin Chest Med 2009;30(3):415–44, vii.

159. Renehan AG, Tyson M, Egger M, et al. Body-mass index and incidence of cancer: a systematic review and meta-analysis of prospective observational studies. Lancet 2008;371(9612):569–78.

160. Renehan AG, Soerjomataram I, Leitzmann MF. Interpreting the epidemiological evidence linking obesity and cancer: a framework for population-attributable risk estimations in Europe. Eur J Cancer 2010;46(14):2581–92.

161. Whitlock G, Lewington S, Sherliker P, et al. Body-mass index and cause-specific mortality in 900 000 adults: collaborative analyses of 57 prospective studies. Lancet 2009;373(9669):1083–96.

162. Henley SJ, Flanders WD, Manatunga A, et al. Leanness and lung cancer risk: fact or artifact? Epidemiology 2002;13(3):268–76.

163. Kabat GC, Miller AB, Rohan TE. Body mass index and lung cancer risk in women. Epidemiology 2007;18(5):607–12.

164. Kabat GC, Kim M, Hunt JR, et al. Body mass index and waist circumference in relation to lung cancer risk in the Women's Health Initiative. Am J Epidemiol 2008;168(2):158–69.

165. Yang L, Yang G, Zhou M, et al. Body mass index and mortality from lung cancer in smokers and nonsmokers: a nationally representative prospective study of 220,000 men in China. Int J Cancer 2009;125(9):2136–43.

166. Leung CC, Lam TH, Yew WW, et al. Lower lung cancer mortality in obesity. Int J Epidemiol 2011; 40(1):174–82.

167. Hecht SS, Seow A, Wang M, et al. Elevated levels of volatile organic carcinogen and toxicant biomarkers in Chinese women who regularly cook at home. Cancer Epidemiol Biomarkers Prev 2010;19(5):1185–92.

168. Wu AH, Fontham ET, Reynolds P, et al. Previous lung disease and risk of lung cancer among lifetime nonsmoking women in the United States. Am J Epidemiol 1995;141(11):1023–32.

169. Skillrud DM, Offord KP, Miller RD. Higher risk of lung cancer in chronic obstructive pulmonary disease. A prospective, matched, controlled study. Ann Intern Med 1986;105(4):503–7.

170. Tockman MS, Anthonisen NR, Wright EC, et al. Airways obstruction and the risk for lung cancer. Ann Intern Med 1987;106(4):512–8.

171. Anthonisen NR, Connett JE, Kiley JP, et al. Effects of smoking intervention and the use of an inhaled anticholinergic bronchodilator on the rate of decline of FEV1. The Lung Health Study. JAMA 1994;272(19):1497–505.

172. Turner MC, Chen Y, Krewski D, et al. Chronic obstructive pulmonary disease is associated with lung cancer mortality in a prospective study of never smokers. Am J Respir Crit Care Med 2007; 176(3):285–90.

173. Loganathan RS, Stover DE, Shi W, et al. Prevalence of COPD in women compared to men around the time of diagnosis of primary lung cancer. Chest 2006;129(5):1305–12.

174. Young RP, Hopkins RJ, Christmas T, et al. COPD prevalence is increased in lung cancer, independent of age, sex and smoking history. Eur Respir J 2009;34(2):380–6.

175. Siemes C, Visser LE, Coebergh JW, et al. C-reactive protein levels, variation in the C-reactive protein gene, and cancer risk: the Rotterdam Study. J Clin Oncol 2006;24(33):5216–22.

176. Parimon T, Chien JW, Bryson CL, et al. Inhaled corticosteroids and risk of lung cancer among patients with chronic obstructive pulmonary disease. Am J Respir Crit Care Med 2007;175(7): 712–9.

177. Yang P, Sun Z, Krowka MJ, et al. Alpha1-antitrypsin deficiency carriers, tobacco smoke, chronic obstructive pulmonary disease, and lung cancer risk. Arch Intern Med 2008;168(10):1097–103.

178. Hubbard R, Venn A, Lewis S, et al. Lung cancer and cryptogenic fibrosing alveolitis. A population-based

cohort study. Am J Respir Crit Care Med 2000; 161(1):5–8.

179. Le Jeune I, Gribbin J, West J, et al. The incidence of cancer in patients with idiopathic pulmonary fibrosis and sarcoidosis in the UK. Respir Med 2007;101(12):2534–40.

180. Mornex JF, Thivolet F, De las Heras M, et al. Pathology of human bronchioloalveolar carcinoma and its relationship to the ovine disease. Curr Top Microbiol Immunol 2003;275:225–48.

181. Syrjänen KJ. Bronchial squamous cell carcinomas associated with epithelial changes identical to condylomatous lesions of the uterine cervix. Lung 1980;158(3):131–42.

182. Chen YC, Chen JH, Richard K, et al. Lung adenocarcinoma and human papillomavirus infection. Cancer 2004;101(6):1428–36.

183. Syrjänen KJ. HPV infections and lung cancer. J Clin Pathol 2002;55(12):885–91.

184. Rezazadeh A, Laber DA, Ghim SJ, et al. The role of human papilloma virus in lung cancer: a review of the evidence. Am J Med Sci 2009;338(1):64–7.

185. Willey JC, Broussoud A, Sleemi A, et al. Immortalization of normal human bronchial epithelial cells by human papillomaviruses 16 or 18. Cancer Res 1991;51(19):5370–7.

186. Castro CY, Ostrowski ML, Barrios R, et al. Relationship between Epstein-Barr virus and lymphoepithelioma-like carcinoma of the lung: a clinicopathologic study of 6 cases and review of the literature. Hum Pathol 2001;32(8):863–72.

187. Brouchet L, Valmary S, Dahan M, et al. Detection of oncogenic virus genomes and gene products in lung carcinoma. Br J Cancer 2005;92(4):743–6.

188. Galateau-Salle F, Bidet P, Iwatsubo Y, et al. Detection of SV40-like DNA sequences in pleural mesothelioma, bronchopulmonary carcinoma and other pulmonary diseases. Dev Biol Stand 1998;94: 147–52.

189. Giuliani L, Jaxmar T, Casadio C, et al. Detection of oncogenic viruses SV40, BKV, JCV, HCMV, HPV and p53 codon 72 polymorphism in lung carcinoma. Lung Cancer 2007;57(3):273–81.

190. Sion-Vardy N, Lasarov I, Delgado B, et al. Measles virus: evidence for association with lung cancer. Exp Lung Res 2009;35(8):701–12.

191. Bando M, Takahashi M, Ohno S, et al. Torque teno virus DNA titre elevated in idiopathic pulmonary fibrosis with primary lung cancer. Respirology 2008;13(2):263–9.

192. Littman AJ, Jackson LA, Vaughan TL. Chlamydia pneumoniae and lung cancer: epidemiologic evidence. Cancer Epidemiol Biomarkers Prev 2005;14(4):773–8.

193. Engels EA, Shen M, Chapman RS, et al. Tuberculosis and subsequent risk of lung cancer in Xuanwei, China. Int J Cancer 2009;124(5):1183–7.

194. Yu YH, Liao CC, Hsu WH, et al. Increased lung cancer risk among patients with pulmonary tuberculosis: a population cohort study. J Thorac Oncol 2011;6(1):32–7.

195. Lavolé A, Wislez M, Antoine M, et al. Lung cancer, a new challenge in the HIV-infected population. Lung Cancer 2006;51(1):1–11.

196. Morris A, Crothers K, Beck JM, et al. An official ATS workshop report: emerging issues and current controversies in HIV-associated pulmonary diseases. Proc Am Thorac Soc 2011;8(1):17–26.

197. Kirk GD, Merlo C, O'Driscoll P, et al. HIV infection is associated with an increased risk for lung cancer, independent of smoking. Clin Infect Dis 2007; 45(1):103–10.

198. Mitsuyasu RT. Non–AIDS-defining malignancies in HIV. Top HIV Med 2008;16(4):117–21.

199. el-Solh A, Kumar NM, Nair MP, et al. An RGD containing peptide from HIV-1 Tat-(65-80) modulates protooncogene expression in human bronchoalveolar carcinoma cell line, A549. Immunol Invest 1997;26(3):351–70.

200. Powles T, Thirwell C, Newsom-Davis T, et al. Does HIV adversely influence the outcome in advanced non-small-cell lung cancer in the era of HAART? Br J Cancer 2003;89(3):457–9.

201. Brock MV, Hooker CM, Engels EA, et al. Delayed diagnosis and elevated mortality in an urban population with HIV and lung cancer: implications for patient care. J Acquir Immune Defic Syndr 2006;43(1):47–55.

202. Engels EA, Brock MV, Chen J, et al. Elevated incidence of lung cancer among HIV-infected individuals. J Clin Oncol 2006;24(9):1383–8.

203. Janerich DT, Thompson WD, Varela LR, et al. Lung cancer and exposure to tobacco smoke in the household. N Engl J Med 1990;323(10):632–6.

204. Hirayama T. Non-smoking wives of heavy smokers have a higher risk of lung cancer: a study from Japan. Br Med J (Clin Res Ed) 1981;282(6259):183–5.

205. Trichopoulos D, Kalandidi A, Sparros L, et al. Lung cancer and passive smoking. Int J Cancer 1981; 27(1):1–4.

206. Hackshaw AK, Law MR, Wald NJ. The accumulated evidence on lung cancer and environmental tobacco smoke. BMJ 1997;315(7114):980–8.

207. Fontham ET, Correa P, Reynolds P, et al. Environmental tobacco smoke and lung cancer in nonsmoking women. A multicenter study. JAMA 1994;271(22):1752–9.

208. National Research Council. Environmental tobacco smoke: measuring exposuresand assessing health effects. Washington, DC: National Academy Press; 1986. p. 337.

209. US Department of Health and Services. Report of the Surgeon General: The Health Consequences of Involuntary Smoking. Washington, DC: DHHS (CDC) 87-8398; 1986.

210. US Environmental Protection Agency, Office of Air and Radiation and Office of Research and Development. Respiratory Health Effects of Passive Smoking: Lung Cancer and Other Disorders. EPA 600-6-90-006F; 1992.

211. Cancer IAfRo. Involuntary smoking, vol. 83. Lyon (France): International Agency for Research on Cancer Monographs; 2002.

212. Cardenas VM, Thun MJ, Austin H, et al. Environmental tobacco smoke and lung cancer mortality in the American Cancer Society's Cancer Prevention Study. II. Cancer Causes Control 1997;8(1):57–64.

213. Nyberg F, Pershagen G. Passive smoking and lung cancer. Accumulated evidence on lung cancer and environmental tobacco smoke. BMJ 1998; 317(7154):347–8 [author reply: 348].

214. Hecht SS, Carmella SG, Murphy SE, et al. A tobacco-specific lung carcinogen in the urine of men exposed to cigarette smoke. N Engl J Med 1993;329(21):1543–6.

215. Pirkle JL, Flegal KM, Bernert JT, et al. Exposure of the US population to environmental tobacco smoke: the Third National Health and Nutrition Examination Survey, 1988 to 1991. JAMA 1996;275(16):1233–40.

216. Thorne S, Malarcher A, Maurice M, et al. Cigarette smoking among adults – United States 2007. MMWR 2008;57:1221–6.

217. Beckett WS. Epidemiology and etiology of lung cancer. Clin Chest Med 1993;14(1):1–15.

218. Luo RX, Wu B, Yi YN, et al. Indoor burning coal air pollution and lung cancer—a case-control study in Fuzhou, China. Lung Cancer 1996;14(Suppl 1): S113–9.

219. Kleinerman RA, Wang Z, Wang L, et al. Lung cancer and indoor exposure to coal and biomass in rural China. J Occup Environ Med 2002;44(4):338–44.

220. Hosgood HD, Boffetta P, Greenland S, et al. In-home coal and wood use and lung cancer risk: a pooled analysis of the International Lung Cancer Consortium. Environ Health Perspect 2010;118(12):1743–7.

221. Lissowska J, Bardin-Mikolajczak A, Fletcher T, et al. Lung cancer and indoor pollution from heating and cooking with solid fuels: the IARC international multicentre case-control study in Eastern/Central Europe and the United Kingdom. Am J Epidemiol 2005;162(4):326–33.

222. Wilkins ET. Air pollution and the London fog of December, 1952. J R Sanit Inst 1954;74(1):1–15 [discussion: 15–21].

223. Pershagen G. Air pollution and cancer. IARC Sci Publ 1990;(104):240–51.

224. Nyberg F, Gustavsson P, Järup L, et al. Urban air pollution and lung cancer in Stockholm. Epidemiology 2000;11(5):487–95.

225. Dockery DW, Pope CA, Xu X, et al. An association between air pollution and mortality in six U.S. cities. N Engl J Med 1993;329(24):1753–9.

226. Pope CA, Burnett RT, Thun MJ, et al. Lung cancer, cardiopulmonary mortality, and long-term exposure to fine particulate air pollution. JAMA 2002;287(9): 1132–41.

227. Cohen BL. How dangerous is low level radiation? Risk Anal 1995;15(6):645–53.

228. Lipsett M, Campleman S. Occupational exposure to diesel exhaust and lung cancer: a meta-analysis. Am J Public Health 1999;89(7):1009–17.

229. Bhatia R, Lopipero P, Smith AH. Diesel exhaust exposure and lung cancer. Epidemiology 1998;9(1):84–91.

230. Driscoll T, Nelson DI, Steenland K, et al. The global burden of disease due to occupational carcinogens. Am J Ind Med 2005;48(6):419–31.

231. Fingerhut M, Nelson DI, Driscoll T, et al. The contribution of occupational risks to the global burden of disease: summary and next steps. Med Lav 2006; 97(2):313–21.

232. Steenland K, Burnett C, Lalich N, et al. Dying for work: The magnitude of US mortality from selected causes of death associated with occupation. Am J Ind Med 2003;43(5):461–82.

233. Steenland K, Loomis D, Shy C, et al. Review of occupational lung carcinogens. Am J Ind Med 1996;29(5):474–90.

234. Hughes JM, Weill H. Potency versus importance in fiber pathogenicity. Am J Ind Med 1994;25(4): 609–10.

235. Doll R. Mortality from lung cancer in asbestos workers. Br J Ind Med 1955;12(2):81–6.

236. Mossman BT, Churg A. Mechanisms in the pathogenesis of asbestosis and silicosis. Am J Respir Crit Care Med 1998;157(5 Pt 1):1666–80.

237. Malignant Mesothelioma Mortality — United States, 1999–2005. MMWR 2009;58(15):393–6.

238. Jones RN, Hughes JM, Weill H. Asbestos exposure, asbestosis, and asbestos-attributable lung cancer. Thorax 1996;51(Suppl 2):S9–15.

239. Egilman D, Reinert A. Lung cancer and asbestos exposure: asbestosis is not necessary. Am J Ind Med 1996;30(4):398–406.

240. Hessel PA, Gamble JF, McDonald JC. Asbestos, asbestosis, and lung cancer: a critical assessment of the epidemiological evidence. Thorax 2005;60(5): 433–6.

241. Weiss W. Asbestosis: a marker for the increased risk of lung cancer among workers exposed to asbestos. Chest 1999;115(2):536–49.

242. Hughes JM, Weill H. Asbestosis as a precursor of asbestos related lung cancer: results of a prospective mortality study. Br J Ind Med 1991;48(4):229–33.

243. Churg A, Wiggs B. Fiber size and number in amphibole asbestos-induced mesothelioma. Am J Pathol 1984;115(3):437–42.

244. Hammond EC, Selikoff IJ, Seidman H. Asbestos exposure, cigarette smoking and death rates. Ann N Y Acad Sci 1979;330:473–90.

245. Frank AL. The epidemiology and etiology of lung cancer. Clin Chest Med 1982;3(2):219–28.

246. Samet JM, Eradze GR. Radon and lung cancer risk: taking stock at the millenium. Environ Health Perspect 2000;108(Suppl 4):635–41.

247. Samet JM. Residential radon and lung cancer: end of the story? J Toxicol Environ Health A 2006;69(7):527–31.

248. Grosche B, Kreuzer M, Kreisheimer M, et al. Lung cancer risk among German male uranium miners: a cohort study, 1946-1998. Br J Cancer 2006;95(9):1280–7.

249. Lubin JH, Boice JD, Edling C, et al. Lung cancer in radon-exposed miners and estimation of risk from indoor exposure. J Natl Cancer Inst 1995;87(11):817–27.

250. Samet JM. Indoor radon and lung cancer: risky or not? J Natl Cancer Inst 1994;86(24):1813–4.

251. Saccomanno G, Huth GC, Auerbach O, et al. Relationship of radioactive radon daughters and cigarette smoking in the genesis of lung cancer in uranium miners. Cancer 1988;62(7):1402–8.

252. Roscoe RJ, Steenland K, Halperin WE, et al. Lung cancer mortality among nonsmoking uranium miners exposed to radon daughters. JAMA 1989;262(5):629–33.

253. Fabrikant JI. Radon and lung cancer: the BEIR IV Report. Health Phys 1990;59(1):89–97.

254. Samet JM, Stolwijk J, Rose SL. Summary: International workshop on residential Rn epidemiology. Health Phys 1991;60(2):223–7.

255. Lubin JH, Boice JD. Lung cancer risk from residential radon: meta-analysis of eight epidemiologic studies. J Natl Cancer Inst 1997;89(1):49–57.

256. Auvinen A, Mäkeläinen I, Hakama M, et al. Indoor radon exposure and risk of lung cancer: a nested case-control study in Finland. J Natl Cancer Inst 1996;88(14):966–72.

257. Alavanja MC, Brownson RC, Lubin JH, et al. Residential radon exposure and lung cancer among nonsmoking women. J Natl Cancer Inst 1994;86(24):1829–37.

258. Létourneau EG, Krewski D, Choi NW, et al. Case-control study of residential radon and lung cancer in Winnipeg, Manitoba, Canada. Am J Epidemiol 1994;140(4):310–22.

259. Cohen BL. Dose-response relationship for radiation carcinogenesis in the low-dose region. Int Arch Occup Environ Health 1994;66(2):71–5.

260. Hei TK, Piao CQ, Willey JC, et al. Malignant transformation of human bronchial epithelial cells by radon-simulated alpha-particles. Carcinogenesis 1994;15(3):431–7.

261. Kelley MJ, McCrory DC. Prevention of lung cancer: summary of published evidence. Chest 2003;123(Suppl 1):50S–9S.

262. Jemal A, Chu KC, Tarone RE. Recent trends in lung cancer mortality in the United States. J Natl Cancer Inst 2001;93(4):277–83.

263. Wiencke JK. DNA adduct burden and tobacco carcinogenesis. Oncogene 2002;21(48):7376–91.

264. Department of Health and Human Services. The Health Benefits of Smoking Cessation: A Report of the Surgeon General, 1990, US DHHS. Public Health Service. Washington, DC, DHHS Pub. No. (CDC) 90–8416.

265. Speizer FE, Colditz GA, Hunter DJ, et al. Prospective study of smoking, antioxidant intake, and lung cancer in middle-aged women (USA). Cancer Causes Control 1999;10(5):475–82.

266. Burns DM. Primary prevention, smoking, and smoking cessation: implications for future trends in lung cancer prevention. Cancer 2000;89(Suppl 11):2506–9.

267. Lange JH, Mastrangelo G, Fadda E, et al. Elevated lung cancer risk shortly after smoking cessation: is it due to a reduction of endotoxin exposure? Med Hypotheses 2005;65(3):534–41.

268. Kumar A, Mallya KB, Kumar JC. Are lung cancers triggered by stopping smoking? Med Hypotheses 2007;68(5):1176–7.

269. Campling BG, Collins BN, Algazy KM, et al. Spontaneous smoking cessation before lung cancer diagnosis. J Thorac Oncol 2011;6(3):517–24.

270. Ebbert JO, Yang P, Vachon CM, et al. Lung cancer risk reduction after smoking cessation: observations from a prospective cohort of women. J Clin Oncol 2003;21(5):921–6.

271. Sporn MB, Dunlop NM, Newton DL, et al. Prevention of chemical carcinogenesis by vitamin A and its synthetic analogs (retinoids). Fed Proc 1976;35(6):1332–8.

272. Kelloff GJ, Sigman CC, Greenwald P. Cancer chemoprevention: progress and promise. Eur J Cancer 1999;35(14):2031–8.

273. Dragnev KH, Stover D, Dmitrovsky E, et al. Lung cancer prevention: the guidelines. Chest 2003;123(Suppl 1):60S–71S.

274. Keith RL. Chemoprevention of lung cancer. Proc Am Thorac Soc 2009;6(2):187–93.

275. Omenn GS. Chemoprevention of lung cancer is proving difficult and frustrating, requiring new approaches. J Natl Cancer Inst 2000;92(12):959–60.

276. Petty TL. The predictive value of spirometry. Identifying patients at risk for lung cancer in the primary care setting. Postgrad Med 1997;101(3):128–30, 133–4, 140.

277. National Lung Screening Trial Research Team, Aberle DR, Adams AM, et al. Reduced Lung-Cancer Mortality with Low-Dose Computed Tomographic Screening. N Engl J Med 2011;365(5):395–409.

Preventing Lung Cancer by Treating Tobacco Dependence

Richard D. Hurt, MD*, Jon O. Ebbert, MD,
J. Taylor Hays, MD, David D. McFadden, MD

KEYWORDS

- Tobacco treatment specialists • Smoking
- Preventing lung cancer

LUNG CANCER

In medicine, no more well-proven association exists than the parallel epidemics of cigarette smoking and lung cancer. This association is evident in the large increase in cigarette use and the parallel epidemic of lung cancer incidence and mortality in the United States. In the early part of the twentieth century, it was observed that lung cancer was an uncommon phenomenon: "On one point, however, there is nearly complete consensus of opinion, and that is that primary malignant neoplasms of the lungs are amongst the rarest forms of disease."[1] This perspective began to change as smoking became prevalent and, by the 1940s, the potential causal relationship between cigarette smoking and lung cancer was postulated.[2] By 1950, reports began more firmly to establish the causal relationship between cigarette smoking and lung cancer.[3] Lung cancer caused by cigarette smoking has been the leading cause of cancer deaths in American men for more than 60 years, and, in 1987, surpassed breast cancer as the leading cause of cancer deaths among American women (**Fig. 1**).

Fig. 1 shows cancer deaths in men and women from 1930 to 2006.[4] Lung cancer accounts for 29% of cancer deaths in American men and 26% of cancer deaths among American women. Tobacco-caused diseases (eg, cardiovascular disease, emphysema, lung cancer) account for an estimated 443,000 deaths each year, making tobacco-caused deaths the leading cause of preventable death in the United States.[5]

CIGARETTES

Tobacco has been used by humans since the earliest recorded history of the Western hemisphere, but cigarettes were not mass produced until the second half of the nineteenth century. Even then, it was not until 1913 when Camel, the first modern cigarette, was introduced and widely promoted by R.J. Reynolds, that consumption of cigarettes greatly increased. Cigarette consumption increased from fewer than 5 billion cigarettes per year in 1905 to more than 17 billion by 1915, and to almost 90 billion by 1925.[6] Per capita consumption continued to increase, and peaked in the 1960s when more than 600 billion cigarettes were consumed in the United States in a single year (**Fig. 2**). Increases in smoking prevalence and per capita consumption of cigarettes were followed by a parallel increase in lung cancer deaths.

In response to convincing evidence establishing a causal relationship between cigarette smoking and lung cancer, the tobacco industry developed a strategy that was made public in *A Frank Statement to Cigarette Smokers*.[7] This statement was printed in newspapers throughout the United States on January 4, 1954, and stated, "We accept an interest in people's health as a basic responsibility, paramount to every other consideration in

Dr Hurt holds a medical education grant from Pfizer Medical Education; Drs Hays and Ebbert hold research grants from Pfizer, Inc; and Drs Hurt and Ebbert serve on an advisory board for GlaxoSmithKline.
Nicotine Dependence Center, Mayo Clinic, 200 First Street Southwest, Rochester, MN 55905, USA
* Corresponding author.
E-mail address: rhurt@mayo.edu

Clin Chest Med 32 (2011) 645–657
doi:10.1016/j.ccm.2011.08.004
0272-5231/11/$ – see front matter © 2011 Elsevier Inc. All rights reserved.

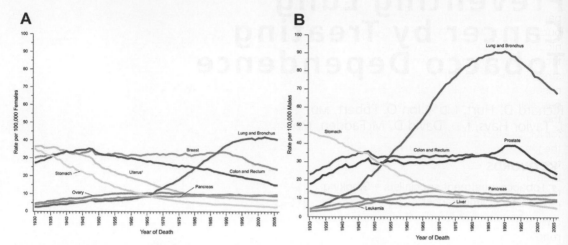

Fig. 1. Age-adjusted cancer death rates for women (*A*) and men (*B*) by site, United States, 1930 to 2006. (*From* Jemal A, Siegel R, Xu J, et al. Cancer statistics, 2010. CA Cancer J Clin 2010;60(5):277–300; with permission. Copyright 2010 American Cancer Society.)

our business." Rather than developing a strategy to protect people's health, the tobacco industry developed a strategy that included "creating doubt about the health charge without actually denying it."[7] In a document entitled *Smoking and Health Proposal*, a marketing executive for Brown & Williamson Tobacco Company succinctly expressed this policy: "Doubt is our product, since it is the best means of competing with 'body of fact' that exists in the minds of the general

public… it is also the means of establishing controversy."[8] In response to the concerns about the health effects of smoking, the tobacco industry introduced filtered cigarettes in the 1950s and, by the 1970s, widely promoted low-tar-low-nicotine cigarettes as a supposedly safe alternative.

Presently, low-tar-low-nicotine cigarettes comprise more than 90% of the cigarette market in the United States. Low-yield cigarettes are created by placing ventilation holes in the filter tipping

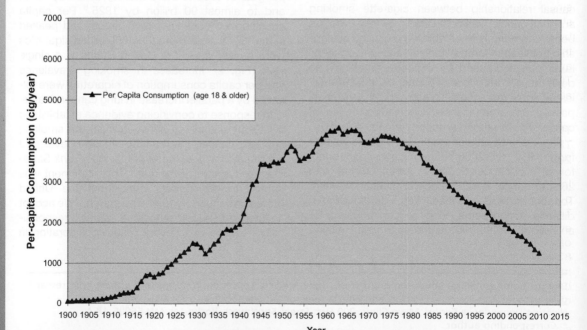

Fig. 2. Per capita consumption (ages 18 years and older) of cigarettes in the United States, 1900 to 2009. (*Courtesy of* David Burns, Centers for Disease Control and Prevention.)

paper so that cigarette smoke pulled through the burning rod is diluted by room air, leading to lower nicotine and tar yields when cigarettes are tested on a standardized smoking machine. Most smokers are unaware of the ventilation holes and misperceive low-yield cigarettes as being less harmful than regular filtered cigarettes. Ironically, the low-yield cigarette design may be responsible for an increased incidence of adenocarcinoma of the lung.[9] This may be because of the compensatory smoking (eg, deeper inhalation and longer breath holding) observed among smokers of low-tar-low-nicotine cigarettes.[10] Despite the implied health claims of low-tar-low-nicotine cigarettes, changing from a higher-yield to a lower-yield cigarette does not reduce the risk of lung cancer. The only way to reduce the risk for lung cancer mortality is to stop smoking. Compared with the never smoker, the relative risk for lung cancer mortality declines from 23.4 to 5.3 after 15 years of abstinence from smoking for men and from 21.1 to 2.4 for women.[11] Recognizing the confusion and potential deception created by low-yield cigarettes, the Federal Trade Commission and Judge Gladys Kessler in the 2006 decision in the Department of Justice case have mandated that cigarette manufacturers can no longer label their products as low-tar-low-nicotine cigarettes.

Although the epidemic of lung cancer and other tobacco-caused diseases in the United States has peaked, it is now spreading throughout the world. In the twenty-first century, an estimated 1 billion smokers will die of tobacco-caused diseases, which sharply contrasts with the 100 million deaths caused by tobacco in the twentieth century.[12] Historians in the future will look back on this period in history and wonder why society allowed this to happen. They will find it difficult to conceive that it was only about money.

THE US PUBLIC HEALTH SERVICE GUIDELINE TREATING TOBACCO USE AND DEPENDENCE 2008 UPDATE

In 2008, the US Public Health Service released a comprehensive update of its 2000 guideline: Treating Tobacco Use and Dependence. This evidence-based guideline was updated by a panel of experts who distilled a literature of more than 8700 peer-reviewed articles using meta-analytical methodology. The guideline emphasizes that tobacco dependence is a chronic medical condition often requiring repeated intervention and multiple attempts to stop. In the United States, 70% of smokers want to stop smoking and 44% attempt to stop smoking every year. However, these efforts are unaided and unsuccessful because only 4% to 7% of smokers who attempt to stop smoking are able to do so on their own.[13] The 2008 guideline notes that substantial progress has been made since the first guideline was published in 1996. The guideline points to the increased coverage of tobacco dependence treatments by health plans, Medicare, and Medicaid. The Joint Commission now requires tobacco dependence interventions for hospitalized smokers with the diagnosis of acute myocardial infarction, congestive heart failure, or community-acquired pneumonia (http://www.jointcommission.org/assets/1/18/A_Comprehensive_Review_of_Development_for_Core_Measures.pdf). In addition, the guideline highlights progress made in disseminating treatment options. Telephone quitlines have been particularly effective in providing wide access to counseling and many quitlines provide nicotine replacement at no cost to the smoker.[14]

Each guideline recommendation is supported by a meta-analysis of scientific studies to provide a strong evidence base that encourages clinicians to advise effective tobacco dependence counseling and medications to their patients who use tobacco. The guideline also recommends that health systems, insurers, and purchasers assist clinicians in making such effective treatments available. In order for this to occur, clinicians and health care delivery systems need to consistently identify and document tobacco use status and treat every tobacco user seen in a health care setting. The guideline recommends that an office-wide system should be implemented to ensure that every patient at every clinic visit is queried about their tobacco use status and it is documented. One easy way to do that is to expand the vital signs to include tobacco use.

Clinicians should encourage every patient willing to make an attempt to stop using tobacco and direct them toward effective counseling and medications. For the patient who is unwilling to set a quit date, the guideline recommends using the technique of motivational interviewing to maintain patient engagement in the treatment process. Even brief tobacco counseling interventions are effective for improving tobacco abstinence outcomes compared with no intervention or self-help materials. Because there is a dose response for counseling interventions, longer or more intensive treatments result in better smoking abstinence outcomes compared with brief behavioral therapy. This finding is true regardless of the format for the counseling intervention (ie, individual, group, or telephone counseling). Two components of counseling, practical counseling and intratreatment support, are especially effective and clinicians should use these when counseling patients to stop tobacco use.

Practical Counseling

This problem-solving and skills training approach is used to help the patient recognize thoughts, behaviors, and situations that may lead to increased smoking or relapse and help the patient identify and practice coping or problem-solving skills to deal with them. Practical counseling also includes providing basic information about the neurobiology of tobacco dependence and withdrawal symptoms that might be experienced.

Intratreatment Support

The clinician engaged with the patient can provide support in a variety of ways, beginning with encouraging the patient to make an attempt to stop. The clinician should communicate in a caring, nonjudgmental manner and also encourage the patient to openly discuss perceived barriers to stopping smoking. Telephone counseling and return visits are a clear demonstration of intratreatment support.

The guideline also recommends that the 7 first-line medications should be used either individually or in combinations. These medications include 5 nicotine medications (nicotine gum, inhaler, lozenge, nasal spray, and patch) and 2 non-nicotine medications (bupropion and varenicline). The guideline highlights that counseling and medication are effective when used by themselves, but the combination of counseling and medication is more effective than either alone. Every patient who is willing to make an attempt to stop smoking should be offered counseling and medications.[13,15]

The guideline emphasizes that telephone quitline counseling is effective with diverse populations and has a broad reach. In the United States, telephone quitlines are available in every state; therefore, both clinicians and health care delivery systems should ensure patient access to quitlines and promote quitline use. The National Quitline number is 1-800-QUITNOW, which connects smokers to a routing system that redirects them to their state quitline service.

In addition, as highlighted in the guideline, counseling and pharmacotherapy are strategies that have proved effective to help smokers stop smoking. Higher taxes for cigarettes and smoke-free workplace policies are 2 effective public health policies that prompt a smoker to make an attempt to stop and often help them stop.

BASIC NEUROBIOLOGY OF TOBACCO DEPENDENCE

A major barrier for most smokers who try to quit is the neurobiology of tobacco dependence driven by the most efficient delivery device of nicotine that exists: the cigarette. Cigarette smoking delivers high concentrations of nicotine to the central nervous system (CNS) within seconds of the first puff. The primary target for nicotine in the CNS is the $\alpha_4\beta_2$ nicotinic acetylcholine receptor, which, when activated by nicotine binding, results in the release of dopamine in the brain's reward center and provides the positive reinforcement seen with cigarette smoking.

Smoking 1 cigarette results in a high level of occupancy of the $\alpha_4\beta_2$ nicotinic acetylcholine receptors in the CNS, and 3 cigarettes almost completely saturates these receptors for as long as 3 hours.[16] Even 1 hour of secondhand smoke (SHS) exposure saturates 19% of the $\alpha_4\beta_2$ receptors and smokers experience a 23% increase in craving with such SHS exposure.[16] Craving results when the receptor occupancy declines with time, and craving reduction requires achieving virtually complete receptor saturation. Clinicians need to understand this important concept that places into context 2 important facts regarding treatment of tobacco use and dependence: (1) the efficient and rapid delivery of nicotine by cigarettes is a key factor in the development of tobacco dependence; (2) nicotine replacement products commonly used to treat tobacco dependence are inefficient in delivering nicotine and deliver much lower concentrations compared with cigarettes.

Nicotine has complex and wide-ranging effects on the CNS. Nicotinic acetylcholine receptors are located in all areas of the human brain and, when stimulated, cause the release of dopamine, norepinephrine, glutamate, vasopressin, serotonin, γ-aminobutyric acid (GABA), β-endorphins, and other neurotransmitters. High concentrations of $\alpha_4\beta_2$ nicotinic acetylcholine receptors exist in the mesolimbic dopamine system and locus ceruleus.[17] The former is important in pleasure and reward and the latter is important for cognitive function. Although not completely understood, upregulation of the high-affinity $\alpha_4\beta_2$ nicotinic acetylcholine receptor is critical for the development of tolerance to, and dependence on, nicotine.[18] Repeated exposure to high concentrations of nicotine causes upregulation of the $\alpha_4\beta_2$ nicotinic acetylcholine receptors, leading to an absolute increase in their numbers.[18,19] Neuroadaptation of the mesolimbic system in smokers and its target neurons in the nucleus accumbens may be longer lasting than previously believed, which could explain the observation that cravings to smoke last for months after a smoker stops smoking.[20]

In laboratory animals, self-administered intravenous nicotine increases the sensitivity of brain reward systems and imprints an indelible memory of its effects in reward systems, an action that seems unique to nicotine among drugs of abuse.[21] This may partially explain the rapid return to former levels of smoking that frequently follows a relapse after a prolonged period of smoking abstinence.

PHARMACOTHERAPY FOR TOBACCO DEPENDENCE
Nicotine Replacement Therapy

One approach to the therapeutic use of nicotine replacement therapy (NRT) for the treatment of tobacco dependence is to determine the patient's level of nicotine exposure. Once the degree of exposure is determined, a nicotine replacement dose approximating the dose the individual receives from smoking can be prescribed. However, several factors make this task difficult. Smokers exposed to the same amount of nicotine through inhaled tobacco smoke have marked interindividual differences in venous nicotine concentrations.[22,23] Further, there are substantial genetically determined variations in nicotine metabolism (ie, slow vs fast metabolizers of nicotine).[24] Cigarette smoking produces initial arterial nicotine concentrations that are several-fold higher than concomitant venous nicotine levels.[25] In addition, nicotine has a short half-life (about 120 minutes) and, with smoking, tends to have peaks and troughs in both venous and arterial concentrations. For these reasons, cotinine, the major metabolite of nicotine, provides a better estimate of nicotine exposure. Although complex algorithms and questionnaires are available to assess the severity of tobacco dependence, simply asking how many cigarettes are smoked per day, and how many minutes after awakening is the first cigarette in the morning, is a practical way to assess the level of tobacco dependence of the smoker. Smoking more than 20 cigarettes per day and smoking within 30 minutes of arising indicates a higher level of dependence.

Cotinine, the major metabolite of nicotine, has a half-life of 18 to 20 hours and is used to quantify an individual's exposure to nicotine over a period of several days. Minor tobacco alkaloids such as nornicotine, anatabine, and anabasine can also be measured in the urine of tobacco users as qualitative assessments of nicotine and tobacco exposure.[26–28] Anabasine is not a metabolic product of nicotine, but is present in the urine of tobacco users and not in the urine of patients using only NRT. Anabasine may be useful in distinguishing abstinent tobacco users who are using NRT from those who are continuing to use tobacco, which has become especially important for adjudicating tobacco abstinence in situations that require

abstinence from tobacco use to pursue advanced medical or surgical therapy, such as lung and/or heart transplantation.

To date, the US Food and Drug Administration (FDA) has approved 5 nicotine replacement products: nicotine gum, nicotine patches, nicotine nasal spray, a nicotine vapor inhaler, and nicotine lozenges. Nicotine gum, patches, and lozenges are available over the counter (OTC), whereas the nasal spray and inhaler are available by prescription only.

In general, physicians who prescribe NRT for tobacco dependence should individualize the dose and duration of treatment and schedule follow-up office visits or telephone calls to monitor patient response. The dose and duration of therapy should be based on the patient's response to treatment, including the subjective relief of withdrawal symptoms and craving.

NRT is divided into 2 groups: short-acting NRT (gum, lozenge, nasal spray, and inhaler) and longer-acting (nicotine patch). If NRT is selected for treatment, combination therapy (nicotine patch and short-acting NRT) is usually preferred rather than monotherapy with a short-acting NRT product. For example, combining ad lib nicotine lozenge therapy with standard-dose nicotine patch therapy yielded an odds ratio of 2.3 compared with placebo for smoking abstinence at 6 months.[29] Short-acting NRT is best used for acute management of nicotine withdrawal symptoms and craving in combination with longer-acting medications such as nicotine patch, bupropion, and/or varenicline.[30]

Nicotine gum is available as an OTC product in 2-mg and 4-mg doses. Patients should be instructed in its proper chew-and-park use and to avoid acidic beverages that lower the intraoral pH, which reduces nicotine absorption. Nicotine gum is most often used in combination with other NRT, bupropion, or varenicline.

The nicotine lozenge is available in the United States as an OTC product. The nicotine lozenge is available in 2-mg and 4-mg doses, with the latter for use in high-dependence smokers (ie, first cigarette of the day <30 minutes after arising).[31] The method of delivery (ie, transbuccal) is similar to that of nicotine gum, and it is most often used in combination with other NRT, bupropion, or varenicline. The newer mini lozenge is smaller and may dissolve more quickly than the original lozenge, which may improve patient adherence to treatment.

Nicotine nasal spray delivers nicotine directly to the nasal mucosa and has been observed to be effective for achieving smoking abstinence as monotherapy.[32] This device delivers nicotine more rapidly than other therapeutic nicotine replacement delivery systems and reduces withdrawal symptoms more quickly than nicotine gum.[33] The reduction in withdrawal symptoms may be partially attributable to the rapidity with which nicotine is absorbed from the nasal mucosa and the resulting arterial venous differences in the plasma concentration of nicotine.[23]

The nicotine vapor inhaler has also been shown to be effective for increasing smoking abstinence as monotherapy.[34] The device delivers nicotine in vapor form that is absorbed across the oral mucosa. Although the device is called an inhaler, this is a misnomer because little of the nicotine vapor reaches the pulmonary alveoli, even with deep inhalation efforts.[35]

Nicotine patch therapy was introduced in 1991 and delivers a steady dose of nicotine for 24 hours after a single application. The once-daily dosing requires little effort on the part of the patient, which enhances compliance. Nicotine patches are available without a prescription in doses of 7, 14, and 21 mg. In almost every randomized clinical trial performed to date, the nicotine patch has been shown to be effective compared with placebo, usually with a doubling of the smoking abstinence rates.

Standard-dose (21 mg/24 hours) nicotine patch therapy achieves a median serum cotinine level of only 54% of the cotinine concentrations achieved through smoking.[22,36] There is a dose response for nicotine patch therapy, particularly among lighter smokers who have lower baseline cotinine concentrations, suggesting that their nicotine replacement needs are more adequately met with standard doses than those of heavier smokers.[37]

Because many patients are underdosed with a standard nicotine patch, studies have been conducted assessing the efficacy of higher doses. Use of high doses of nicotine patch therapy (ie, doses>21 mg/d) are appropriate for heavy smokers, those who previously failed standard-dose patch therapy, and/or those whose nicotine withdrawal symptoms are not relieved sufficiently with standard-dose therapy.[38] This approach is especially important for heavy smokers because they are significantly underdosed with standard-dose patch therapy.[22] High-dose nicotine patch therapy has been shown to be safe and well tolerated in patients who smoke more than 20 cigarettes per day.[22] The 2008 USPHS Guideline Panel concluded that high-dose nicotine patch therapy (>21 mg/d) did not seem to produce more benefit than that of standard-dose nicotine patch therapy, although the recent Cochrane meta-analysis did show a small but significant benefit for higher-dose NRT.[39] The panel

concluded that, if the patient is highly dependent, the clinician may consider higher than the FDA-recommended dose and that higher doses have been shown to be effective in highly dependent smokers. The panel also notes that there is no evidence of increased cardiovascular risk with any of the NRT medications.

Smoking rate can be used to determine the initial nicotine patch dose roughly at a dose of 1 mg of nicotine to each cigarette smoked per day (CPD). Thus, fewer than 10 CPD warrants a dose between 7 and 14 patches; 10 to 20 CPD, a 14-mg to 21-mg dose; 21 to 40 CPD, a 21-mg to 42-mg dose; and more than 40 CPD, a dose of 42 mg/d or more. Adequacy of the initial dose is determined by assessing the patient's withdrawal symptom and craving relief.

Where available, clinicians can use serum cotinine concentrations to tailor the nicotine patch dose so that it approaches 100% replacement. A baseline cotinine concentration is obtained while the smoker is smoking at the usual rate. An initial nicotine patch dose based on the baseline cotinine concentration is prescribed. A 14-mg to 21-mg nicotine patch dose should be prescribed if the baseline cotinine is less than 200 mg/mL, a 21-mg to 42-mg dose for a baseline cotinine of 200 to 300 mg/mL, and a dose of more than 42 mg if the baseline cotinine is greater than 300 mg/mL. After the patient reaches steady state (>3 days of nicotine patch therapy and not smoking), the serum cotinine concentration is rechecked and the replacement dose is adjusted to achieve a steady-state cotinine level that approaches the baseline level (ie, 100% replacement). Higher percentage replacement has been shown to reduce nicotine withdrawal symptoms,[22] but the efficacy for long-term smoking abstinence of such an approach has not been clearly established.[22,38,40] Smokers who did not get adequate relief of withdrawal symptoms from a single nicotine patch dose on a prior attempt should be considered for a higher nicotine patch dose plus supplemental short-acting NRT.

After initiation of nicotine patch therapy on the stop date, the patient should have a follow-up visit or a telephone counseling session within the first 2 weeks and periodically thereafter. Abstinence from smoking during the first 2 weeks of patch therapy has been shown to be highly predictive of long-term abstinence.[37,41] Thus, the first 2 weeks after treatment initiation are critical in setting the stage for long-term smoking abstinence. Alterations in therapy at follow-up depend on relief of withdrawal symptoms and craving and how well the patient is maintaining smoking abstinence. If the patient continues to smoke at all during the first 2 weeks, the treatment plan needs to be changed either by changing the nicotine patch dose, adding additional pharmacotherapy, or intensifying behavioral counseling. Nicotine patch doses should be increased for patients experiencing pronounced withdrawal symptoms such as irritability, anxiety, loss of concentration, or craving, or for patients who do not achieve 100% replacement based on the second serum cotinine concentration. A standard course of nicotine patch therapy is for 8 weeks, and it is safe, but 24 weeks of nicotine patch therapy not only increases smoking abstinence rates at 6 and 12 months but also reduces the risk of smoking lapses and increases the recovery from smoking lapses compared with 8 weeks of therapy.[42] Thus, the optimal length of treatment has not been determined, but longer-term treatment (>14 weeks) seems to provide benefit compared with standard lengths of treatment when combining nicotine patch and nicotine gum.[42] Further, long-term treatment up to 6 months with triple combination therapy (nicotine patch, bupropion, and nicotine inhaler) seems superior to a standard-dose nicotine patch therapy given for a 10-week period.[43]

NON-NICOTINE MEDICATIONS
Bupropion Sustained Release

Bupropion is a monocyclic antidepressant that inhibits the reuptake of both norepinephrine and dopamine.[43] Dopamine release in the mesolimbic system and the nucleus accumbens is believed to be the basis for the reinforcing properties of nicotine and other drugs of addiction.[44,45] The efficacy of bupropion in treating smokers is hypothesized to stem from its dopaminergic activity on the pleasure and reward pathways in the mesolimbic system and nucleus accumbens. Bupropion also has been shown to have an antagonist effect on nicotinic acetylcholine receptors.[46] Thus, its mechanism of action likely is multifactorial.

Bupropion sustained release (SR) has been shown to be effective and exhibits a significant dose-response effect.[47] In addition, weight gain attenuation occurs during the treatment phase for subjects continuously abstinent while receiving the 300 mg/d dose. However, the attenuation of weight gain does not persist at 1-year follow-up for smokers who received short-term treatment (7 weeks). Weight gain attenuation has been observed with 52 weeks of bupropion SR compared with subjects who received placebo, and the weight gain attenuation in these subjects persisted for the 1-year follow-up after the medication

was discontinued.[48] Bupropion SR has also been shown to be effective in populations of smokers including those with coronary artery disease, chronic obstructive pulmonary disease (COPD), or those who have previously failed to achieve long-term smoking abstinence after an initial course of bupropion SR.[49–51] Treatment with bupropion SR alone or in combination with the nicotine patch resulted in a significantly higher long-term rate of abstinence from smoking than did use of either the nicotine patch alone or placebo.[52] The 2008 USPHS guideline recommends the combined used of bupropion SR and nicotine patch therapy.

Varenicline

Varenicline is a partial nicotine agonist/antagonist that selectively binds to the $\alpha_4\beta_2$ nicotinic acetylcholine receptor. Varenicline both blocks nicotine from binding to the receptor (antagonist effect)[53] and partially stimulates (agonist effect) receptor-mediated activity leading to the release of dopamine, which reduces craving and nicotine withdrawal symptoms. Varenicline is not metabolized but it is excreted virtually unchanged in the urine and has a half-life of approximately 17 hours.

Pivotal trials in healthy smokers comparing varenicline 1 mg twice daily with placebo or bupropion SR have shown[54,55] that varenicline is more effective than placebo or bupropion SR, with end-of-treatment (12 weeks) continuous smoking abstinence rates during weeks 9 to 12 of 44% versus 30% for bupropion SR and 18% for placebo. The end-of-treatment 7-day point prevalence smoking abstinence rates were approximately 50% for varenicline versus 35% for bupropion SR and 20% for placebo. An additional 12 weeks of varenicline has been shown to be effective in maintaining smoking abstinence in smokers who had stopped smoking after 12 weeks of open-label varenicline treatment.[56] In this study, 70% of subjects treated with varenicline continuously were abstinent from smoking from weeks 13 to 24 compared with 50% assigned to placebo ($P<.001$). More recently, varenicline has shown efficacy in smokers with cardiovascular disease[57] and COPD,[58] the latter with a striking end-of-treatment odds ratio of 8.4 for active varenicline compared with placebo.

Varenicline is initiated at a dose of 0.5 mg once daily for 3 days, then 0.5 mg twice daily for 4 days. The target quit date is day 8, when the maintenance dose of 1 mg twice daily begins. Length of treatment should be at least 12 weeks and can be extended for an additional 12 weeks.

From a practical standpoint, we frequently recommend longer treatment of abstinent smokers who are not secure and are concerned about smoking relapse. Varenicline treatment of 12 months has been shown to be safe.[59]

Nausea is the most frequent adverse effect of varenicline and was reported by approximately 30% of the subjects in the clinical trials. Nausea was most often mild to moderate, and participant dropouts related to nausea were infrequent (<3%). Vivid dreams (~15%) are the next most common adverse event, but do not often lead to discontinuation of the medication. In February 2008, the FDA issued a public health advisory because of postmarketing surveillance reports of suicidal thoughts and aggressive or erratic behavior in people who had taken varenicline. In addition, some case reports have suggested that varenicline could exacerbate psychiatric symptoms in individuals with severe mental illness, so these types of patients should be monitored carefully when on varenicline. A more recent large study showed that past history of depression in smokers taking varenicline to stop smoking did not lead to new or worsening depression symptoms compared with smokers without a past history of depression.[60]

COMBINATION PHARMACOTHERAPY

The 2008 USPHS guideline states that certain combinations of first-line medications have been shown to be more effective than monotherapy. Long-term (>14 weeks) nicotine patch therapy combined with nicotine gum or nicotine nasal spray, nicotine patch therapy plus nicotine inhaler, and nicotine patch therapy plus bupropion SR are cited as examples. Combining bupropion with the nicotine inhaler provides a better treatment effect than either alone.[61] However, the expert panel points out that the use of combinations of medications may be based on considerations other than smoking abstinence. Withdrawal symptom control is an important consideration, as is patient past experience and/or preference. Whether the superiority of combination therapy is caused by the use of 2 types of delivery systems or to the 2 delivery systems tending to produce higher blood nicotine levels remains unclear. Combination pharmacotherapy or higher-dose NRT more effectively relieves nicotine withdrawal symptoms, especially in more dependent smokers. We frequently use 3 or more pharmacologic agents at the same time, a practice that is now being verified in clinical trials.[43]

CLINICAL DECISION MAKING SURROUNDING PHARMACOTHERAPY

Clinical decision making for medication selection and dosing is based on the published literature but also on clinical experience. It has long been recognized by clinicians that there are limitations to standard-dose or fixed-dose regimens, with most drugs used in clinical practice today. As a result, clinicians use their clinical skills and knowledge of pharmacotherapy to individualize drug dosing for patients. These same skills and knowledge should be applied to medications used to treat tobacco dependence. Much of this clinical decision making is based on the patient's past experience with pharmacotherapy and the patient's preference.

Although each of the FDA-approved medications has been shown to be effective compared with placebo in randomized clinical trials, we rarely use short-acting NRT (nicotine gum, nicotine inhaler, nicotine lozenge, or nicotine nasal spray) alone. The exception is for the patient who previously stopped smoking using a short-acting NRT as monotherapy, and in certain special situations, such as pregnancy. The same would be true for monotherapy with nicotine patches, bupropion, or varenicline. From a practical standpoint, we view nicotine patch therapy, bupropion SR, or varenicline as the foundation on which to begin building a patient's pharmacotherapeutic regimen and may use one of these longer-acting medications either as monotherapy or in combination with a short-acting NRT product. Depending on the patient's past experience and desires, we may use nicotine patch therapy in combination with bupropion SR. A short-acting NRT product is usually added to any regimen as needed to control withdrawal symptoms or cravings. Because varenicline and bupropion have different mechanisms of action, we sometimes use them in combination, particularly in smokers who have previously stopped smoking using bupropion monotherapy but struggled during the process. A pilot study of this combination showed excellent efficacy and suggests that the combination of bupropion and varenicline was well tolerated.[30]

For patients with more severe tobacco dependence, such as those treated in our Residential Treatment Program, we commonly use combination therapy and often use 3 or more products simultaneously.[58] For patients with a partial response to initial medication therapy (ie, decreased smoking rate but not abstinent from smoking), further tailoring of the medication regimen maybe be necessary to reach the desired therapeutic goal of smoking abstinence. For example, if a patient has reduced smoking using varenicline 1 mg twice daily and has tolerated the medication without substantial nausea, we may increase the dose to 1 mg 3 times daily. Another situation requiring creativity (ie, the art of medicine) is a smoker who has stopped smoking using nicotine patch therapy and a short-acting NRT but notices increased withdrawal symptoms in the early evening. Adding a 14-mg patch in the late afternoon may decrease evening withdrawal. We have used nicotine patch therapy in our Residential Treatment Program for smokers who want to start varenicline at admission.[62] Because patients stop smoking on admission to our Residential Treatment Program and varenicline requires several days to reach steady-state concentrations, withdrawal symptoms are poorly controlled during the initiation of varenicline treatment. Thus, we are better able to control nicotine withdrawal symptoms that may be disruptive to their treatment experience.

Patients frequently ask, "How long do I need to stay on these medications after I stop smoking?" The answer is usually "As long as it takes." Recent trials have shown better smoking abstinence outcomes at 12 months after 24 weeks of treatment of both nicotine patch therapy or varenicline.[42,56]

TOBACCO TREATMENT SPECIALISTS

In the past 20 years, clinicians have been encouraged to actively treat tobacco dependence. Brief interventions were promoted using 4 A's then the 5 A's (Ask, Advise, Assess, Assist, and Arrange). Brief interventions by physicians have been shown to be effective, but there is a dose response for behavioral counseling. Overall, engagement by clinicians in the provision of brief interventions has been limited.[63] Despite the evidence that more intensive interventions are more effective, they are rarely provided except by clinicians who have special expertise in treating tobacco dependence.

A growing number of clinicians have developed the specialized knowledge and skills required to effectively treat tobacco dependence. Despite this growing expertise among physicians, the time they are able to devote to tobacco dependence interventions remains limited in most health care settings. As a result, a new model of care using trained and certified Tobacco Treatment Specialists (TTS) has developed.[64] This is a new and growing part of the health care team. Certified TTS typically hold a Bachelor's or Master's degree in a health care or related field such as counseling

or social work. TTS serve several important roles in the health care team: (1) primary care providers can refer tobacco users to a TTS, especially those patients who have failed previous treatments; (2) TTS are agents for disseminating new treatment approaches; (3) TTS provide advocacy for effective treatment of tobacco users and policy changes that promote use of effective treatments; (4) TTS can spearhead quality improvement efforts in tobacco dependence treatment; (5) specialists such as TTS legitimize dissemination within their primary professions.[64] The US Public Health Service Guideline 2008 Update defines TTS as health care providers from various professional backgrounds who view tobacco dependence treatment as a primary professional role. In addition to having the knowledge, skills, and ability to provide treatment through modalities across a range of intensities, TTS contribute to tobacco control efforts by (1) providing a resource to nonspecialists in treating tobacco dependence; (2) developing, implementing, and evaluating procedures for treating tobacco dependence in the office, clinic, or hospital; and (3) developing and evaluating innovative strategies to increase effectiveness in the use of tobacco dependence treatment. TTS are trained in the breadth of interventions for treating tobacco dependence, including motivational interviewing techniques. Thus, TTS are not constrained to provide treatment to those already motivated to stop smoking but also help unmotivated smokers to move through the change process toward an attempt to stop smoking. Health care providers with counseling backgrounds are ideally suited to be trained as TTS, but they would then need to work under the supervision of a prescribing physician. Trained and certified practitioners, such as physician assistants and nurse practitioners, may be trained as TTS and are able to be more independent because they have prescribing capabilities in most states in the United States. They also are able to bill independently of a physician and may care for patients in both the outpatient and inpatient areas. Labeling tobacco dependence treatment as a clinical activity rather than a prevention effort helps to promote TTS who are then viewed as being essential to developing an adequate system of treatment of tobacco dependence.[64]

TTS offer intensive treatment interventions or services in a medical setting or through telephone quitlines. They are able to provide cost-effective and more intensive interventions than physicians by providing comprehensive consultations, multiple counseling sessions, and group interventions. Working in concert with physicians,

TTS can provide a unique referral resource for the physician who then can practice with the 2 As and an R (ask, advise, and refer) approach to treating tobacco users. This model fits well with the time constraints common in modern medical practice. TTS may be useful for developing, evaluating, and implementing changes in the office or clinic to increase the rate of tobacco user identification and triage. Because tobacco dependence treatment is their primary professional role, TTS possess the skills, knowledge, and training to provide effective intervention across a range of intensities.

LOW-DOSE COMPUTED TOMOGRAPHY SCREENING FOR LUNG CANCER VERSUS PAYING FOR TREATING TOBACCO DEPENDENCE

Until recently, lung cancer screening for cigarette smokers had never been convincingly shown to reduce mortality. Data suggesting the potential for a survival benefit began to emerge with studies evaluating the use of low-dose computed tomography (LDCT) for this purpose. With funding from the National Cancer Institute (NCI), the National Lung Screening Trial (NLST) began recruitment for what would be the largest study ever comparing the effectiveness of LDCT and standard chest radiograph (CXR) for reducing lung cancer mortality. Recruitment began in September 2002 and 53,454 subjects were recruited in more than 30 sites across the United States. Enrolled subjects were men or women who had to be 55 to 74 years of age and either be an active smoker with a history of smoking greater than or equal to 30 pack-years or be a former smoker who had quit smoking in the previous 15 years. LDCT scans were conducted at baseline and at 2 annual follow-up examinations. The primary endpoint was lung cancer mortality. Secondary endpoints of overall mortality, lung cancer incidence, screening-related and treatment-related mortality, and health care use were also evaluated.[65]

The results from NLST show a 20% (95% confidence interval [CI], 6.8–26.7; $P = .004$) reduction in lung cancer mortality in the LDCT group compared with the CXR group.[66] A 6% (CI 1.2–13.6; $P = .02$) reduction in all-cause mortality was also observed in the LDCT group compared with the CXR group. Study subjects were informed by letter of the study findings, with recommendations to the CXR group to talk to their health providers about having an evaluation with LDCT.

Decreasing mortality from lung cancer remains a critical health care priority, but preventing lung cancer through the promotion of smoking abstinence needs to remain sharply in focus. However, findings from the Lung Screening Study (LSS),[67,68] the previously conducted NLST feasibility study, suggest that a normal LDCT result may decrease the motivation to achieve smoking abstinence. Among younger participants (≤64 years), an abnormal screening result was significantly associated with becoming more ready to stop smoking, whereas a normal result was associated with becoming less ready to stop smoking ($P = .02$).[69] These observations underscore the importance of engaging in ongoing discussions with all patients about the importance of smoking abstinence for the prevention of lung cancer. We urge that current smokers who ask to undergo LDCT screening be required to undergo treatment for tobacco dependence before receiving LDCT screening, especially because treating tobacco dependence is among the most cost-effective interventions in all of medicine.[70] Indeed, the NLST investigators noted that "The cost-effectiveness of low-dose CT screening must be considered in the context of competing interventions, particularly, smoking cessation."[66] The NLST investigators indicate that analyses of cost-effectiveness and quality of life are being conducted.

SUMMARY

The US Public Health Service Guideline 2008 Update emphasizes tobacco use as a chronic medical disorder, highlights both behavioral counseling and the use of the 7 approved medications, and points out the usefulness, efficacy, and reach of telephone quitlines. Although providing evidence-based treatment of tobacco-dependent patients is a challenge for busy physicians, a team approach including trained and certified TTS provides an efficient treatment model. TTS represent a new and growing part of the health care team and could expand the collective tobacco treatment expertise in the medical setting. Effective tobacco dependence treatment frequently requires tailoring, and often intensifying, of the interventions, both counseling and pharmacotherapy, to meet the needs of the individual patient. Although the report of LDCT screening reducing lung cancer mortality is an important advance, stopping smoking not only reduces the risk of lung cancer but a myriad of other cancers, cardiovascular disease, stroke, peripheral vascular disease, and many others. Treating tobacco dependence is one of the most cost-effective therapies in medicine and it deserves adequate reimbursement for it to be more widely available.

REFERENCES

1. Aldler I. Primary malignant growths of the lung. Primary malignant growths of the lungs and bronchi. London, Bombay (India), Calcutta (India): Longmans, Green and Co; 1912. p. 1–12.

2. Ochsner A, DeBakey M. Carcinoma of the lung. Arch Surg 1941;42:209–58.

3. Wynder EL, Graham EA. Tobacco smoking as a possible etiologic factor in bronchiogenic carcinoma; a study of 684 proved cases. J Am Med Assoc 1950;143(4):329–36.

4. Jemal A, Siegel R, Xu J, et al. Cancer statistics, 2010. CA Cancer J Clin 2010;60(5):277–300.

5. Centers for Disease Control and Prevention. Tobacco use, targeting the nation's leading killer at a glance 2011. Chronic disease prevention and health promotion 2011. Available at: http://www.cdc.gov/chronicdisease/resources/publications/aag/pdf/2011/Tobacco_AAG_2011_508.pdf. Accessed April 20, 2011.

6. McNally W. The tar in cigarette smoke and its possible effects. Am J Cancer 1932;162:1502–14.

7. Hurt RD, Robertson CR. Prying open the door to the tobacco industry's secrets about nicotine: the Minnesota Tobacco Trial. JAMA 1998;280(13):1173–81.

8. Smoking and health proposal. UCSF Legacy Tobacco Documents Library, Brown & Williamson Collection; 1969. Available at: http://legacy.library.ucsf.edu/tid/ypb72d00. Accessed April 20, 2011.

9. Janssen-Heijnen ML, Coebergh JW, Klinkhamer PJ, et al. Is there a common etiology for the rising incidence of and decreasing survival with adenocarcinoma of the lung? Epidemiology 2001;12(2):256–8.

10. Kozlowski LT, Goldberg ME, Yost BA, et al. Smokers' misperceptions of light and ultra-light cigarettes may keep them smoking. Am J Prev Med 1998;15(1):9–16.

11. US Department of Health and Human Services. A report of the surgeon general. Washington, DC: Public Health Service, Centers for Disease Control, Office on Smoking and Health; 1990.

12. Peto R, Lopez AD. The future worldwide health effects of current smoking patterns. In: Koop CE, Pearson CE, Schwarz MR, editors. Critical issues in global health. New York: Jossey-Bass; 2000. Available at: http://www.cdc.gov/chronicdisease/resources/publications/aag/pdf/2011/Tobacco_AAG_2011_508.pdf. Accessed August 8, 2011.

13. Fiore MC, Jaen C, Baker TB, et al. Treating tobacco use and dependence: 2008 update U.S. Surgeon General, Clinical Practice Guideline. Availabe at: http://www.surgeongeneral.gov/tobacco/treating_tobacco_use08.pdf.

14. Swartz SH, Cowan TM, Klayman JE, et al. Use and effectiveness of tobacco telephone counseling and nicotine therapy in Maine. Am J Prev Med 2005;29(4):288–94.

15. Fiore M, Jaen C, Baker T, et al. A clinical practice guideline for treating tobacco use and dependence: 2008 update. A U.S. Public Health Service report. Am J Prev Med 2008;35(2):158–76.

16. Brody AL, Mandelkern MA, London ED, et al. Effect of secondhand smoke on occupancy of nicotinic acetylcholine receptors in brain. Arch Gen Psychiatry 2011;68:953–60.

17. Watkins SS, Koob GF, Markou A. Neural mechanisms underlying nicotine addiction: acute positive reinforcement and withdrawal. Nicotine Tob Res 2000;2(1):19–37.

18. Balfour D. The neurochemical mechanisms underlying nicotine tolerance and dependence. In: Pratt JA, editor. The biological basis of drug tolerance and dependence. London: Academic Press; 1991. p. 121–51.

19. Perry D, Davila-Garcia M, Stockmeier C. Increased nicotine receptors in brains from smokers: membrane binding and autoradiography studies. J Pharmacol Exp Ther 1999;289(3):1545–52.

20. Hope BT, Nagarkar D, Leonard S, et al. Long-term upregulation of protein kinase A and adenylate cyclase levels in human smokers. J Neurosci 2007;27(8):1964–72.

21. Kenny PJ, Markou A. Conditioned nicotine withdrawal profoundly decreases the activity of brain reward systems. J Neurosci 2005;25(26):6208–12.

22. Dale LC, Hurt RD, Offord KP, et al. High-dose nicotine patch therapy. Percentage of replacement and smoking cessation. JAMA 1995;274(17):1353–8.

23. Gourlay SG, Benowitz NL. Arteriovenous differences in plasma concentration of nicotine and catecholamines and related cardiovascular effects after smoking, nicotine nasal spray, and intravenous nicotine. Clin Pharmacol Ther 1997;62(4):453–63.

24. Ho MK, Mwenifumbo JC, Al Koudsi N, et al. Association of nicotine metabolite ratio and CYP2A6 genotype with smoking cessation treatment in African-American light smokers. Clin Pharmacol Ther 2009;85(6):635–43.

25. Henningfield JE, Stapleton JM, Benowitz NL, et al. Higher levels of nicotine in arterial than in venous blood after cigarette smoking. Drug Alcohol Depend 1993;33(1):23–9.

26. Jacob P 3rd, Yu L, Shulgin AT, et al. Minor tobacco alkaloids as biomarkers for tobacco use: comparison of users of cigarettes, smokeless tobacco, cigars, and pipes. Am J Public Health 1999;89(5):731–6.

27. Moyer TP, Charlson JR, Enger RJ, et al. Simultaneous analysis of nicotine, nicotine metabolites, and tobacco alkaloids in serum or urine by tandem mass spectrometry, with clinically relevant metabolic profiles. Clin Chem 2002;48(9):1460–71.

28. Jacob P 3rd, Hatsukami D, Severson H, et al. Anabasine and anatabine as biomarkers for tobacco use during nicotine replacement therapy. Cancer Epidemiol Biomarkers Prev 2002;11(12):1668–73.

29. Piper ME, Smith SS, Schlam TR, et al. A randomized placebo-controlled clinical trial of 5 smoking cessation pharmacotherapies. Arch Gen Psychiatry 2009; 66(11):1253–62.

30. Ebbert JO, Severson HH, Croghan IT, et al. A randomized clinical trial of nicotine lozenge for smokeless tobacco use. Nicotine Tob Res 2009; 11(12):1415–23.

31. Shiffman S, Dresler CM, Hajek P, et al. Efficacy of a nicotine lozenge for smoking cessation. Arch Intern Med 2002;162(11):1267–76.

32. Schneider NG, Olmstead R, Mody FV, et al. Efficacy of a nicotine nasal spray in smoking cessation: a placebo-controlled, double-blind trial. Addiction 1995;90(12):1671–82.

33. Hurt RD, Offord KP, Croghan IT, et al. Temporal effects of nicotine nasal spray and gum on nicotine withdrawal symptoms. Psychopharmacology (Berl) 1998;140(1):98–104.

34. Leischow S, Nilsson F, Franzon M, et al. Efficacy of the nicotine inhaler as an adjunct to smoking cessation. Am J Health Behav 1996;20(5):364–71.

35. Bergstrom M, Nordberg A, Lunell E, et al. Regional deposition of inhaled 11C-nicotine vapor in the human airway as visualized by positron emission tomography. Clin Pharmacol Ther 1995;57(3):309–17.

36. Hurt RD, Dale LC, Offord KP, et al. Serum nicotine and cotinine levels during nicotine-patch therapy. Clin Pharmacol Ther 1993;54(1):98–106.

37. Hurt RD, Dale LC, Fredrickson PA, et al. Nicotine patch therapy for smoking cessation combined with physician advice and nurse follow-up. One-year outcome and percentage of nicotine replacement. JAMA 1994;271(8):595–600.

38. Hughes JR, Lesmes GR, Hatsukami DK, et al. Are higher doses of nicotine replacement more effective for smoking cessation? Nicotine Tob Res 1999;1(2): 169–74.

39. Stead LF, Perera R, Bullen C, et al. Nicotine replacement therapy for smoking cessation. Cochrane Database of Systemic Reviews 2008;1:CD000146.

40. Jorenby DE, Smith SS, Fiore MC, et al. Varying nicotine patch dose and type of smoking cessation counseling. JAMA 1995;274(17):1347–52.

41. Kenford SL, Fiore MC, Jorenby DE, et al. Predicting smoking cessation. Who will quit with and without the nicotine patch. JAMA 1994;271(8):589–94.

42. Schnoll RA, Patterson F, Wileyto EP, et al. Effectiveness of extended-duration transdermal nicotine therapy: a randomized trial. Ann Intern Med 2010; 152(3):144–51.

43. Steinberg MB, Greenhaus S, Schmelzer AC, et al. Triple-combination pharmacotherapy for medically ill smokers: a randomized trial. Ann Intern Med 2009;150(7):447–54.

44. Clarke PB. Nicotine dependence–mechanisms and therapeutic strategies. Biochem Soc Symp 1993; 59:83–95.

45. Pontieri FE, Tanda G, Orzi F, et al. Effects of nicotine on the nucleus accumbens and similarity to those of addictive drugs. Nature 1996;382(6588):255–7.

46. Fryer JD, Lukas RJ. Noncompetitive functional inhibition at diverse, human nicotinic acetylcholine receptor subtypes by bupropion, phencyclidine, and ibogaine. J Pharmacol Exp Ther 1999;288(1): 88–92.

47. Hurt RD, Sachs DP, Glover ED, et al. A comparison of sustained-release bupropion and placebo for smoking cessation. N Engl J Med 1997;337(17): 1195–202.

48. Hays JT, Hurt RD, Rigotti NA, et al. Sustained-release bupropion for pharmacologic relapse prevention after smoking cessation. a randomized, controlled trial. Ann Intern Med 2001;135(6):423–33.

49. Gonzales DH, Nides MA, Ferry LH, et al. Bupropion SR as an aid to smoking cessation in smokers treated previously with bupropion: a randomized placebo-controlled study. Clin Pharmacol Ther 2001;69(6):438–44.

50. Tashkin D, Kanner R, Bailey W, et al. Smoking cessation in patients with chronic obstructive pulmonary disease: a double-blind, placebo-controlled, randomised trial. Lancet 2001;357(9268):1571–5.

51. Tonstad S, Farsang C, Klaene G, et al. Bupropion SR for smoking cessation in smokers with cardiovascular disease: a multicentre, randomised study. Eur Heart J 2003;24(10):946–55.

52. Jorenby DE, Leischow SJ, Nides MA, et al. A controlled trial of sustained-release bupropion, a nicotine patch, or both for smoking cessation. N Engl J Med 1999;340(9):685–91.

53. Rollema H, Chambers LK, Coe JW, et al. Pharmacological profile of the alpha4beta2 nicotinic acetylcholine receptor partial agonist varenicline, an effective smoking cessation aid. Neuropharmacology 2007;52(3):985–94.

54. Jorenby DE, Hays JT, Rigotti NA, et al. Efficacy of varenicline, an alpha4beta2 nicotinic acetylcholine receptor partial agonist, vs placebo or sustained-release bupropion for smoking cessation: a randomized controlled trial. JAMA 2006;296(1):56–63.

55. Gonzales D, Rennard SI, Nides M, et al. Varenicline, an alpha4beta2 nicotinic acetylcholine receptor partial agonist, vs sustained-release bupropion and placebo for smoking cessation: a randomized controlled trial. JAMA 2006;296(1):47–55.

56. Tonstad S, Tonnesen P, Hajek P, et al. Effect of maintenance therapy with varenicline on smoking cessation: a randomized controlled trial. JAMA 2006; 296(1):64–71.

57. Rigotti NA, Pipe AL, Benowitz NL, et al. Efficacy and safety of varenicline for smoking cessation in patients with cardiovascular disease: a randomized trial. Circulation 2010;121(2):221–9.

58. Tashkin DP, Rennard S, Hays JT, et al. Effects of varenicline on smoking cessation in patients with mild to moderate COPD: a randomized controlled trial. Chest 2011;139(3):591–9.

59. Williams CR, Fiore MC, Jaen C, et al. A clinical practice guideline for treating tobacco use and dependence: 2008 update. A U.S. Public Health Service report. Am J Prev Med 2008;35(2):158–76.

60. McClure JB, Swan GE, Jack L, et al. Mood, side-effects and smoking outcomes among persons with and without probable lifetime depression taking varenicline. J Gen Intern Med 2009;24(5):563–9.

61. Croghan IT, Hurt RD, Dakhil SR, et al. Randomized comparison of a nicotine inhaler and bupropion for smoking cessation and relapse prevention. Mayo Clin Proc 2007;82(2):186–95.

62. Ebbert JO, Burke MV, Hays JT, et al. Combination treatment with varenicline and nicotine replacement therapy. Nicotine Tob Res 2009;11(5):572–6.

63. Quinn VP, Hollis JF, Smith KS, et al. Effectiveness of the 5-As tobacco cessation treatments in nine HMOs. J Gen Intern Med 2009;24(2):149–54.

64. Hughes J. Tobacco treatments specialists: a new profession. J Smoking Cessation 2007;2(Suppl):2–7.

65. Aberle DR, Berg CD, Black WC, et al. The National Lung Screening Trial: overview and study design. Radiology 2011;258(1):243–53.

66. National Lung Screening Trial Research Team. Reduced lung-cancer mortality with low-dose computed tomographic screening. N Engl J Med 2011; 365(5):395–409.

67. Gohagan J, Marcus P, Fagerstrom R, et al. Baseline findings of a randomized feasibility trial of lung cancer screening with spiral CT scan vs chest radiograph: the Lung Screening Study of the National Cancer Institute. Chest 2004;126(1):114–21.

68. Gohagan JK, Marcus PM, Fagerstrom RM, et al. Final results of the Lung Screening Study, a randomized feasibility study of spiral CT versus chest X-ray screening for lung cancer. Lung Cancer 2005;47(1): 9–15.

69. Taylor KL, Cox LS, Zincke N, et al. Lung cancer screening as a teachable moment for smoking cessation. Lung Cancer 2007;56(1):125–34.

70. Croghan IT, Offord KP, Evans RW, et al. Cost-effectiveness of treating nicotine dependence: the Mayo Clinic experience. Mayo Clin Proc 1997;72(10): 917–24.

Screening for Lung Cancer

David E. Midthun, MD

KEYWORDS

- Computed tomography screening • Randomized trials
- Screen bias • Nodule evaluation • Mortality reduction

Screening for lung cancer works! Given the high incidence and lethality of lung cancer, an effective screening test for lung cancer has long been desired. The recently published National Lung Screening Study (NLST), a prospective, randomized controlled trial (RCT), has shown that screening with low-dose spiral computed tomography (LDSCT) results in mortality reduction, in other words, fewer deaths from lung cancer.[1,2] There is much to be learned about who may benefit from screening computed tomography (CT) and who may not benefit. Despite finding more cancers and more early stage cancers, previous randomized trials of screening with chest radiography (CXR) and sputum cytology did not result in fewer deaths from lung cancer in comparison with no screening or screening at a lesser frequency. Early studies showed CT had promise as a much more sensitive test than CXR in detecting lung cancer. Debate ensued as to whether the apparent survival benefit demonstrated with CT in nonrandomized studies proved effectiveness, because the appropriate measure of screening benefit would be a decrease in cancer mortality. The debate was further intensified by the recognition that CT screening frequently results in the detection of pulmonary nodules that often require follow-up or further evaluation. There will likely be age and quantity-of-smoking criteria for which screening will be recommended and reimbursed. Until those recommendations are available, it is best to discuss the potential benefits and risks of CT screening with each patient at risk who is interested in being screened.

THE PROBLEM

The unfortunately persistent smoking prevalence rate suggests that the problem of lung cancer will have a secure presence for several decades. The current clinical management of patients with lung cancer too often begins with detection at the time of symptomatic presentation. Symptoms are usually an indication that the lung cancer is in an advanced stage. Early detection is preferred, but until now no test has proven efficacy as a screening test for lung cancer. Prevention is key; however, improving outcomes from lung cancer will result from early detection and more effective treatment. The present 5-year survival of 16% for lung cancer pales in comparison with 5-year survivals of 88% for breast cancer, 65% for colon cancer, and 100% for prostate cancer, respectively.[3] Part of the reason lung cancer has lagged so far behind in survival is that there has been no established screening test. An effective screening tool has thus been greatly anticipated.

SCREENING

The results of the NLST are the first confirmation that any screening test can reduce deaths from lung cancer. The most recent edition of the American Cancer Society (ACS) Guidelines for the early detection of cancer state: "At present neither the ACS, nor any other medical/scientific organization, recommends testing for early lung cancer detection in asymptomatic individuals."[4] The NLST will likely have game-changing impact on this recommendation. But why hasn't screening been recommended when it was already known that screening with CXR or CT led to the detection of more cancers, more early-stage cancers, and marked improvement in survival? The answer lies within issues introduced by screening—each of those measures are necessary outcomes but together remain insufficient to show efficacy from screening.

The author has nothing to disclose.

Mayo Clinic, Division of Pulmonary and Critical Care Medicine, 200 1st Street Southwest, Rochester, MN 55905, USA
E-mail address: midthun.david@mayo.edu

Clin Chest Med 32 (2011) 659–668
doi:10.1016/j.ccm.2011.08.014
0272-5231/11/$ – see front matter © 2011 Elsevier Inc. All rights reserved.

Use of a screening test introduces biases that are inherent in screening. The most significant of these are lead time, length time, and overdiagnosis bias. Lead-time bias occurs when a cancer is detected earlier than it would have been in the absence of screening, yet even with appropriate intervention, the natural history of disease is not changed. As the measure of time between detection and death, apparent survival is lengthened, suggesting benefit. However, true survival is something that cannot be measured—that is, the time from disease onset to eventual death, whether that is due to lung cancer or not. In the situation of lead-time bias, apparent survival is improved by applying a screening test, but mortality remains unchanged. A patient with cancer would appear to live longer simply because the disease was detected earlier, but this is not necessarily an indication of a change in the natural history. An example would be an aggressive cancer that originates from one cell at time zero, results in the onset of symptoms and is detected at year 4, and leads to the patient's death at 5 years. Survival from diagnosis in this case would be 1 year. Applying a screening tool such as CXR might lead to detection and intervention at year 2. Even if intervention did not change the course of the cancer and death occurred at year 5, survival is now 3 years from diagnosis. Survival time tripled with screening, yet death resulted at the same time it would have without screening. Although lengthening apparent survival is desired, it is not sufficient proof of benefit from screening.

Length-time bias describes an apparent improvement in survival, when that improvement is actually due to selective detection of cancers with a less progressive course while missing cancers that have the most rapidly progressive course. Application of a screening tool at specified intervals would have a higher likelihood of detecting a cancer with a more indolent course than one with a more rapid course that presents with symptoms between screenings. The result is the demonstration of an apparent improvement in survival, though the better outcome reflects the more indolent cancers found with screening. CT screening is most likely to detect peripheral nodular cancers, and these are more likely to be adenocarcinomas with a more favorable outcome than, for example, small cell lung cancers that tend to be central and aggressive, and unlikely to be found by periodic CT screening.

An overdiagnosis cancer is a true cancer but one the patient would have died *with* rather than died *from*. Overdiagnosis bias is an extreme form of length-time bias in which indolent lung cancers are detected that would not have altered the expected survival when compared with the normal population. Patients with overdiagnosed lung cancers would have died of a cause other than lung cancer; were it not for screening, these lung cancers may have gone undetected. The natural history of these cancers does not need to be altered with detection and treatment, as they were not destined to do harm.

In summary, because of these biases inherent in screening, survival would be expected to be more favorable even if earlier detection and intervention did not alter the course of disease. For this reason, the apparent improvement in survival demonstrated in observational CT-screening studies was not proof that it saved lives. Mortality reduction, rather than survival improvement, is the ultimate measure of a screening tool's effectiveness, and needs to be demonstrated by performance of RCTs. The RCT has been accepted as the best scientific method for determining the effectiveness of screening and for other medical-practice interventions.[5]

CHEST RADIOGRAPHY AND SPUTUM CYTOLOGY

The National Cancer Institute supported 3 prospective randomized trials evaluating screening for lung cancer in the 1970s at 3 sites: Johns Hopkins, Memorial Sloan-Kettering, and Mayo Clinic.[6–10] These studies involved more than 30,000 men, current or former smokers, who were older than 45 years. Screening at Memorial Sloan-Kettering and Johns Hopkins showed no change in mortality rate of lung cancer by adding sputum cytology every 4 months to annual CXR screening, when compared with the use of annual CXR alone. The 5-year survival in these two studies was nearly 35%, considerably above the historical average at the time of 13%, but was simply the result of screen bias.[7,8]

After prevalence screening to exclude cancer was performed, the Mayo Lung Project (MLP) compared sputum cytology and CXR every 4 months with standard care, which at the time was the recommendation for these tests annually. In the more frequently screened group 206 cancers were detected, of which 46% were resectable, whereas 160 cancers were detected in the control group with only 32% resectable.[9] However, the anticipated shift from detection of cancers at advanced stage to cancers at earlier stage was not seen. Unresectable lung cancer was identified in 112 participants in the group screened every 4 months compared with 109 in the control group. In the MLP the screened group had a 5-year survival of 35% compared with 15%

in the control group, yet the mortality of 3.2 per 1000 person-years in the screened group was not statistically different from the mortality of 3.0 per 1000 person-years in the control group.[10] This lack of mortality reduction in all 3 of the NCI-sponsored studies essentially failed to prove benefit from screening for lung cancer, and drew the line on screening until now. Moreover, a slight increase in mortality resulting from more frequent screening compared with less frequent screening was subsequently shown by meta-analysis, suggesting that screening actually resulted in more harm than good.[11] The results of the Prostate, Lung, Colon, and Ovary (PLCO) screening trial that investigated CXR versus no screening for lung cancer are still awaited, but the NLST essentially renders these results irrelevant.[12]

CT SCREENING: SINGLE-ARM, OBSERVATIONAL STUDIES

The most sensitive imaging modality for detecting pulmonary nodules is CT scanning. CT was put into clinical use back in the mid 1970s, so why has it taken so long to be used for lung cancer screening? Conventional chest CT required radiation dosages and image-acquisition times that were impractical for screening purposes. The development of LDSCT greatly reduced the radiation dose and the scan time, making LDSCT a feasible screening tool. Conventional CT images are obtained at 140 to 300 mA and are performed over many minutes using multiple breath holds. By contrast, LDSCT images may be completed in 15

seconds during a single breath hold, using at only 20 to 50 mA. LDSCT is comparable in sensitivity and specificity of lung nodule detection with conventional CT mode.

Studies from Japan created excitement in suggesting the viability of LDSCT as a tool for early lung cancer detection. The first report was from Kaneko and colleagues,[13] who screened 1369 high-risk participants with both LDSCT and chest radiography. CT detected 15 cases of peripheral lung cancer while 11 of these were missed on chest radiography. Of the non–small cell carcinomas identified, an amazing 93% were stage I. Sone and colleagues[14] authored the second report in the literature, with 3958 participants screened with both LDSCT and CXR. Only 4 lung cancers were detected by CXR whereas 19 were seen on CT; 84% were stage I at resection. In the United States, CT-screening efforts were led by Henschke and colleagues[15] with the Early Lung Cancer Action Project (ELCAP). This study enrolled 1000 high-risk participants (based on smoking history) and screened with both LDSCT and CXR; initial results were reported in 1999. A total of 27 prevalence lung cancers (ie, present on the baseline scan) were detected by CT; only 7 of those were seen by CXR. At surgery, 23 of the 27 (85%) malignancies were stage IA. **Tables 1** and **2** summarize the baseline and incident findings of these and other observational studies using LDSCT and CXR.

In each of these early studies, CT detected about 4 times more lung cancers than did CXR. Several additional single-arm observational studies

---

Table 1
Observational CT-screening studies: prevalence cancers and nodules detected

Study/Authors[Ref.]	No. of Participants	CT Collimation (mm)	No. of CT-Detected Lung Cancers	Surgical Stage I A/B	Number Missed on CXR	Participants with Noncalcified Nodules
Kaneko et al[13]	1369	10	15 (1.1%)	14 (93%)	11 (73%)	588 (17%)
Sone et al[14]	3967	10	19 (0.48%)	16 (84%)	15 (79%)	217 (5%)
ELCAP[15]	1000	10	27 (2.7%)	23 (85%)	20 (74%)	233 (23%)
Mayo[16]	1520	5	31 (2.0%)	22 (71%)	a	782 (51%)
Diederich et al[17]	817	5	12 (1.5%)	7 (58%)	a	350 (43%)
Pastorino et al[18]	1035	10	11 (1.1%)	6 (55%)	a	199 (19%)
Nawa et al[32]	7956	10	36 (.45%)	31 (86%)	a	2099 (26%)
McWilliams et al[29]	561	7 (36%) 1.25 (60%)	10 (1.8%)	7 (70%)	a	431 (46%)
IELCAP[20]	31,567	1.25–10	405 (1.3)	85%[b]	a	4186 (13%)[c]

[a] CXR not performed.
[b] Only pooled prevalence and incidence clinical stage information reported.
[c] Not reported for nodules <5 mm.

Table 2
Observational CT-screening studies: incidence cancers detected

Study/Authors[Ref.]	No. of Participants	No. of CT-Detected Lung Cancers	Surgical Stage I	Scans with Newly Detected Noncalcified Nodules	Interval Cancers
Sobue et al[18]	1611	22 (1.4%)	18 (82%)	721 (9%)	—
ELCAP[19]	841	7 (0.8%)	3 (43%)	63 (5%)	2
Mayo[16]	1478	34 (2.3%)	17 (61%)	9%–13%	3
Diederich et al[17]	668	10 (1.5%)	7 (70%)	13%	5
Pastorino et al[18]	1035	11 (1.1%)	11 (100%)	10%	—
Nawa et al[32]	5568	4 (0.07%)	4 (100%)	148 (3%)[a]	—
IELCAP[20]	27456	74 (0.27%)	85%[b]	1460 (5%)[c]	5

[a] Only nodules ≥8 mm reported.
[b] Only pooled prevalence and incidence clinical stage information reported.
[c] Not reported for nodules <5 mm.

reported similar results with LDSCT in the United States, Germany, Italy, and Japan.[16–21] The reported survival results from these studies were promising; however, by design they were insufficient to show that CT screening saved lives. To highlight this point, Bach and colleagues[22] applied a validated lung cancer prediction model to 3 prospective single-arm observational studies of CT screening combining 3246 participants. CT screening found 3 times the number of expected cancers, resulted in 10 times the expected number of resections (109 of 144 cancers were resectable), and identified more than the expected number of advanced stage cancers. The 4-year actual survival was 94% for participants with surgical stage I cancers, yet CT screening did not result in a predicted reduction in the expected number of deaths from lung cancer. Of note, the 95% confidence intervals within the Bach article[22] would not have been able to detect a reduction in lung cancer mortality as large as 30%. These results emphasized the need to evaluate the effectiveness of screening by mortality reduction rather than survival improvement.

CT SCREENING: RANDOMIZED CONTROLLED TRIALS

Several RCTs of CT screening are under way or have been completed (**Table 3**). The NLST is by far the largest of these; it included 53,454 participants who were current or former heavy smokers (the equivalent of a pack per day for 30 years) aged 55 to 74 years. Participants who had quit smoking had to have done so within 15 years of enrollment, and participants could not have had a previous CT scan within 18 months of enrollment. Participants were randomized between LDSCT and CXR at baseline, year 1, and year 2, and then followed for a median of 6.5 years.[2] The study was designed to have 90% power to detect a 21% reduction in mortality.

A positive CT-screening result in the NLST was defined as the finding of a noncalcified nodule of at least 4 mm. Twenty-seven percent of participants randomized to LDSCT screening had a positive baseline scan, of which 96% were false positive (ie, not lung cancer). In the CXR screening arm, a positive baseline study was found in 9%, of which 95% were false positives. In the LDSCT arm of the NLST there were 649 cancers that were detected by CT screening, 44 interval cancers (identified during the screening period but not detected by screening), and 367 diagnosed during follow-up post screening.[1] In the CXR arm there were 279 cancers detected by CXR screening, 137 interval cancers, and 525 diagnosed during follow-up post screening. Among cancers detected by CXR, 47.6% were stage I and 43.2% were stage III or IV. By contrast, within the LDSCT arm, 63% of lung cancers diagnosed from a positive screening test were Stage I, and 29.8% were Stages III or IV. This finding demonstrated that CT resulted in a shift in stage at diagnosis from advanced disease to early stage. By late October 2010, 354 deaths from lung cancer had occurred among those in the LDSCT arm versus 442 deaths among those in the CXR arm, corresponding to a 20.3% mortality reduction with CT screening.[1] Overall mortality in the CT-screening arm was reduced by 6.7% ($P = .02$) over the CXR arm, but this was not significant after excluding deaths from lung cancer. The number needed to treat (ie, the number of high-risk participants needed to be screened to save one life from lung cancer) was 320.

Table 3
Randomized, controlled CT-screening studies

Study[Ref.]	Participants	Noncalcified Nodules (%)	CT Collimation (mm)	No. of Cancers Detected by Screening	Surgical Stage I (%)	Lung Cancer Deaths
NELSON[22]	CT: 7557	50.5	1	70 (0.9%)	63.9	—
	None: —	—	—	—	—	—
ITALUNG[23]	CT: 1613	30[a]	3	20 (1.5%)	47.6	—
	None: 1593	—		—	—	—
DLSCT[24]	CT: 2052	29	3	17 (0.8%)	53	—
	None: 2052	—		—	—	—
Lung Screening Study[25]	CT: 1660	25.8[b]	5	40 (2.4%)	48	—
	CXR: 1658	8.7[b]	—	20 (1.2%)	40	—
Depiscan[26]	CT: 330	45.2	1–1.5	8	37.5	—
	CXR: 285	7.4	—	1	100	—
DANTE[27]	CT: 1276	27.5	5	60 (0.5%)	55	20 (1.6%)
	None: 1196	—	—	34 (0.3%)	35	20 (1.7%)
NLST[1]	CT: 26722	27.3[b]	≤2.5	649	63	356 (1.3%)
	CXR: 26732	9.2	—	279	47.6	443 (1.7%)

[a] Reported as positive if a nodule ≥5 mm was detected.
[b] Reported as positive if a nodule ≥4 mm was detected.

The Dutch-Belgian randomized lung cancer screening trial known as the NELSON trial is ongoing. Information was reported for the 7557 participants randomized to receive CT screening.[23] More than 50% of the participants had one or more nodules identified at baseline. Seventy cancers were diagnosed at the baseline examination, resulting in a prevalence rate of 0.9%; 64% of these cancers were stage I. The second round of CT screening identified an additional 57 cancers in 54 participants; 74% were surgical stage I cancers. No information from the NELSON study has been provided thus far for the control group or regarding mortality.

The ITALUNG study is under way in Italy, wherein 3206 participants have been randomized to LDSCT versus no screening.[24] The baseline CT was positive (defined as a pulmonary nodule ≥5 mm) in 426 (30.3%) of 1406 subjects. Twenty-one prevalence lung cancers were diagnosed in 20 participants (prevalence 1.5%); 10 (47.6%) were stage I. Control group findings have not yet been reported. The Danish Lung Cancer Screening Trial (DLCST) randomized 4104 participants to CT versus no screening.[25] Among those who received CT screening, there were 17 cancers found at baseline (prevalence rate of 0.8%); 9 (53%) were stage I, and 8 (47%) were stage III or IV. No information has been provided on the control group.

Two small RCTs of CT screening have also reported data on both the screened and the control group. The Lung Screening Study was the pilot study to determine feasibility of the NLST. A total of 1660 subjects were randomized to the LDSCT arm and 1658 to the CXR arm.[26] In the CT arm the rate of cancer detection on the baseline scan was 1.9%, and for year 1 was 0.57%. In the CXR arm the rate of cancer detection at baseline was 0.45%, and for year 1 was 0.68%. No mortality information was presented for the study; however, the finding of a nearly twofold higher number of advanced stage cancers in the CT arm suggested there was not likely to be any mortality benefit from CT screening. The Depiscan study performed in France randomized 621 participants between CT and CXR.[27] One or more nodules were seen in 152 (45%) of 336 subjects receiving CT with 8 lung cancers identified, whereas only one cancer was detected in the CXR arm.

The DANTE trial is under way in Europe, and enrolled 2472 participants who were randomized between CT versus no CT (following a baseline CXR) with the plan to screen annually for 4 years.[28] After a mean of 33 months follow-up, lung cancer was detected in 60 participants in the CT arm versus 34 in the control group. Stage I cancers represented 60% of the cancers in the CT-screening group compared with only 15% in the controls. No mortality data have been published from this study. Results for these smaller RCTs may be additive to the NLST and may help define the population(s) for whom CT screening is appropriate, as well as the frequency with which screening should be performed.

POTENTIAL PROBLEMS WITH CT SCREENING

Now that LDSCT has been shown to reduce mortality, the problems of CT screening are recognized as manageable. A few major concerns raised include the issues of false-positive scans, benign nodule resections, overdiagnosis, and the effect of radiation, as well as cost.

In the Mayo CT study, baseline scanning revealed one or more noncalcified nodules in 51% of the participants; after 4 annual scans 74% of the participants had one or more nodules.[16] In the ELCAP study, 23% of the participants had a nodule at baseline.[20] The ELCAP study used a single detector scanner with 10-mm collimation (slice thickness) and increments of 5 mm of overlap. The Mayo study used a multidetector scanner with 5-mm slice width and a 3.75-mm reconstruction interval. In the study by Diederich and colleagues,[17] noncalcified pulmonary nodules were detected in 43% of the participants; this study also used 5-mm collimation. A Canadian study showed that the number of participants with one or more nodules increased from 36% to 60% when scan slice thickness was reduced from 7 mm to 1.25 mm.[29] These data indicate that the frequency of nodule detection is a function of slice thickness rather than the geographic location of screening. In response to this high rate of false-positive results, many researchers decide to call a scan "negative" if the largest nodule detected is less than 4 or 5 mm.[2,21,23] Doing this serves to reduce the number of false positives; however, this is at the cost of increasing the number of false negatives. This author would recommend against calling a nodule of any size, even very small, "negative," as it gives the wrong information; one should be able to convey lack of immediate concern for a tiny nodule without completely ignoring it. The consequence to calling tiny nodules "negative" will be to miss lung cancers and increase the number of false negatives (Fig. 1). Regarding this point, in one study 18% of cancers identified were actually first detected when less than 4 mm.[30]

Overdiagnosis is the detection of a true cancer, but one that grows so slowly as to not compete with comorbidities for the eventual cause of death. Data from the observational CT-screening studies indicate that such tumors, which have long tumor doubling times, contribute to the apparent survival improvement observed with LDSCT screening. A study from Japan reported tumor doubling times ranging from 662 to 1486 days, with a mean of

880 days.[31] Nawa and colleagues[32] found that 23 of 40 (58%) prevalence cancers in a CT-screened population were found in subjects who were never smokers, suggesting that CT screening may identify a different population of lung cancers than nonscreened patients presenting with clinical symptoms. Volume doubling times were retrospectively calculated in the Mayo CT-screening study; 13 of 48 (27%) screening-detected cancers exhibited slow doubling times that were more than 400 days.[33] These relatively indolent cancers are often nonsolid radiographically, appearing as either pure ground-glass opacities (GGOs) or as partly solid. GGOs require a different approach than solid nodules.[34] GGOs may demonstrate stability for several years and then show evidence of change, thus violating the conventional 2-year "no change" rule indicating a solid nodule is benign (Fig. 2). GGOs may not grow in diameter, yet development of invasion may be evident as they become partially solid. Positron emission tomography (PET) is often falsely negative in GGOs and partly solid lesions. Concern for overdiagnosis is diminished, knowing that mortality is reduced with screening—even if nonlethal cancers are detected, lives saved through screening indicate that enough fast-growing cancers are found to make it worthwhile.

Surgery for nodules eventually found to be benign could be considered by some as having been unnecessary, but is part of the physical and financial cost of screening for lung cancer. In the Mayo CT-screening study, 18% of participants who underwent procedures performed were found to have a benign histology.[35] Similarly, in the study by Diederich and colleagues, the DANTE study, and the NLST study, benign nodules represented 20%, 22%, and 27% of resections, respectively.[1,17,36] Overall, CT-screening studies report benign nodule resection rates of between 15% and 30%. In the absence of a perfectly sensitive, noninvasive test, some benign nodules will be removed when showing growth, change in density characteristics, or avidity on PET imaging. However, the desire is clearly to keep benign resections to a minimum. The literature suggests that focused screening programs have done this better than usual practice, which is a concern with the anticipation of a generalized recommendation to screen high-risk patients. Recent surgical series report that benign nodules comprise as many as 50% to 86% of resected nodules.[37–39] This rate of benign resections is simply too high. Reducing the removal of benign nodules can be achieved in many circumstances by careful evaluation through review of old images, followed by serial examinations, or evaluating larger nodules

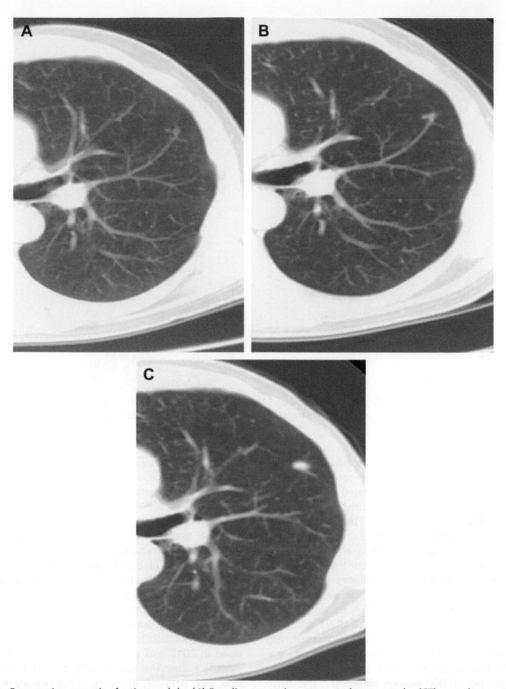

Fig. 1. Progressive growth of a tiny nodule. (*A*) Baseline screening computed tomography (CT) scan demonstrates a 2-mm nodule in the left upper lobe. (*B*) Follow-up CT scan at 1 year demonstrates slight growth to 3 mm. (*C*) Follow-up CT scan at 2 years demonstrates further growth to 6 mm. At resection, the nodule was a stage IA adenocarcinoma. If the nodule had been deemed "negative" on the baseline CT scan, it would have been a false negative.

with PET or needle biopsy. Published nodule guidelines can assist in these evaluations.[40,41]

One other concerning issue is that diagnostic radiation associated with CT screening may actually cause some lung cancers. Radiation absorption is expressed as an effective dose in Sievert (Sv) or millisieverts (mSv) for dose distributions that are nonhomogeneous, as in x-ray radiation (1 mSv =

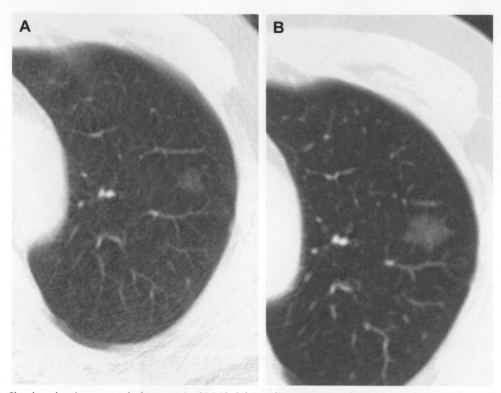

Fig. 2. Slowly enlarging ground-glass opacity (GGO). (*A*) Baseline screening chest CT scan shows a 13-mm GGO. (*B*) Follow-up chest CT scan after 5 years demonstrates slow growth to 20 mm. Limited resection revealed a stage I adenocarcinoma in situ.

1 mGy). The average effective dose for a CT of the chest is about 7 mSv.[42] Women are estimated to have a higher risk of cancer-related mortality than men with similar levels of exposure.[43] Age at radiation exposure is also a factor. The number of CT scans of the chest that would be required to cause one radiation-induced cancer is estimated to be 720 for 40-year-old women and 1566 scans for 40-year-old men. Older age reduces the eventual risk; for 60-year-old persons, one cancer would be induced for every 1090 CT scans for women and 2080 CT scans for men.[44] The NLST investigators estimated that the radiation risk from screening 55-year-old smokers results in 1 to 3 lung cancer deaths per 10,000 screened and 0.3 new breast cancers per 10,000 women screened.[1] This harm from screening highlights the importance of having proven cancer mortality reduction through an RCT.

SUMMARY

Proof of mortality reduction has been shown with mammography for breast cancer and with fecal occult blood testing for colon cancer, and CT screening for lung cancer can now be added to that list; CT screening saves lives. Results of the nonrandomized trials provided insufficient evidence to move CT screening from the realm of personal choice to a matter of health policy. Due to the frequency and lethality of lung cancer, a 20% reduction in deaths certainly provides some long-awaited good news. The response of the ACS and US Preventive Services Task Force in making recommendations for CT screening in public policy is also anticipated. More information is forthcoming from the NLST regarding quality of life, smoking behavior, health care use, and cost effectiveness of screening.[1] Further studies such as the UK Lung Screen trial will define the appropriate population to screen. This study is set to open in 2012 and will use a validated method to calculate absolute risk of lung cancer based on age, sex, smoking duration, family history of lung cancer, history of nonpulmonary malignant tumor, history of pneumonia, and occupational exposure to asbestos.[45] What is a clinician to do in the meantime? The decision to case-find lung cancer with screening requires a discussion between the physician and the patient of the risks and potential benefits. Despite the potential harm in biopsies and surgery performed for benign lesions as well as the potential risks of radiation, the mortality reduction demonstrated in the NLST suggests that screening benefit outweighs the risk. Use of a risk-prediction model may identify individuals at comparable or even higher risk for lung cancer who would benefit from CT screening even though they do not fit the age and pack-year criteria of the NLST. A celebratory response to mortality reduction from screening must not diminish the focus on primary prevention through encouraging smoking cessation, promoting avoidance of smoking initiation, and limiting passive smoke exposure.

REFERENCES

1. The National Lung Screening Trial Research Team. Reduced lung-cancer mortality with low-dose computed tomographic screening. N Engl J Med 2011;365:395–409.
2. National Lung Screening Trial Research Team, Aberle DR, Berg CD, et al. The National Lung Screening Trial: overview and study design. Radiology 2011;258:243–53.
3. Jemal A, Siegel R, Xu J, et al. Cancer statistics, 2010. CA Cancer J Clin 2010;60:277–300.
4. Smith R, Cokkinides V, Brooks D, et al. Cancer screening in the United States, 2010: a review of current American Cancer Society guidelines and issues in cancer screening. CA Cancer J Clin 2010;60:99–119.
5. Strauss GM. Screening for lung cancer. Surg Oncol Clin N Am 1999;8:747–74.
6. Frost JK, Ball WC, Levin ML, et al. Early lung cancer detection: results of the initial (prevalence) radiologic and cytologic screening in the Johns Hopkins Study. Am Rev Respir Dis 1984;130:549–54.
7. Tockman MS. Survival and mortality from lung cancer in a screened population: the Johns Hopkins Study. Chest 1986;89:324S–6S.
8. Flehinger BJ, Melamed MR, Zaman MB, et al. Early lung cancer detection: results of the initial (prevalence) radiologic and cytologic screening in the Memorial Sloan-Kettering study. Am Rev Respir Dis 1984;130:555–60.
9. Fontana RS, Sanderson DR, Taylor WF, et al. Early lung cancer detection: results of the initial (prevalence) radiologic and cytologic screening in the Mayo Clinic Study. Am Rev Respir Dis 1984;130:561–5.
10. Fontana RS, Sanderson DR, Woolner LB, et al. Screening for lung cancer: a critique of the Mayo Lung Project. Cancer 1991;67:1155–64.
11. Manser R, Wright G, Hart D, et al. Surgery for early stage non-small cell lung cancer. Cochrane Database Syst Rev 2005;1:CD004699.
12. Hocking WG, Hu P, Oken MM, et al, PLCO Project Team. Lung cancer screening in the randomized Prostate, Lung, Colorectal, and Ovarian (PLCO) Cancer Screening Trial. J Natl Cancer Inst 2010;102:722–31.
13. Kaneko M, Eguchi K, Ohmatsu H, et al. Peripheral lung cancer: screening and detection with low-dose spiral CT versus radiography. Radiology 1999;201:798–802.
14. Sone S, Takashima S, Li F, et al. Mass screening for lung cancer with mobile spiral computed tomography scanner. Lancet 1998;351:1242–5.
15. Henschke CI, McCauley DI, Yankelevitz DF, et al. Early Lung Cancer Action Project: overall design and findings from baseline screening. Lancet 1999;354:99–105.
16. Swensen SJ, Jett JR, Hartman TE, et al. CT screening for lung cancer: five-year prospective experience. Radiology 2005;235:259–65.
17. Diederich S, Wormanns D, Semik M, et al. Screening for early lung cancer with low-dose spiral CT: prevalence in 817 asymptomatic smokers. Radiology 2002;222:773–81.
18. Pastorino U, Bellomi M, Landoni C, et al. Early lung cancer detection with spiral CT and positron emission tomography in heavy smokers: two-year results. Lancet 2003;362:593–7.
19. Sobue T, Moriyama N, Kaneko M, et al. Screening for lung cancer with low-dose helical computed tomography: anti-lung cancer association project. J Clin Oncol 2002;20:911–20.
20. Henschke CI, Naidich DP, Yankelevitz DF, et al. Early Lung Cancer Action Project: initial findings on repeat scanning. Cancer 2001;92:153–9.
21. The International Early Lung Cancer Action Program Investigators. Survival of patients with stage I lung cancer detected on CT screening. N Engl J Med 2006;355:1763–71.
22. Bach P, Jett J, Pastorino U, et al. Computed tomography screening and lung cancer outcomes. JAMA 2007;297:953–61.
23. van Klaveren RJ, Oudkerk M, Prokop M, et al. Management of lung nodules detected by volume CT scanning. N Engl J Med 2009;361:2221–9.
24. Lopes Pegna A, Picozzi G, Mascalchi M, et al, ITALUNG Study Research Group. Design, recruitment and baseline results of the ITALUNG trial for lung cancer screening with low-dose CT. Lung Cancer 2009;64:34–40.
25. Pedersen JH, Ashraf H, Dirksen A, et al. The Danish randomized lung cancer CT screening trial–overall design and results of the prevalence round. J Thorac Oncol 2009;4:608–14.
26. Gohagan J, Marcus P, Fagerstrom R, et al, Writing Committee, Lung Screening Study Research Group. Baseline findings of a randomized feasibility trial of lung cancer screening with spiral CT scan vs chest radiograph: the Lung Screening Study of the National Cancer Institute. Chest 2004;126:114–21.
27. Blanchon T, Brechot J, Grenier PA, et al, "Depiscan" Group. Baseline results of the Depiscan study: a French randomized pilot trial of lung cancer

screening comparing low dose CT scan (LDCT) and chest X-ray (CXR). Lung Cancer 2007;58:50–8.

28. Infante M, Lutman FR, Cavuto S, et al, DANTE Study Group. Lung cancer screening with spiral CT: baseline results of the randomized DANTE trial. Lung Cancer 2008;59:355–63.

29. McWilliams A, Mayo J, MacDonald S, et al. Lung cancer screening: a different Paradigm. Am J Respir Crit Care Med 2003;168:1167–73.

30. McWilliams AM, Mayo JR, Ahn MI, et al. Lung cancer screening using multi-slice thin-section computed tomography and autofluorescence bronchoscopy. J Thorac Oncol 2006;1:61–8.

31. Aoki T, Nakata H, Watanabe H, et al. Evolution of peripheral lung adenocarcinomas: CT findings correlated with histology tumor doubling time. AJR Am J Roentgenol 2000;174:763–8.

32. Nawa T, Nakagawa T, Suzushi S, et al. Lung cancer screening using low-dose spiral CT: results of baseline and 1-year follow-up studies. Chest 2002;122:15–20.

33. Lindell RM, Hartman TE, Swensen SJ, et al. Five-year lung cancer screening experience: CT appearance, growth rate, location, and histologic features of 61 lung cancers. Radiology 2007;242:555–62.

34. Godoy MC, Naidich DP. Subsolid pulmonary nodules and the spectrum of peripheral adenocarcinomas of the lung: recommended interim guidelines for assessment and management. Radiology 2009; 253:606–22.

35. Crestanello JA, Allen MS, Jett JR, et al. Thoracic surgical operations in patients enrolled in a computed tomographic screening trial. J Thorac Cardiovasc Surg 2004;128:254–9.

36. Infante M, Chiesa G, Solomon D, et al, DANTE Study Group. Surgical procedures in the DANTE trial, a randomized study of lung cancer early detection with spiral computed tomography: comparative analysis in the screening and control arm. J Thorac Oncol 2011;6:327–35.

37. Grogan EL, Jones DR, Kozower BD, et al. Identification of small lung nodules: technique of radiotracer-guided thoracoscopic biopsy. Ann Thorac Surg 2008;85:S772–7.

38. Chen W, Chen L, Yang S, et al. A novel technique for localization of small pulmonary nodules. Chest 2007; 131:1526–31.

39. Cardillo G, Regal M, Sera F, et al. Videothoracoscopic management of the solitary pulmonary nodule: a single-institution study on 429 cases. Ann Thorac Surg 2003;75:1607–11.

40. MacMahon H, Austin JH, Gamsu G, et al, Fleischner Society. Guidelines for management of small pulmonary nodules detected on CT scans: a statement from the Fleischner Society. Radiology 2005;237: 395–400.

41. Gould MK, Fletcher J, Iannettoni MD, et al. American College of Chest Physicians. Evaluation of patients with pulmonary nodules: when is it lung cancer? ACCP evidence-based clinical practice guidelines (2nd edition). Chest 2007;132:108S–30S.

42. National Research Council. Committee to assess health risks from exposure to low levels of ionizing radiation. Health Risks from Exposure to low levels of Ionizing Radiation: BEIR-VII. Washington, DC: National Academy of Sciences; 2005.

43. Mettler F, Huda W, Yoshizumi T, et al. Effective doses in radiology and diagnostic nuclear medicine: a catalog. Radiology 2008;248:254–63.

44. Smith-Bindman R, Lipson J, Marcus R, et al. Radiation dose associated with common computed tomography examinations and the associated lifetime attributable risk of cancer. Arch Intern Med 2009;169:2078–86.

45. Baldwin DR, Duffy SW, Wald NJ, et al. UK Lung Screen (UKLS) nodule management protocol: modelling of a single screen randomized controlled trial of low-dose CT screening for lung cancer. Thorax 2011;66(4):308–13.

Pathology of Lung Cancer

William D. Travis, MD

KEYWORDS

- Pathology • Lung cancer • Pathologic classification

CLASSIFICATION

Worldwide, lung cancer is the most common cause of major cancer incidence and mortality in men, whereas in women it is the third most common cause of cancer incidence and the second most common cause of cancer mortality.[1] In 2010 the American Cancer Society estimated that lung cancer would account for more than 222,520 new cases in the United States during 2010 and 157,300 cancer deaths.[2] Although lung cancer incidence in the United States began to decline in men in the early 1980s,[3] it seems to have plateaued in women.[2]

Lung cancer can be diagnosed pathologically either by a histologic or cytologic approach.[4–8] The new International Association for the Study of Lung Cancer (IASLC)/American Thoracic Society (ATS)/European Respiratory Society (ERS) Lung Adenocarcinoma Classification has made major changes in how lung adenocarcinoma is diagnosed.[5,7,9] It will significantly alter the structure of the previous 2004 World Health Organization (WHO) classification of lung tumors (**Box 1**). Not only does it address classification in resection specimens (see **Box 1**), but it also makes recommendations applicable to small biopsies and cytology specimens, for diagnostic terms and criteria for other major histologic subtypes in addition to adenocarcinoma (**Table 1**). The 4 major histologic types of lung cancer are squamous cell carcinoma, adenocarcinoma, small cell carcinoma, and large cell carcinoma.[6] These major types can be subclassified into more specific subtypes such as lepidic predominant subtype of adenocarcinoma or the basaloid variant of large cell carcinoma.[6] More detailed reviews of the pathology, cytology, and molecular biology of lung cancer can be found elsewhere.[5–7,10–18]

Although lung cancer can be divided into many subtypes, historically the most important distinction was between small cell lung carcinoma (SCLC) and non–small cell lung carcinoma (NSCLC).[6] This situation is because of the major clinical differences in presentation, metastatic spread, and response to therapy. However, in the past decade, there has been a major transformation in the approach to diagnosis of NSCLC, so now more attention is given to its precise classification in small biopsies and cytology.[5,7,9,19] Because 70% of lung cancers present in advanced stages, most patients are unresectable and the diagnosis is based on small biopsies and cytology. The main reason for this new importance to classify NSCLC further is because the choice of therapies now is dependent on histology. For example, patients with adenocarcinomas and NSCLC not otherwise specified (NSCLC-NOS) are eligible for *EGFR* tyrosine kinase inhibitors (TKIs) if an *EGFR* mutation is present[20–24]; they are also eligible for either pemetrexed-based[25–28] or bevacizumab-based regimens.[29] In contrast, if the diagnosis is squamous cell carcinoma, patients are not eligible for these therapies. The implications of these new therapeutic paradigms for lung cancer classification are profound and are outlined in this review.

PREINVASIVE LESIONS

The pathology of preinvasive lesions for lung cancer has attracted increasing interest in recent years because of the growing importance of early detection of lung cancer using screening of high-risk patients by fluorescence bronchoscopy[30,31] and by spiral or helical computed tomography (CT).[32,33] In addition, the concepts of preinvasive lesions have evolved over the past several

Department of Pathology, Memorial Sloan Kettering Cancer Center, 1275 York Avenue, New York, NY 10065, USA

E-mail address: traviswm@mskcc.org

Clin Chest Med 32 (2011) 669–692

doi:10.1016/j.ccm.2011.08.005

0272-5231/11/$ – see front matter © 2011 Elsevier Inc. All rights reserved.

Box 1
Histologic classification of lung cancer[a]

- **Preinvasive lesions**
  - Squamous dysplasia/carcinoma in situ (CIS)
  - Atypical adenomatous hyperplasia (AAH)
  - Adenocarcinoma in situ (AIS) (nonmucinous, mucinous, or mixed nonmucinous/mucinous)
  - Diffuse idiopathic pulmonary neuroendocrine cell hyperplasia (DIPNECH)
- **Squamous cell carcinoma**
  - Variants
    - Papillary
    - Clear cell
    - Small cell (probably should be discontinued)
    - Basaloid
- **Small cell carcinoma**
  - Combined small cell carcinoma
- **Adenocarcinoma**
  - Minimally invasive adenocarcinoma (MIA) (≤3 cm lepidic predominant tumor with ≤5 mm invasion)
    - nonmucinous, mucinous, mixed mucinous/nonmucinous
  - Invasive adenocarcinoma
    - Lepidic predominant (formerly nonmucinous bronchioloalveolar carcinoma (BAC) pattern, with >5 mm invasion)
    - Acinar predominant
    - Papillary predominant
    - Micropapillary predominant
    - Solid predominant with mucin
  - Variants of invasive adenocarcinoma
    - Invasive mucinous adenocarcinoma (formerly mucinous BAC)
    - Colloid
    - Fetal (low and high grade)
    - Enteric
- **Large cell carcinoma**
  - Variants
  - Large cell neuroendocrine carcinoma (LCNEC)
    - Combined LCNEC
  - Basaloid carcinoma
  - Lymphoepithelioma-like carcinoma

- Clear cell carcinoma
- Large cell carcinoma with rhabdoid phenotype
- **Adenosquamous carcinoma**
- **Sarcomatoid carcinomas**
  - Pleomorphic carcinoma
  - Spindle cell carcinoma
  - Giant cell carcinoma
  - Carcinosarcoma
  - Pulmonary blastoma
  - Other
- **Carcinoid tumor**
  - Typical carcinoid (TC)
  - Atypical carcinoid (AC)
- **Carcinomas of salivary gland type**
  - Mucoepidermoid carcinoma
  - Adenoid cystic carcinoma
  - Epimyoepithelial carcinoma

[a] Modified from the 2004 WHO Classification[6] and the 2011 IASLC/ATS/ERS Classification of Lung Adenocarcinoma.[10] This classification primarily addresses histology in resected specimens.

decades, with none mentioned in the 1967 WHO classification of lung tumors[34] and only bronchial squamous dysplasia and CIS in the 1981 WHO histologic classification of lung tumors.[35] In the 1999 WHO classification 2 new lesions were described: AAH and DIPNECH, and these were maintained in the 2004 WHO classification.[6,36] So in the 1999 and 2004 WHO classification, there were only 3 preinvasive lesions. Now, in the 2011 IASLC/ATS/ERS Classification of Lung Adenocarcinoma, AIS was added as a new preinvasive lesion for adenocarcinoma (see **Box 1**).[5]

Squamous Dysplasia and CIS

Bronchial carcinogenesis is conceptualized as a multistep process involving transformation of the normal bronchial mucosa through a continuous spectrum of lesions, including basal cell hyperplasia, squamous metaplasia, dysplasia, and CIS.[6,36–38] Associated with the morphologic changes are a series of molecular events that accumulate as the squamous lesions progress through increasing dysplasia to CIS and invasive squamous cell carcinoma. Such changes include allelic loss at the 3p

Table 1
Proposed IASLC/ATS/ERS classification for small biopsies/cytology

2004 WHO Classification	Small Biopsy/Cytology: IASLC/ATS/ERS

Adenocarcinoma
  Mixed subtype
  Acinar
  Papillary
  Solid
	Morphologic adenocarcinoma patterns clearly present:
	Adenocarcinoma, describe identifiable patterns present (including micropapillary pattern not included in 2004 WHO classification)
	If pure lepidic growth: mention an invasive component cannot be excluded in this small specimen

No 2004 WHO counterpart:
  most are solid
  adenocarcinomas
	Morphologic adenocarcinoma patterns not present (supported by special stains):
	Non–small cell carcinoma, favor adenocarcinoma

BAC (nonmucinous)	Adenocarcinoma with lepidic pattern (if pure, add note: an invasive component cannot be excluded)
BAC (mucinous)	Mucinous adenocarcinoma (describe patterns present)
Fetal	Adenocarcinoma with fetal pattern
Mucinous (colloid)	Adenocarcinoma with colloid pattern
Signet ring	Adenocarcinoma with (describe patterns present) and signet ring features
Clear cell	Adenocarcinoma with (describe patterns present) and clear cell features

Squamous Cell Carcinoma
  Papillary
  Clear cell
  Small cell
  Basaloid
	Morphologic squamous cell patterns clearly present:
	Squamous cell carcinoma

No 2004 WHO counterpart	Morphologic squamous cell patterns not present (supported by stains): Non–small cell carcinoma, favor squamous cell carcinoma
Small cell carcinoma	Small cell carcinoma
Large cell carcinoma	Non–small cell carcinoma, not otherwise specified (NOS)
LCNEC	Non–small cell carcinoma with NE morphology (positive NE markers), possible LCNEC
Large cell carcinoma with NE morphology	Non–small cell carcinoma with NE morphology (negative NE markers): see comment Comment: This is a non–small cell carcinoma in which LCNEC is suspected, but stains failed to show NE differentiation
Adenosquamous carcinoma	Morphologic squamous cell and adenocarcinoma patterns present: Non–small cell carcinoma, NOS (comment that glandular and squamous components are present) Comment: this could represent adenosquamous carcinoma
No counterpart in 2004 WHO classification	Morphologic squamous cell or adenocarcinoma patterns not present but immunostains favor separate favor glandular and adenocarcinoma component Non–small cell carcinoma, NOS (specify the results of the immunohistochemical stains and the interpretation) Comment: this could represent adenosquamous carcinoma
Sarcomatoid carcinoma	Poorly differentiated NSCLC with spindle or giant cell carcinoma (mention if adenocarcinoma or squamous carcinoma are present)

From Travis WD, Brambilla E, Noguchi M, et al. The new IASLC/ATS/ERS international multidisciplinary lung adenocarcinoma classification. J Thorac Oncol 2011;6:247.

region, which is an early event found in 78% of preinvasive bronchial lesions.[38] Followed by a series of other molecular events such as loss of heterozygosity at 9p21 (p16), 17p loss (hyperplasia), telomere activation, telomerase reactivation, retinoic acid receptor (RAR) β loss (mild dysplasia), p53 mutation, vascular endothelial growth factor overexpression (moderate dysplasia), p16 inactivation, Bcl-2 overexpression, and cyclin D1 and E overexpression (CIS).[38]

Squamous dysplasia may be mild, moderate, or severe depending on the severity of cytologic atypia and the thickness of the abnormality within the bronchial epithelium.[6,36,37] CIS shows full thickness involvement of the epithelium by marked cytologic atypia. There is a continuum of morphologic changes, but these categories can be separated with good reproducibility.[39] Care must be taken not to confuse dysplasia with reactive atypia associated with inflammation or granulation tissue. CIS with involvement of submucosal glands must also be separated from microinvasive squamous cell carcinoma.[6,36,37]

AAH and AIS

AIS is now added to AAH as a new preinvasive lesion for lung adenocarcinoma.

AAH

AAH is a bronchioloalveolar proliferation that resembles but falls short of criteria for BAC, nonmucinous type (**Fig. 1**).[5,6,37,38,40–42] AAH is most commonly encountered as an incidental histologic finding in a lung cancer resection specimen.[36,43,44]

The incidence of AAH varies from 5.7% to 21.4% depending on extent of the search and the criteria used for the diagnosis.[44–47] Most lesions of AAH are less than 5 mm in diameter and frequently they are multiple.[44,45] Histologically AAH consists of a focal proliferation of slightly atypical cuboidal to low columnar epithelial cells along alveoli and respiratory bronchioles (see **Fig. 1**). Slight thickening of alveolar septa may be present.

AAH must be separated from a variety of lesions, the most important of which is the nonmucinous AIS, MIA, or lepidic predominant

adenocarcinoma (LPA).[48] This distinction can be difficult because there is considerable overlap in the morphologic features between AAH and the lepidic pattern of adenocarcinoma.[36,43,49,50] There are currently no data to show that patients with lung cancer and AAH have any different prognosis from those without AAH.[51]

AIS

In the new IASLC/ATS/ERS adenocarcinoma classification AIS is defined as a glandular proliferation measuring 3 cm or less that has pure lepidic growth lacking invasion (**Fig. 2**).[5] In most cases the tumor cells are nonmucinous, with a proliferation of type II pneumocytes or Clara cells, but rarely are they mucinous consisting of tall columnar goblet cells having abundant apical mucin. If these lesions are completely resected, patients have been reported to have 100% 5-year disease-free survival (DFS).[52–59] By CT these lesions typically consist of a ground-glass nodule if nonmucinous and a solid nodule if mucinous AIS.[5]

DIPNECH

DIPNECH is a rare condition in which the peripheral airways are diffusely involved by neuroendocrine (NE) cell hyperplasia and tumorlets (**Box 2, Fig. 3**).[60,61] The clinical presentation resembles interstitial lung disease manifest by airway obstruction caused by bronchiolar fibrosis in approximately half of the patients.[60,61] The remaining patients typically present with multiple incidentally discovered pulmonary nodules, often found during follow-up for an extrathoracic malignancy. Because carcinoid tumors are frequently found in patients with DIPNECH and the tumors are often multiple, this is believed to represent

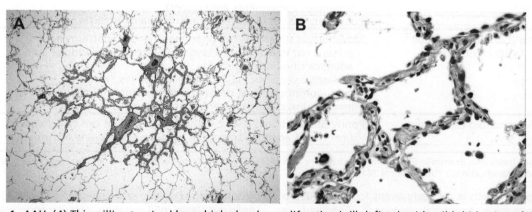

Fig. 1. AAH. (*A*) This millimeter-sized bronchioloalveolar proliferation is ill defined, with mild thickening of the alveolar walls (hematoxylin-eosin, original magnification ×20). (*B*) The alveolar walls show mild fibrous thickening and the hyperplastic pneumocytes show minimal atypia and there are gaps between the cells (hematoxylin-eosin, original magnification ×400).

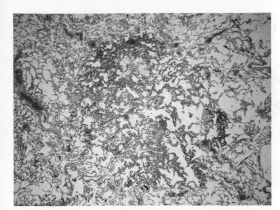

Fig. 2. Nonmucinous AIS. This circumscribed nonmucinous tumor grows purely with a lepidic pattern. No foci of invasion or scarring are seen.

a preinvasive lesion for carcinoid tumors.[6,61] There is a distinctive CT appearance consisting of centrilobular nodules and pulmonary nodules, which correspond to the tumorlets and carcinoid tumors, respectively. Furthermore, in patients who present with clinical manifestations of interstitial lung disease, the CT can be normal or it can show mosaic perfusion from air trapping, bronchial wall thickening, and bronchiectasis.[61,62]

SQUAMOUS CELL CARCINOMA

Squamous cell carcinoma accounts for approximately 20% of all lung cancers in the United States.[63] Historically, two-thirds of squamous cell carcinomas presented as central lung tumors, whereas many among the remaining third are peripheral.[64,65] However, recent reports document that an increasing percentage of squamous cell carcinomas are found in the periphery, exceeding 50% in some studies.[66] The morphologic features that suggest squamous differentiation include intercellular bridging, squamous pearl formation, and individual cell keratinization (**Fig. 4**). In well-differentiated tumors these features are readily apparent; however, in poorly differentiated tumors they are difficult to find.[67] Squamous cell carcinoma arises most often segmental bronchi and involvement of lobar and mainstem bronchus occurs by extension.[68] Squamous cell carcinoma can have papillary, clear cell, small cell,[69] and basaloid subtypes.[36] However, this subtyping needs updating because it does not address well the morphologic spectrum of appearances of lung squamous cell carcinoma and it does not allow for meaningful correlations with clinical, prognostic, or molecular features. For example, the

---

Box 2
The spectrum of NE lung proliferations and tumors

1. NE cell hyperplasia and tumorlets
   a. NE cell hyperplasia
      i. NE cell hyperplasia associated with fibrosis or inflammation
      ii. NE cell hyperplasia adjacent to carcinoid tumors
      iii. Diffuse idiopathic NE cell hyperplasia with or without airway fibrosis/obstruction
   b. Tumorlets (less than 0.5 cm)
2. Tumors with NE morphology
   a. TC (0.5 cm or larger)
   b. AC
   c. LCNEC
      Combined large cell NE carcinoma[a]
   d. Small cell carcinoma
      Combined small cell carcinoma[a]
3. Non–small cell carcinomas with NE differentiation (NED)
4. Other tumors with NE properties
   a. Pulmonary blastoma
   b. Primitive neuroectodermal tumor
   c. Desmoplastic round cell tumor
   d. Carcinomas with rhabdoid phenotype
   e. Paraganglioma

[a] The histologic type of the other component of non–small cell carcinoma should be specified.
Modified from Travis WD, Brambilla E, Müller-Hermelink HK, et al. Pathology and Genetics: Tumors of the Lung, Pleura, Thymus and Heart. Lyon (France): IARC, 2004. p. 20; and Travis WD. Lung tumors with neuroendocrine differentiation. Eur J Cancer 2009; 45;(Suppl 1):252.

---

small cell variant probably should be discarded, because most of these cases would better be classified as basaloid variants and the term small cell creates confusion with true small cell carcinoma. Papillary squamous cell carcinomas often show a pattern of exophytic endobronchial growth.[70,71]

Several articles have proposed alternative approaches to subclassifying pulmonary squamous cell carcinomas.[66,72,73] These approaches include recognition of an alveolar space-filling

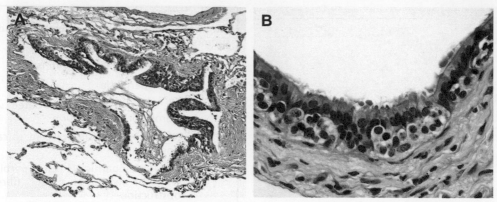

Fig. 3. DIPNECH. (*A*) This bronchiole shows mild fibrotic thickening of the wall and increased numbers of NE cells in the mucosa (hematoxylin-eosin, original magnification ×200). (*B*) At the base of the mucosa are numerous round to oval NE cells with small nuclei and clear cytoplasm (hematoxylin-eosin, original magnification ×400).

variant, which corresponds to favorable prognosis.[66,73] Funai and colleagues[66] reported 5 cases with 100% disease-free survival, and Watanabe and colleagues[73] found that an alveolar space-filling ratio of 70% or more also had a 100% disease-free survival. However, this pattern occurs in only a few cases and is more often seen only focally; in a study from North America prognostic significance could not be shown.[74] Maeshima and colleagues[72] defined minimal tumor cell nests as large (>6 tumor cells), small (2–5 cells), and single cell. In this study the single-cell infiltrating tumors had the worst prognosis. Also tumors associated with a background of usual interstitial pneumonia and lymph node metastases had a poor prognosis. Further work is needed to develop a more practical approach

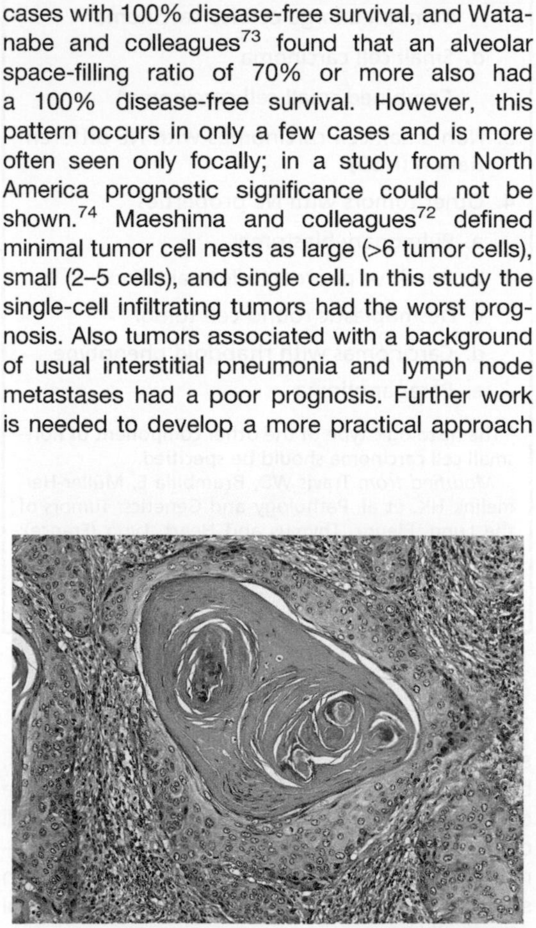

Fig. 4. Squamous cell carcinoma. These tumor cells have abundant eosinophilic keratinized cytoplasm and form nests and keratin pearls characteristic of squamous differentiation (hematoxylin-eosin, original magnification ×200).

to subclassification of squamous cell carcinoma and to identify better histologic predictors of prognosis.

ADENOCARCINOMA

Adenocarcinomas represent 38% of all lung cancers in the United States.[63,75] The 2011 IASLC/ATS/ERS lung adenocarcinoma classification recommends multiple major changes (see **Box 1**).[5,7,9,19] First, it is recommended to no longer use the term BAC because the tumors formerly classified under this term are now classified into 5 different tumors. Second, there are new concepts of AIS (see preinvasive lesions) and MIA. Third, it is recommended to no longer use the term mixed subtype, but rather to use comprehensive histologic subtyping to estimate the percentage of histologic patterns in 5% increments within a tumor with final classification according to the predominant subtype. Fourth, tumors with a predominant component formerly called nonmucinous BAC should be classified as LPA. Fifth, micropapillary adenocarcinoma is recognized as a new subtype with a poor prognosis. Sixth, invasive mucinous adenocarcinoma is the term recommended for those tumors formerly classified as mucinous BAC. Sixth, specific terminology and diagnostic criteria are proposed for tumors in small biopsies and cytology specimens along with recommendations for strategic management of tissue and *EGFR* - mutation testing in patients with advanced adenocarcinoma.[5,7,9,19]

ADENOCARCINOMA CLASSIFICATION IN RESECTED SPECIMENS
MIA

MIA was introduced as a lepidic predominant tumor measuring 3 cm or less that has 5 mm or less of an invasive component (**Fig. 5**).[5] Limited data suggest patients with MIA have a near 100% 5-year disease-free survival.[5,59] Although few articles use the same criteria,[59,76] multiple studies support this concept[77,78] Most of these cases are nonmucinous, but rarely mucinous cases may occur.[5] By CT nonmucinous MIA typically shows a ground-glass nodule with a solid component measuring 5 mm or less. However, mucinous MIA presents as a solid nodule on CT.[5]

Invasive Adenocarcinoma

Classification of overtly invasive adenocarcinomas is now made according to the predominant subtype. This classification is best determined after using comprehensive histologic subtyping to estimate the percentages of the various histologic subtypes within a tumor in a semiquantitative fashion in 5% to 10% increments. LPA consists of tumors formerly classified as mixed subtype tumors containing a predominant lepidic growth pattern of type II pneumocytes or Clara cells (formerly known as nonmucinous BAC) that have an invasive component greater than 5 mm (**Fig. 6**A–C). The other major subtypes include acinar (see **Fig. 6**D), papillary (see **Fig. 6**E), micropapillary (see **Fig. 6**F), and solid with mucin-predominant adenocarcinomas (see **Fig. 6**G, H). The micropapillary predominant subtype is a new addition as a result of the observation in multiple studies that it is associated with poor prognosis in early-stage adenocarcinomas (see **Fig. 3**).[5,76,79,80] Signet ring and clear cell carcinoma subtypes are no longer regarded as histologic subtypes, but they are now documented as cytologic features whenever present with a comment about the percentage identified. Although clear and signet ring cell cytologic

changes are seen mostly in the solid subtype, they can also be seen in acinar or papillary patterns as well.[81,82]

By CT there is a good correlation between amount of the ground-glass component and lepidic growth on biopsy versus the solid component on CT and the invasive components by biopsy.[76] However, few studies have addressed this issue according to the new classification.

Adenocarcinoma Variants

The variants of lung adenocarcinoma consist of invasive mucinous adenocarcinoma (formerly mucinous BAC), colloid adenocarcinoma, fetal adenocarcinoma, and enteric adenocarcinoma.[5] Invasive mucinous adenocarcinomas (formerly mucinous BAC) are separated from the nonmucinous invasive adenocarcinomas because of the frequent association with *KRAS* mutation, lack of thyroid transcription factor 1 (TTF-1), and frequent multicentric lung lesions. Histologically these tumors show varying amounts of lepidic, acinar, papillary, or micropapillary growth consisting of columnar cells with abundant apical mucin and small basally oriented nuclei (**Fig. 7**).[5] CT findings frequently show localized or multifocal consolidation with air bronchograms forming nodules and lobar consolidation.

Prognosis of Adenocarcinoma Subtypes in Resected Specimens

Few studies have evaluated prognosis of the adenocarcinoma subtypes according to the precise criteria and terminology of the new classification. However, multiple studies have reported 100% 5-year DFS for tumors that

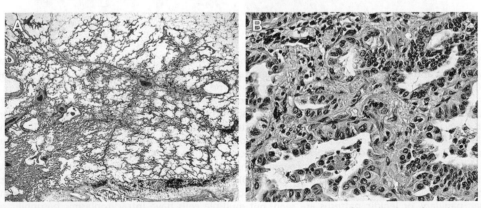

Fig. 5. Nonmucinous MIA. (*A*) This adenocarcinoma tumor consists primarily of lepidic growth with a small (<0.5 cm) area of invasion (*bottom left*) (hematoxylin-eosin, original magnification ×1). (*B*) From the area of invasion, these acinar glands are invading in the fibrous stroma (hematoxylin-eosin, original magnification ×200).

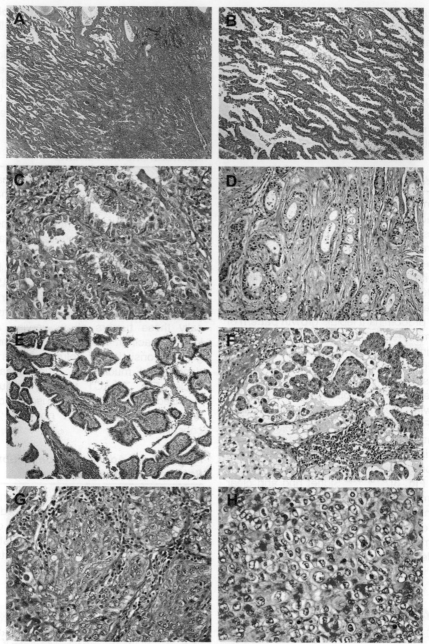

Fig. 6. Major histologic patterns of invasive adenocarcinoma. (*A*) Lepidic predominant pattern with mostly lepidic growth (*left*) and an area of invasive acinar adenocarcinoma (*right*) (hematoxylin-eosin, original magnification ×100). (*B*) Lepidic pattern consists of a proliferation type II pneumocytes and Clara cells along the surface alveolar walls (hematoxylin-eosin, original magnification ×200). (*C*) Area of invasive acinar adenocarcinoma (same tumor as in *6A, B*) (hematoxylin-eosin, original magnification ×400). (*D*) Acinar adenocarcinoma composed of round to oval malignant glands invading a fibrous stroma (hematoxylin-eosin, original magnification ×200). (*E*) Papillary adenocarcinoma consists of malignant cuboidal to columnar tumor cells growing on the surface of fibrovascular cores (hematoxylin-eosin, original magnification ×100). (*F*) Micropapillary adenocarcinoma consists of small papillary clusters of glandular cells growing within this airspace, most of which do not show fibrovascular cores (hematoxylin-eosin, original magnification ×200). (*G*) Solid adenocarcinoma with mucin consisting of sheets of tumor cells with abundant cytoplasm and mostly vesicular nuclei with several conspicuous nucleoli. No acinar, papillary, or lepidic patterns are seen, but multiple cells have intracytoplasmic basophilic globules that suggest intracytoplasmic mucin (hematoxylin-eosin, original magnification ×400). (*H*) Solid adenocarcinoma with mucin. Numerous intracytoplasmic droplets of mucin are highlighted with this mucicarmine stain (original magnification ×400).

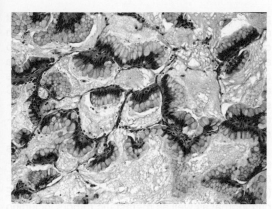

Fig. 7. Invasive mucinous adenocarcinoma. This area of invasive mucinous adenocarcinoma shows a pure lepidic growth. The tumor consists of columnar cells filled with abundant mucin in the apical cytoplasm and small basal oriented nuclei (hematoxylin-eosin, original magnification ×200).

would be classified as AIS in the new classification.[52–59] Although the specific criteria for MIA proposed in the new classification were not used in previous studies, data from multiple studies suggest that these tumors also have a 100% or near 100% 5-year DFS.[58,59,78,83]

In a study of 514 stage I adenocarcinomas reported by Yoshizawa and colleagues,[76] 3 groups of tumors were identified according to grades of clinical behavior: (1) low-grade AIS and MIA with 100% 5-year DFS; (2) intermediate-grade nonmucinous lepidic predominant, papillary predominant, and acinar predominant with 90%, 83%, and 84% 5-year DFS, respectively; and (3) high-grade invasive mucinous adenocarcinoma, colloid predominant, solid predominant, and micropapillary predominant with 75%, 71%, 70%, and 67% 5-year DFS, respectively. Similar results were found in 2 independent datasets.[84,85] This finding was confirmed by Kadota and colleagues[84] in a separate dataset of 540 stage I lung adenocarcinomas in which there was 100% DFS for AIS and MIA, 97% for lepidic predominant, 87% for acinar, 80% for papillary, 59% for micropapillary, and 69% for solid with a 62% 3-year DFS for invasive mucinous and colloid adenocarcinoma. In a Japanese cohort of 432 patients that included some higher stage patients (250 Stage IA, 88 1B, 30 IIA, 13 IIB, 26 IIIA, 4 IIIB, and 15 IV), 5-year DFS was 100% for AIS and MIA, 89% for lepidic predominant, 67% for papillary, 59% for acinar, 61% for solid predominant, and 17% for micropapillary, with 80% for invasive mucinous adenocarcinoma.[85]

Potential Impact of Classification on TNM Staging

There are 2 major ways the new lung adenocarcinoma classification affects TNM staging. First, comprehensive histologic subtyping provides a useful way to compare multiple lung adenocarcinomas by providing a detailed way to assess whether the 2 tumors represent metastasis versus synchronous or metachronous primaries. The distribution of percentages of the histologic components is one of multiple morphologic features in addition to cytologic and stromal characteristics that have been shown to correlate highly with molecular and clinical approaches to making this distinction.[86–88] Whether or not a second tumor is classified as a separate primary or an intrapulmonary metastasis can significantly alter TNM staging and patient management, particularly for separate lobe or contralateral tumors.

Second, it is possible that in invasive lung adenocarcinomas with a prominent lepidic component comprehensive histologic subtyping may help to determine the size of the invasive component, and this may be more predictive of survival than total tumor size as suggested in several studies reporting that the invasive size is an independent prognostic factor.[76,77] The invasive tumor size can be estimated by subtracting the percentage of the lepidic component from the total gross size. These data suggest that, similar to breast cancer, the size T factor for early lung adenocarcinomas may be best determined by the size of the invasive component rather than the total tumor size. This finding also needs to be studied by CT to determine if prognosis is best predicted according to the size of the solid component rather than total tumor size including the ground-glass component.[5] It is hoped that sufficient data can be accumulated before the next TNM revision to address this issue.

ADENOCARCINOMA CLASSIFICATION IN SMALL BIOPSIES AND CYTOLOGY

For the first time in lung cancer classification formal criteria for diagnosis of lung cancer in small biopsies and cytology were proposed by the new IASLC/ATS/ERS lung adenocarcinoma classification (see **Table 1**).[5] Because 70% of lung cancers present in advanced stages and are unresectable, they are diagnosed in these small specimens. These new criteria were driven by the need to separate adenocarcinoma from squamous cell carcinoma because of the therapeutic implications based on histology. Patients who have either adenocarcinoma, NSCLC, favor adenocarcinoma, or NSCLC-NOS rather than squamous cell carcinoma are eligible at the moment for 3 therapeutic options. Patients with advanced stage lung adenocarcinoma with 1 of these histologic diagnoses should be tested for *EGFR* mutation, and if the result is positive, EGFR TKI therapy has predictive benefit for response rate and progression-free survival.[20–23] Furthermore, it has been shown that in patients with adenocarcinoma or NSCLC-NOS, histology is a strong predictor of response to pemetrexed in patients who have advanced lung cancer.[25–28] In addition patients with squamous cell carcinoma are at risk for life-threatening hemorrhage in contrast to those with adenocarcinoma.[29]

For tumors that show clear morphologic features of adenocarcinoma or squamous cell carcinoma, these standard terms are used. However, if the tumor shows only a carcinoma with no clear squamous or glandular features (NSCLC-NOS), a minimal immunohistochemical workup is recommended using a single adenocarcinoma marker and squamous marker, which should allow for classification of most tumors. The best markers for adenocarcinoma and squamous cell carcinoma are TTF-1 and p63, respectively.[5] In a tumor that shows no clear squamous or glandular morphology, but the staining results favor adenocarcinoma (ie, TTF-1 positive, p63 negative), the tumor should be classified as NSCLC, favor adenocarcinoma (**Fig. 8**). Likewise, the stains in such a tumor favor squamous cell carcinoma, the diagnosis would be NSCLC, favor squamous cell carcinoma (**Fig. 9**). Then for tumors for which there is clear differentiation by light microscopy or special stains, or if the results are conflicting, the diagnosis remains NSCLC-NOS. Cytology is another powerful tool in subclassifying poorly differentiated NSCLC. In some cases, it may be easier to classify the tumor based on cytology than biopsy.[4,7] It is recommended to avoid use of the term nonsquamous carcinoma and state the specific diagnosis in precise terms as outlined earlier.[5] Also use of the term NSCLC should be minimized and instead the specific diagnosis of adenocarcinoma or squamous cell carcinoma should be used whenever possible.[5]

The approach to interpretation of small biopsies and cytology must include considerations of diagnoses other than NSCLC, such as NE tumors (carcinoid, small cell carcinoma, or large cell NE carcinoma) as well as metastatic tumors including metastatic malignant melanoma, breast cancer, or prostate cancer.[7] Therefore if the initial evaluation does not clearly point to adenocarcinoma or squamous cell carcinoma, some of these other diagnoses may need to be considered.

Because the diagnosis of NSCLC-NOS was encouraged by previous WHO classifications, because of the lack of any clinical reason to be more precise, in studies of advanced NSCLC, this diagnosis has been made in 20% to 40% of cases, and some data suggest its use has been increasing.[27,89]

However, with the new IASLC/ATS/ERS criteria and use of immunohistochemistry as well as cytology correlation, the percentage of NSCLC diagnosed as NSCLC-NOS should be less than 5% of cases.[4,7]

EGFR Mutation Testing

In the new IASLC/ATS/ERS lung adenocarcinoma classification, there is a clinical recommendation that *EGFR* mutation testing be performed in advanced lung adenocarcinomas because of the

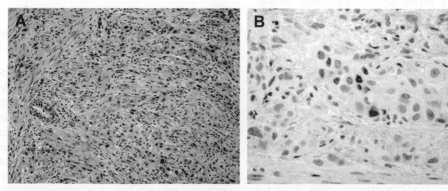

Fig. 8. Non–small cell carcinoma, favor adenocarcinoma. (*A*) This carcinoma shows no clear squamous or glandular differentiation (hematoxylin-eosin, original magnification ×200). (*B*) The diffuse positive TTF-1 staining allows for the diagnosis of non–small cell carcinoma, favor adenocarcinoma (hematoxylin-eosin, original magnification ×200).

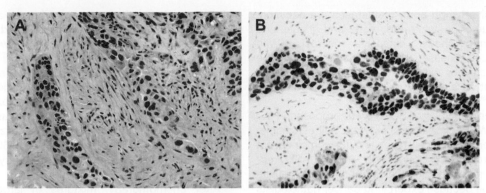

Fig. 9. Non–small cell carcinoma, favor squamous cell carcinoma. (*A*) This carcinoma shows no clear squamous or glandular differentiation (hematoxylin-eosin, original magnification ×200). (*B*) The diffuse positive p63 staining and negative TTF-1 staining (*not shown*) allows for the diagnosis of non–small cell carcinoma, favor squamous cell carcinoma (immunohistochemistry for p63, original magnification ×200).

predictive benefit of *EGFR* mutation with treatment by EGFR TKIs as described earlier.[5] *EGFR* mutation testing should be performed for all patients with a pathologic diagnosis of: (1) adenocarcinoma, (2) NSCLC, favor adenocarcinoma, and (3) NSCLC-NOS. This recommendation has major implications for tissue management and pathologic diagnosis.

Multidisciplinary Strategy Needed to Obtain and Process Small Biopsies and Cytology

Each institution needs to develop a multidisciplinary strategy to manage these small pieces of tissue from (1) obtaining the specimen, (2) processing it in the pathology laboratory, (3) providing material to the molecular diagnostic laboratory, and (4) getting the results back into a pathology report and into the medical record.[5,7] This process requires ongoing communication between specialists to ensure optimal management of tissues and efficient reporting of results. One of the central aspects of this process that affects radiologists, pulmonologists, or surgeons is the need to obtain sufficient tissue not only for diagnosis but also for molecular studies. To achieve this goal, biopsy procedures should be designed to result either in a core biopsy or a cell block from tissue samples obtained for cytology.[5,90] Cytology specimens such as pleural fluids should also be processed to generate cell blocks so immunostaining and molecular studies can be performed.

Use Minimal Stains to Maximize Tissue for Molecular Testing

Pathologists should minimize the amount of tissue used for making the diagnosis, including use of as

few special stains as possible.[5,7] This strategy is necessary to preserve as much tissue as possible for molecular testing. One helpful approach is to cut multiple unstained slides from the block after initial review in cases that are potential candidates for molecular testing, so the block is cut only once and valuable tissue is not lost during the process of facing the block multiple times.[7] This strategy includes tumors that are either clearly adenocarcinoma or those with NSCLC-NOS patterns on hematoxylin and eosin stain that require special stains. If adenocarcinoma is suspected, by performing only a TTF-1 stain, if the result is positive, it would confirm not only the adenocarcinoma diagnosis but also a pulmonary origin. If by morphology the tumor could be either adenocarcinoma or squamous cell carcinoma, it may be best to perform 1 adenocarcinoma (ie, TTF-1) and 1 squamous (ie, p63) marker as recommended in the new classification.[5] Limited additional stains may be considered for the small percentage of cases that cannot be classified after this initial panel.[5,7]

SMALL CELL CARCINOMA

SCLC comprises 14% of all lung cancers, and more than 30,000 new cases are diagnosed per year in the United States.[63,75] Approximately two-thirds of SCLC present as a perihilar mass. SCLC typically are situated in a peribronchial location with infiltration of the bronchial submucosa and peribronchial tissue. Bronchial obstruction is usually caused by circumferential compression, although rarely endobronchial lesions can occur. Because the diagnosis is usually established on transbronchial biopsy or cytology, is it unusual to encounter SCLC as a surgical specimen.

Extensive lymph node metastases are common. The tumor is white-tan, soft, and friable and frequently shows extensive necrosis. With advanced disease, the bronchial lumen may be obstructed by extrinsic compression. SCLC may present as a solitary coin lesion in up to 5% of cases.[91,92]

Three subtypes of SCLC were proposed in the 1981 WHO classification: (1) oat cell carcinoma, (2) intermediate cell type, and (3) combined oat cell carcinoma.[35] However, in 1988 the IASLC recommended dropping the category of intermediate cell type because expert lung cancer pathologists could not reproduce this subclassification and significant differences in survival could not be shown. They also recommended adding the category of mixed small cell/large cell carcinoma because these patients seemed to have a worse prognosis than other patients with SCLC.[93] The category of combined SCLC was retained for SCLC with a mixture of adenocarcinoma or squamous cell carcinoma.[93] The 1999 WHO classification discarded the category of mixed small cell/large cell carcinoma because there were data indicating problems in reproducibility for this subtype and lack of confirmation that these patients had a worse prognosis.[36,94] Therefore in the 2004 WHO classifications there are only 2 types of SCLC: SCLC (with pure SCLC histology) and combined SCLC (with a mixture of any non–small cell type) (see **Box 2**).[6]

SCLC has a distinctive histologic appearance. The tumor cells are small and have a round to fusiform shape, scant cytoplasm, finely granular nuclear chromatin, and absent or inconspicuous nucleoli (**Fig. 10**).[6] Nuclear molding and smearing

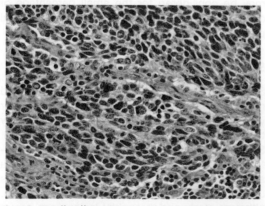

Fig. 10. Small cell carcinoma. This tumor is composed of small cells with scant cytoplasm, finely granular chromatin, and frequent mitoses. Nucleoli are absent (hematoxylin-eosin, original magnification ×400).

of nuclear chromatin as a result of crush artifact may be conspicuous. There is usually extensive necrosis and mitotic rates are high, with an average of 80 mitoses per 2 mm^2 area.[6,95,96] The growth pattern usually consists of diffuse sheets, but rosettes, peripheral palisading, organoid nesting, streams, ribbons, and rarely, tubules or ductules may be present.[97] Basophilic encrustation of vessel walls, also known as the Azzopardi effect, is often seen in necrotic areas.[97] SCLC is reliably diagnosed in small biopsies and cytology specimens.

After chemotherapy, mixtures of large cell, squamous, giant cell, or adenocarcinoma may be seen in 15% to 45% of SCLC.[98–100]

Combined SCLC

The frequency of combined SCLC depends on the extent of histologic sampling but most studies report this occurs in less than 10% of cases. A combination of SCLC and large cell carcinoma (see **Fig. 8**) is found in about 4% to 6% of cases.[93] Approximately 1% to 3% of SCLC may be combined with adenocarcinoma or squamous cell carcinoma.[93,94,99,101] The amount of the non–small cell component is not important for adenocarcinoma or squamous cell carcinoma so long as the histology is clear. However, for combined small cell and large cell carcinoma at least 10% of large cells is required to make the diagnosis.[6,95,96] SCLC can also be associated with spindle cell carcinoma,[102,103] giant cell carcinoma,[103] and carcinosarcoma.[104] However, there are no consistent data to suggest that there is any significant difference in clinical features, prognosis, and response to therapy compared with patients with pure SCLC.[94,101]

Although immunohistochemistry is useful in the diagnosis of SCLC, the most important stain is a good-quality hematoxylin and eosin stain that is not too thick or overstained. The diagnosis can be established without immunostains in most cases and it is needed only in problematic cases. A pancytokeratin antibody such as AE1/AE3 is useful to confirm that the tumor is a carcinoma rather than a lymphoid lesion and the most useful NE markers include CD56, chromogranin and synaptophysin, which are best used as a panel. TTF-1 expression is found in 70% to 80% of SCLC.[6,96,105–109] However, because extrapulmonary small cell carcinomas can express TTF-1, this stain should not be used to determine the primary site of small cell carcinomas.[110] The proliferation rate by Ki-67 staining is high, averaging 70% to 90%.[111]

Clinical features and prognosis

SCLC has distinctive clinical properties, with an aggressive clinical course, frequent wide-spread metastases at presentation, common paraneoplastic syndromes, and responsiveness to chemotherapy.[112]

With combination chemotherapy (etoposide/cisplatin) and chest radiotherapy, for patients with limited-stage disease, the median survival is 15 months and 5-year survival is 10%.[112]

Differential diagnosis

Separation of SCLC from large cell carcinoma or LCNEC requires the application of a constellation of criteria including cell size, nucleoli, nuclear/cytoplasmic (N/C) ratio, nuclear chromatin, nucleoli, nuclear molding, cell shape (fusiform vs polygonal), and hematoxylin vascular staining (**Table 2**).[108,113] There is a continuum of cell size between SCLC and large cell carcinoma,[113] but the cells of SCLC usually are about the diameter of 2 to 3 small resting lymphocytes.[6] Vollmer[113] showed that the size of cells of SCLC also seems greater in larger biopsy specimens. This finding explains why the tumor cells of SCLC seem larger in well-fixed open biopsies than in transbronchial biopsy specimens.

Disagreement among expert lung cancer pathologists over the distinction between SCLC and NSCLC may occur in up to 5% to 7% of cases.[114–116] In the study by Roggli and colleagues,[115] agreement for the diagnosis of SCLCs for all 5 observers was 93% and for at least 4 of 5

observers it was 98%. In problem cases it can be helpful to try to achieve a consensus approach among other pathology colleagues. If a consensus diagnosis cannot be reached locally, it may be appropriate to refer the case for extramural consultation. For problematic cases in small biopsy specimens, it can be helpful to evaluate any cytology specimens that may have been taken at the time of bronchoscopy because the morphology by cytology may be more diagnostic than in the biopsy specimen.

Crush artifact is common in small biopsy specimens and this can complicate evaluation for diagnosis. Whereas most tumors showing dense sheets of small blue cells turn out to be SCLC, this artifact can also be seen in carcinoid tumors, lymphocytic infiltrates, or poorly differentiated NSCLC. However, even in crushed specimens, some preserved tumor cells with morphology compatible with SCLC should be seen to confirm the diagnosis. Immunohistochemical markers can be of assistance in crushed specimens, because SCLC may show positive staining for cytokeratin, chromogranin, CD56, synaptophysin, TTF-1, and a high proliferation index with Ki-67.[117,118] Up to 10% of SCLC may be negative for a panel of NE markers if the workup includes CD56. So if all other morphologic features are present the diagnosis of SCLC can be rendered even with negative NE markers.[119]

If keratin staining is negative in a suspected SCLC, one should be careful to exclude other possibilities such as chronic inflammation,

---

Table 2
Light microscopic features for distinguishing small cell carcinoma and large cell NE carcinoma

Histologic Feature	Small Cell Carcinoma	LCNEC
Cell size	Smaller (less than diameter of 3 lymphocytes)	Larger
N/C ratio	Higher	Lower
Nuclear chromatin	Finely granular, uniform	Coarsely granular or vesicular Less uniform
Nucleoli	Absent or faint	Often (not always) present May be prominent or faint
Nuclear molding	Characteristic	Less prominent
Fusiform	Common	Uncommon
Polygonal with ample pink cytoplasm	Uncharacteristic	Characteristic
Nuclear smear	Frequent	Uncommon
Basophilic staining of vessels and stroma	Occasional	Rare

Data from Travis WD. Neuroendocrine lung tumors. Path Case Rev 2006;11:235–42; and Vollmer RT. The effect of cell size on the pathologic diagnosis of small and large cell carcinomas of the lung. Cancer 1982;50:1380–3.

lymphoma, primitive neuroectodermal tumor, or small round cell sarcoma.[5,7] There is no immunohistochemical or molecular marker that reliably distinguishes SCLC from non-SCLC.[120,121] However, in a poorly differentiated tumor that is TTF-1–negative and NE-marker– negative but diffusely positive for p63, the diagnosis of basaloid carcinoma or basaloid variant of squamous cell carcinoma is favored.[122] Nevertheless, the primary criteria for separating SCLC from NSCLC are based on light microscopy (see **Box 2**).[6]

LARGE CELL CARCINOMA

Large cell carcinoma comprised 3% of all lung carcinomas in a recent report of the US National Cancer Institute (NCI) Surveillance, Epidemiology, and End Results (SEER) data.[75] This finding is a decrease from 9% reported in the SEER monograph for 1983 to 1987.[63] The SEER data include unresectable tumors that would have been diagnosed on small biopsies or cytology as well as resected tumors; other recent surgical series also report a frequency of approximately 3%.[123,124] These tumors are mostly found in the lung periphery, although they may be centrally located. By gross examination they frequently appear as large necrotic tumors. Large cell carcinoma is a diagnosis of exclusion, where the presence of squamous cell or glandular differentiation needs to be excluded by light microscopy. Histologically the tumors usually consist of sheets and nests of large polygonal cells with vesicular nuclei and prominent nucleoli (**Fig. 11**).[6] In the separation from solid adenocarcinoma with mucin, there

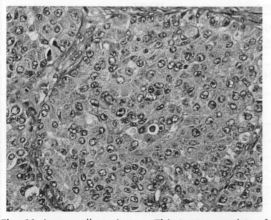

Fig. 11. Large cell carcinoma. This tumor consists of sheets and nests of large cells with abundant cytoplasm and vesicular nuclei with prominent nucleoli (hematoxylin-eosin, original magnification ×400).

should be less than 5 mucin positive cells in at least 2 high power fields.[6]

The diagnosis of large cell carcinoma cannot be made without a resection specimen.[6] This situation is because in small biopsies and cytology, the presence of an adenocarcinoma or squamous cell carcinoma component cannot be excluded. There is considerable confusion in the literature on this topic, because tumors have been classified as large cell carcinoma in both pathology as well as clinical publications in which the data were based on small biopsy specimens rather than resections.[27,125] According to the 2011 IASLC/ATS/ERS lung adenocarcinoma classification, in small biopsy specimens, these tumors would now be classified as NSCLC-NOS if evaluated by light microscopy alone.[5,6] If immunostains are performed, some of these tumors might be reclassified as NSCLC favor adenocarcinoma or NSCLC favor squamous cell carcinoma and a small percentage would remain as NSCLC-NOS.[5,6]

It has been known for decades that electron microscopy (EM) of large cell carcinoma frequently reveals features of adenocarcinoma or squamous differentiation.[126–128] Similar observations are being made using immunohistochemistry, in which studies of large cell carcinomas express adenocarcinoma (TTF-1) or squamous (p63) markers and some have suggested these tumors should now be reclassified.[125,129] A small percentage of these tumors may also harbor mutations such as KRAS that are associated with adenocarcinoma. However, this information by immunohistochemistry or mutation testing does not add any new information beyond what we have known for decades with EM: (1) tumors classified as large cell carcinoma by light microscopy consist of a heterogeneous group of poorly differentiated tumors most of which share properties (EM, immunohistochemistry, or molecular) of adenocarcinoma, some have squamous features, a smaller percentage have both, and a small subset remains a null phenotype or truly undifferentiated large cell carcinoma. How to resolve this issue needs to be addressed in the upcoming revision of the WHO classification. Regardless of whether the decision is to lump (keep large cell carcinoma close to the current definition) or to split (reclassify most large cell carcinomas according to immunohistochemistry), this decision is arbitrary in the absence of any clinical trial data to compare clinical properties, such as different outcomes or response to therapy, relative to the other major lung cancer histologic subtypes. One option may be to retain the diagnosis of large cell carcinoma based on traditional criteria, but add a comment about the immunophenotype that may reflect adenocarcinoma or squamous cell carcinoma differentiation.

Several variants of large cell carcinoma are recognized in the 2004 WHO histologic classification of lung cancer (see **Box 1**). These variants include LCNEC,[6,130,131] basaloid carcinoma,[132] lymphoepithelial-like carcinoma,[133,134] clear cell carcinoma,[135] and large cell carcinoma with rhabdoid phenotype.[136,137] LCNEC is discussed below.

LCNEC

LCNEC comprises approximately 3% of resected lung cancers.[109] LCNEC is a high-grade non–small cell NE carcinoma that differs from AC and small cell carcinoma (see **Table 2**). Histologic criteria include: (1) NE morphology: organoid, palisading, trabecular, or rosette-like growth patterns (**Fig. 12**); (2) non–small cell cytologic features: large size, polygonal shape, low N/C ratio, coarse or vesicular nuclear chromatin, and frequent nucleoli; (3) high mitotic rate (11 or more per 2 mm^2) with a mean of 60 mitoses per 2 mm^2; (4) frequent necrosis; and (5) at least 1 positive NE immunohistochemical marker or NE granules by EM (see **Fig. 12**B).[6,131] It is difficult to diagnose LCNEC based on small biopsy specimens such as needle or bronchoscopic biopsy specimens because it is usually difficult to be certain of the NE morphology without a substantial sampling of the tumor. However, recently criteria were proposed to diagnose LCNEC based on cytology.[138] The term large cell carcinoma, with NE morphology, can be used for tumors resembling LCNEC by light microscopy but lacking proof of NED by EM or immunohistochemistry.[6] The term combined LCNEC is used for those tumors associated with other histologic types of NSCLC such as adenocarcinoma or squamous cell carcinoma (see **Box 1**).[6] A variety of criteria must be used to separate SCLC from LCNEC (see **Table 2**).

Clinical features

Patients with LCNEC have a median age of 62 years (range 33–87 years) and they are typically heavy cigarette smokers.[131] Patients with LCNEC have a poor prognosis. Travis and colleagues[130] found the 5-year and 10-year survival for LCNEC is 27% and 11%, respectively, with a significantly worse prognosis than patients with AC. Iyoda and colleagues[139] found a 35.3% and 31.7% 5-year and 10-year survival, respectively, for LCNEC. Iyoda and colleagues[139] also found a worse survival for LCNEC compared with classic large cell carcinoma ($P = .031$), whereas Jiang and colleagues[140] found a worse survival for LCNEC compared with non–small cell carcinomas ($P = .046$). However, it has not been possible to show a difference in survival between LCNEC and SCLC.[130,141] Surgical resection should be performed if possible; however, it remains to be proved whether adjunctive radiation or chemotherapy is effective. Iyoda and colleagues[139] found no significant difference between the age, sex, smoking history, tumor size, and survival for patients with large cell carcinoma with NE morphology compared with those with LCNEC, although the mitotic rate was higher ($P = .0071$). A recent analysis of the NCI SEER data suggested overall survival and lung cancer specific survival rates for patients with LCNEC after surgical resection without radiation therapy were similar to those for patients who had other large cell carcinoma and better

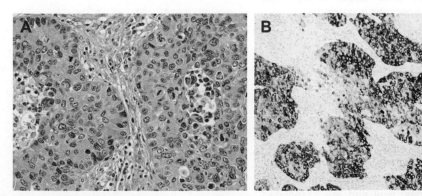

Fig. 12. LCNEC. (*A*) Peripheral palisading and rosette-like structures give this tumor an NE morphologic appearance. The tumor cells have abundant cytoplasm with large hyperchromatic nuclei. Some of the nuclei show vesicular chromatin or prominent nucleoli. Mitoses are frequent (hematoxylin-eosin, original magnification ×400). (*B*) The tumor cells are diffusely positive for synaptophysin (immunohistochemistry for synaptophysin, original magnification ×200).

than for those patients with SCLC, although the differences were not significant on multivariate analysis.[142]

If immunohistochemistry is performed on non–small cell carcinomas lacking NE morphology, positive staining can be found in 10% to 20% of cases. Similarly NE granules can be found in up to 10% of cases by EM. Such tumors are called non–small cell carcinomas (adenocarcinoma, squamous cell carcinoma, or large cell carcinoma) with neuroendocrine differentiation (NSCLC-NED).[36,131] The clinical significance of the diagnosis of NSCLC-NED is not known. Iyoda and colleagues[139] found that the tumor size of large cell carcinoma with NED (LCC-ND) was larger than that for LCNEC ($P = .0033$), but the survival was not different from patients with LCNEC. Whether these tumors are responsive to SCLC chemotherapy regimens[143,144] or whether expression of NE markers may be an unfavorable prognostic factor[145–152] remains to be determined.

ADENOSQUAMOUS CARCINOMA

Adenosquamous carcinoma accounts for 0.6% to 2.3% of all lung cancers[153–157] and it is defined as a lung carcinoma having at least 10% squamous cell and adenocarcinoma by light microscopy.[36] Similar to large cell carcinoma enormous confusion has been introduced by use of immunostains. The current WHO definition recognizes this tumor if the 10% of squamous and adenocarcinoma components are diagnosable by light microscopy. This diagnosis should be made only if the adenocarcinoma and squamous components are both recognizable by light microscopy and not purely by immunohistochemistry. This diagnosis may be suspected, but cannot be made by small biopsy or cytology, because a resection specimen is needed.

CARCINOMAS WITH PLEOMORPHIC, SARCOMATOID, OR SARCOMATOUS ELEMENTS

Sarcomatoid carcinomas comprise 0.3% of all invasive lung malignancies.[63] This group of lung carcinomas is poorly differentiated and expresses a spectrum of pleomorphic, sarcomatoid, and sarcomatous elements.[158] Pleomorphic carcinomas tend to be large, peripheral tumors that often invade the chest wall and are associated with a poor prognosis.[158] Because of the prominent histologic heterogeneity of this tumor, adequate sampling is important and should consist of at least 1 section per centimeter of the tumor diameter. Pleomorphic carcinomas should have at least a 10% component of a spindle cell or giant cell component, and frequently other histologic types such as adenocarcinoma or squamous cell carcinoma (**Fig. 13**) are present.[6,158]

If the tumor has a pure giant cell or spindle cell pattern the term giant cell or spindle cell carcinoma, respectively, can be used. Giant cell carcinoma consists of huge bizarre pleomorphic and multinucleated tumor giant cells.[6,158] The cells are often dyscohesive and infiltrated by inflammatory cells, particularly neutrophils. This tumor is defined by light microscopy, but immunohistochemistry, particularly for epithelial markers such as keratin, can be helpful in confirming epithelial differentiation.[6,158] The diagnosis of pleomorphic carcinoma cannot be made based on small biopsies or cytology; a resection specimen is required to identify the criteria outlined earlier.

Carcinosarcoma and Pulmonary Blastoma

Carcinosarcoma is a tumor composed of a mixture of carcinoma and sarcoma that should show heterologous elements such as malignant cartilage, bone, or skeletal muscle according to the 2004 WHO classification.[6,158] Pulmonary blastomas are composed of a glandular component that resembles well-differentiated fetal adenocarcinoma and a primitive sarcomatous component. Fetal adenocarcinoma is no longer regarded as the epithelial pattern of pulmonary blastoma, but rather as a variant of adenocarcinoma.[6,158]

TYPICAL AND ATYPICAL CARCINOID

Carcinoid tumors account for 1% to 2% of all invasive lung malignancies.[63] Approximately 50%

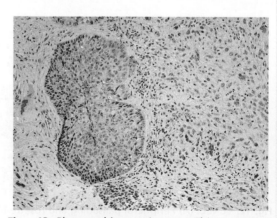

Fig. 13. Pleomorphic carcinoma. This tumor is composed of squamous cell carcinoma (*left*) and an malignant spindle cell proliferation (*right*) (hematoxylin-eosin, original magnification ×200).

of patients are asymptomatic at presentation.[96,112,159] Typical carcinoid (TC) and atypical carcinoid (AC) occur at any age, with an average of 45 to 55 years, and there is no sex predilection. They are the most common lung tumor in childhood.[160] Symptoms include hemoptysis in 18%, postobstructive pneumonitis in 17%, and dyspnea in 2% of patients. Paraneoplastic syndromes include the carcinoid syndrome, Cushing syndrome.[96,112]

The primary approach to treatment of pulmonary carcinoids is surgical resection.[161,162] Patients with TC have an excellent prognosis and rarely die of tumor.[96,112] The finding of metastases should not be used as a criterion for distinguishing TC from AC because 5% to 20% of TCs have regional lymph node involvement.[161,162]

Compared with TCs, ACs have a larger tumor size, a higher rate of metastases, and the survival is significantly reduced. The mortality reported in most series is approximately 30%, ranging from 27% to 47%.[96,112]

Carcinoid tumors may be central, with a frequent polypoid endobronchial component. Peripheral carcinoids are usually found in the subpleural parenchyma. Both TCs and ACs are characterized histologically by an organoid growth pattern and uniform cytologic features consisting of moderate eosinophilic, finely granular cytoplasm with nuclei possessing a finely granular chromatin pattern (**Fig. 14, Table 3**). Nucleoli are inconspicuous in

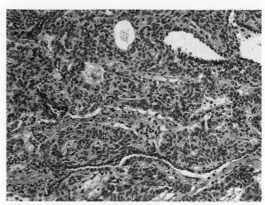

Fig. 14. Typical carcinoid. This tumor is growing in organoid nests and consists of uniform medium-sized cells with a moderate amount of eosinophilic cytoplasm (hematoxylin-eosin, original magnification ×200).

most TCs, but they may be more prominent in ACs. A variety of histologic patterns may occur in both ACs and TCs, including spindle cell, trabecular, palisading, rosette-like, papillary, sclerosing papillary, glandular, and follicular patterns.[131] The tumor cells of pulmonary carcinoid tumors may have oncocytic, acinic cell–like, signet ring, mucin-producing, or melanocytic features.[131]

ACs are defined as carcinoid tumors with mitoses between 2 and 10 per 2 mm² area of viable tumor (10 high power fields in certain microscopes) or the presence of necrosis (**Fig. 15**).[130]

Table 3
Typical and atypical carcinoid: distinguishing features

Histologic or Clinical Feature	Typical Carcinoid	Atypical Carcinoid
Histologic patterns: organoid, trabecular, palisading and spindle cell	Characteristic	Characteristic
Mitoses	Absent or <2 per 2 mm² area of viable tumor (10 high power fields on some microscopes)	2–10 per 2 mm² or area of viable tumor (10 high power fields on some microscopes)
Necrosis	Absent	Characteristic, usually focal or punctate
Nuclear pleomorphism, hyperchromatism	Usually absent, not sufficient by itself for diagnosis of AC	Often present
Regional lymph node metastases at presentation (%)	5–15	40–48
Distant metastases at presentation (%)	Rare	20
Survival at 5 years (%)	90–95	50–60
Survival at 10 years (%)	90–95	35

Data from Colby TV, Koss MN, Travis WD. Tumors of the lower respiratory tract; Armed Forces Institute of Pathology fascicle, third series. Washington, DC: Armed Forces Institute of Pathology, 1995 . p. 295; and Travis WD. Pathology of lung cancer. Clin Chest Med 2002;23:77.

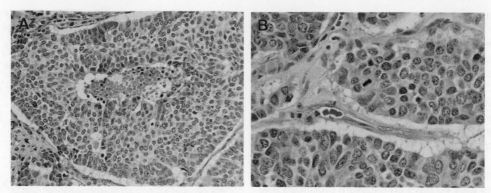

Fig. 15. Atypical carcinoid. (*A*) Punctate foci of necrosis are present in the center of several organoid nests of uniform tumor cells. This feature is characteristic of atypical carcinoids (hematoxylin-eosin, original magnification ×200). (*B*) The tumor cells are uniform, with moderate spindle-shaped cytoplasm, and the nuclear chromatin is finely granular. A single mitosis is present (*center*) (hematoxylin-eosin, original magnification ×800).

The presence of features such as pleomorphism, vascular invasion, and increased cellularity is not so helpful in separating TC from AC. In TC necrosis is absent and mitotic figures are rare (<2 per 2 mm^2) (see **Table 3**).[130,131] The necrosis in AC usually consists of small foci centrally located within organoid nests of tumor cells; uncommonly the necrosis may form larger confluent zones.

Carcinoid tumors stain for NE markers such as chromogranin, synaptophysin, and CD56. A low proliferation rate (≤5%) is seen in TC by Ki-67 staining compared with AC, in which it is usually between 5% and 20%.[111,163] In small crushed biopsies Ki-67 staining can be helpful to separate TC or AC from the high-grade LCNEC or SCLC, which have high proliferation rates.[111,163]

SUMMARY

This article reviews current concepts in pathologic classification of lung cancer based on the 2004 WHO classification of lung tumors and the 2011 IASLC/ATS/ERS classification of lung adenocarcinoma. AIS is now added to the other preinvasive lesions that include squamous dysplasia/CIS, AAH, and DIPNECH. Major changes in lung disease diagnosis have now resulted from the new IASLC/ATS/ERS classification including: (1) the term BAC is no longer used because tumors formerly classified under this term fall into 5 different places in this classification; (2) new concepts of AIS and MIA have been introduced; (3) comprehensive histologic subtyping is recommended for evaluation of invasive lung adenocarcinomas with classification according to the predominant subtype; (4) micropapillary adenocarcinoma is introduced as a new subtype with a poor prognosis; (5) for tumors previously classified as mixed subtype with a predominant

component formerly called nonmucinous BAC, the term LPA is recommended and the term mixed subtype is discontinued; (6) tumors formerly classified as mucinous BAC are now classified as invasive mucinous adenocarcinoma (formerly mucinous BAC). The topic of lung cancer diagnosis in small biopsies and cytology is now addressed for the first time with an official standardized classification in which specific terminology and diagnostic criteria are proposed along with recommendations for strategic management of tissue and *EGFR* mutation testing in patients with advanced adenocarcinoma. The pathology of other lung cancers is also discussed such as large cell carcinoma, sarcomatoid carcinomas, and NE tumors, including small cell carcinoma and large cell NE carcinoma, as well as typical and atypical carcinoid tumors.

REFERENCES

1. Jemal A, Bray F, Center MM, et al. Global cancer statistics. CA Cancer J Clin 2011;61:69–90.
2. Jemal A, Siegel R, Xu J, et al. Cancer statistics, 2010. CA Cancer J Clin 2010;60:277–300.
3. Travis WD, Lubin J, Ries L, et al. United States lung carcinoma incidence trends: declining for most histologic types among males, increasing among females. Cancer 1996;77:2464–70.
4. Rekhtman N, Brandt SM, Sigel CS, et al. Suitability of thoracic cytology for new therapeutic paradigms in non-small cell lung carcinoma: high accuracy of tumor subtyping and feasibility of EGFR and KRAS molecular testing. J Thorac Oncol 2011;6:451–8.
5. Travis WD, Brambilla E, Noguchi M, et al. The new IASLC/ATS/ERS international multidisciplinary lung adenocarcinoma classification. J Thorac Oncol 2011;6:244–85.

6. Travis WD, Brambilla E, Müller-Hermelink HK, et al. Pathology and genetics: tumours of the lung, pleura, thymus and heart. Lyon (France): IARC; 2004.

7. Travis WD, Rekhtman N. Pathological diagnosis and classification of lung cancer in small biopsies and cytology: strategic management of tissue for molecular testing. Semin Respir Crit Care Med 2011;32:22–31.

8. Nizzoli R, Tiseo M, Gelsomino F, et al. Accuracy of fine needle aspiration cytology in the pathological typing of non-small cell lung cancer. J Thorac Oncol 2011;6:489–93.

9. Travis WD, Brambilla E, Van Schil P, et al. Paradigm shifts in lung cancer as defined in the new IASLC/ATS/ERS lung adenocarcinoma classification. Eur Respir J 2011;38:239–43.

10. Brambilla E, Gazdar A. Pathogenesis of lung cancer signalling pathways: roadmap for therapies. Eur Respir J 2009;33:1485–97.

11. Dacic S. Molecular diagnostics of lung carcinomas. Arch Pathol Lab Med 2011;135:622–9.

12. Gomperts BN, Spira A, Massion PP, et al. Evolving concepts in lung carcinogenesis. Semin Respir Crit Care Med 2011;32:32–43.

13. Dowell J, Minna JD. Small-cell lung cancer: translational research enroute to therapeutic advances. Oncology (Williston Park) 2008;22:1493–5.

14. Travis WD. Classification of lung cancer. Semin Roentgenol 2011;46:178–86.

15. Wallace WA. The challenge of classifying poorly differentiated tumours in the lung. Histopathology 2009;54:28–42.

16. Idowu MO, Powers CN. Lung cancer cytology: potential pitfalls and mimics–a review. Int J Clin Exp Pathol 2010;3:367–85.

17. Saad RS, Silverman JF. Respiratory cytology: differential diagnosis and pitfalls. Diagn Cytopathol 2010;38:297–307.

18. Siddiqui MT. Pulmonary neuroendocrine neoplasms: a review of clinicopathologic and cytologic features. Diagn Cytopathol 2010;38:607–17.

19. Travis WD, Rekhtman N, Riley GJ, et al. Pathologic diagnosis of advanced lung cancer based on small biopsies and cytology: a paradigm shift. J Thorac Oncol 2010;5:411–4.

20. Mok TS, Wu YL, Thongprasert S, et al. Gefitinib or carboplatin-paclitaxel in pulmonary adenocarcinoma. N Engl J Med 2009;361:947–57.

21. Mitsudomi T, Morita S, Yatabe Y, et al. Gefitinib versus cisplatin plus docetaxel in patients with non-small-cell lung cancer harbouring mutations of the epidermal growth factor receptor (WJTO G3405): an open label, randomised phase 3 trial. Lancet Oncol 2010;11:121–8.

22. Maemondo M, Inoue A, Kobayashi K, et al. Gefitinib or chemotherapy for non-small-cell lung cancer with mutated EGFR. N Engl J Med 2010;362:2380–8.

23. Zhou C, Wu YL, Chen G, et al. Efficacy results from the randomized phase III OPTIMAL (CTONG 0802) study comparing first-line erlotinib versus carboplatin (CBDCA) plus gemcitabine (GEM) in Chinese advanced non-small cell lung cancer (NSCLC) patients (PTS) with EGFR activating mutations. Ann Oncol 2010;21:LBA13.

24. Rosell R, Gervais R, Vergnenegre A, et al. Erlotinib versus chemotherapy (CT) in advanced non-small cell lung cancer (NSCLC) patients (p) with epidermal growth factor receptor (EGFR) mutations: interim results of the European Erlotinib Versus Chemotherapy (EURTAC) phase III randomized trial [abstract]. J Clin Oncol 2011;29:7503.

25. Ciuleanu T, Brodowicz T, Zielinski C, et al. Maintenance pemetrexed plus best supportive care versus placebo plus best supportive care for non-small-cell lung cancer: a randomised, double-blind, phase 3 study. Lancet 2009;374:1432–40.

26. Scagliotti G, Hanna N, Fossella F, et al. The differential efficacy of pemetrexed according to NSCLC histology: a review of two phase III studies. Oncologist 2009;14:253–63.

27. Scagliotti GV, Parikh P, von PJ, et al. Phase III study comparing cisplatin plus gemcitabine with cisplatin plus pemetrexed in chemotherapy-naive patients with advanced-stage non-small-cell lung cancer. J Clin Oncol 2008;26:3543–51.

28. Scagliotti G, Brodowicz T, Shepherd FA, et al. Treatment-by-histology interaction analyses in three phase III trials show superiority of pemetrexed in nonsquamous non-small cell lung cancer. J Thorac Oncol 2011;6:64–70.

29. Johnson DH, Fehrenbacher L, Novotny WF, et al. Randomized phase II trial comparing bevacizumab plus carboplatin and paclitaxel with carboplatin and paclitaxel alone in previously untreated locally advanced or metastatic non-small-cell lung cancer. J Clin Oncol 2004;22:2184–91.

30. Ishizumi T, McWilliams A, MacAulay C, et al. Natural history of bronchial preinvasive lesions. Cancer Metastasis Rev 2010;29:5–14.

31. Edell E, Lam S, Pass H, et al. Detection and localization of intraepithelial neoplasia and invasive carcinoma using fluorescence-reflectance bronchoscopy: an international, multicenter clinical trial. J Thorac Oncol 2009;4:49–54.

32. Aberle DR, Berg CD, Black WC, et al. The National Lung Screening Trial: overview and study design. Radiology 2011;258:243–53.

33. Aberle DR, Adams AM, Berg CD, et al. Baseline characteristics of participants in the Randomized National Lung Screening Trial. J Natl Cancer Inst 2010;102:1771–9.

34. Travis WD. Lung. In: Henson DE, Albores-Saavedra J, editors. Pathology of incipient neoplasia. 3rd edition. New York: Oxford University Press; 2001. p. 295–318.

35. World Health Organization. Histological typing of lung tumors. 2nd edition. Geneva (Switzerland): World Health Organization; 1981.

36. Travis WD, Colby TV, Corrin B, et al, In collaboration with L.H. Sobin and pathologists from 14 countries. Histological Typing of Lung and Pleural Tumors. 3rd edition. Berlin: Springer; 1999.

37. Travis WD, Brambilla E. Pathology of lung preneoplasia. In: Hirsch FR, Bunn PA, Kato H, et al, editors. Textbook of prevention and detection of early lung cancer; International Association for the Study of Lung Cancer. 1st edition. London and New York: Taylor & Francis; 2006. p. 75–89.

38. Lantuejoul S, Salameire D, Salon C, et al. Pulmonary preneoplasia–sequential molecular carcinogenetic events. Histopathology 2009;54:43–54.

39. Nicholson AG, Perry LJ, Cury PM, et al. Reproducibility of the WHO/IASLC grading system for pre-invasive squamous lesions of the bronchus: a study of inter-observer and intra-observer variation. Histopathology 2001;38:202–8.

40. Noguchi M. Stepwise progression of pulmonary adenocarcinoma–clinical and molecular implications. Cancer Metastasis Rev 2010;29:15–21.

41. Yoo SB, Chung JH, Lee HJ, et al. Epidermal growth factor receptor mutation and p53 overexpression during the multistage progression of small adenocarcinoma of the lung. J Thorac Oncol 2010;5: 964–9.

42. Ruffini E, Bongiovanni M, Cavallo A, et al. The significance of associated pre-invasive lesions in patients resected for primary lung neoplasms. Eur J Cardiothorac Surg 2004;26:165–72.

43. Kitamura H, Kameda Y, Ito T, et al. Atypical adenomatous hyperplasia of the lung. Implications for the pathogenesis of peripheral lung adenocarcinoma. Am J Clin Pathol 1999;111:610–22.

44. Miller RR. Bronchioloalveolar cell adenomas. Am J Surg Pathol 1990;14:904–12.

45. Weng SY, Tsuchiya E, Kasuga T, et al. Incidence of atypical bronchioloalveolar cell hyperplasia of the lung: relation to histological subtypes of lung cancer. Virchows Arch A Pathol Anat Histopathol 1992;420:463–71.

46. Carey FA, Wallace WA, Fergusson RJ, et al. Alveolar atypical hyperplasia in association with primary pulmonary adenocarcinoma: a clinicopathological study of 10 cases. Thorax 1992;47: 1041–3.

47. Nakanishi K. Alveolar epithelial hyperplasia and adenocarcinoma of the lung. Arch Pathol Lab Med 1990;114:363–8.

48. Mori M, Chiba R, Tezuka F, et al. Papillary adenoma of type II pneumocytes might have malignant potential. Virchows Arch 1996;428:195–200.

49. Mori M, Chiba R, Takahashi T. Atypical adenomatous hyperplasia of the lung and its differentiation from adenocarcinoma. Characterization of atypical cells by morphometry and multivariate cluster analysis. Cancer 1993;72:2331–40.

50. Ritter JH. Pulmonary atypical adenomatous hyperplasia. A histologic lesion in search of usable criteria and clinical significance. Am J Clin Pathol 1999;111:587–9.

51. Suzuki K, Nagai K, Yoshida J, et al. The prognosis of resected lung carcinoma associated with atypical adenomatous hyperplasia: a comparison of the prognosis of well-differentiated adenocarcinoma associated with atypical adenomatous hyperplasia and intrapulmonary metastasis. Cancer 1997;79:1521–6.

52. Watanabe S, Watanabe T, Arai K, et al. Results of wedge resection for focal bronchioloalveolar carcinoma showing pure ground-glass attenuation on computed tomography. Ann Thorac Surg 2002; 73:1071–5.

53. Sakurai H, Dobashi Y, Mizutani E, et al. Bronchioloalveolar carcinoma of the lung 3 centimeters or less in diameter: a prognostic assessment. Ann Thorac Surg 2004;78:1728–33.

54. Vazquez M, Carter D, Brambilla E, et al. Solitary and multiple resected adenocarcinomas after CT screening for lung cancer: histopathologic features and their prognostic implications. Lung Cancer 2009;64:148–54.

55. Yamato Y, Tsuchida M, Watanabe T, et al. Early results of a prospective study of limited resection for bronchioloalveolar adenocarcinoma of the lung. Ann Thorac Surg 2001;71:971–4.

56. Yoshida J, Nagai K, Yokose T, et al. Limited resection trial for pulmonary ground-glass opacity nodules: fifty-case experience. J Thorac Cardiovasc Surg 2005;129:991–6.

57. Koike T, Togashi K, Shirato T, et al. Limited resection for noninvasive bronchioloalveolar carcinoma diagnosed by intraoperative pathologic examination. Ann Thorac Surg 2009;88:1106–11.

58. Noguchi M, Morikawa A, Kawasaki M, et al. Small adenocarcinoma of the lung. Histologic characteristics and prognosis. Cancer 1995;75:2844–52.

59. Yim J, Zhu LC, Chiriboga L, et al. Histologic features are important prognostic indicators in early stages lung adenocarcinomas. Mod Pathol 2007;20:233–41.

60. Aguayo SM, Miller YE, Waldron JA Jr, et al. Brief report: idiopathic diffuse hyperplasia of pulmonary neuroendocrine cells and airways disease. N Engl J Med 1992;327:1285–8.

61. Davies SJ, Gosney JR, Hansell DM, et al. Diffuse idiopathic pulmonary neuroendocrine cell hyperplasia: an under-recognised spectrum of disease. Thorax 2007;62:248–52.

62. Koo CW, Baliff JP, Torigian DA, et al. Spectrum of pulmonary neuroendocrine cell proliferation: diffuse

idiopathic pulmonary neuroendocrine cell hyperplasia, tumorlet, and carcinoids. AJR Am J Roentgenol 2010;195:661–8.

63. Travis WD, Travis LB, Devesa SS. Lung cancer [Published erratum appears in Cancer 1995 Jun 15;75(12):2979]. Cancer 1995;75:191–202.

64. Tomashefski JF Jr, Connors AF Jr, Rosenthal ES, et al. Peripheral vs central squamous cell carcinoma of the lung. A comparison of clinical features, histopathology, and survival. Arch Pathol Lab Med 1990;114:468–74.

65. Colby TV, Koss MN, Travis WD. Tumors of the lower respiratory tract; Armed Forces Institute of Pathology fascicle, third series. Washington, DC: Armed Forces Institute of Pathology; 1995.

66. Funai K, Yokose T, Ishii G, et al. Clinicopathologic characteristics of peripheral squamous cell carcinoma of the lung. Am J Surg Pathol 2003;27:978–84.

67. Carlile A, Edwards C. Poorly differentiated squamous carcinoma of the bronchus: a light and electron microscopic study. J Clin Pathol 1986; 39:284–92.

68. Melamed MR, Zaman MB, Flehinger BJ, et al. Radiologically occult in situ and incipient invasive epidermoid lung cancer: detection by sputum cytology in a survey of asymptomatic cigarette smokers. Am J Surg Pathol 1977;1:5–16.

69. Churg A, Johnston WH, Stulbarg M. Small cell squamous and mixed small cell squamous–small cell anaplastic carcinomas of the lung. Am J Surg Pathol 1980;4:255–63.

70. Dulmet-Brender E, Jaubert F, Huchon G. Exophytic endobronchial epidermoid carcinoma. Cancer 1986;57:1358–64.

71. Sherwin RP, Laforet EG, Strieder JW. Exophytic endobronchial carcinoma. J Thorac Cardiovasc Surg 1962;43:716–30.

72. Maeshima AM, Maeshima A, Asamura H, et al. Histologic prognostic factors for small-sized squamous cell carcinomas of the peripheral lung. Lung Cancer 2006;52:53–8.

73. Watanabe Y, Yokose T, Sakuma Y, et al. Alveolar space filling ratio as a favorable prognostic factor in small peripheral squamous cell carcinoma of the lung. Lung Cancer 2011;73(2):217–21.

74. Yousem SA. Peripheral squamous cell carcinoma of lung: patterns of growth with particular focus on airspace filling. Hum Pathol 2009;40:861–7.

75. Altekruse SF, Kosary CL, Krapcho M, et al. SEER cancer statistics review, 1975-2007. National Cancer Institute; 2010. Available at: http://seer.cancer.gov/csr/1975_2007/. Accessed December 12, 2010.

76. Yoshizawa A, Motoi N, Riely GJ, et al. Impact of proposed IASLC/ATS/ERS classification of lung adenocarcinoma: prognostic subgroups and implications for further revision of staging based on

analysis of 514 stage I cases. Mod Pathol 2011; 24:653–64.

77. Borczuk AC, Qian F, Kazeros A, et al. Invasive size is an independent predictor of survival in pulmonary adenocarcinoma. Am J Surg Pathol 2009;33: 462–9.

78. Suzuki K, Yokose T, Yoshida J, et al. Prognostic significance of the size of central fibrosis in peripheral adenocarcinoma of the lung. Ann Thorac Surg 2000;69:893–7.

79. Miyoshi T, Satoh Y, Okumura S, et al. Early-stage lung adenocarcinomas with a micropapillary pattern, a distinct pathologic marker for a significantly poor prognosis. Am J Surg Pathol 2003;27: 101–9.

80. Tsutsumida H, Nomoto M, Goto M, et al. A micropapillary pattern is predictive of a poor prognosis in lung adenocarcinoma, and reduced surfactant apoprotein A expression in the micropapillary pattern is an excellent indicator of a poor prognosis. Mod Pathol 2007;20:638–47.

81. Cohen PR, Yoshizawa A, Motoi N, et al. Signet ring cell features (SRCF) in lung adenocarcinoma: a cytologic feature or a histologic subtype? Mod Pathol 2010;23:400A.

82. Deshpande CG, Yoshizawa A, Motoi N, et al. Clear cell change in lung adenocarcinoma: a cytologic change rather than a histologic variant. Mod Pathol 2009;22:352A.

83. Sakurai H, Maeshima A, Watanabe S, et al. Grade of stromal invasion in small adenocarcinoma of the lung: histopathological minimal invasion and prognosis. Am J Surg Pathol 2004;28:198–206.

84. Kadota K, Suzuki K, D'Angelo SP, et al. Validation of the proposed IASLC/American Thoracic Society (ATS)/European Respiratory Society (ERS) international multidisciplinary classification of lung adenocarcinoma (ADC). J Thorac Oncol 2011;6:244–85.

85. Yoshizawa A, Sumiyoshi S, Moreira AL, et al. Validation of the IASLC/ATS/ERS lung adenocarcinoma (ADC) classification and use of comprehensive histologic subtyping (CHS) for architectural grading in 432 Japanese patients. Mod Pathol 2011;24:429A.

86. Girard N, Deshpande C, Azzoli CG, et al. Use of epidermal growth factor receptor/Kirsten rat sarcoma 2 viral oncogene homolog mutation testing to define clonal relationships among multiple lung adenocarcinomas: comparison with clinical guidelines. Chest 2010;137:46–52.

87. Girard N, Deshpande C, Lau C, et al. Comprehensive histologic assessment helps to differentiate multiple lung primary nonsmall cell carcinomas from metastases. Am J Surg Pathol 2009;33:1752–64.

88. Girard N, Ostrovnaya I, Lau C, et al. Genomic and mutational profiling to assess clonal relationships between multiple non-small cell lung cancers. Clin Cancer Res 2009;15:5184–90.

89. Ou SH, Zell JA. Carcinoma NOS is a common histologic diagnosis and is increasing in proportion among non-small cell lung cancer histologies. J Thorac Oncol 2009;4:1202–11.

90. Solomon SB, Zakowski MF, Pao W, et al. Core needle lung biopsy specimens: adequacy for EGFR and KRAS mutational analysis. AJR Am J Roentgenol 2010;194:266–9.

91. Kreisman H, Wolkove N, Quoix E. Small cell lung cancer presenting as a solitary pulmonary nodule. Chest 1992;101:225–31.

92. Gephardt GN, Grady KJ, Ahmad M, et al. Peripheral small cell undifferentiated carcinoma of the lung. Clinicopathologic features of 17 cases. Cancer 1988;61:1002–8.

93. Hirsch FR, Matthews MJ, Aisner S, et al. Histopathologic classification of small cell lung cancer. Changing concepts and terminology. Cancer 1988;62:973–7.

94. Fraire AE, Johnson EH, Yesner R, et al. Prognostic significance of histopathologic subtype and stage in small cell lung cancer. Hum Pathol 1992;23:520–8.

95. Nicholson SA, Beasley MB, Brambilla E, et al. Small cell lung carcinoma (SCLC): a clinicopathologic study of 100 cases with surgical specimens. Am J Surg Pathol 2002;26:1184–97.

96. Travis WD. Advances in neuroendocrine lung tumors. Ann Oncol 2010;21(Suppl 7):vii65–71.

97. Azzopardi JG. Oat-cell carcinoma of the bronchus. J Pathol Bacteriol 1959;78:513–9.

98. Bégin P, Sahai S, Wang NS. Giant cell formation in small cell carcinoma of the lung. Cancer 1983;52:1875–9.

99. Sehested M, Hirsch FR, Osterlind K, et al. Morphologic variations of small cell lung cancer. A histopathologic study of pretreatment and post-treatment specimens in 104 patients. Cancer 1986;57:804–7.

100. Bepler G, Neumann K, Holle R, et al. Clinical relevance of histologic subtyping in small cell lung cancer. Cancer 1989;64:74–9.

101. Mangum MD, Greco FA, Hainsworth JD, et al. Combined small-cell and non-small-cell lung cancer. J Clin Oncol 1989;7:607–12.

102. Tsubota YT, Kawaguchi T, Hoso T, et al. A combined small cell and spindle cell carcinoma of the lung. Report of a unique case with immunohistochemical and ultrastructural studies. Am J Surg Pathol 1992;16:1108–15.

103. Fishback NF, Travis WD, Moran CA, et al. Pleomorphic (spindle/giant cell) carcinoma of the lung. A clinicopathologic correlation of 78 cases. Cancer 1994;73:2936–45.

104. Sümmermann E, Huwer H, Seitz G. Carcinosarcoma of the lung, a tumour which has a poor prognosis and is extremely rarely diagnosed preoperatively. Thorac Cardiovasc Surg 1990;38:247–50.

105. Folpe AL, Gown AM, Lamps LW, et al. Thyroid transcription factor-1: immunohistochemical evaluation in pulmonary neuroendocrine tumors. Mod Pathol 1999;12:5–8.

106. Sturm N, Rossi G, Lantuejoul S, et al. Expression of thyroid transcription factor-1 in the spectrum of neuroendocrine cell lung proliferations with special interest in carcinoids. Hum Pathol 2002;33:175–82.

107. Sturm N, Lantuejoul S, Laverriere MH, et al. Thyroid transcription factor 1 and cytokeratins 1, 5, 10, 14 (34betaE12) expression in basaloid and large-cell neuroendocrine carcinomas of the lung. Hum Pathol 2001;32:918–25.

108. Travis WD. Neuroendocrine lung tumors. Path Case Rev 2006;11:235–42.

109. Travis WD. Lung tumours with neuroendocrine differentiation. Eur J Cancer 2009;45(Suppl 1):251–66.

110. Agoff SN, Lamps LW, Philip AT, et al. Thyroid transcription factor-1 is expressed in extrapulmonary small cell carcinomas but not in other extrapulmonary neuroendocrine tumors. Mod Pathol 2000;13:238–42.

111. Pelosi G, Rodriguez J, Viale G, et al. Typical and atypical pulmonary carcinoid tumor overdiagnosed as small-cell carcinoma on biopsy specimens: a major pitfall in the management of lung cancer patients. Am J Surg Pathol 2005;29:179–87.

112. Krug LM, Pietanza MC, Kris MG, et al. Small cell and other neuroendocrine tumors of the lung. In: DeVita VT, Lawrence TS, Rosenberg SA, editors. DeVita, Hellman and Rosenberg's cancer, principles and practice of oncology. 9th edition. Philadelphia: Wolters Kluwer; Lippincott Williams & Wilkins; 2011. p. 848–70.

113. Vollmer RT. The effect of cell size on the pathologic diagnosis of small and large cell carcinomas of the lung. Cancer 1982;50:1380–3.

114. Vollmer RT, Ogden L, Crissman JD. Separation of small-cell from non-small-cell lung cancer. The Southeastern Cancer Study Group pathologists' experience. Arch Pathol Lab Med 1984;108:792–4.

115. Roggli VL, Vollmer RT, Greenberg SD, et al. Lung cancer heterogeneity: a blinded and randomized study of 100 consecutive cases. Hum Pathol 1985;16:569–79.

116. Travis WD, Gal AA, Colby TV, et al. Reproducibility of neuroendocrine lung tumor classification. Hum Pathol 1998;29:272–9.

117. Marchevsky AM, Chuang MT, Teirstein AS, et al. Problems in the diagnosis of small cell carcinoma of the lungs by fiberoptic bronchoscopy. Cancer Detect Prev 1984;7:253–60.

118. Travis WD, Garg K, Franklin WA, et al. Bronchioloalveolar carcinoma and lung adenocarcinoma: the

clinical importance and research relevance of the 2004 World Health Organization pathologic criteria. J Thorac Oncol 2006;1:S13–9.

119. Hiroshima K, Iyoda A, Shida T, et al. Distinction of pulmonary large cell neuroendocrine carcinoma from small cell lung carcinoma: a morphological, immunohistochemical, and molecular analysis. Mod Pathol 2006;19:1358–68.

120. Souhami RL, Beverley PC, Bobrow LG. Antigens of small-cell lung cancer. First International Workshop. Lancet 1987;2:325–6.

121. Tome Y, Hirohashi S, Noguchi M, et al. Preservation of cluster 1 small cell lung cancer antigen in zinc-formalin fixative and its application to immunohistological diagnosis. Histopathology 1990;16:469–74.

122. Maleki Z. Diagnostic issues with cytopathologic interpretation of lung neoplasms displaying high-grade basaloid or neuroendocrine morphology. Diagn Cytopathol 2011;39:159–67.

123. Sun Z, Aubry MC, Deschamps C, et al. Histologic grade is an independent prognostic factor for survival in non-small cell lung cancer: an analysis of 5018 hospital- and 712 population-based cases. J Thorac Cardiovasc Surg 2006;131:1014–20.

124. Sawabata N, Asamura H, Goya T, et al. Japanese Lung Cancer Registry Study: first prospective enrollment of a large number of surgical and nonsurgical cases in 2002. J Thorac Oncol 2010; 5:1369–75.

125. Rossi G, Marchioni A, Milani M, et al. TTF-1, cytokeratin 7, 34betaE12, and CD56/NCAM immunostaining in the subclassification of large cell carcinomas of the lung. Am J Clin Pathol 2004; 122:884–93.

126. Churg A. The fine structure of large cell undifferentiated carcinoma of the lung. Evidence for its relation to squamous cell carcinomas and adenocarcinomas. Hum Pathol 1978;9:143–56.

127. Horie A, Ohta M. Ultrastructural features of large cell carcinoma of the lung with reference to the prognosis of patients. Hum Pathol 1981;12:423–32.

128. Kodama T, Shimosato Y, Koide T, et al. Large cell carcinoma of the lung–ultrastructural and immunohistochemical studies. Jpn J Clin Oncol 1985;15: 431–41.

129. Carvalho L. Reclassifying bronchial-pulmonary carcinoma: differentiating histological type in biopsies by immunohistochemistry. Rev Port Pneumol 2009;15:1101–19.

130. Travis WD, Rush W, Flieder DB, et al. Survival analysis of 200 pulmonary neuroendocrine tumors with clarification of criteria for atypical carcinoid and its separation from typical carcinoid. Am J Surg Pathol 1998;22:934–44.

131. Travis WD, Linnoila RI, Tsokos MG, et al. Neuroendocrine tumors of the lung with proposed criteria for large-cell neuroendocrine carcinoma.

An ultrastructural, immunohistochemical, and flow cytometric study of 35 cases. Am J Surg Pathol 1991;15:529–53.

132. Moro-Sibilot D, Lantuejoul S, Diab S, et al. Lung carcinomas with a basaloid pattern: a study of 90 cases focusing on their poor prognosis. Eur Respir J 2008;31:854–9.

133. Chang YL, Wu CT, Shih JY, et al. Unique p53 and epidermal growth factor receptor gene mutation status in 46 pulmonary lymphoepithelioma-like carcinomas. Cancer Sci 2011;102:282–7.

134. Chang YL, Wu CT, Shih JY, et al. New aspects in clinicopathologic and oncogene studies of 23 pulmonary lymphoepithelioma-like carcinomas. Am J Surg Pathol 2002;26:715–23.

135. Katzenstein AL, Prioleau PG, Askin FB. The histologic spectrum and significance of clear-cell change in lung carcinoma. Cancer 1980;45:943–7.

136. Cavazza A, Colby TV, Tsokos M, et al. Lung tumors with a rhabdoid phenotype. Am J Clin Pathol 1996; 105:182–8.

137. Izquierdo-Garcia FM, Moreno-Mata N, Herranz-Aladro ML, et al. Lung carcinoma with rhabdoid component. A series of seven cases associated with uncommon types of non-small cell lung carcinomas and alveolar entrapment. Histol Histopathol 2010;25:1287–95.

138. Wiatrowska BA, Krol J, Zakowski MF. Large-cell neuroendocrine carcinoma of the lung: proposed criteria for cytologic diagnosis. Diagn Cytopathol 2001;24:58–64.

139. Iyoda A, Hiroshima K, Toyozaki T, et al. Clinical characterization of pulmonary large cell neuroendocrine carcinoma and large cell carcinoma with neuroendocrine morphology. Cancer 2001;91:1992–2000.

140. Jiang SX, Kameya T, Shoji M, et al. Large cell neuroendocrine carcinoma of the lung: a histologic and immunohistochemical study of 22 cases. Am J Surg Pathol 1998;22:526–37.

141. Beasley MB, Thunnissen FB, Brambilla E, et al. Pulmonary atypical carcinoid: predictors of survival in 106 cases. Hum Pathol 2000;31:1255–65.

142. Varlotto JM, Medford-Davis LN, Recht A, et al. Should large cell neuroendocrine lung carcinoma be classified and treated as a small cell lung cancer or with other large cell carcinomas? J Thorac Oncol 2011;6:1050–8.

143. Graziano SL, Mazid R, Newman N, et al. The use of neuroendocrine immunoperoxidase markers to predict chemotherapy response in patients with non-small-cell lung cancer. J Clin Oncol 1989;7: 1398–406.

144. Gazdar AF, Kadoyama C, Venzon D, et al. Association between histological type and neuroendocrine differentiation on drug sensitivity of lung cancer cell lines. J Natl Cancer Inst Monogr 1992;13:191–6.

145. Berendsen HH, de Leij L, Poppema S, et al. Clinical characterization of non-small-cell lung cancer tumors showing neuroendocrine differentiation features. J Clin Oncol 1989;7:1614–20.

146. Kibbelaar RE, Moolenaar KE, Michalides RJ, et al. Neural cell adhesion molecule expression, neuroendocrine differentiation and prognosis in lung carcinoma. Eur J Cancer 1991;27:431–5.

147. Schleusener JT, Tazelaar HD, Jung SH, et al. Neuroendocrine differentiation is an independent prognostic factor in chemotherapy-treated nonsmall cell lung carcinoma. Cancer 1996;77:1284–91.

148. Addis BJ. Neuroendocrine differentiation in lung carcinoma [editorial]. Thorax 1995;50:113–5.

149. Kiriakogiani-Psaropoulou P, Malamou-Mitsi V, Martinopoulou U, et al. The value of neuroendocrine markers in non-small cell lung cancer: a comparative immunohistopathologic study. Lung Cancer 1994;11:353–64.

150. Linnoila RI, Piantadosi S, Ruckdeschel JC. Impact of neuroendocrine differentiation in non-small cell lung cancer. The LCSG experience. Chest 1994; 106:367S–71S.

151. Carles J, Rosell R, Ariza A, et al. Neuroendocrine differentiation as a prognostic factor in non-small cell lung cancer. Lung Cancer 1993; 10:209–19.

152. Skov BG, Sorensen JB, Hirsch FR, et al. Prognostic impact of histologic demonstration of chromogranin A and neuron specific enolase in pulmonary adenocarcinoma. Ann Oncol 1991;2: 355–60.

153. Fitzgibbons PL, Kern WH. Adenosquamous carcinoma of the lung: a clinical and pathologic study of seven cases. Hum Pathol 1985;16:463–6.

154. Ishida T, Kaneko S, Yokoyama H, et al. Adenosquamous carcinoma of the lung. Clinicopathologic and immunohistochemical features. Am J Clin Pathol 1992;97:678–85.

155. Naunheim KS, Taylor JR, Skosey C, et al. Adenosquamous lung carcinoma: clinical characteristics, treatment, and prognosis. Ann Thorac Surg 1987; 44:462–6.

156. Sridhar KS, Raub WA Jr, Duncan RC, et al. The increasing recognition of adenosquamous lung carcinoma (1977-1986). Am J Clin Oncol 1992;15: 356–62.

157. Takamori S, Noguchi M, Morinaga S, et al. Clinicopathologic characteristics of adenosquamous carcinoma of the lung. Cancer 1991;67:649–54.

158. Travis WD. Sarcomatoid neoplasms of the lung and pleura. Arch Pathol Lab Med 2010;134:1645–58.

159. Asamura H, Kameya T, Matsuno Y, et al. Neuroendocrine neoplasms of the lung: a prognostic spectrum. J Clin Oncol 2006;24:70–6.

160. Lack EE, Harris GB, Eraklis AJ, et al. Primary bronchial tumors in childhood. A clinicopathologic study of six cases. Cancer 1983;51:492–7.

161. Naalsund A, Rostad H, Strom EH, et al. Carcinoid lung tumors–incidence, treatment and outcomes: a population-based study. Eur J Cardiothorac Surg 2011;39:565–9.

162. Rea F, Rizzardi G, Zuin A, et al. Outcome and surgical strategy in bronchial carcinoid tumors: single institution experience with 252 patients. Eur J Cardiothorac Surg 2007;31:186–91.

163. Iyoda A, Hiroshima K, Moriya Y, et al. Pulmonary large cell neuroendocrine carcinoma demonstrates high proliferative activity. Ann Thorac Surg 2004; 77:1891–5.

Preinvasive Lesions of the Bronchus

M. Patricia Rivera, MD

KEYWORDS

- Preinvasive lesions • Lung cancer
- Carcinoma of the bronchus
- Autofluorescence bronchoscopy

Although the incidence of lung cancer is less common than breast and prostate cancers, lung cancer is the leading cause of cancer death worldwide.[1] The 5-year survival for a patient newly diagnosed with non–small cell lung cancer (NSCLC) remains approximately 16%.[1] This dismal survival is mainly caused by diagnosis late in the stage of the disease. In contrast to the poor survival of patients with locally advanced or advanced NSCLC, the prognosis for patients with stage 0 (carcinoma in situ [CIS]) or resected stage IA disease (tumor <2 cm without lymph node or extrathoracic spread) is much better, with a reported 5-year survival of more than 70%.[2,3]

Several groups of patients are at an especially high risk for the development of lung cancer. Patients with a resected stage I lung cancer have a risk of developing a second primary lung cancer at a rate of approximately 4% per year.[4] Similarly, about 4% of patients with head and neck cancer develop a primary lung cancer within 5 years.[5] Family history of a first-degree relative with lung cancer has also been shown to increase the risk for lung cancer in smokers (odds ratio = 5.3).[6] More than 80% of lung cancers are associated with cigarette smoking; since the 1950s, tobacco smoking has been known as one of the strongest risk factors for lung cancer. Tobacco smoking is not only associated with an increased incidence of lung cancer but also with metaplasia and dysplasia of the bronchial epithelial cells, changes that are thought to be the first steps in lung carcinogenesis.[7]

A seminal concept for lung cancer risk has been the demonstration that cigarette smoke creates a field of injury, whereby long-term exposure to carcinogens causes diffuse injury to an organ.[8] A proposed progression model of carcinogenesis in the bronchial epithelium has been described for squamous cell carcinoma[9–13] whereby invasive carcinoma develops through transitions from metaplasia, dysplasia, and CIS to overt malignancy.

HISTOLOGIC CLASSIFICATION OF PREINVASIVE BRONCHIAL LESIONS

The pathology of preinvasive lesions for lung cancer has been a topic of increased interest because of the importance of screening and early detection of lung cancer using modern screening technologies, such as fluorescence bronchoscopy and computed tomography of the chest.[14] Since its revision in 2004, the World Health Organization (WHO) classification of lung tumors has included squamous dysplasia and CIS as forms of preinvasive lung lesions.[15] Metaplasia may be recognized as a thicker epithelium with basal zone regenerative activity lacking dysplasia. Squamous dysplasia may be mild, moderate, or severe, depending on the severity of cytologic atypia and the thickness of the abnormality within the bronchial epithelium.[15] In mild dysplasia, there is mildly increased thickness and mild pleomorphism, cellular disarray in the lower one-third of the bronchial epithelium, and mitotic figures are absent. Moderate dysplasia reveals moderately increased thickness and pleomorphism, cellular disarray is noted in the lower two-thirds of the epithelium, and mitotic figures are seen in the lower third of the epithelium. In severe dysplasia, there is markedly increased thickness and marked pleomorphism, cellular disarray extends to the upper third of the epithelium, and the mitotic figures are confined to the lower two-thirds. CIS

Division of Pulmonary and Critical Care Medicine, Department of Medicine, University of North Carolina at Chapel Hill, 4133 Bioinformatics Building, Mason Farm Road, CB # 7020, Chapel Hill, NC 27516, USA
E-mail address: mprivera@med.unc.edu

Clin Chest Med 32 (2011) 693–702
doi:10.1016/j.ccm.2011.08.008
0272-5231/11/$ – see front matter © 2011 Elsevier Inc. All rights reserved.

demonstrates extension of cellular disarray to the epithelial surface with mitotic figures present throughout the full thickness of the epithelium.[14]

A unique lesion, angiogenic squamous dysplasia (ASD), a lesion that consists of capillary blood vessels closely juxtaposed to and projecting into metaplastic or dysplastic squamous bronchial epithelium, has been described.[16] Keith and colleagues[16] reported that ASD was found in 34% of smokers without lung cancer. In 45% of the patients, the lesion was found to persist at 1 year after the initial diagnosis. The presence of this lesion in smokers suggests that aberrant patterns of microvascularization may occur at an early stage in bronchial carcinogenesis.[16]

DIAGNOSIS OF PREINVASIVE/EARLY STAGE LUNG CANCER

If moderate or severe dysplasia and CIS are premalignant lesions, then early detection may offer improvement in survival. Conventional white light bronchoscopy (WLB) is limited in its ability to detect preinvasive lesions. This limitation fueled research that led to the development of autofluorescence bronchoscopy (AFB) to improve the detection of dysplasia and CIS more than that achieved using WLB alone.[17,18] Dysplastic lesions, CIS, and invasive carcinoma have different autofluorescence properties.[19] The reasons for this difference are poorly understood but seem to be related to changes in extracellular matrix components. The light-induced fluorescence endoscopy (LIFE) system (Xillix Technologies Corp, Vancouver, BC, Canada) generates blue light from a helium-cadmium laser (at 442 nm) to illuminate the tissue. Low-intensity autofluorescence is then captured by a photomultiplier camera and split into 2 images (green and red wavelengths) that are simultaneously but separately sent to a computer imaging board. The 2 images are then processed into a pseudoimage that can be viewed on a monitor.[18] Because of the reduced green autofluorescence in abnormal areas, normal bronchial epithelium seems green, whereas abnormal areas in the bronchial epithelium seem reddish-brown on the monitor.[19] A ratio measurement has the advantage that it corrects for distance, angle, and intensity of excitation light.[19] One early study measured the red/green ratio by averaging the fluorescence from the total field and compared the resulting ratio with an average of red/green ratios from normal bronchial areas. In this study, which involved 238 lesions, dysplastic lesions had a ratio ranging between 1 and 3 times more than normal, whereas the ratio for CIS was 2 to 5 times that of normal.[17]

The initial study comparing WLB with WLB plus AFB in 94 subjects (53 patients with known or suspected malignancy and 41 volunteers) claimed an improvement from about 50% to 73% in sensitivity for the WLB plus AFB group with a specificity of 94% by both strategies.[18] In the same study, 15% of patients with known lung cancer were found to have CIS at other sites. In addition, 13% of former smokers were found to have CIS and 6% had severe dysplasia. The study demonstrated an improved detection of dysplasia and CIS using the WLB plus AFB combination in volunteers and patients with cancer. Other investigators have reported similar improvement of WLB plus AFB versus WLB alone for the detection of preinvasive lesions.[20–25] In these studies, the relative sensitivity of WLB plus AFB for the detection of preinvasive lesions ranged from 1.2 to 5.0.[20–25] In a subsequent multicenter trial of 173 subjects with a total of 700 lesions, AFB plus AFB with the LIFE device resulted in a 2.71 increase in the relative sensitivity for the detection of moderate dysplasia, severe dysplasia, CIS, and invasive carcinoma compared with WLB alone.[26] A study by Kurie and colleagues[27] on the effectiveness of the LIFE system failed to show any improvement of the LIFE unit in the detection of squamous metaplasia or dysplasia over WLB bronchoscopy alone. However, this study examined only 39 patients who were current or former smokers and did not include any former or current patient with cancer. In addition, the study was limited by the lack of statistical power because of small patient numbers. Based on overall results, the US Food and Drug Administration approved the LIFE system for use as an adjunct to WLB for the detection of preinvasive endobronchial lesions in high-risk patients.

In addition to the LIFE device, the Storz D-light (Karl Storz Endoscopy-America, Inc, CA, USA) system and the Pentax SAFE-1000 (Pentax Asahi Optical Co, Tokyo, Japan) system are also approved fluorescence devices to be used in addition to WLB for the detection of preinvasive lesions. The Storz D-light system uses dual fluorescence and blue reflectance; thus, suspicious lesions seem blue-brown against a green background. The SAFE-1000 system uses green fluorescence; suspicious lesions seem to be dark green lesions against a lighter green background.[3]

Classification of Bronchoscopic Findings

Bronchoscopic findings describing mucosal abnormalities are classified by both pathologic and visual criteria. The pathology of the mucosal lesions should be classified using an 8-point

Table 1
Histopathologic coding of endobronchial lesions

Histology Negative		Histology Positive	
Code Number	Description	Code Number	Description
1	Normal	5	Moderate/severe dysplasia
2	Inflammation	6	CIS
3	Hyperplasia/metaplasia	7	Microinvasive carcinoma
4	Mild Dysplasia	8	Invasive carcinoma

Adapted from Lam S, Kennedy T, Unger M, et al. Localization of bronchial intraepithelial neoplastic lesions by fluorescence bronchoscopy. Chest 1998;113:696–2.

coding system described by Lam and colleagues,[26] which is outlined in **Table 1**. During WLB inspection, it is recommended that a 3-point visual classification system be used to grade the abnormal-seeming endobronchial area.[26] Areas without any visual abnormality should be classified as class I. Areas of nonspecific erythema, swelling, trauma, or thickening should be defined as class II. Nodular/polypoid lesions or severe thickening of the bronchial mucosa should be classified as class III (**Table 2**). Under AFB inspection, findings should be categorized using 1 of 3 classes: class I, normal fluorescence (normal-seeming green areas); class II, abnormal fluorescence, benign (ill-defined areas of slight brown or brownish-red discoloration, endoscopic trauma, bronchitis, or pathology codes 2.0–3.0 lesions); and class III, abnormal fluorescence, suspicious (definite brownish-red appearance, pathology code 4.0 or greater lesions).[26] It is recommended that all class III lesions should be biopsied.[26] Progression from class I, II, and III correlates with advancement from normal mucosa to various degrees of dysplasia and finally invasive carcinoma.[19]

PREVALENCE OF PREINVASIVE BRONCHIAL LESIONS

In a study published by Auerbach and colleagues[10] 50 years ago, preinvasive lesions in the bronchial epithelium were reported to be a "frequent finding"[10] in male smokers and male patients with lung cancer. Given the limitations in the diagnostic techniques used and because all atypical lesions were defined as CIS, the prevalence of preinvasive lesions was not well defined. One important change since the publication of Auerbach's study has been the classification of preinvasive lesions to include varying degrees of dysplasia. In addition, improvement in diagnostic technologies, such as fluorescence bronchoscopy, has facilitated the study of preinvasive

lesions. Although the studies are limited and many are small in numbers of subjects studied, we now have a better understanding of how frequently these lesions are found in high-risk patients. In a study of 511 volunteer smokers who underwent fluorescence bronchoscopy, Lam and colleagues[28] reported a prevalence rate of 40% for mild dysplasia, 14% for moderate dysplasia, 6.5% for severe dysplasia, and 1.8% for CIS. A large European multicenter study of 1173 smokers (>20 pack-years, 916 men) comparing WLB with WLB plus AFB reported an overall prevalence of preinvasive lesions of 3.9%, a much lower prevalence rate than previously reported.[29] In this study, the highest prevalence of preinvasive lesions was noted in patients with abnormal sputum cytology and normal chest radiography (11.1%), patients with a history of resected lung cancer (6.7%), and in patients with a clinical suspicion for lung cancer (4.6%).[29] In a study by Paris and colleagues,[30] 241 patients at high risk for lung cancer (history of resected lung cancer, history of resected head and neck cancer, >30 pack-year smoking history, exposure to occupational respiratory carcinogens) underwent

Table 2
3-point visual identification system of normal and abnormal bronchoscopic findings

Class	Description
I Normal	No visual abnormality
II Abnormal	Inflammation, trauma, granulation tissue, hyperplasia, metaplasia, or mild dysplasia
III Suspicious	Moderate or severe dysplasia, CIS, or invasive carcinoma

Adapted from Lam S, Kennedy T, Unger M, et al. Localization of bronchial intraepithelial neoplastic lesions by fluorescence bronchoscopy. Chest 1998;113:696–2.

AFB. The overall prevalence of high-grade preinvasive lesions (severe dysplasia and CIS) was 9%. Multivariate analysis revealed significant and independent associations between high-grade lesions and (1) active smoking, relative to former smokers; (2) the presence of synchronous invasive lung cancer; (3) duration of asbestos exposure; and (4) exposure to other occupational carcinogens. The risk of having a high-grade preinvasive lesion ranged from 0.2% to 90.4% and was related to the number of risk factors for lung cancer within the individual patient.[30]

GENETIC ALTERATIONS IN PREMALIGNANT ENDOBRONCHIAL LESIONS

Human lung carcinoma has been shown to harbor several distinct genetic alterations; these include activating mutations in the K-ras oncogene, inactivating point mutations in the p53 tumor suppressor gene, aneuploidy, and loss of large regions of DNA or loss of heterozygosity (LOH), typically found on regions of chromosomes 3, 5, and 9.[31] Although the frequency and type of alterations of many of these genes are well established in overt carcinomas, it is less clear whether these genetic changes occur in precancerous lesions and when they develop in the process of lung carcinogenesis.[32]

As noted earlier, the concept of field cancerization is now well appreciated.[8] The first morphologic changes occurring in bronchial epithelium are metaplasia and dysplasia, and the number of these lesions increases in a dose-dependent manner with the number of cigarettes smoked.[7] However, only a small number of these lesions progress to invasive cancer and some may regress spontaneously or after smoking cessation.

The bronchial tree may contain a multitude of genetic alterations from carcinogen exposure in tobacco smokers. It has been reported that K-ras oncogene mutations are associated with smoking,[33] and there is evidence that molecular changes may persist in the lungs of former smokers for many years.[34] In the evolution of

squamous cell carcinoma, abnormal p53 staining occurs as early as in the squamous metaplasia/dysplasia stage.[32,35,36] The reported frequencies are 15% to 25% in metaplasia, 25% to 35% in dysplasia, and 60% to 70% in CIS.[37,38] To date, there is no information on how these high frequencies of abnormal p53 staining correlate with risk for progression.

Several studies have demonstrated chromosomal abnormalities/allelic loss (LOH) in preinvasive squamous lesions in the bronchus. One early report found LOH at chromosome 3 in all 9 dysplastic lesions investigated, whereas p53 abnormalities in immunohistochemical staining and LOH at the p53 locus on chromosome 17 were found in 7 of the 9 lesions.[39] These findings have been confirmed in subsequent studies, indicating that LOH at 3p is especially frequent in premalignant lesions and can sometimes be detected in histologically normal bronchial epithelium.[40–44] In one of these studies, a total of 253 biopsies were obtained from 54 subjects.[42] Five of 11 (45%) former smokers versus 22 of 25 (88%) current smokers had LOH at 3p14 ($P = .01$), but no difference was found for LOH at 9p or 17p. An increase in LOH at 17p was suggested in heavier smokers: 0 of 11 (0%) of light smokers and 6 of 23 (26%) of heavy smokers (greater than 30 pack-years) were positive ($P = .15$, Fisher's exact test, and $P = .06$ Chi²-test).[42] The ranges of frequencies of LOH in current smokers across the spectrum of histologies from normal tissue to carcinoma are listed in **Table 3**.

There are several reports investigating LOH in preinvasive lesions in the bronchus and in normal lung tissue using AFB.[41,42,45] In one study, LIFE was used to localize areas with suspected morphologic changes.[42] Six patients were followed with sequential biopsies over a time period of maximally 4 years, and these biopsies were analyzed for LOH on 3p (unknown gene), 5q (APC), and 9p (p16^MTS1). The full histologic spectrum of bronchogenic changes was available for study; normal, metaplastic, dysplastic, CIS,

Table 3
Summary of LOH findings in lung lesions from smokers

Histology	3p14 (%)	3p21 (%)	9p21 (%)	17p13 (%)
Normal	0–5	15–20	10–30	0
Metaplasia/dysplasia	5–50	15–20	10–30	5–15
CIS	75–90	40–60	70–80	40–50
Carcinoma	90–100	80–100	80–90	40–60

Data from Refs.[39–44]

microinvasive, and overt cancer cells were obtained by manual microdissection. Frequent changes at all chromosomal loci were found, with increasing incidence following the severity of the morphologic changes. The main finding in these studies was that LOH at 3p is already detectable in lung metaplasia and even in histologically normal lung tissue from current smokers, but LOH at 17p13 and 9p21 is less frequently seen in these tissues.[41,45] With the exception of one case, none of the tissues obtained from lifetime nonsmokers harbored any changes in the investigated chromosomal regions. However, the average age of the nonsmokers was significantly lower than the average age of the smokers in both studies so that a possible age effect cannot be excluded.

Abnormal DNA content, or aneuploidy, is another common feature of premalignant lung lesions, although it has been less well studied than LOH. Aneuploidy can be found at the earliest abnormal morphologic stages in bronchial epithelium and has even been reported in apparently normal tissue.[46] In this study, the prevalence of abnormal DNA ploidy in normal bronchial epithelium was 5% in nonsmokers and 43% in current tobacco smokers.

NATURAL HISTORY OF PREINVASIVE BRONCHIAL LESIONS

Although a progression model from metaplasia to dysplasia to CIS to squamous cell carcinoma of the lung has been described,[9–13] the exact proportion of patients with dysplasia or CIS who will progress to invasive carcinoma is unknown.

The mechanism of progression or regression as well as the risk and rate of progression of preinvasive lesions to carcinoma has only been reported in a small number of highly selected patients. Several studies have followed patients with preinvasive lesions longitudinally using AFB.[30,47–55] Most of the studies have enrolled small numbers of patients (<50) and have used different inclusion criteria, different treatment criteria, and different time periods of follow-up, including short duration (<3 years) of follow-up, making it difficult to draw definitive conclusions.[56] In addition, the WHO criteria for diagnosis and classification of preinvasive lesions have changed twice recently, making the analysis of older studies difficult.[56] The distinction between severe dysplasia and CIS is often challenging.[57] Some studies combine severe dysplasia and CIS, thus, making the long-term outcome of the separate lesions difficult to interpret. In addition, in some studies, CIS and invasive carcinoma were combined end-points, further

compromising the study of the natural history of CIS.[49,58] Because preinvasive lesions are often small,[59] they may be completely removed when an endobronchial biopsy is performed.[47] This suggests that the results of previous studies of the natural history of preinvasive lesions may have been compromised by the diagnostic biopsy itself.[56]

When the data from all the studies reporting on the natural history of preinvasive lesions are combined, there is a general consensus that such lesions may progress to invasive squamous cell carcinoma, that the progression rate is variable, and that the risk is much higher for high-grade lesions than low-grade lesions.[30,47–55] Progression from a preinvasive lesion to overt carcinoma is reported to vary from 7% to 75% depending on the grade of the initial lesion.[47–55,59] Low-grade lesions (hyperplasia, metaplasia, mild to moderate dysplasia) are reported to have a low risk of progression and are more likely to regress to normal or remain stable.[47,54,56,59–61]

Bota and colleagues[47] reported progression from hyperplasia and metaplasia to mild or moderate dysplasia in about 30% of patients, with progression to CIS reported in about 2%. Breuer and colleagues[49] reported a much higher rate of progression (9%) from metaplasia to CIS or invasive cancer. Progression from mild or moderate dysplasia to persistent severe dysplasia requiring treatment is reported to occur in about 3.5% of cases. In a study by Hoshino and colleagues,[54] only 1 of 88 lesions (1.1%) with mild or moderate dysplasia progressed to squamous cell carcinoma. George and colleagues[61] found that none of the lesions with mild or moderate dysplasia progressed to CIS or cancer during a follow-up period of 12 to 85 months.

Approximately 59% to 70% of lesions with severe dysplasia are noted to spontaneously regress on follow-up evaluation.[47,49,50,52–55,58] In one study, a small number of severe dysplastic lesions (2/19) that had regressed on follow-up evaluation had recurred (2/19). About 41% of severe dysplastic lesions progress to CIS or overt carcinoma. In contrast, 78% to 87% of CIS lesions remain high-grade lesions, reoccur despite endobronchial therapy, or progress to invasive cancer.[47,50–53] More than 50% of CIS lesions are reported to progress to overt cancer within 3 months of the diagnosis.[47]

Predictive Factors for Progression of Preinvasive Lesions

Several studies have documented an association between high-grade premalignant lesions (severe dysplasia and CIS) and previous cancers of the bronchus or head and neck and occupational exposure to asbestos or other carcinogens.[29,30] This group is made up of patients who may warrant closer follow-up with AFB when preinvasive lesions are identified. The number of suspicious lesions at the time of the baseline AFB has been reported to predict progression to cancer in high-risk patients.[62] In a study by Pasic and colleagues,[62] 46 high-risk patients (previous resected lung cancer, head and neck cancer, or abnormal sputum cytology) underwent baseline AFB and the baseline AFB score was correlated to outcome (development of cancer). In a follow-up period of 12 to 80 months, 24% of the patients had developed squamous cell carcinoma of the lung. Progression to carcinoma was noted in all 5 patients (100%) who had 3 or more suspicious lesions, 5 of 10 patients (50%) who had 2 suspicious lesions, and 1 of 12 (8%) patients with 1 suspicious lesion.

Molecular alterations in preinvasive lesions have been reported to predict progression to cancer. Salaün and colleagues[50] followed 23 severe dysplasia and 31 CIS lesions over a period of 12 years. In the whole group of lesions as well as in the CIS group, 3p LOH was strongly associated with progression ($P<.0001$ and $P = .02$, respectively). Molecular follow-up analysis of preinvasive lesions reveals that molecular alterations (LOH 3p, 5q, and 9p) can persist in dysplastic and CIS lesions for several months or years.[63] Regression of the molecular abnormality usually predicts regression of a dysplastic lesion or CIS to a lower-grade lesion. Conversely, the persistence of the genetic alteration or the appearance of additional genomic damage over time at the same bronchial site was associated with the progression to cancer.[45] Alterations in p53 and *FHIT* genes have also been reported to be associated with the progression to invasive cancer.[63,64]

TREATMENT OF PREINVASIVE ENDOBRONCHIAL LESIONS

Because severe dysplasia and CIS have been shown to have a higher risk for progression, it has been recommended that these lesions be treated with local therapy. Several endobronchial therapies may be effective in treating these high-grade preinvasive lesions (severe dysplasia and CIS) while preserving lung function, including photodynamic therapy (PDT), brachytherapy, electrocautery, cryotherapy, and Nd:YAG laser-therapy, although there is limited experience with most of these interventions.[65–69]

PDT combines the interaction of a photosensitizer with narrow bandwidth light, which results in tumor death in the presence of oxygen.[3] Complete response rates ranging from 46% to 95% have been reported. Favorable response rates (>85%) are noted in lesions that are less than 1 cm in size and in lesions whereby the margin can be clearly defined bronchoscopically.[66,70–73] In a study by Lam and colleagues,[74] 102 patients with occult squamous cell carcinoma (stage 0, IA, and IB) were treated with PDT. In this study, complete response rate was 78% (95% confidence interval, 7%–87%). About 44% of the patients had a recurrence of tumor on follow-up, with a long-term response rate of 43%. Recurrence of tumor after treatment occurred at a median of 2.8 years (range 0.1–10.0 years).[74] Imamura and colleagues[75] studied 29 patients with occult carcinoma of the bronchus who were treated with PDT. Overall complete response was 64%; recurrence rate was 36%, resulting in a long-term response rate of 41%.[75] Again, smaller lesion size (in this study, <3 cm) was associated with complete response.[75] In a study of 58 patients with early bronchogenic carcinoma, the complete response rate following PDT was 84%. Recurrence after the first treatment was 39%, with a median time to recurrence of 4.1 years.[76] PDT seems to be an effective treatment of occult squamous cell carcinoma, with a complete response rate of about 75% and a recurrence rate of about 30%. For lesions less than 1 cm in size, the complete response rate is greater than 90%. It is important to note, however, that there are limited data on the role of PDT in patients with occult or early stage lung cancer who are candidates for surgery.[3] In a study of patients with severe dysplasia and CIS monitored using repeated AFB over a period of 12 years, 14 of 54 lesions (25%) progressed to cancer after treatment. In 6 of these, the cancer developed at the site of the original CIS; in the remaining 8 cases, invasive cancer occurred at another site. The time between first bronchoscopy and invasive cancer diagnosis ranged from 3 months to 49 months.[50]

Electrocautery performed bronchoscopically uses high-frequency electrical current that generates heat to coagulate and vaporize tumor tissue.[68] One study evaluating the treatment of 13 patients with early lung cancer with electrocautery resulted in a complete response rate of 80% with no recurrence at follow-up (median duration of follow-up was 21 months with a range of 16–43 months).[68]

Cryotherapy, using nitrous oxide–driven cryoprobes, exerts its effects from selective cellular necrosis caused by tissue freezing and the elimination of vascularization.[65] In a study of 35 patients with histologically defined CIS treated with cryotherapy,[65] a complete histologic response was noted in 32 of 35 patients (91%) at 1 month and lasted a full year. At 2 years, 62% of the patients were noted to be disease free and 50% were still alive and disease free at 4 years. In 2 patients, recurrence was noted at 1 month; following a second treatment with cryotherapy, survival was 36 months and 50 months, respectively. One patient had progression with metastatic disease.[65]

Brachytherapy requires the placement of a radioactive source via a catheter inserted through the bronchoscope and placed within or near the endobronchial lesion. Local radiation is then delivered.[3] Marsiglia and colleagues[77] treated 34 patients with early stage lung cancer with brachytherapy and reported a complete response rate of 85% at 2 years after treatment. Perol and colleagues[67] reported complete and 1-year response rates of 83% and 75%, respectively, in a study of 19 patients with early stage lung cancer.

Nd:YAG laser uses direct thermal ablation of tissue in endobronchial malignancy.[69] It has been used extensively to provide palliative therapy to patients with obstructing airway lesions, but its role in the treatment of early stage bronchial lesions is well defined.[3] In one study of 22 patients with early stage lung cancer treated with Nd:YAG laser, a complete response rate of 100% was reported; however, no long-term follow-up data were provided.[69]

SUMMARY

Lung cancer remains one of the most lethal diseases known to human kind, not only because of its high incidence rate but, more importantly, because of its high mortality rate. By far, the strongest risk for lung cancer is tobacco smoking, which has been linked not only to the development of lung cancer but also to preinvasive lesions (metaplasia, dysplasia, and CIS) in the bronchial epithelium. It has been proposed that the development of lung cancer in the bronchial epithelium occurs through a stepwise fashion with progression from preinvasive lesions to overt carcinoma. Given that lung cancer mortality is linked to the stage of disease at the time of diagnosis, detection and treatment of high-grade preinvasive lesions may result in improved outcome for selected patients. AFB has been shown to increase the diagnostic yield of preinvasive lesions when compared with WLB alone. The prevalence and natural history of preinvasive lesions is not well known but we do know that certain patients are at higher risk for harboring such lesions. High-grade lesions are more likely to progress to overt carcinoma. Several therapeutic options are available for the treatment of preinvasive lesions, with favorable results reported in lesions less than 2 cm. Molecular alterations in preinvasive lesions have been reported; in particular, 3p LOH is associated with a higher risk of progression to invasive carcinoma.

Our understanding of preinvasive lesions in the bronchial epithelium is limited by several issues. These issues include small numbers of studies, small numbers and heterogeneity of the patients enrolled, inconsistent pathologic classification of the lesions, and difficulty differentiating severe dysplasia from CIS. In addition, preinvasive lesions may be biopsied off during bronchoscopy, further confounding our understanding of their natural history and, thus, recommendations regarding the appropriate treatment and follow-up of these lesions are not well standardized.

One area of significant interest is the role of molecular alterations in preinvasive lesions and how these alterations may help predict which lesions will indeed progress, thereby improving our understanding of how and when to treat and how long to follow patients found to have such lesions. Clearly, more studies incorporating molecular analysis are needed.

REFERENCES

1. Jemal A, Siegel R, Xu J, et al. Cancer statistics 2010. CA Cancer J Cin 2010;60:277–300.
2. Goldstraw P, Crowley J, Chansky K, et al. The IASLC Lung Cancer Staging Project: proposals for the revision of the TNM stage groupings in the forthcoming (seventh) edition of the TNM classification of malignant tumors. J Thorac Oncol 2007;2:706–14.
3. Kennedy TC, McWilliams A, Edell E, et al. Bronchial intraepithelial neoplasia/early central airways lung cancer. ACCP evidence-based clinical practice guidelines (2nd edition). Chest 2007;132:221S–33S.
4. Thomas P, Rubinstein L. Cancer recurrence after resection: T1 N0 non-small cell lung cancer. Lung Cancer Study Group. Ann Thorac Surg 1990;49: 242–6.
5. Deleyiannis FW, Thomas DB. Risk of lung cancer among patients with head and neck cancer. Otolaryngol Head Neck Surg 1997;116:630–6.
6. Samet JM, Humble CG, Pathak DR. Personal and family history of respiratory disease and lung cancer risk. Am Rev Respir Dis 1986;134:466–70.
7. Auerbach O, Hammond EC, Garfinkel L. Changes in bronchial epithelium in relation to cigarette smoking, 1955-1960 vs. 1970-1977. N Engl J Med 1979;300: 381–5.

8. Slaughter DP, Southwick HW, Smejkal W. Field cancerization in oral stratified squamous epithelium: clinical implications of multicentric origin. Cancer 1954;6:963–8.

9. Saccomanno G, Archer VE, Auerbach O, et al. Development of carcinoma of the lung as reflected in exfoliated cells. Cancer 1974;33:256–70.

10. Auerbach O, Stout AP, Hammond EC, et al. Changes in bronchial epithelium in relation to cigarette smoking and in relation to lung cancer. N Engl J Med 1961;265:253–67.

11. Auerbach O, Saccomanno G, Kuschner M, et al. Histologic findings in the tracheobronchial tree of uranium miners and non-miners with lung cancer. Cancer 1978;42:483–9.

12. Colby TV, Koss MN, Travis WD. Tumors of the lower respiratory tract. (atlas of tumor pathology 3rd series). Washington, DC: Armed Forces Institute of Pathology Fascicle; 1995.

13. Carter D. Pathology of early squamous cell carcinoma of the lung. Pathol Annu 1978;13(pt 1): 131–47.

14. Travis WD. Pathology of lung cancer. Clin Chest Med 2002;23:65–81.

15. Brambilla E, Travis WD, Colby TV, et al. The new World Health Organization classification of lung tumours. Eur Respir J 2001;18:1059–68.

16. Keith RL, Miller YE, Gemmill RM, et al. Angiogenic squamous dysplasia in bronchi of individuals at high risk for lung cancer. Clin Cancer Res 2000;6: 1616–25.

17. Lam S, Hung JY, Kennedy SM, et al. Detection of dysplasia and carcinoma in situ by ratio fluorometry. Am Rev Respir Dis 1992;146:1458–61.

18. Lam S, MacAulay C, Hung J, et al. Detection of dysplasia and carcinoma in situ with a lung imaging fluorescence endoscope device. J Thorac Cardiovasc Surg 1993;105:1035–40.

19. Hung J, Lam S, LeRiche JC, et al. Autofluorescence of normal and malignant bronchial tissue. Lasers Surg Med 1991;11:99–105.

20. Hirsch FR, Prindiville SA, Miller YE, et al. A randomized study of fluorescence bronchoscopy versus white light bronchoscopy for early detection of lung cancer in high risk patients. J Natl Cancer Inst 2000;93:1385–91.

21. Vermylen P, Pierard P, Verhest A, et al. Detection of preneoplastic lesions with fluorescence bronchoscopy [abstract]. Eur Respir J 1997;10:425S.

22. Venmans BT, Smit EF, Postmus P, et al. Results of two-years' experience with fluorescence bronchoscopy in detection of preinvasive bronchial neoplasia. Diagn Ther Endosc 1999;5:77–84.

23. Van Res MT, Schramel FM, Elberts JR, et al. The clinical value of lung imaging fluorescence endoscopy for detecting synchronous lung cancer. Lung Cancer 2001;32:13–8.

24. Yokomise H, Yanagihara K, Fukuse T, et al. Clinical experience with lung-imaging fluorescence endoscope (LIFE) in patients with lung cancer. J Bronchol 1997;4:205–8.

25. Ikeda N, Honda H, Katsumi T, et al. Early detection of bronchial lesions using lung imaging fluorescence endoscope. Diagn Ther Endosc 1999;5:85–90.

26. Lam S, Kennedy T, Unger M, et al. Localization of bronchial intraepithelial neoplastic lesions by fluorescence bronchoscopy. Chest 1998;113: 696–702.

27. Kurie JM, Lee JS, Morice RC, et al. Autofluorescence bronchoscopy in the detection of squamous metaplasia and dysplasia in current and former smokers. J Natl Cancer Inst 1998;90:991–5.

28. Lam S, LeRiche JC, Zheng Y. Sex-related differences in bronchial epithelial changes associated with tobacco smoking. J Natl Cancer Inst 1999;91: 691–6.

29. HäuBinger K, Becher H, Stanzel F, et al. Autofluorescence bronchoscopy with white light bronchoscopy compared with white light bronchoscopy alone for the detection of precancerous lesions: a European randomized controlled multicenter trial. Thorax 2005;60:496–503.

30. Paris C, Benichou J, Bota S, et al. Occupational and nonoccupational factors associated with high grade bronchial pre-invasive lesions. Eur Respir J 2003;21: 332–41.

31. Devereux TR, Taylor JA, Barrett JC. Molecular mechanisms of lung cancer. Interaction of environmental and genetic factors. Chest 1996;109:14S–9S.

32. Gazdar AF, Bader S, Hung J, et al. Molecular genetic changes found in human lung cancer and its precursor lesions. Cold Spring Harbor Symposium. Quant Biol 1994;59:565–72.

33. Slebos RJ, Hruban RH, Dalesio O, et al. Relationship between K-ras oncogene activation and smoking in adenocarcinoma of the human lung. J Natl Cancer Inst 1991;83:1024–7.

34. Westra WH, Slebos RJ, Offerhaus GJ, et al. K-ras oncogene activation in lung adenocarcinomas from former smokers. Evidence that K-ras mutations are an early and irreversible event in the development of adenocarcinoma of the lung. Cancer 1993;72: 432–8.

35. Sozzi G, Miozzo M, Donghi R, et al. Deletions of 17p and p53 mutations in preneoplastic lesions of the lung. Cancer Res 1992;52:6079–82.

36. Franklin WA, Gazdar AF, Haney J, et al. Widely dispersed p53 mutation in respiratory epithelium. A novel mechanism for field carcinogenesis. J Clin Invest 1997;100:2133–7.

37. Walker C, Robertson LJ, Myskow MW, et al. p53 expression in normal and dysplastic bronchial epithelium and in lung carcinomas. Br J Cancer 1994;70:297–303.

38. Bennett WP, Colby TV, Travis WD, et al. p53 protein accumulates frequently in early bronchial neoplasia. Cancer Res 1993;53:4817–22.

39. Sundaresan V, Ganly P, Hasleton P, et al. p53 and chromosome 3 abnormalities, characteristic of malignant lung tumours, are detectable in preinvasive lesions of the bronchus. Oncogene 1992;7:1989–97.

40. Hung J, Kishimoto Y, Sugio K, et al. Allele-specific chromosome 3p deletions occur at an early stage in the pathogenesis of lung carcinoma. JAMA 1995;273:558–63.

41. Wistuba II, Lam S, Behrens C, et al. Molecular damage in the bronchial epithelium of current and former smokers. J Natl Cancer Inst 1997;89:1366–73.

42. Mao L, Lee JS, Kurie JM, et al. Clonal genetic alterations in the lungs of current and former smokers. J Natl Cancer Inst 1997;89:857–62.

43. Miozzo M, Sozzi G, Musso K, et al. Microsatellite alterations in bronchial and sputum specimens of lung cancer patients. Cancer Res 1996;56:2285–8.

44. Fong KM, Biesterveld EJ, Virmani A, et al. FHIT and FRA 3B #p14.2 allele loss are common in lung cancer and preneoplastic bronchial lesions and are associated with cancer-related FHIT cDNA splicing alteration. Cancer Res 1997;57:2256–67.

45. Thiberville L, Payne P, Vielkinds J, et al. Evidence of cumulative gene losses with progression of premalignant epithelial lesions to carcinoma of the bronchus. Cancer Res 1995;55:5133–9.

46. Barsky SH, Roth MD, Kleerup EC, et al. Histopathologic and molecular alterations in bronchial epithelium in habitual smokers of marijuana, cocaine, and/or tobacco. J Natl Cancer Inst 1998;90:1198–205.

47. Bota S, Auliac J-B, Paris C, et al. Follow-up of bronchial precancerous lesions and carcinoma in situ using fluorescence endoscopy. Am J Respir Crit Care Med 2001;164:1688–93.

48. Loewen G, Natarajan N, Tan D, et al. Autofluorescence bronchoscopy for lung cancer surveillance based on risk assessment. Thorax 2007;62:335–40.

49. Breuer RH, Pasic A, Smith EF, et al. The natural course of preneoplastic lesions in bronchial epithelium. Clin Cancer Res 1982;42:4241–7.

50. Salaün M, Sesboüé R, Moreno-Swirc S, et al. Molecular predictive factors for progression of high grade preinvasive bronchial lesions. Am J Respir Crit Care Med 2008;177:880–6.

51. Venmans B, van Boxem A, Smit E, et al. Outcome of bronchial carcinoma in-situ. Chest 2000;117:1572–6.

52. Moro-Sibilot D, Fievet F, Jeanmart M, et al. Clinical prognostic indicators of high-grade pre-invasive bronchial lesions. Eur Respir J 2004;24:24–9.

53. Salaün M, Bota S, Thiberville L. Long-term follow-up of severe dysplasia and carcinoma in-situ of the bronchus. J Thorac Oncol 2009;4:1187–8.

54. Hoshino H, Shibuya K, Chiyo M, et al. Biologic features of bronchial squamous dysplasia followed by autofluorescence bronchoscopy. Lung Cancer 2004;46:187–96.

55. Pasic A, van Vliet E, Breur R, et al. Smoking behavior does not influence the natural course of pre-invasive lesions of the bronchial mucosa. Lung Cancer 2004;45:153–4.

56. Banerjee AK. Preinvasive lesions of the bronchus. J Thorac Oncol 2009;4:545–51.

57. Venmans B, van der Linden J, Elbers J. Observer variability in histopathological reporting of bronchial biopsy specimens: influence on the results of autofluorescence bronchoscopy in detection of bronchial neoplasia. J Bronchol 2004;46:187–96.

58. Jeanmart M, Lantuejoul S, Fievet F, et al. Value of immunohistochemical markers in preinvasive bronchial lesions in risk assessment of lung cancer. Clin Cancer Res 2003;9:2195–203.

59. Woolner LB, Fontana RS, Cortese DA, et al. Roentgenographically occult lung cancer: pathologic findings and frequency of multicentricity during a 10-year period. Mayo Clin Proc 1984;59:453–66.

60. Ishizumi T, McWilliams A, MacAulay C, et al. Natural history of bronchial preinvasive lesions. Cancer Metastasis Rev 2010;29:5–14.

61. George P, Banerjee A, Read C, et al. Surveillance for the detection of early lung cancer in patients with bronchial dysplasia. Thorax 2007;62:43–50.

62. Pasic A, Vonk-Noordegraaf A, Risse EK, et al. Multiple suspicious lesions detected by autofluorescence bronchoscopy predict malignant development in the bronchial mucosa in high risk patients. Lung Cancer 2003;41:295–301.

63. Sozzi G, Oggionni M, Alasio L, et al. Molecular changes track recurrence and progression of bronchial precancerous lesions. Lung Cancer 2002;37:267–70.

64. Ponticiello A, Barra E, Giana U, et al. p53 immunohistochemistry can identify bronchial dysplastic lesions proceeding to lung cancer: a prospective study. Eur Respir J 2000;15:547–52.

65. Deygas N, Froudarakis M, Ozenne G, et al. Cryotherapy in early superficial bronchogenic carcinoma. Chest 2001;120:26–31.

66. Lam S. Photodynamic therapy of lung cancer. Semin Oncol 1994;21(Suppl):15–9.

67. Perol M, Caliandro R, Pommier P, et al. Curative irradiation of limited endobronchial carcinomas with high-dose rate brachytherapy: results of a pilot study. Chest 1997;111:1417–23.

68. Van Boxem TJ, Venmans BJ, Schramel FM, et al. Radiographically occult lung cancer treated with fiberoptic bronchoscopic electrocautery: a pilot study of a simple and inexpensive technique. Eur Respir J 1998;11:169–72.

69. Cavaliere S, Foccoli P, Toninelli C, et al. Nd-YAG laser therapy in lung cancer: an 11 year experience with 2,253 applications in 1,585 patients. J Bronchol 1994;1:105–11.

70. McCaughan JS Jr, Williams TE. Photo dynamic therapy for endobronchial malignant disease: a prospective fourteen-year study. J Thorac Cardio-vasc Surg 1997;114:940–7.

71. Hayata Y, Kato H, Tanaka C, et al. Hematopor-phyrin derivative and laser photoradiation in the treatment of lung cancer. Chest 1982;81: 269–77.

72. Kato H, Okunaka T, Shimatani H. Photodynamic therapy for early stage bronchogenic carcinoma. J Clin Laser Med Surg 1996;14:235–8.

73. Kato H. Photodynamic therapy for lung cancer: a review of 19 years' experience. J Photochem Photobiol B 1998;42:96–9.

74. Lam S, Haussinger K, Leroy M, et al. Photodynamic therapy (PDT) with Photofrin, a treatment with curative potential for early stage superficial lung cancer [abstract]. In: 34th Annual Meeting of the American Society of Clinical Oncology. Los Angeles (CA), May 17–19, 1998.

75. Imamura S, Kusunoki Y, Takifuji N, et al. Photody-namic therapy and/or external beam radiation therapy for roentgenologically occult lung cancer. Cancer 1994;73:1608–14.

76. Edell ES, Cortese DA. Bronchoscopic phototherapy with hematoporphyrin derivative for treatment of localized bronchogenic carcinoma: a 5-year experi-ence. Mayo Clin Proc 1993;68:685–90.

77. Marsiglia H, Baldyrou P, Lartigau E, et al. High-dose rate brachytherapy as sole modality for early-stage endobronchial carcinoma. Int J Radiat Oncol Biol Phys 2000;47:665–72.

Molecular Biology of Lung Cancer: Clinical Implications

Jill E. Larsen, PhD, John D. Minna, MD*

KEYWORDS

- Lung cancer • Gene mutation • Lung carcinogenesis
- Genome-wide analysis

Lung cancer is the leading cause of cancer-related death in men and women in the United States, accounting for approximately 28% of total cancer deaths in 2010 despite comprising only approximately 15% of new cancer cases.[1] Decades of research have contributed to our understanding that lung cancer is a multistep process involving genetic and epigenetic alterations, through which resulting DNA damage transforms normal lung epithelial cells into lung cancer.[2,3] It is not known whether all lung epithelial cells or only a subset of these cells (such as pulmonary epithelial stem cells or their immediate progenitors) are susceptible to full malignant transformation. In addition, while the tumor-initiating cell may have only a handful of mutations, as the tumor expands cells may acquire additional mutations.[4] Smoking damages the entire respiratory epithelium and thus "field cancerization" or "field defects" (molecular changes) are observed in histologically normal lung epithelium, as well as a variety of histologic preneoplastic/premalignant lesions, which also harbor molecular abnormalities common to the adjacent tumor.[5] The culmination of these changes leads to lung cancers exhibiting all the "hallmarks of cancer," including self-sufficiency of growth signals, insensitivity to growth-inhibitory (antigrowth) signals, evasion of programmed cell death (apoptosis), limitless replicative potential, sustained

angiogenesis, and tissue invasion and metastasis.[6,7] Lung cancer is a heterogeneous disease clinically, biologically, histologically, and molecularly. Understanding the molecular causes of this heterogeneity, which might reflect changes occurring in different classes of epithelial cells or different molecular changes occurring in the same target lung epithelial cells, is the focus of current research. Identifying the genes and pathways involved, determining how they relate to the biological behavior of lung cancer, and their utility as diagnostic and therapeutic targets are important basic and translational research issues. Thus, current information on the key molecular steps in lung cancer pathogenesis and their timing in preneoplasia, primary cancer, and metastatic disease and the clinical implications is the subject of this review.

MOLECULAR EPIDEMIOLOGY AND ETIOLOGY

The two main types of lung cancer, non–small cell lung cancer (NSCLC) (representing 80%–85% of cases) and small cell lung cancer (SCLC) (representing 15%–20%) are identified based on histologic, clinical, and neuroendocrine characteristics. NSCLC and SCLC also differ molecularly, with many genetic alterations exhibiting subtype specificity. NSCLC can be further histologically subdivided into adenocarcinoma, squamous carcinoma,

This research was supported by: National Cancer Institute Lung Cancer Specialized Program of Research Excellence (SPORE) (P50CA70907), Department of Defense VITAL (W81XWH0410142) and PROSPECT (W81XWH0710306), NASA NSCOR (NNJ05HD36G) and by the Office of Science (BER) U.S. Department of Energy, Grant Number DEAI02-05ER64068. J.E.L. is supported by an NH&MRC Biomedical Fellowship (494511). Hamon Center for Therapeutic Oncology Research, Simmons Cancer Center, 6000 Harry Hines Boulevard, University of Texas Southwestern Medical Center, Dallas, TX 75390-8593, USA
* Corresponding author.
E-mail address: john.minna@utsouthwestern.edu

large-cell carcinoma (including large-cell neuroendocrine lung cancers), bronchoalveolar lung cancer, and mixed histologic types (eg, adenosquamous carcinoma). Common molecular differences between these major NSCLC subtypes and between NSCLC and SCLC are outlined in **Table 1**. These differences, as well as advances in both conventional and targeted therapy, signify the importance of stratifying NSCLC tumors by subtype for prognostic and predictive purposes and molecular studies.[8]

Worldwide approximately 85% of lung cancers are caused by carcinogens present in tobacco smoke, whereas 15% to 25% of lung cancer cases occur in lifetime "never smokers" (less than 100 cigarettes in a lifetime). These etiologic differences are associated with distinct differences in tumor-acquired molecular changes, and are discussed later in this review.[9,10] Although the general public associates lung cancer with smoking because of the number of lung cancer cases overall, lung cancer occurring in lifetime never smokers is also a huge public health problem. Likewise, more than 50% of newly diagnosed lung cancers in the United States occur in "former smokers" who have changed their lifestyle but for whom the damage caused by past smoking still leads to the development of lung cancer. Thus, it is important to identify the nonsmoking-related etiology of lung cancer arising in never smokers as well as methods to identify which former smokers are most likely to develop clinically evident lung cancer.

Genetic Susceptibility to Lung Cancer

There has been intense study of inherited predisposition to lung cancer, including study of polymorphisms associated with lung cancer risk (reviewed in Refs.[11,12]) and familial linkage studies. In 2008, 3 independent genome-wide association studies identified that single-nucleotide polymorphism (SNP) variations at 15q24-q25.1 were associated with an increased risk of both nicotine dependence and developing lung cancer.[13–15] This locus includes genes encoding nicotinic acetylcholine receptor (nAChR) subunits (CHRNA5, CHRNA3, and CHRNB4). More recently, 2 meta-analyses have provided further evidence that variation at 15q25.1, 5p15.33, and 6p21.33 influences lung cancer risk.[16,17] It has not yet been elucidated whether there is a mechanistic association with these nAChR polymorphisms and nicotine addiction, carcinogenic derivatives of nicotine exposure, or the effect of nicotine acting on nAChRs known to be expressed in lung epithelial cells.[18–26] In addition, a genome-wide linkage study of pedigrees containing multiple generations of lung cancer

from the Genetic Epidemiology of Lung Cancer Consortium mapped a familial susceptibility locus to 6q23-25.[27,28] A member of the regulator of G-protein signaling (RGS) family, RGS17, was identified as a potential causal gene within this locus where common variants were associated with familial, but not sporadic lung cancer[29]; however, it is likely that more than one genetic locus in the 6q region is influencing susceptibility.

Lung Cancer in Never Smokers

Never-smoking lung cancers represent a distinct epidemiologic, clinical, and molecular disease from smoking lung cancers. If considered independently, never-smoking lung cancers comprise the seventh most common cause of cancer death.[30] Never-smoking lung cancer occurs more frequently in women and East Asians, has a peak incidence at a younger age, targets the distal airways, is usually adenocarcinoma, and frequently has acquired epidermal growth factor receptor (EGFR) mutations, making it very responsive to EGFR-targeted therapies.[9,31–36] **Table 2** outlines the molecular differences between smoking and never-smoking lung cancers.

Human Papilloma Virus–Mediated Lung Cancer

Human papilloma virus (HPV), an established human carcinogen (for both uterine cervical and head and neck cancer), has been proposed to play a role in lung cancer pathogenesis; however, published data remain controversial. The presence of HPV oncoproteins E6 and E7 leads to inactivation of tumor suppressors p53 and Rb, respectively.[37,38] A meta-analysis of 53 publications comprising 4508 cases found a mean incidence of HPV-positive lung cancer of 25%, detected in all subtypes of lung cancer.[39] Geographically, European and American studies had a lower incidence of 15% to 17% whereas Asian lung cancer cases reported a mean incidence of 38%. In an effort to overcome sample and detection limitations of earlier studies, a recent case-control study of approximately 400 lung cancer patients of European descent, representing the largest study to date, found no evidence of an association between HPV and lung cancer.[40] While HPV will likely be primarily found in lung cancer arising in Asian populations, the detection of oncogenic variants of HPV in some tumors and the wealth of knowledge of the role of HPV oncoproteins suggest that a subset of lung cancer will have HPV infection as a major etiologic feature. It will be important to characterize other molecular alterations in these lung cancers and how they respond to various therapies, given the differences in response of head and neck cancer associated with HPV from EGFR-targeted therapy.

MOLECULAR CHANGES IN LUNG CARCINOGENESIS: THERAPEUTIC IMPLICATIONS FROM BOTH ONCOGENIC CHANGES AND THE CELLULAR ADAPTATIONS NECESSARY TO TOLERATE THESE CHANGES

Characterization of the molecular changes in lung cancer and associated preneoplastic cells is becoming increasingly well defined, aided immeasurably by the continued advancement of both clinical and genomic tools. Improved detection and sampling of clinical samples using, for example, fluorescent bronchoscopy, endobronchial ultrasonography, and laser capture microdissection techniques, enables precise analysis of abnormal epithelial cells. Introduction of high-resolution and high-throughput genomic tools (described in more detail later in this article) has facilitated the identification and characterization of key molecular changes—often involving oncogenes and tumor suppressor genes (TSGs)—and, importantly, the associated "tumor cell acquired vulnerabilities" that accompany these oncogenotype changes (**Fig. 1**). The key new concept that applies to many cancers, including lung cancer, is that with the genetic and epigenetic changes that occur during carcinogenesis the cancer becomes both dependent ("addicted") to the continued presence/function of these changes and also must make other cellular adaptations, including mutations to minimize the "oncogene stress" induced by these changes. While mutated oncogenic proteins themselves are therapeutic targets (see later discussion of mutant EGFR), the other cellular adaptations that are present in tumor but not normal cells also become cancer-specific therapeutic targets. The cancer needs both the oncogenic changes and the cellular adaptations to tolerate the oncogenic changes—that is, the oncogenic changes are "synthetically lethal" with the adaptation changes. Thus, both of these are potential therapeutic targets that can be discovered by genome-wide functional approaches such as siRNA library screening (see later discussion). Together, these advances promote our understanding of the development and progression of lung cancer, which is of fundamental importance for improving the prevention, early detection, and treatment of this disease. Ultimately these findings need to be translated to the clinic by using molecular alterations as biomarkers for early detection and risk assessment, targets for prevention, signatures for personalizing prognosis and therapy

selection for each patient, and therapeutic targets to selectively kill or inhibit the growth of lung cancer.

Technologic Revolution Has Allowed Genome-Wide Analyses of Molecular Changes Occurring in Lung Cancer

Chronic exposure to carcinogens in tobacco smoke propels genetic and epigenetic damage, which can result in lung epithelial cells steadily acquiring growth and/or survival advantages. Malignant transformation is characterized by genetic instability, which can exist at the chromosomal level (with large-scale loss or gain of genomic material, translocations, and microsatellite instability), at the nucleotide level (with single or several nucleotide base changes), or in the transcriptome (with altered gene expression). Abnormalities are typically targeted to proto-oncogenes, TSGs, DNA repair genes, and other genes that can promote outgrowth of affected cells. Activation of telomerase (the telomere-lengthening enzyme required for cell immortality) and disruption or escape from apoptotic pathways are other common events in cancer cells. Over the past 5 to 10 years there has been a revolution in technologies that can be applied to determining all of the genetic and epigenetic changes in lung cancer as well as other cancers. These techniques include genome-wide mRNA expression profiles, genome-wide DNA copy-number variation changes, genome-wide DNA methylation changes, MicroRNA (miRNA) changes, and mass spectroscopy proteomics analyses. The recent application of "next-generation" (NexGen) sequencing technologies has led to the first genome-wide mutational analyses of lung cancers in comparison with normal germline DNA.[41–43] These analyses have demonstrated a huge number of mutations occurring in lung cancers arising in smokers, many changes that do not alter the coding sequences, and many changes that are idiotypic to the particular tumor (see later discussion in the section "Genomics: Tools for Identification, Prediction, and Prognosis"). Within the next several years there will be similar data on perhaps 1000 lung cancers, which will provide an unprecedented amount of information. The key issues will be to determine which of these mutations are "actionable" (ie, provide a guide for targeting therapy), which are "passenger" and which are "driver" mutations, how frequent the mutations are, how the mutations are related to other molecular changes (eg, in the epigenome and miRNAs), and which mutations provide information to identify important subgroups ("molecular portraits") of lung cancer that provide prognostic (survival information independent of therapy) and/or predictive (survival

Table 1
Common genetic alterations found in lung cancer

Gene	SCLC (%)	NSCLC (%)			References
		All	Adenocarcinoma	Squamous Cell	
Oncogenic Alterations					
Mutation					
BRAF	Rare	1–3	1–5	Rare	400,401
EGFR	Rare	~20	10–40	Rare	96,400,402–404
ErbB2 (HER2)	Rare	2	4	Rare	400,405
KRAS	Rare	10–30	15–35	<5	400,406–408
MET	13	21	14	12	12
PIK3CA	Rare	1–5	<5	<5	57,385,409,410
Amplification					
EGFR	Rare	20–30	15	30	12
ErbB2 (HER2)	5–30	2–23	6	2	12,405,411,412
MDM2	—	6–24	14	22	390,413
MET	—	7–21	20	21	414,415
MYC	18–30	8–22	—	—	130,416–418
NKX2-1 (TITF1)	Rare	12–30	10–15	3–15	12,74,93
PIK3CA	~5	9–17	6	33–36	12,385
Increase in protein expression					
CRK	—	8–30	8–30	—	419
BCL2	75–95	10–35	—	—	408,420,421
CCND1	0	43	35–55	30–35	396,422
CD44	Rare	Common	3	48	423
c-KIT	46–91	Rare	—	—	424–430
EGFR	Rare	50–90	40–65	60–85	100–103,408
ErbB2 (HER2)	<10	20–35	16–38	6–16	405,408,427, 431–433
MYC	10–45	<10	—	—	133,434–436
PDGFRA	65	2–100	100	89	437–440
Tumor-Suppressing Alterations					
Mutation					
CDKN2A (p16)	<1	10–40	—	—	408
LKB1	Rare	30–40	30–60	5–30	186,187,189, 441,442
p53	75–90	50–60	50–70	60–70	408,443–445
PTEN	15–20	<10	—	—	408
Rb	80–100	20–40	—	—	408,446–448
Deletion/LOH					
CDKN2A (p16)	37	75–80	—	—	72,395,449
FHIT	100	55–75	—	—	72,449,450
p53	86–93	74–86	—	—	72,449
Rb	93	62	—	—	72,449
Loss of protein expression					
CAV1	95	24	—	—	451
CDKN2A (p14ARF)	65	40–50	—	—	391,392, 395,452

(continued on next page)

Table 1
(*continued*)

Gene	SCLC (%)	NSCLC (%)			References
		All	Adenocarcinoma	Squamous Cell	
CDKN2A (p16)	3–37	30–79	~55	60–75	72,449
FHIT	80–95	40–70	—	—	72,408,449
PTEN	—	25–74	77	70	389,452
Rb	90	15–60	23–57	6–14	72
TUSC2 (FUS1)	100	82	79	87	453
Tumor-Acquired DNA Methylation					
APC	15–26	24–96	—	—	172,173,454
CAV1	93	9	—	—	451
CDH1	60 40	20–35	—	—	173,454–456
CDH13	15–20	45	—	—	172,173
CDKN2A (p14ARF)	nd	6–8	—	—	173
CDKN2A (p16)	5, 0	15–41	21–36	24–33	296,457,458
DAPK1	nd	16–45	—	—	173,298,454
FHIT	64	37	—	—	172,173
GSTP1	16	7–15	—	—	173,459
MGMT	16	10–30	—	—	173,454
PTEN	—	26	24	30	389
RARβ	45–70	40–43	—	—	172,173,460
RASSF1A	72–85	15–45	31	43	169,173,175, 297,454,461
SEMA3B	nd	41–50	46	47	169,170
TIMP3	nd	19–26	—	—	173
Telomeres					
Telomerase activity	75–100	50–80	65–85	80–90	261–263, 408,462
Chromosomal Aberrations					
EML4-ALK fusion	—	2–13	—	—	136
Large-scale loss	1p, 3p, 4p, 4q, 5q, 8p, 10q, 13q, 17p	3p, 5q, 8p, 9p, 13q, 17p, 18q, 19p, 19q, 21q, 22q	2q, 3p, 4q, 8p, 9p, 9q, 10p, 10q, 13q, 15q, 18, 20	3p, 4q, 9p, 10p, 10q, 18, 20	63,64,90,449, 463–466
Focal deletions	—	2q22.1, 3p14.2, 3q25.1, 5q11.2, 7q11.22, 7q34, 9p23, 9p21.3, 10q23.31, 11q11, 13q12.11, 13q14.2, 13q32.2, 18q23, 21p11.2			74,84,86
Large-scale gain	3q, 5p, 8q, 18q	1q, 3q, 5p, 6p, 7p, 7q, 8q, 20p, 20q	5p, 7p, 7q, 8q, 11q, 19, 20q	2q, 3q, 5p, 7, 8q, 11q, 13q, 19, 20q	63,64,90,449, 463–466
Focal amplifications	—	1p36.32, 1p34.3, 1q32.2, 1q21.2, 2p24.3, 2q11.2, 2q31.1, 3q26.31, 5p15.33, 5p15.31, 5p14.3, 5q31.3, 6p21.1, 7p11.2, 8p12, 8q21.13, 8q24.21, 10q24.1, 10q26.3, 11q13.3, 12p12.1, 12q13.2, 12q14.1, 12q15, 14q13.3, 14q32.13, 16q22.2, 17q12, 18q12.1, 19q12, 19q13.33, 20q13.32, 22q11.21			74,84,86

Abbreviations: LOH, loss of heterozygosity; nd, not determined.

Table 2
Molecular differences between smoking and never-smoking lung cancers

Gene	Never Smoking	Smoking
TP53 mutations—overall	Less common	More common
TP53 mutations—G:C to T:A mutations	Less common	More common
KRAS mutations	Less common (0%–7%)	More common (30%–43%)
EGFR mutations	More common (45%)	Less common (7%)
STK11 mutations	Less common	More common
EML4-ALK fusions	More common	Less common
HER2 mutations	More common	Less common
Methylation index	Low	High
p16 methylation	Less common	More common
APC methylation	Less common	More common
Loss of hMSH2 expression	Common (40%)	Rare (10%)

Data from Refs.[9,35,36]

information dependent on the administration of specific therapies) utility. Of course this will require large-scale multidisciplinary and international collaboration to unite clinically annotated with molecularly annotated lung cancer specimens. Examples of this are the United States National Cancer Institute (NCI) "The Cancer Genome Anatomy" Program (TCGA), the NCI Lung Cancer Mutation Consortium (LCMC), as well as international lung cancer sequencing consortiums. A key component of this is to be able to perform mutation testing of clinically available materials (such as formalin-fixed paraffin embedded [FFPE] specimens) in a timely fashion using clinical laboratory practices (Clinical Laboratory Improvement Amendments certified laboratory methods). Recently, the NCI's LCMC performed such a study on more than 800 lung adenocarcinoma tumor specimens, examining mutations in established lung cancer driver genes (*EGFR, KRAS, BRAF, HER2, AKT1, NRAS, PIK3CA, MEK1, EML4-ALK, MET* amplification). Mutations in at least one of these genes were found in approximately 60% of tumor specimens, and greater than 90% were "exclusive": only one mutation was found in a particular tumor.[44] **Table 1** describes the current state of our knowledge of the common genetic alterations found in lung cancer. A key element will be to make this information accessible and understandable to patients and physicians who are not expert in cancer genomics. An example of how patients and their physicians can interface with these data is the "My Cancer Genome" Web site established by the Vanderbilt Cancer Center (http://www.vicc.org/mycancergenome/).

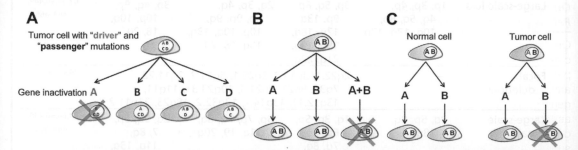

Fig. 1. Oncogene addiction and synthetic lethality in targeting acquired tumor cell vulnerability. (*A*) Oncogene addiction. A tumor cell contains many abnormalities in oncogenes and tumor suppressor genes (TSGs); however, while some gene mutations may be critical for tumor cell survival ("driver" mutations), other gene mutations are not ("passenger" mutations). Inactivation of a critical "driver" gene in a tumor cell will result in cell death or differentiation into a normal phenotype. Inactivation of noncritical "passenger" mutations, however, will not affect the tumor cell. (*B*) Synthetic lethality arises when inactivation of two of more genes (A + B) leads to cell death, whereas inactivation of either gene alone does not affect viability of the cell as the remaining gene acts in a compensatory manner. (*C*) Synthetic lethality to target tumor cells. If a tumor cell has a nondrugable oncogene or inactivation of a TSG (Gene A), the cell will be vulnerable to inactivation of Gene B whereas a normal cell will not, thus creating a second therapeutic target in addition to targeting the "driver" mutation. (*Data from* Refs.[94,375,376])

Genetic Instability: Chromosomal Aberration and Loss of Heterozygosity

Like many solid tumors, genomic instability is a hallmark of lung cancer.[3] Mapping high-level amplifications and deletions in copy number throughout the cancer genome has led to the identification of many oncogenes and TSGs.[45–62] Many genetic alterations have been associated with lung cancer, with the more frequently observed changes including aneuploidy, specific allelic loss at 3p, 4q, 9p, and 17p, and gain at 1q, 3q, 5p, and 17q.[63–65] In addition, genetic alterations in several genes have been implicated in lung cancer development, including activation of MYC, RAS, EGFR, NKX2-1, ERBB2, SOX2, BCL2, FGFR2, and CRKL as well as inactivation of RB1, CDKN2A, STK11, and FHIT.[3,63,65–80]

Identification of the genetic alterations that occur in tumors has long been an important approach to understanding tumorigenesis. Early techniques to analyze the cancer genome involved cytogenetic karyotyping, loss of heterozygosity (LOH), and microsatellite analyses, followed later by comparative genomic hybridization (CGH) using metaphase spreads or fluorescence in situ hybridization (FISH). These techniques identified multiple numeric and structural chromosomal alterations in the cancer genome; however, the shift of CGH into a microarray-based format improved on previous techniques by providing high-resolution detection of copy-number gain and loss.[56,79,81–92] Thus, due to low resolution of earlier cytogenetic and CGH techniques that made it difficult to identify focal aberrations and the causal genes critical for tumorigenesis, aberrant loci/genes in lung carcinogenesis continue to be defined.[75–80]

Oncogenes and Growth Stimulatory Pathways, and Targeted Therapeutics

Oncogene activation occurs in probably all lung cancers (typically by gene amplification, overexpression, point mutation, or DNA rearrangements), and can result in persistent upregulation of mitogenic growth signals that induce cell growth as well as "oncogene addiction" whereby the cell becomes dependent on this aberrant oncogenic signaling for survival (see **Table 1**).[48,50–52,56,58,60,62,74,93,94] In lung cancer, commonly activated oncogenes include EGFR, ERBB2, MYC, KRAS, MET, CCND1, CDK4, MET, EML4-ALK fusion, and BCL2. These "driver" oncogenes or oncogene "addictions" represent acquired conditional (on the oncogene) vulnerabilities in lung cancer cells, and present as significant therapeutic targets by offering specificity of killing tumor cells but not normal cells. Oncogenic signaling pathways commonly found in lung cancer and potential targeted therapies are summarized in **Figs. 2–5** and **Table 3**, (see also the article elsewhere in this issue by Gettinger at al.).

Epidermal growth factor receptor signaling in lung cancer

The ErbB family of tyrosine kinase receptors includes 4 members, namely EGFR, ErbB-2 (HER2), ErbB-3, and ErbB-4, with ability to form homodimers and heterodimers and to bind different ligands leading to receptor activation (see **Fig. 2**).[95] EGFR exhibits overexpression or aberrant activation in 50% to 90% of NSCLCs; therefore, much effort has been focused on the development of targeted inhibitors for this molecule.[96] Initial research used monoclonal antibodies that target the extracellular domain, but this was supplanted by the development of small molecules that inhibit intracellular EGFR tyrosine kinase activity: EGFR tyrosine kinase inhibitors (TKIs). In 2004, a significant advancement was made in the treatment of NSCLC following the observation that somatic mutations in the kinase domain of EGFR strongly correlated with sensitivity to EGFR TKIs.[50,51] Exquisite sensitivity and marked tumor response has since been shown with EGFR TKIs (such as erlotinib and gefitinib) and antibodies (such as cetuximab) in EGFR mutant tumors[50–52,97,98]—an example of oncogene addiction in lung cancer whereby tumors initiated through EGFR mutation-activation of EGF signaling rely on continued EGF signaling for survival. Mutant EGFRs (either by exon 19 deletion or exon 21 L858R mutation) show an increased amount and duration of EGFR activation compared with wild-type receptors,[50] and have preferential activation of the phosphoinositide 3-kinase (PI3K)/AKT and STAT3/STAT5 pathways rather than the RAS/RAF/MEK/MAPK pathway.[98] EGFR mutations are particularly prevalent in certain patient subgroups: adenocarcinoma histology, women, never smokers, and East Asian ethnicity.[52,99–103] Resistance to TKI therapy has been associated with EGFR exon-20 insertions or a secondary T790M mutation, KRAS mutation, or amplification of the MET proto-oncogene[104–109] where MET activates the PI3K pathway through phosphorylation of ERBB3, independent of EGFR and ERBB2.[109] Of importance, these investigators found that inhibition of MET signaling can restore sensitivity to TKIs.[109] In lung adenocarcinomas, activated mutant EGFR has been shown to induce levels of interleukin (IL)-6, leading to activation of STAT3.[110] IL-6 also plays an important role by activation of JAK family tyrosine kinases,[111] which in turn activate multiple pathways through signaling molecules such as STAT3, MAPK, and PI3K.[112]

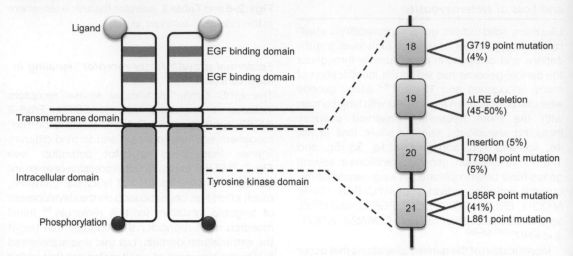

Fig. 2. EGFR mutations found in lung cancer. Activating mutations, which are found with increased frequency in certain subsets of lung cancer patients, occur as 3 different types of somatic mutations—deletions, insertions, and missense point mutations—and are located in exons 19 to 21, which code for the tyrosine kinase domain of EGFR.[50,51] Mutant EGFRs (either by exon 19 deletion or exon 21 L858R mutation) show an increased amount and duration of EGFR activation compared with wild-type receptors,[50] and have preferential activation of the PI3K/AKT and STAT3/STAT5 pathways rather than the RAS/RAF/MEK/MAPK pathway.[98] EGFR mutant tumors are initially highly sensitive to EGFR tyrosine kinase inhibitors (TKIs)[50–52]; however, despite an initial response, patients treated with EGFR TKIs eventually develop resistance to TKIs, which is linked (in approximately 50% of tumors) to the acquiring of a second mutation at T790M in exon 20.[107,108,377–380] Of interest, the presence of the T790M mutation in a primary lung cancer that had not been treated with EGFR TKIs, however, suggests that this resistance mutation may develop with tumor progression and not necessarily as a response to treatment.[381] (*Data from* Gazdar AF. Activating and resistance mutations of EGFR in non-small-cell lung cancer: role in clinical response to EGFR tyrosine kinase inhibitors. Oncogene 2009;28(Suppl 1):S24–31; and Mitsudomi T, Kosaka T, Yatabe Y. Biological and clinical implications of EGFR mutations in lung cancer. Int J Clin Oncol 2006;11(3):190–8.)

The RAS/RAF/MEK/MAPK pathway signaling in lung cancer

Activation of the RAS/RAF/MEK/MAPK pathway occurs frequently in lung cancer (see **Fig. 3**), most commonly via activating mutations in KRAS, which occur in approximately 20% of lung cancers, particularly adenocarcinomas.[113,114] In lung cancer, 90% of mutations are located in *KRAS* (80% in codon 12 and the remainder in codons 13 and 61), with *HRAS* and *NRAS* mutations only occasionally documented.[115] Mutation results in constitutive activation of downstream signaling pathways such as PI3K and MAPK, rendering KRAS mutant tumors independent of EGFR signaling, and therefore resistant to EGFR TKIs as well as chemotherapy.[97,106,116] KRAS mutations are mutually exclusive with EGFR and ERBB2 mutations, and are primarily observed in lung adenocarcinomas of smokers.[97,117] The prevalence and importance of KRAS in lung tumorigenesis make it an attractive therapeutic target. Two unsuccessful approaches were farnesyltransferase inhibitors, to inhibit posttranslational processing

and membrane localization of RAS proteins, and antisense oligonucleotides against RAS.[113] More recently, efforts have been centered on downstream effectors of RAS signaling: RAF kinase and mitogen-activated protein kinase (MAPK) kinase (MEK).[113,118] BRAF is the direct effector of RAS, and although commonly mutated in melanoma (~70%), mutations are rare in lung cancer (~3%), predominantly in adenocarcinoma, and mutually exclusive to EGFR and KRAS mutations.[119–122] Strategies to inhibit RAF kinase include degradation of *RAF1* mRNA through antisense oligodeoxyribonucleotides, and inhibition of kinase activity with multikinase inhibitors such as sorafenib. Several MEK inhibitors have commenced phase 2 testing in lung cancer patients, and are listed in **Table 3**. Attempts to directly inhibit or perturb mutant KRAS continue with the advent of whole-genome approaches. Synthetic lethal siRNA screens have identified small interfering RNAs (siRNAs) that specifically kill human lung cancer cells with KRAS mutations in vitro.[123–125] In addition, combination of anti-KRAS strategies (such as

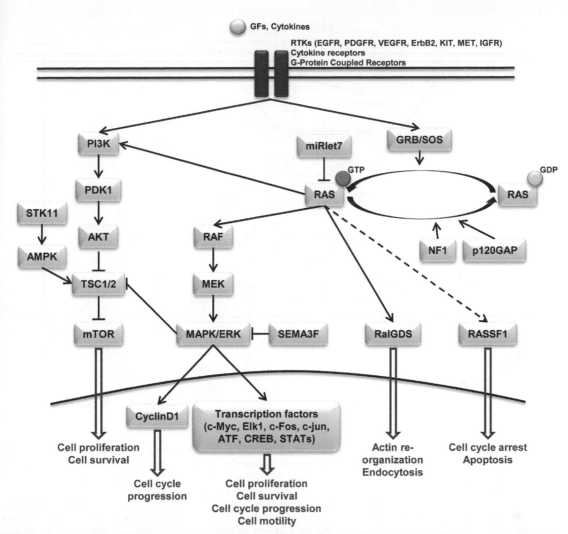

Fig. 3. The RAS/RAF/MEK/MAPK pathway. The RAS proto-oncogene family (*KRAS*, *HRAS*, *NRAS*, and *RRAS*) encode 4 highly homologous 21-kDa membrane-bound proteins involved in signal transduction. Proteins encoded by the RAS genes exist in two states: an active state, in which guanosine triphosphate (GTP) is bound to the molecule, and an inactive state, whereby the GTP has been cleaved to guanosine diphosphate (GDP).[382] Activating point mutations can confer oncogenic potential through a loss of intrinsic GTPase activity, resulting in an inability to cleave GTP to GDP. This process can initiate unchecked cell proliferation through the RAS/RAF/MEK/MAPK pathway, downstream of the EGFR signaling pathway.[383] Ras signaling also activates the PI3K/AKT pathway (leading to cell growth, proliferation, and survival), RalGDS, and RASSF1. (*Data from* Herbst RS, Heymach JV, Lippman SM. Lung cancer. N Engl J Med 2008;359(13):1367–80; and Harris TJ, McCormick F. The molecular pathology of cancer. Nat Rev Clin Oncol 2010;7(5):251–65.)

depletion with short-hairpin RNAs [shRNAs]) with other targeted drugs has shown potential therapeutic utility.[126–128]

MYC

One of the major downstream effectors of the RAS/RAF/MEK/MAPK pathway is the MYC proto-oncogene (see **Fig. 3**). In normal conditions this transcription factor functions to keep tight control of cellular proliferation; however, aberrant expression through amplification or overexpression is commonly found in lung cancer.[129,130] MYC proto-oncogene members (MYC, MYCN, and MYCL) are targets of RAS signaling and key regulators of numerous downstream pathways such as cell proliferation,[131] whereby enforced Myc expression drives the cell cycle in an autonomous fashion. It can also sensitize cells to apoptosis through activation of the mitochondrial apoptosis pathway; thus, Myc-driven tumorigenesis often requires coexpression of antiapoptotic BCL2 proteins.[132] Activation of MYC members often

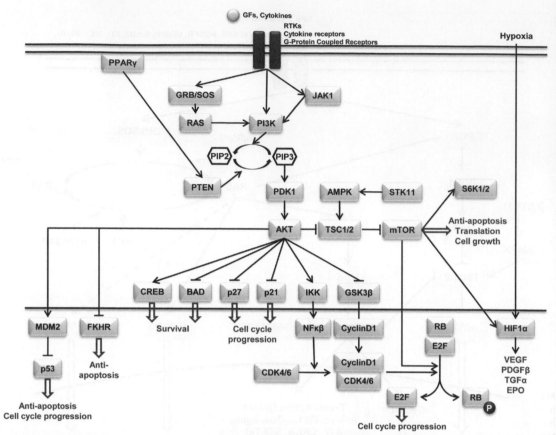

Fig. 4. The PI3K/AKT/mTOR pathway. Downstream targets of AKT are involved in cell growth, angiogenesis, cell metabolism, protein synthesis, and suppression of apoptosis directly or via the activation of mTOR. Activation of the PI3K/AKT pathway can occur through the binding of the SH2-domains of p85, the regulatory subunit of phosphatidylinositol 3-kinase (PI3K), to phosphotyrosine residues of activated receptor tyrosine kinases such as EGFR.[143] Alternatively, activation can occur via binding of PI3K to activated RAS. Mutation and, more commonly, amplification of *PIK3CA*, which encodes the catalytic subunit of PI3K, occur most commonly in squamous cell carcinomas.[56,90,384,385] AKT, a serine/threonine kinase that acts downstream from PI3K, can also have mutations that lead to pathway activation. One of the primary effectors of AKT is mTOR, a serine/threonine kinase involved in regulating proliferation, cell-cycle progression, mRNA translation, cytoskeletal organization, and survival.[386] The tumor suppressor PTEN, which negatively regulates the PI3K/AKT pathway via phosphatase activity on phosphatidylinositol 3,4,5-trisphosphate (PIP3), a product of PI3K,[387] is commonly suppressed in lung cancer by inactivating mutations or loss of expression.[388,389]

occurs through gene amplification. MYC is most frequently activated in NSCLC,[133] whereas the other 2 members, MYCN and MYCL along with MYC, are usually activated in SCLC.[64,134]

EML4-ALK Fusion Proteins

In 2007, a novel fusion gene with transforming ability was reported in a small subset of NSCLC patients.[135] Formed by the inversion of two closely located genes on chromosome 2p, fusion of PTK echinoderm microtubule-associated protein like-4 (EML4) with anaplastic lymphoma kinase (ALK), a transmembrane tyrosine kinase, yields the EML4-ALK fusion protein. The fusion results in constitutive oligomerization, leading to persistent

mitogenic signaling and malignant transformation. A recent meta-analysis of 13 studies encompassing 2835 tumors reported that the EML4-ALK fusion protein is present in 4% of NSCLCs.[136] *EML4-ALK* fusions are found exclusive of *EGFR* and *KRAS* mutations, and occur predominantly in adenocarcinomas and never or light smokers. Tumors with EML4-ALK fusions exhibit dramatic clinical responses to ALK-targeted therapy,[137–141] and the ALK inhibitor crizotinib (PF-02341066) has now entered a phase 3 clinical trial.

The PI3K/AKT/mTOR pathway

PI3Ks are lipid kinases that regulate cellular processes such as proliferation, survival, adhesion,

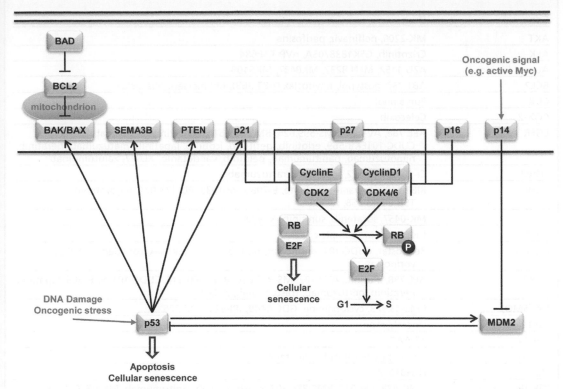

Fig. 5. The p53 and RB pathways. Regulation of p53 can occur through the MDM2 oncogene, which reduces p53 levels through degradation by ubiquitination. MDM2 can in turn be inhibited by the tumor suppressor p14^ARF, an isoform of *CDKN2A*. As such, the genes that encode MDM2 and p14^ARF are commonly altered in lung cancer through amplification and loss of expression, respectively.[390–392] The CDKN2A/RB1 pathway controls G1 to S phase cell-cycle progression. RB acts as a tumor suppressor by acting with E2F proteins to repress transcription of genes necessary for the G1-S phase transition. RB is inhibited by hyperphosphorylation by CDK-CCND1 complexes (complexes between CDK4 or CDK6 and CCND1), and in turn, formation of CDK-CCND1 complexes can be inhibited by the p16 isoform of CDNK2A.[393] Nearly all constituents of the CDKN2A/RB pathway have been shown to be altered in lung cancer through mutations (*CDK4* and *CDKN2A*), deletions (*RB1* and *CDKN2A*), amplifications (*CDK4* and *CCDN1*), methylation silencing (*CDKN2A* and *RB1*), and phosphorylation (RB).[394–399]

and motility.[142] The PI3K/AKT/mTOR pathway is a downstream signaling pathway of several receptor tyrosine kinases, such as EGFR, and can also be activated via binding of PI3K to activated RAS.[143] In lung tumorigenesis, activation of the PI3K/AKT/mTOR pathway occurs early in pathogenesis, generally through mutations in PI3K or PTEN as well as EGFR or KRAS, amplification of *PIK3CA*, PTEN loss, or activation of AKT,[144] and results in cell survival through inhibition of apoptosis (see **Fig. 4**). The pathway has two negative regulators: the tumor suppressor gene, *PTEN*, and the TSC1/TSC2 complex, which act upstream and downstream of AKT, respectively. The serine/threonine kinase mTOR, a downstream effector of AKT, is an important intracellular signaling enzyme in the regulation of cell growth, motility, and survival in tumor cells.[145] Targeted therapies to the PI3K/AKT/mTOR pathway (such as LY294002 and rapamycin) have shown significant efficacy in both

NSCLC and SCLC cells with activated AKT signaling.[146–148]

SOX2 and NKX2-1 (TITF1): lung cancer lineage–dependent oncogenes

Genome-wide screens for DNA copy-number changes in primary NSCLCs has led to the identification of recurrent, histologic subtype-specific focal amplification at 14q13.3 (adenocarcinoma) and 3q26.33 (squamous cell carcinoma).[74,75,80,93,149] Functional analysis identified *NKX2-1* (also termed *TITF1*) and *SOX2* as the respective targets of these amplifications. *NKX2-1* encodes a lineage-specific transcription factor essential for branching morphogenesis in lung development and the formation of type II pneumocytes—the cells lining lung alveoli.[150,151] Initial studies reported on the oncogenic role of *NKX2-1* in lung adenocarcinoma[74,93,149,152]; however, recent in vivo data suggest it also has a tumor-suppressive role.[153] *SOX2* amplification

Table 3
Targeted therapies against oncogenic pathways in lung cancer

Gene	Drug
AKT	MK-2206, nelfinavir, perifosine
ALK	Crizotinib, GSK1838705A, nVP-TAE684
Aurora kinase	AZD 1152, MLN 8237, MK0457, MK5108
BCL2	ABT-737, gossypol, navitoclax (ABT-263), oblimersen, obatoclax
CDK	Purvalanol
COX-2	Celecoxib
EGFR	AEE 788, AV-412, BMS-599,626, BMS-690,514, canertinib, cetuximab, CUDC-101EKB-569, erlotinib, gefitinib, icotinib, lapatinib, matuzumab, neratinib, nimotuzumab, panitumumab, pelitinib, vandetanib, XL647, zalutumumab
ErbB2	CI-1033, HKI-272, lapatinib, trastuzumab
FGFR	BIBF 1120, brivanib alaninate, E-7080, FP-1039, PD-173,074, regorafenib, TSU-68TKI-258, XL999
FLT-3	MK-0457, sorafenib, sunitinib, XL999
FUS1	fus1 liposome complex
HDACs	Belinostat, CUDC-101, entinostat, panobinostat, pivanex, romidepsin, SB939, vorinostat
HER2	AEE 788, afatinib, AV-412, BMS-599,626, BMS-690,514, CUDC-101, EKB-569, lapatinib, neratinib, pertuzumab, trastuzumab, XL647,
Hh (SMO)	BMS-33,923, cyclopamine, GDC-0449, IPI-926, LDE 225
HIF1	Oncothyreon
HSP70	17-AAG
HSP90	Alvespimycin, retaspimycin, tanespimycin
IAPs	HGS01029
IGF-1R	AMG 479, BIIB022, BMS-754,807, cixutumumab, figitumumab, MK-0646, OSI906
c-KIT	AMG-706, axitinib, cediranib, dasatinib, imatinib, motesanib, pazopanib, regorafenib, sorafenib, sunitinib, vatalanib
MDM2	JNJ-26,854,165, RO5045337
MEK	AS 703,026, AZD6244 (selumetinib), AZD8330, GDC-0973, GSK1120212, PD325901, RDEA119, sorafenib
c-MET	AMG 102, AMG 208, ARQ197, crizotinib, foretinib, GSK1363089, PF-04,217,903, PHA-665,752, SCH900105, SGX523, SU11274, XL184
mTOR	AZD 8055, BEZ235, everolimus, OSI 027, PX-866, ridaforolimus, sirolimus/rapamycin, temsirolimus
Notch (γ-secretase)	MK0752, MRK-003, PF03084014, RO 4,929,097
p53	p53 peptide vaccine, PRIMA-1
PARP	AG014699, iniparib, olaparib, veliparib
PDGFR	AMG-706, axitinib, BIBF 1120, cediranib, dasatinib, E7080, imatinib, IMC-3G3, linifanib, motesanib, pazopanib, ramucirumab, regorafenib, sorafenib, sunitinib, TKI-258, TSU-68, vatalanib, XL999
PI3K	BEZ235, BGT226, GDC-0941, LY294002, PX-866, XL147, XL765
PPARγ	BSI-201, CS 7017, olaparib
Proteasome	Bortezomib, carfilzomib, CEP-18,770, MLN9708, salinosporamide A
RAF	AZ628, GSK2118436, ISIS 5132, regorafenib, sorafenib, XL281
RAS	Lonafarnib, ISIS 2503 (H-Ras), tipifarnib
SRC/BCR-ABL	AZD0530, dasatinib, imatinib, KX2-391, XL999
telomerase	Imetelstat, sodium meta-arsenite
TGF-β	Trabedersen
TRAIL	Apomab, conatumumab, dulanermin, lexatumumab, mapatumumab, rhApo2L
VEGF	Aflibercept, bevacizumab
VEGFR	Adnectin, AEE 788, axitinib, BIBF 1120, BMS-690,514, brivanib alaninate, cediranib, E7080, foretinib, linifanib, motesanib, neovasat, pazopanib, ramucirumab, regorafenib, sorafenib, sunitinib, tivozanib, TKI-258, TSU-68, vandetanib, vatalanib, XL184, XL647, XL999

was identified specifically in squamous cell carcinomas and is required for normal esophageal squamous development.[75,80] Amplification of tissue-specific transcription factors in cancer has been previously observed in prostate cancer (AR),[154] melanoma (MITF),[155] and breast cancer (ESR1).[156] These findings have led to the development of a "lineage-dependency" concept in tumors[157] whereby the survival and progression of a tumor is dependent on continued signaling through a specific lineage pathway (ie, abnormal expression of pathways involved in normal cell development) rather than continued signaling through the pathway of oncogenic transformation as seen with oncogene addiction.[94]

Tumor-Suppressor Genes and Growth-Inhibitory Pathways

Loss of TSG function is an important step in lung carcinogenesis, and usually results from inactivation of both alleles with LOH inactivating one allele through chromosomal deletion or translocation, and point mutation, epigenetic, or transcriptional silencing inactivating the second allele.[158,159] Commonly inactivated TSGs in lung cancer include TP53, RB1, STK11, CDKN2A, FHIT, RASSF1A, and PTEN.

The p53 pathway
TP53 (17p13) encodes a phosphoprotein that prevents accumulation of genetic damage in daughter cells. In response to cellular stress, p53 induces the expression of downstream genes such as cyclin-dependent kinase (CDK) inhibitors, which regulate cell-cycle checkpoint signals, causing the cell to undergo G1 arrest and allowing DNA repair or apoptosis (see **Fig. 5**).[159] p53 inactivating mutations are the most common alterations in lung cancer, whereby 17p13 frequently demonstrates hemizygous deletion and mutational inactivation in the remaining allele.[160–162] Some point mutations in TP53 confer a gain-of-function phenotype leading to increased aggressiveness of lung cancer.[163] Due to the prevalence of p53 inactivating mutations in human cancers, large-scale efforts have been focused on therapeutic strategies to restore normal p53 function. Such efforts include reintroduction of wild-type p53 using gene therapy, pharmacologic rescue of mutant p53 with small-molecule agents and peptides, blocking of MDM2 expression, inhibiting MDM2 ubiquitin ligase activity, and targeting the p53-MDM2 interaction with small-molecule inhibitors. In vivo restoration of p53 expression in a subpopulation of tumor cells has been achieved with p53 gene therapy for lung cancer patients.[164]

The CDKN2A/RB pathway
The CDKN2A-RB1 pathway controls G1 to S phase cell-cycle progression (see **Fig. 5**). Hypophosphorylated retinoblastoma (RB) protein, encoded by RB1, halts the G1/S phase transition by binding to the transcription factor E2F1, and was the first tumor-suppresser gene identified in lung cancer.[165,166] Absent or mutant RB protein is found in approximately 90% of SCLCs compared with only 10% to 15% of NSCLCs, whereas abnormalities in p16 (encoded by CDKN2A) and an upstream regulator of RB phosphorylation are predominantly found in NSCLCs.[167]

Chromosome 3p TSGs
Loss of one copy of chromosome 3p is one of the most frequent and early events in human cancer, found in 96% of lung tumors and 78% of lung preneoplastic lesions.[168] Mapping of this loss identified several genes with functional tumor-suppressing capacity, including FHIT (3p14.2), RASSF1A, TUSC2 (also called FUS1), semaphorin family members SEMA3B and SEMA3F (all at 3p21.3), and RARβ (3p24). In addition to LOH or allele loss, some of these 3p genes (FHIT, RASSF1A, SEMA3B, and RARβ) often exhibit decreased expression in lung cancer cells by means of epigenetic mechanisms such as promoter hypermethylation.[169–173] Furthermore, FHIT, RASSF1A, TUSC2, and SEMA3B will reduce growth when reintroduced into lung cancer cells. FHIT, located in the most common fragile site in the human genome (FRA3B), has been shown to induce apoptosis in lung cancer.[174] RASSF1A can induce apoptosis, as well as stabilize microtubules and affect cell-cycle regulation.[175] The tumor-suppressing effect of TUSC2 is thought to occur via inhibition of protein tyrosine kinases such as EGFR, PDGFR, c-Abl, c-Kit, and AKT[176] as well as inhibition of MDM2-mediated degradation of p53.[177] The candidate TSG SEMA3B encodes a secreted protein that can decrease cell proliferation and induce apoptosis when reexpressed in lung, breast, and ovarian cancer cells[169,170,178,179] in part, by inhibiting the AKT pathway.[180] Another family member, SEMA3F, may inhibit vascularization and tumorigenesis by acting on VEGF and ERK1/2 activation,[181,182] and RARβ exerts its tumor-suppressing function by binding retinoic acid, thereby limiting cell growth and differentiation.

STK11 (LKB1)
The serine/threonine kinase STK11 (also called LKB1) functions as a TSG by regulating cell polarity, motility, differentiation, metastasis, and metabolism.[183] Germline-inactivating mutations of STK11 cause Peutz-Jeghers syndrome,[184] but somatic

inactivation through point mutation and frequent deletion on 19p13 occurs in approximately 30% of lung cancers, ranking it the third most commonly mutated gene in lung adenocarcinoma after p53 and RAS.[119,185,186] STK11 mutations often correlate with KRAS activation and result in the promotion of cell growth.[187] Its tumor-suppressing effect is thought to function, in part, through inhibition of the mTOR pathway via adenosine monophosphate–activated protein kinase (AMPK) (see **Fig. 3**).[188] STK11 inactivation appears to be particularly prevalent in NSCLC while rare in SCLCs, and inactivating mutations are more common in tumors from males and smokers, and in poorly differentiated adenocarcinomas.[78,185–187,189] Mutation in both *KRAS* and *STK11* appears to confer increased sensitivity to MEK inhibition in NSCLC cell lines in comparison with either mutation alone.[190]

Lung Cancer Stem Cells: Detection, Signaling Pathways, and Therapeutic Targeting

The cancer stem cell (CSC) model hypothesizes there is a population of rare, stemlike tumor cells capable of self-renewing and undergoing asymmetric division, thereby giving rise to differentiated progeny that comprise the bulk of the tumor.[191–193] Although the first evidence for CSCs (also termed tumor-initiating cells) was reported in acute myeloid leukemia,[194] support for their existence in solid tumors, including lung cancer, is becoming increasingly common.[137,139,195–199] Several cell-surface biomarkers have been reported for the detection and isolation of putative lung CSCs (**Table 4**). Of interest, it is becoming apparent that in addition to significant variability of the utility of CSC biomarkers between different solid tumor types, no single biomarker can reliably detect CSCs in tumors from the same tissue, possibly reflecting tumor heterogeneity. Regulation of CSCs in lung cancer is likely by the Hedgehog (Hh), Wnt, and Notch stem cell signaling pathways (**Fig. 6**).[200] Important in normal lung development, specifically progenitor cell development and pulmonary organogenesis, these pathways are now also being studied as regards their role in tumor development. Increased signaling of the Hh pathway results in activation of the transcription-regulating GLI oncogenes (GLI1, GLI2, and GLI3),[201–203] and persistent activation is found in both SCLC and NSCLC.[204,205] The Wnt pathway has critical roles in organogenesis, cancer initiation and progression, and maintenance of stem cell pluripotency. In NSCLC, studies have found dysregulation of Wnt pathway members such as Wnt1, Wnt2 and Wnt7a, as well as upregulation of Wnt pathway agonists (Dvl proteins, LEF1, and Ruvb11) and underexpression or silencing of antagonists (WIF-1, sFRP1, CTNNBIP1, and WISP2).[206–212] Notch signaling is important the determination of in cell fate, but can also promote and maintain survival in many human cancers.[213–216] These signaling pathways are thought to be involved in the regulation of stem/progenitor cell self-renewal and maintenance, and while normally a tightly regulated process, genes that comprise these pathways are often mutated in human cancers,[217–219] leading to abnormal activation of downstream effectors.

Clinical implications

CSCs are thought to have higher resistance than the bulk tumor cells to cytotoxic therapies and radiotherapy. Thus, while conventional treatment strategies may initially "debulk" the primary tumor through elimination of differentiated tumor cells, the small population of CSCs eventually regenerates the tumor, giving rise to recurrence. In lung cancer, evidence of this increased resistance has been shown in primary tumors[199] and lung cancer

Table 4
Published putative markers for the isolation of lung cancer stem cells

Sample Type	Tumor Type	Marker/Property for CSC Isolation	References
Cell lines	NSCLC	Hoechst exclusion	198,467
		Chemoresistance	468
		ALDH activity	196,469,470
		CD133+	195
	SCLC	ALDH activity	469
		CD133+	471
		uPAR	472
Tumor tissue	NSCLC	Hoechst exclusion	198
		ALDH activity	469
		CD133+	137,195,199
	SCLC	CD133+	199

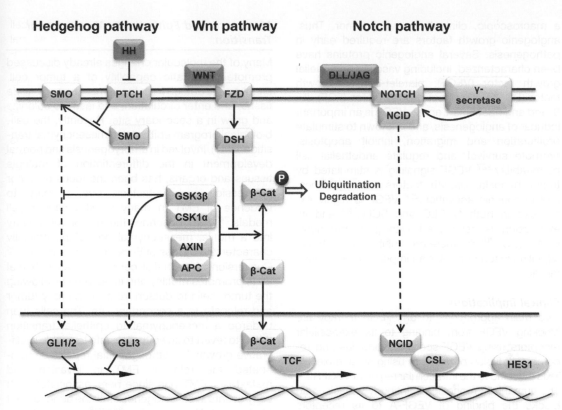

Fig. 6. Stem cell self-renewal pathways and therapeutic strategies to block these pathways in cancer. Notch, Wnt, and Hedgehog (Hh) are stem cell self-renewal pathways that are often deregulated and aberrantly activated in lung cancer, thus representing key therapeutic targets. The hedgehog pathway signals through Hh ligands binding to the Patched (PTCH) receptor and inhibiting its repression of Smoothened (SMO), allowing SMO activation, which results in nuclear translocation of GLI transcription factors. Wnt signaling functions through Wnt ligands binding to the Frizzled (FZD) receptor and signaling through disheveled (DSH), leading to the stabilization of β-catenin. In the absence of Hh or Wnt ligands, GSK3 phosphorylates GLI1/2 and β-catenin, respectively, resulting in ubiquitination and degradation. Notch signaling functions through Notch ligands (DLL and JAG) binding to the Notch receptor, which results in the cleavage of Notch intracellular binding domain (NICD) by γ-secretase, enabling it to translocate to the nucleus, bind to CLS transcription factors, and activate transcription. Some components of the pathways are omitted (*dashed lines*) for simplicity. (*Data from* Sun S, Schiller JH, Spinola M, et al. New molecularly targeted therapies for lung cancer. J Clin Invest 2007;117(10):2740–50; and Larsen JE, Spinola M, Gazdar AF, et al. An overview of the molecular biology of lung cancer. In: Pass HI, Carbone DP, Johnson DH et al, editors. Principles and practice of lung cancer: the official reference text of the International Association for the Study of Lung Cancer (IASLC). 4th edition. Philadelphia: Lippincott Williams & Wilkins; 2010. p. 59–74.)

mouse xenografts.[137] Approaches to specifically treating the CSC population include selective targeting using CSC detection molecules, sensitization of CSCs to conventional therapies and differentiation therapies, and inhibition of signaling pathways important to CSCs such as Hh, Wnt, and Notch signaling pathways, and telomerase, an important enzyme in normal stem cell function that is activated in most lung cancers (see later discussion). In lung, progress toward the latter approach has been shown in lung cancer cells.[204,220] Inhibition of the Hh pathway has been demonstrated with cyclopamine, a naturally occurring inhibitor of SMO, which has led to the development of synthetic oral inhibitors that

show clinical activity in basal cell carcinoma.[221] Inhibition of the Notch signaling pathway shows potential with γ-secretase inhibitors. Several inhibitors have shown efficacy in NSCLC,[222,223] and a phase 2 trial using a γ-secretase inhibitor as second-line therapy has commenced. Lastly, analysis of CSC biomarkers as diagnostic and prognostic biomarkers has recently shown clinical utility.[196,224–226]

Angiogenesis and the Tumor Microenvironment

Angiogenesis is one of the hallmarks of cancer, essential for a microscopic tumor to expand into a macroscopic, clinically relevant tumor. Thus, angiogenic growth factors are required early in pathogenesis. Several angiogenic proteins have been characterized, including vascular endothelial growth factor (VEGF), platelet-derived growth factor (PDGF), fibroblast growth factor (FGF), IL-8, and angiopoietins 1 and 2. VEGF is an important inducer of angiogenesis, and is known to stimulate proliferation and migration, inhibit apoptosis, promote survival, and regulate endothelial cell permeability.[227] VEGF signaling is stimulated by tumor hypoxia, growth factors and cytokines, and oncogenic activation.[228] VEGF is highly expressed in both NSCLC and SCLC[229] and its expression is associated with poor prognosis in NSCLC,[230–232] therefore inhibition of VEGF signaling in tumor cells is an important therapeutic target.

Clinical implications

Two main approaches to anti-VEGF therapy are blocking VEGF from binding to its extracellular receptors using VEGF-specific antibodies and recombinant fusion proteins, or using small-molecule TKIs that bind to the intracellular region of VEGFR.[233] The humanized monoclonal antibody bevacizumab blocks the binding of VEGF-A to its receptors VEGFR1 and VEGFR1, and is now approved for use in some solid cancers, including lung.[234] It is interesting that VEGF expression does not always correlate with response to bevacizumab,[235] one possible reason for which could be SNPs in *VEGF*. Numerous SNPs have been reported in *VEGF*, with some being associated with lower plasma levels of VEGF,[236] better outcome in NSCLC[237] or, recently, response to bevacizumab.[238]

The tumor microenvironment describes the complex and dynamic milieu of stromal cells, endothelial cells, innate cells, and lymphoblasts that surround tumor cells. Cells that comprise the tumor microenvironment interact both with each other and with tumor cells, and as a consequence they can affect tumor growth, invasion, and metastasis.[239] This concept supports the "seed and soil" hypothesis proposed by Stephen Paget in 1889,[240] who observed that the patterns of organ metastasis were a result of favorable conditions between metastatic tumor cells (the "seed") and the organ microenvironment (the "soil"). Modulation of critical tumor microenvironment biomarkers could improve current treatment of lung cancers. For example, hypoxia is associated with an increased risk of metastasis and increased resistance to radiotherapy and possible chemotherapy. Inhibition of HIF1α, a master transcription factor activated in response to hypoxia, or VEGFR, a target of HIF1α, can increase sensitivity to radiotherapy.[241,242]

Metastasis and Epithelial to Mesenchymal Transition

Many of the molecular changes already discussed promote metastatic capability of a tumor cell, enabling it to detach from the primary tumor, invade tissue, and enter circulation, and lastly to colonize and grow in a secondary site. Recently, the cell-biological program epithelial to mesenchymal transition (EMT), involved in embryogenesis and normal development in the differentiation of multiple tissues and organs, has been the focus of tumor progression and metastasis due, in part, to evidence of EMT in many in vitro cancer cell models.[243] EMT describes the loss of cell polarity into a motile, mesenchymal phenotype typically characterized by loss of E-cadherin expression.[244] Conversion of epithelial cells to a mesenchymal state promotes motility and invasiveness, allowing the tumor cells to detach from the primary tumor and relocate to a secondary site. The cells then undergo a mesenchymal to epithelial transition (MET) to revert to an epithelial state to enable proliferative growth.[245] Although initial reports demonstrated the role of EMT in invasion and metastasis, EMT has since been associated with early events in carcinogenesis,[246] the acquirement of stem cell–like properties,[246–248] and resistance to cell death, senescence, and conventional chemotherapies.[245] In lung cancer, mesenchymal markers and EMT inducers (eg, Vimentin, Twist, and Snail) have been shown to be strong prognostic markers.[249–251] EMT has also been linked to resistance to EGFR TKIs,[252,253] and COX-2 and LKB1 have been implicated in promoting EMT in lung cancer.[254–256] The miR-200 family of miRNAs is an important negative regulator of EMT,[257–260] and is discussed later in this article.

Activation of Telomerase in Lung Cancer Pathogenesis

Activation of telomerase, the telomere-lengthening enzyme, in premalignant cells prevents loss of telomere ends beyond critical points and is essential for cell immortality. Although silenced in normal cells, telomerase is activated in greater than 80% of NSCLCs and almost uniformly in SCLCs (see **Table 1**).[261–263]

Clinical implications

The prevalence of activated telomerase in cancer cells has made it an attractive target for therapeutic inhibition. Inhibition of telomerase in such cells leads to telomere shortening and ultimately either cellular senescence or apoptosis.[264,265] Approaches to telomerase inhibition include using antisense oligonucleotides that bind to human telomerase RNA[265] (such as imetelstat, which has started phase 2 trials[266]) and immunotherapy, whereby a patient's own immune system is stimulated with a vaccine to recognize tumor cells containing a major histocompatibility complex presenting hTERT peptide on the cell surface.[267,268]

EPIGENETIC CHANGES IN LUNG CARCINOGENESIS
Methylation and Histone Modification

Epigenetic events can lead to changes in gene expression without any changes in DNA sequence and therefore, importantly, are potentially reversible.[269] Aberrant promoter hypermethylation is an epigenetic change that occurs early in lung tumorigenesis, resulting in silencing of gene transcription, and is therefore a common method for inactivation of TSGs in lung cancer (see **Table 1**).[270] Such methods include genes involved in tissue invasion, DNA repair, detoxification of tobacco carcinogens, and differentiation. The prevalence of promoter methylation has been reported to differ between smokers and never smokers. Promoter methylation of *p16*, *MGMT*, *RASSF1*, *MTHFR*, and *FHIT* was significantly higher among smokers than never smokers whereas promoter methylation of *RASSF2*, *TNFRSF10C*, *BHLHB5*, and *BOLL* was more common in never smokers.[271–275] Recent advances in whole-genome microarray profiling have allowed researchers to globally study DNA methylation patterns in lung cancer—the lung cancer epigenome or methylome—and indicate that the role of methylation in lung tumorigenesis may have been underestimated.[276–285] Initial genome-wide studies analyzed the effect on gene expression following treatment of lung cancer cell lines with demethylating agents (such as 5-azacytidine); however, development of methylation-specific microarrays enables epigenomic analysis of tumor specimens.[276–281]

Clinical implications
Aberrant methylation occurs early in lung cancer pathogenesis and can be detected in circulating DNA; thus many studies have investigated the utility of methylation status in lung cancer for risk assessment, early detection, disease progression, and prognosis (reviewed in Refs.[286,287]). **Table 5** summarizes published candidate early detection, and prognostic and predictive methylation biomarkers, where hypermethylation of *p16*, *APC*, *FHIT*, *RASSF1A*, *DAPK*, and *CDH1* are being repeatedly reported as potential prognostic markers.[288–302]

DNA is methylated by DNA methyltransferases (DNMTs), which are responsible for both de novo and maintenance of preexisting methylation in

Table 5
DNA methylation as a biomarker in lung cancer

Early Detection	Prognostic Marker	Predictive Marker
APC	APC	SFN (14-3-3 sigma)
CDH13	CDH1	
DAPK1	CDH13	
DNMT1	CXCL12	
FHIT	DAPK1	
GATA5	DLEC1	
GSTP1	EPB41L3 (DAL-1)	
MAGEA1	ESR1	
MAGEB2	FHIT	
MGMT	IGFBP-3	
p16	MGMT	
PAX5-b	MLH1	
RARβ2	MSH2	
RASSF1A	p16	
RASSF5	PYCARD (ASC)	
RUNX3	PTEN	
TCF21	RASSF1A	
	RRAD	
	RUNX3	
	SPARC	
	TIMP3	
	TMS1	
	TSLC1	
	WIF1	

Data from Refs.[286,287,473]

a cell.[303] Histone modification is another mechanism for epigenetic control of gene transcription whereby histone deacetylation results in condensing of chromatin, resulting in transcriptionally inactive DNA. Inhibitors of DNMTs or histone deacetylases (HDACs) resulting in pharmacologic restoration of expression of epigenetically silenced genes comprises an exciting targeted therapeutic approach, and shows promise in lung cancer (see **Table 3**).[304,305]

MicroRNA-Mediated Regulation of Lung Cancer

miRNAs are a class of nonprotein-encoding small RNAs capable of regulating gene expression by either direct cleavage of a targeted mRNA or inhibiting translation by interacting with the 3′ untranslated region (UTR) of a target mRNA. miRNAs commonly have multiple target genes, therefore a single miRNA can often affect multiple cellular processes. Furthermore, an mRNA may be targeted by more than one miRNA, resulting in a complex network of molecular pathways to elucidate. Aberrant expression of miRNAs has been found to play an important role in the pathogenesis of cancer as either oncogenes or TSGs.[306–316] Microarray-based analyses of miRNA expression have identified many lung cancer–associated miRNAs,[313,314,317–328] and a review of experimentally validated miRNAs has been published previously.[329] One of the most widely studied lung cancer–associated miRNAs is the *let-7* miRNA family. Functioning as a tumor suppressor, it has been shown to regulate N-RAS, K-RAS, MYC, and HMGA2[330–332] via binding to the let-7 binding sites in their respective 3′ UTRs.[330,333] It is frequently underexpressed in lung tumors, particularly NSCLC, compared with normal lung, and decreased expression has also been associated with poor prognosis.[313,318] Induction of *let-7* miRNA expression has been found to inhibit in vitro growth[313,331,334,335] and reduce tumor development in a murine model of lung cancer.[335,336] Other miRNAs that exhibit tumor-suppressing effects in lung cancer include *miR-29a/b/c*, *miR-34a/b/c*, *miR-16*, and *miR-126*,[318–321,337,338] and recently, *miR-128b* was reported to be a direct regulator of EGFR with frequent LOH occurring in NSCLC cell lines.[322] Oncogenic miRNAs found to be overexpressed in lung cancer include the *miR-17-92* cluster of 7 miRNAs (that target PTEN, E2F1-3, and BIM), *miR-21* (suggested to be positively regulated by the EGFR signaling pathway, specifically EGFR mutations), *miR-93*, *miR-98*, *miR-197*, *miR-221/222*, and *miR-155*.[314,323,327,328] In addition, *hsa-miR-146b*, *miR-155*, and *miR-21* have been reported to be strong predictors of poor prognosis in lung cancer.[318,326,339,340] Recent evidence shows a strong link between miRNAs and invasion and metastasis, with several miRNAs found to regulate key regulators of EMT, a process central to cancer metastasis.[258–260,341] These regulators include *miR-10b* (through inhibition of *HOXD10*), *miR-126*, and the miRNA-200 family (which inhibit EMT inducers ZEB1 and ZEB2).[257–259,320,341]

Clinical implications

There is currently a strong research focus on miRNAs as potential diagnostic and prognostic biomarkers, and as therapeutic targets. Restoration of aberrantly expressed miRNAs can be achieved in vitro and in vivo using miRNA mimics (for underexpressed miRNAs) or miRNA inhibitors (termed antisense oligonucleotides or antagomirs) (for overexpressed miRNAs).[342–346] miRNA profiles for histologic[347,348] and prognostic[318,326,337,338,340] classification of lung tumors and detection of miRNAs in peripheral blood and sputum[349–351] illustrate the potential of miRNAs as diagnostic and early detection biomarkers in lung cancer. In addition, concurrent inhibition or overexpression of miRNAs with conventional therapies has resulted in an increased response to EGFR TKIs and radiotherapy.[327,352] These studies illustrate the immense potential of miRNAs in therapeutics development; however, limitations in pharmacokinetics, delivery, and toxicity need to be addressed.[353,354]

THE SEARCH FOR NEW BIOMARKERS: TOOLS AND MODEL SYSTEMS
Genomics: Tools for Identification, Prediction, and Prognosis

Genetic and epigenetic mechanisms underlying lung cancer development and progression continue to emerge, spearheaded by the development of technologies allowing genome-wide analysis of DNA copy number, mutations, gene expression, SNPs, and methylation.

Transcriptome profiling

Profiling the lung cancer transcriptome has imparted biologically and clinically relevant information such as novel dysregulated genes and pathways and gene signatures that can predict patient prognosis, response to treatment, and histology (reviewed in Refs.[355–357]). In an effort to overcome limitations of sample size and heterogeneity in previous studies, a multisite, blinded validation study of 442 lung adenocarcinomas comprehensively examined whether the mRNA profile of primary tumors robustly predicts patient outcome either alone or in combination with clinicopathological factors.[358] This study developed several models (or signatures) which, for the most part, predicted outcome better than current clinical methods. A recent critical review of published prognostic signatures in lung cancer, however, found little evidence of any published signature being ready for clinical application due, for the most part, to problems with study design and analysis.[359] The role of expression of the 48 nuclear receptors (and later their coregulators) has been studied in lung cancer and has been found to provide as good or better prognostic information than other mRNA expression signatures.[360] Because the nuclear receptors are also targets for therapeutic manipulation (via hormone agonists and antagonists), the expression of nuclear receptor patterns in individual lung cancers may also provide insight for targeted therapy. Despite complexities of mRNA profiling, the success of prognostic signatures in breast cancer, as seen with Oncotype DX,[361] impels further research efforts.

Genome-wide copy-number profiling

High-resolution mapping of copy-number alterations in the lung cancer genome has been able to identify single genes as targets of genomic gain or loss through improved definition of known aberrant regions or by identification of focal alterations undetectable with earlier technology.[74–76,79,80,83,84,86] A large-scale analysis of 371 primary lung adenocarcinomas identified 57 significant recurrent copy-number alterations, of which 31 were focal events and many were new lung cancer loci[74]; for example, amplification at 14q13.3 was reported as the most common event targeting the transcription factor *NKX2-1*, discussed earlier. Similar studies in NSCLC and squamous cell carcinoma cohorts have identified other novel "drivers" of lung carcinogenesis.[75,76,79,80]

Genome-wide sequencing of lung cancers

Large-scale sequencing and SNP analyses have also led to the identification of novel somatic mutations in the lung cancer genome.[13–15,119] In a screen of 188 lung adenocarcinomas, Ding and colleagues[119] identified somatic mutations in putative oncogenes (*ERBB4*, *KDR*, *FGFR4*, *EPHA3*) and TSGs (*NF1*, *RB1*, *ATM*, and *APC*). A major breakthrough has come with the development of "next-generation" (also termed second-generation) DNA sequencing technologies, which enable sequencing of expressed genes ("transcriptomes"), known exons ("exomes"), and complete genomes of tumors.[362] Data analysis can detect point mutations, insertions/deletions, copy-number alterations, translocations, and nonhuman sequences. Comparison of a primary lung NSCLC of adenocarcinoma histology with adjacent normal tissue identified many somatic mutations at an estimated rate of about 18 per megabase, including more than 50,000 single nucleotide variants.[41] Sequencing of an SCLC cell line revealed more than 22,000 somatic substitutions[42] while another study that sequenced an SCLC cell line and a neuroendocrine lung cancer cell line found a higher rate of somatic and germline rearrangements in the SCLC cell line.[43] Sequencing of the coding exons of approximately 1500 genes across 441 tumors, including 134 lung, found that lung adenocarcinomas and squamous cell carcinomas displayed high protein-altering mutation rates,[363] perhaps indicating the inherent heterogeneity found in lung tumors compared with tumors from other tissues. One hurdle in second-generation sequencing is storage and analysis of the immense amount of data that is produced and separating biologically meaningful data from noise. However, the potential insight we will have into cancer genomes and its applicability to diagnostic sampling brings us even closer to the goal of "personalized medicine."

Genome-wide functional (siRNA, shRNA library) screening

"Synthetic lethal" screens using RNAi (siRNAs and shRNA libraries) technology have allowed unbiased, genome-wide approaches to identification of genes whose perturbation can selectively kill lung cancer cells (see **Fig. 1**). The ability to identify "synthetic lethality" associated with oncogenic changes in tumor cells has particular utility in identifying new therapeutic targets or molecules to treat traditionally hard to target tumors, such as those with oncogenic KRAS. siRNA and shRNA screens have identified genes whose perturbation can selectively sensitize NSCLC cell lines to sublethal doses of chemotherapeutic agents,[364] sensitize KRAS mutant cells to targeted drugs,[126–128] suppress tumorigenicity in cells with specific gene dysregulation such as oncogenic KRAS[123–125,365] or aberrant EGFR,[366,367] or identify novel genes critical for tumorigenic processes such as metastasis.[368]

Public databases and bioinformatics

Although the challenges in gathering reliable and clinically and pathologically annotated data are not trivial, high-throughput technologies and publicly stored genome-wide databases related to lung cancer are resources with the potential to drive a global collaborative effort in identifying new targets for lung cancer diagnostics and therapeutics. At present, and within the near future, all lung cancer investigators will have access to all of the genome-wide studies performed on lung cancers with the attached clinical annotation. This information will allow independent confirmation on the role of the different molecular changes for prognosis, prediction, and targeting of therapy. With these tools researchers have enhanced ability to correlate patient subsets with augmented sensitivity to conventional or targeted therapeutics, distinguish driver versus passenger mutations, and better focus the design on novel therapeutic targets.

In Vitro and In Vivo Model Systems

While genome-wide approaches have the capacity of identifying novel genes or interactions in relation to lung cancer, the functional relevance of these findings needs to be elucidated using preclinical model systems, namely in vitro models (such as tumor cell lines or immortalized human bronchial epithelial cells) and in vivo xenograft and transgenic mouse models of lung carcinogenesis. Experimental disease models play a crucial role in developing our understanding of lung carcinogenesis. Lung cancer cell lines and xenografts provide one set of important models. However, because of the genetic complexity of lung cancers they will usually have hundreds if not thousands of genetic/epigenetic changes. By contrast, two much simpler and equally valuable models, particularly to study the progression of lung carcinogenesis, are immortalized human bronchial epithelial cells (HBECs) and genetically engineered mouse models (GEMMs). These systems provide methods to reduce the inherent complexity and heterogeneity of the lung cancer genome, and allow characterization of single or sequential genetic alterations in relation to the development, maintenance, and progression of lung cancer.

HBECs are derived from primary human airway epithelial cells and immortalized with either viral oncoproteins (such as SV40 early region) and hTERT[369] or overexpression of Cdk4 and Htert.[260,370] Stepwise transformation of these cells can be studied by the introduction of defined genetic manipulations commonly found in lung cancer.[371,372]

GEMMs allow the study of lung cancer pathogenesis with defined changes in the setting of the whole organism. GEMMs were critical in developing our understanding of oncogene dependence,[94] as observed in conditional

Table 6
Conditional genetically engineered mouse models of lung cancer

Genetic Manipulation[a]	Histopathology of Lungs	Metastasis	References
BRAF^{V600E}	Adenocarcinoma	—	474
EGFR^{L858R} or ^{Del}	Adenocarcinoma with BAC features	—	475,476
EGFR^{T790M} or $^{T790M+L858R}$ or $^{T790M+Del}$	Adenocarcinoma	—	477,478
EGFRvIII	Adenocarcinoma	None	479
EML4/ALK	Adenocarcinoma with BAC features	—	480
HER2^{YVMA}	Adenosquamous	Yes	481
Kras^{D12}	Adenocarcinoma	None	482
Kras^{V12}	Adenocarcinoma	Lymph node, kidney	483
Kras^{D12} + HIF2α	—	Yes	484
Kras^{D12} + Ink4a/Arf$^{-/-}$	Adenocarcinoma	None	441
Kras^{D12} + p16$^{Ink4a-/-}$	Adenocarcinoma	Yes	441
Kras^{D12} + p53$^{L/L-}$	Adenocarcinoma	Yes	441
Kras^{D12} + p53$^{F/F}$	Adenocarcinoma	Yes	485
Kras^{D12} + p53$^{R270H/F}$	Adenocarcinoma	—	485
Kras^{D12} + p53$^{R172H/F}$	Adenocarcinoma	—	485
Kras^{D12} + PTEN$^{\Delta5/\Delta5}$	Adenocarcinoma	—	486
Kras^{D12} + Lkb1$^{L/L}$ or $^{L/-}$	Squamous cell, adenosquamous, large cell	Yes (lymph node, skeletal)	441
Kras^{D12} + Lkb1$^{L/+}$ or $^{-}$	Adenocarcinoma	Yes (lymph node, skeletal)	441
PIK3CA^{H1047R}	Adenocarcinoma with BAC features	—	128
p16$^{Ink4a-/-}$ + p53$^{L/L}$	—	None	441
p53$^{\pm}$	Adenocarcinoma	—	487
p53$^{F/F}$	Adenocarcinoma	—	488
p53$^{R172H/+}$ or $^{R172H/-}$	Adenocarcinoma	—	487
p53$^{R270H/+}$ or $^{R270H/-}$	Adenocarcinoma, squamous cell	—	487
p53$^{F/F}$ + Rb$^{F/F}$	SCLC	Yes	488

Abbreviation: BAC, bronchioloalveolar.
[a] Germline null allele; L or F, conditional knockout allele.

$Kras^{D12}$-induced lung adenocarcinomas, where switching off the driving oncogene was sufficient to induce tumor regression even in the presence of other nondriving oncogenic alterations.[373] Ensuing research has characterized several conditional lung tumor–inducing combinations of oncogenic activations in mice (summarized in **Table 6**), which have been used to test new targeted therapies, improve effectiveness of conventional chemotherapies, identify biomarkers and imaging strategies for early detection, and study disease relapse and metastasis.[374]

SUMMARY

This review outlines some of the significant molecular alterations known to be involved in the initiation and/or progression of lung cancer. Continued development of targeted therapies for the treatment of lung cancer is dependent on our increased understanding of involved molecules and pathways. Cancer genome analyses are identifying hundreds to thousands of candidate targets, but these all require molecular and clinical validation. Furthermore, it is becoming increasingly apparent that targeting a single molecule will not be enough, due to the nonlinearity of pathways involved in carcinogenesis. Rather, targeting multiple molecules at once to combat the interconnective and complex signaling pathways will improve efficacy. Recent next-generation sequencing efforts are revealing that the lung cancer genome is mutated at a high rate, likely contributing to the known heterogeneity of these tumors and explaining the lack of identifying effective conventional and targeted therapies that have a universal effect in lung cancer. Systematic understanding of the molecular basis of lung cancer through comprehensive characterization of aberrations in the cancer genome and their functionality will provide the means to evaluate their use in diagnosis, prognosis, and therapy. Integration of clinical and biological factors will ultimately lead to improved detection, diagnosis, treatment, and prognosis of lung cancer by achieving "personalized medicine," the selection of the best treatment for each patient based on tumor-associated biomarkers.

ACKNOWLEDGMENTS

The authors thank the many current and past members of the Minna lab for their contributions to lung cancer translational research and especially our long-term collaborator Dr Adi Gazdar. Also, the authors apologize to other investigators for omission of any references.

REFERENCES

1. Jemal A, Siegel R, Xu J, et al. Cancer statistics, 2010. CA Cancer J Clin 2010;60(5):277–300.
2. Wistuba II, Gazdar AF. Lung cancer preneoplasia. Annu Rev Pathol 2006;1:331–48.
3. Sekido Y, Fong KM, Minna JD. Progress in understanding the molecular pathogenesis of human lung cancer. Biochim Biophys Acta 1998;1378(1):F21–59.
4. Nowell PC. The clonal evolution of tumor cell populations. Science 1976;194(4260):23–8.
5. Dakubo GD, Jakupciak JP, Birch-Machin MA, et al. Clinical implications and utility of field cancerization. Cancer Cell Int 2007;7:2.
6. Hanahan D, Weinberg RA. The hallmarks of cancer. Cell 2000;100(1):57–70.
7. Hanahan D, Weinberg RA. Hallmarks of cancer: the next generation. Cell 2011;144(5):646–74.
8. Gazdar AF. Should we continue to use the term non-small-cell lung cancer? Ann Oncol 2010; 21(Suppl 7):vii225–9.
9. Sun S, Schiller JH, Gazdar AF. Lung cancer in never smokers–a different disease. Nat Rev Cancer 2007; 7(10):778–90.
10. Scagliotti GV, Longo M, Novello S. Nonsmall cell lung cancer in never smokers. Curr Opin Oncol 2009;21(2):99–104.
11. Risch A, Plass C. Lung cancer epigenetics and genetics. Int J Cancer 2008;123(1):1–7.
12. Herbst RS, Heymach JV, Lippman SM. Lung cancer. N Engl J Med 2008;359(13):1367–80.
13. Amos CI, Wu X, Broderick P, et al. Genome-wide association scan of tag SNPs identifies a susceptibility locus for lung cancer at 15q25.1. Nat Genet 2008;40(5):616–22.
14. Hung RJ, McKay JD, Gaborieau V, et al. A susceptibility locus for lung cancer maps to nicotinic acetylcholine receptor subunit genes on 15q25. Nature 2008;452(7187):633–7.
15. Thorgeirsson TE, Geller F, Sulem P, et al. A variant associated with nicotine dependence, lung cancer and peripheral arterial disease. Nature 2008;452(7187):638–42.
16. Rafnar T, Sulem P, Besenbacher S, et al. Genome-wide significant association between a sequence variant at 15q15.2 and lung cancer risk. Cancer Res 2011;71(4):1356–61.
17. Broderick P, Wang Y, Vijayakrishnan J, et al. Deciphering the impact of common genetic variation on lung cancer risk: a genome-wide association study. Cancer Res 2009;69(16):6633–41.
18. Le Marchand L, Derby KS, Murphy SE, et al. Smokers with the CHRNA lung cancer-associated variants are exposed to higher levels of nicotine equivalents and a carcinogenic tobacco-specific nitrosamine. Cancer Res 2008;68(22):9137–40.
19. Spitz MR, Amos CI, Dong Q, et al. The CHRNA5-A3 region on chromosome 15q24-25.1 is a risk factor

both for nicotine dependence and for lung cancer. J Natl Cancer Inst 2008;100(21):1552–6.

20. Shiraishi K, Kohno T, Kunitoh H, et al. Contribution of nicotine acetylcholine receptor polymorphisms to lung cancer risk in a smoking-independent manner in the Japanese. Carcinogenesis 2009; 30(1):65–70.

21. Saccone SF, Hinrichs AL, Saccone NL, et al. Cholinergic nicotinic receptor genes implicated in a nicotine dependence association study targeting 348 candidate genes with 3713 SNPs. Hum Mol Genet 2007;16(1):36–49.

22. Weiss RB, Baker TB, Cannon DS, et al. A candidate gene approach identifies the CHRNA5-A3-B4 region as a risk factor for age-dependent nicotine addiction. PLoS Genet 2008;4(7):e1000125.

23. Stevens VL, Bierut LJ, Talbot JT, et al. Nicotinic receptor gene variants influence susceptibility to heavy smoking. Cancer Epidemiol Biomarkers Prev 2008;17(12):3517–25.

24. Bierut LJ, Stitzel JA, Wang JC, et al. Variants in nicotinic receptors and risk for nicotine dependence. Am J Psychiatry 2008;165(9):1163–71.

25. Paliwal A, Vaissiere T, Krais A, et al. Aberrant DNA methylation links cancer susceptibility locus 15q25.1 to apoptotic regulation and lung cancer. Cancer Res 2010;70(7):2779–88.

26. Liu Y, Liu P, Wen W, et al. Haplotype and cell proliferation analyses of candidate lung cancer susceptibility genes on chromosome 15q24-25.1. Cancer Res 2009;69(19):7844–50.

27. Bailey-Wilson JE, Amos CI, Pinney SM, et al. A major lung cancer susceptibility locus maps to chromosome 6q23-25. Am J Hum Genet 2004; 75(3):460–74.

28. Amos CI, Pinney SM, Li Y, et al. A susceptibility locus on chromosome 6q greatly increases lung cancer risk among light and never smokers. Cancer Res 2010;70(6):2359–67.

29. You M, Wang D, Liu P, et al. Fine mapping of chromosome 6q23-25 region in familial lung cancer families reveals RGS17 as a likely candidate gene. Clin Cancer Res 2009;15(8):2666–74.

30. Parkin DM, Bray F, Ferlay J, et al. Global cancer statistics, 2002. CA Cancer J Clin 2005;55(2): 74–108.

31. Tan YK, Wee TC, Koh WP, et al. Survival among Chinese women with lung cancer in Singapore: a comparison by stage, histology and smoking status. Lung Cancer 2003;40(3):237–46.

32. Nordquist LT, Simon GR, Cantor A, et al. Improved survival in never-smokers vs current smokers with primary adenocarcinoma of the lung. Chest 2004; 126(2):347–51.

33. Toh CK, Gao F, Lim WT, et al. Never-smokers with lung cancer: epidemiologic evidence of a distinct disease entity. J Clin Oncol 2006;24(15):2245–51.

34. Janjigian YY, McDonnell K, Kris MG, et al. Pack-years of cigarette smoking as a prognostic factor in patients with stage IIIB/IV nonsmall cell lung cancer. Cancer 2010;116(3):670–5.

35. Subramanian J, Govindan R. Lung cancer in never smokers: a review. J Clin Oncol 2007;25(5):561–70.

36. Rudin CM, Avila-Tang E, Harris CC, et al. Lung cancer in never smokers: molecular profiles and therapeutic implications. Clin Cancer Res 2009; 15(18):5646–61.

37. Werness BA, Levine AJ, Howley PM. Association of human papillomavirus types 16 and 18 E6 proteins with p53. Science 1990;248(4951):76–9.

38. Dyson N, Howley PM, Munger K, et al. The human papilloma virus-16 E7 oncoprotein is able to bind to the retinoblastoma gene product. Science 1989; 243(4893):934–7.

39. Klein F, Kotb WF, Petersen I. Incidence of human papilloma virus in lung cancer. Lung Cancer 2009;65(1):13–8.

40. Koshiol J, Rotunno M, Gillison ML, et al. Assessment of human papillomavirus in lung tumor tissue. J Natl Cancer Inst 2011;103(6):501–7.

41. Lee W, Jiang Z, Liu J, et al. The mutation spectrum revealed by paired genome sequences from a lung cancer patient. Nature 2010;465(7297):473–7.

42. Pleasance ED, Stephens PJ, O'Meara S, et al. A small-cell lung cancer genome with complex signatures of tobacco exposure. Nature 2010; 463(7278):184–90.

43. Campbell PJ, Stephens PJ, Pleasance ED, et al. Identification of somatically acquired rearrangements in cancer using genome-wide massively parallel paired-end sequencing. Nat Genet 2008; 40(6):722–9.

44. Kris MG, Johnson BE, Kwiatkowski DJ, et al. Identification of driver mutations in tumor specimens from 1000 patients with lung adenocarcinoma: the NCI's lung cancer mutation consortium (LCMC) [abstract CRA7506]. J Clin Oncol 2011;29(Suppl).

45. Fleming TP, Saxena A, Clark WC, et al. Amplification and/or overexpression of platelet-derived growth factor receptors and epidermal growth factor receptor in human glial tumors. Cancer Res 1992;52(16):4550–3.

46. Heinrich MC, Corless CL, Duensing A, et al. PDGFRA activating mutations in gastrointestinal stromal tumors. Science 2003;299(5607):708–10.

47. Lin CR, Chen WS, Kruiger W, et al. Expression cloning of human EGF receptor complementary DNA: gene amplification and three related messenger RNA products in A431 cells. Science 1984;224(4651):843–8.

48. Merlino GT, Xu YH, Ishii S, et al. Amplification and enhanced expression of the epidermal growth factor receptor gene in A431 human carcinoma cells. Science 1984;224(4647):417–9.

49. Ullrich A, Coussens L, Hayflick JS, et al. Human epidermal growth factor receptor cDNA sequence and aberrant expression of the amplified gene in A431 epidermoid carcinoma cells. Nature 1984; 309(5967):418–25.

50. Lynch TJ, Bell DW, Sordella R, et al. Activating mutations in the epidermal growth factor receptor underlying responsiveness of non-small-cell lung cancer to gefitinib. N Engl J Med 2004;350(21): 2129–39.

51. Paez JG, Janne PA, Lee JC, et al. EGFR mutations in lung cancer: correlation with clinical response to gefitinib therapy. Science 2004;304(5676):1497–500.

52. Pao W, Miller V, Zakowski M, et al. EGF receptor gene mutations are common in lung cancers from "never smokers" and are associated with sensitivity of tumors to gefitinib and erlotinib. Proc Natl Acad Sci U S A 2004;101(36):13306–11.

53. Semba K, Kamata N, Toyoshima K, et al. A v-erbB-related protooncogene, c-erbB-2, is distinct from the c-erbB-1/epidermal growth factor-receptor gene and is amplified in a human salivary gland adenocarcinoma. Proc Natl Acad Sci U S A 1985; 82(19):6497–501.

54. Stephens P, Hunter C, Bignell G, et al. Lung cancer: intragenic ERBB2 kinase mutations in tumours. Nature 2004;431(7008):525–6.

55. Shayesteh L, Lu Y, Kuo WL, et al. PIK3CA is implicated as an oncogene in ovarian cancer. Nat Genet 1999;21(1):99–102.

56. Massion PP, Kuo WL, Stokoe D, et al. Genomic copy number analysis of non-small cell lung cancer using array comparative genomic hybridization: implications of the phosphatidylinositol 3-kinase pathway. Cancer Res 2002;62(13):3636–40.

57. Samuels Y, Wang Z, Bardelli A, et al. High frequency of mutations of the PIK3CA gene in human cancers. Science 2004;304(5670):554.

58. Friend SH, Bernards R, Rogelj S, et al. A human DNA segment with properties of the gene that predisposes to retinoblastoma and osteosarcoma. Nature 1986;323(6089):643–6.

59. Kamb A, Gruis NA, Weaver-Feldhaus J, et al. A cell cycle regulator potentially involved in genesis of many tumor types. Science 1994;264(5157):436–40.

60. Nobori T, Miura K, Wu DJ, et al. Deletions of the cyclin-dependent kinase-4 inhibitor gene in multiple human cancers. Nature 1994;368(6473):753–6.

61. Li J, Yen C, Liaw D, et al. PTEN, a putative protein tyrosine phosphatase gene mutated in human brain, breast, and prostate cancer. Science 1997; 275(5308):1943–7.

62. Steck PA, Pershouse MA, Jasser SA, et al. Identification of a candidate tumour suppressor gene, MMAC1, at chromosome 10q23.3 that is mutated in multiple advanced cancers. Nat Genet 1997; 15(4):356–62.

63. Fong KM, Kida Y, Zimmerman PV, et al. Loss of heterozygosity frequently affects chromosome 17q in non-small cell lung cancer. Cancer Res 1995;55(19):4268–72.

64. Fong KM, Sekido Y, Minna JD. Molecular pathogenesis of lung cancer. J Thorac Cardiovasc Surg 1999;118(6):1136–52.

65. Sekido Y, Fong KM, Minna JD. Molecular genetics of lung cancer. Annu Rev Med 2003;54:73–87.

66. Zimmerman PV, Hawson GA, Bint MH, et al. Ploidy as a prognostic determinant in surgically treated lung cancer. Lancet 1987;2(8558):530–3.

67. Fong KM, Zimmerman PV, Smith PJ. Correlation of loss of heterozygosity at 11p with tumour progression and survival in non-small cell lung cancer. Genes Chromosomes Cancer 1994;10(3):183–9.

68. Fong KM, Zimmerman PV, Smith PJ. Microsatellite instability and other molecular abnormalities in non-small cell lung cancer. Cancer Res 1995; 55(1):28–30.

69. Fong KM, Zimmerman PV, Smith PJ. Tumor progression and loss of heterozygosity at 5q and 18q in non-small cell lung cancer. Cancer Res 1995;55(2):220–3.

70. Fong KM, Kida Y, Zimmerman PV, et al. MYCL genotypes and loss of heterozygosity in non-small-cell lung cancer. Br J Cancer 1996;74(12): 1975–8.

71. Fong KM, Zimmerman PV, Smith PJ. KRAS codon 12 mutations in Australian non-small cell lung cancer. Aust N Z J Med 1998;28(2):184–9.

72. Virmani AK, Fong KM, Kodagoda D, et al. Allelotyping demonstrates common and distinct patterns of chromosomal loss in human lung cancer types. Genes Chromosomes Cancer 1998;21(4):308–19.

73. Geradts J, Fong KM, Zimmerman PV, et al. Loss of Fhit expression in non-small-cell lung cancer: correlation with molecular genetic abnormalities and clinicopathological features. Br J Cancer 2000;82(6):1191–7.

74. Weir BA, Woo MS, Getz G, et al. Characterizing the cancer genome in lung adenocarcinoma. Nature 2007;450(7171):893–8.

75. Bass AJ, Watanabe H, Mermel CH, et al. SOX2 is an amplified lineage-survival oncogene in lung and esophageal squamous cell carcinomas. Nat Genet 2009;41(11):1238–42.

76. Weiss J, Sos ML, Seidel D, et al. Frequent and focal FGFR1 amplification associates with therapeutically tractable FGFR1 dependency in squamous cell lung cancer. Sci Transl Med 2010;2(62):62ra93.

77. Sanchez-Cespedes M, Ahrendt SA, Piantadosi S, et al. Chromosomal alterations in lung adenocarcinoma from smokers and nonsmokers. Cancer Res 2001;61(4):1309–13.

78. Gill RK, Yang SH, Meerzaman D, et al. Frequent homozygous deletion of the LKB1/STK11 gene in

non-small cell lung cancer. Oncogene 2011;30: 3784–91.

79. Kim YH, Kwei KA, Girard L, et al. Genomic and functional analysis identifies CRKL as an oncogene amplified in lung cancer. Oncogene 2010;29(10): 1421–30.

80. Yuan P, Kadara H, Behrens C, et al. Sex determining region Y-Box 2 (SOX2) is a potential cell-lineage gene highly expressed in the pathogenesis of squamous cell carcinomas of the lung. PLoS One 2010;5(2):e9112.

81. Jiang F, Yin Z, Caraway NP, et al. Genomic profiles in stage I primary non small cell lung cancer using comparative genomic hybridization analysis of cDNA microarrays. Neoplasia 2004;6(5):623–35.

82. Kim TM, Yim SH, Lee JS, et al. Genome-wide screening of genomic alterations and their clinico-pathologic implications in non-small cell lung cancers. Clin Cancer Res 2005;11(23):8235–42.

83. Shibata T, Uryu S, Kokubu A, et al. Genetic classification of lung adenocarcinoma based on array-based comparative genomic hybridization analysis: its association with clinicopathologic features. Clin Cancer Res 2005;11(17):6177–85.

84. Tonon G, Wong KK, Maulik G, et al. High-resolution genomic profiles of human lung cancer. Proc Natl Acad Sci U S A 2005;102(27):9625–30.

85. Wikman H, Nymark P, Vayrynen A, et al. CDK4 is a probable target gene in a novel amplicon at 12q13.3-q14.1 in lung cancer. Genes Chromosomes Cancer 2005;42(2):193–9.

86. Zhao X, Weir BA, LaFramboise T, et al. Homozygous deletions and chromosome amplifications in human lung carcinomas revealed by single nucleotide polymorphism array analysis. Cancer Res 2005;65(13):5561–70.

87. Choi JS, Zheng LT, Ha E, et al. Comparative genomic hybridization array analysis and real-time PCR reveals genomic copy number alteration for lung adenocarcinomas. Lung 2006;184(6): 355–62.

88. Choi YW, Choi JS, Zheng LT, et al. Comparative genomic hybridization array analysis and real time PCR reveals genomic alterations in squamous cell carcinomas of the lung. Lung Cancer 2007; 55(1):43–51.

89. Zhu H, Lam DCL, Han KC, et al. High resolution analysis of genomic aberrations by metaphase and array comparative genomic hybridization identifies candidate tumour genes in lung cancer cell lines. Cancer Lett 2007;255(1–2):303–14.

90. Garnis C, Lockwood WW, Vucic E, et al. High resolution analysis of non-small cell lung cancer cell lines by whole genome tiling path array CGH. Int J Cancer 2006;118(6):1556–64.

91. Dehan E, Ben-Dor A, Liao W, et al. Chromosomal aberrations and gene expression profiles in non-

small cell lung cancer. Lung Cancer 2007;56(2): 175–84.

92. Girard N, Ostrovnaya I, Lau C, et al. Genomic and mutational profiling to assess clonal relationships between multiple non-small cell lung cancers. Clin Cancer Res 2009;15(16):5184–90.

93. Kwei KA, Kim YH, Girard L, et al. Genomic profiling identifies TITF1 as a lineage-specific oncogene amplified in lung cancer. Oncogene 2008;27(25): 3635–40.

94. Weinstein IB. Cancer. Addiction to oncogenes—the Achilles heal of cancer. Science 2002;297(5578): 63–4.

95. Normanno N, Bianco C, Strizzi L, et al. The ErbB receptors and their ligands in cancer: an overview. Curr Drug Targets 2005;6(3):243–57.

96. Hirsch FR, Varella-Garcia M, Bunn PA Jr, et al. Epidermal growth factor receptor in non-small-cell lung carcinomas: correlation between gene copy number and protein expression and impact on prognosis. J Clin Oncol 2003;21(20):3798–807.

97. Eberhard DA, Johnson BE, Amler LC, et al. Mutations in the epidermal growth factor receptor and in KRAS are predictive and prognostic indicators in patients with non-small-cell lung cancer treated with chemotherapy alone and in combination with erlotinib. J Clin Oncol 2005;23(25):5900–9.

98. Sordella R, Bell DW, Haber DA, et al. Gefitinib-sensitizing EGFR mutations in lung cancer activate anti-apoptotic pathways. Science 2004;305(5687): 1163–7.

99. Shigematsu H, Lin L, Takahashi T, et al. Clinical and biological features associated with epidermal growth factor receptor gene mutations in lung cancers. J Natl Cancer Inst 2005;97(5):339–46.

100. Rusch V, Baselga J, Cordon-Cardo C, et al. Differential expression of the epidermal growth factor receptor and its ligands in primary non-small cell lung cancers and adjacent benign lung. Cancer Res 1993;53(10 Suppl):2379–85.

101. Franklin WA, Veve R, Hirsch FR, et al. Epidermal growth factor receptor family in lung cancer and premalignancy. Semin Oncol 2002;29(1 Suppl 4): 3–14.

102. Herbst RS. Review of epidermal growth factor receptor biology. Int J Radiat Oncol Biol Phys 2004;59(2 Suppl):21–6.

103. Fujino S, Enokibori T, Tezuka N, et al. A comparison of epidermal growth factor receptor levels and other prognostic parameters in non-small cell lung cancer. Eur J Cancer 1996;32A(12):2070–4.

104. Gazdar AF. Activating and resistance mutations of EGFR in non-small-cell lung cancer: role in clinical response to EGFR tyrosine kinase inhibitors. Oncogene 2009;28(Suppl 1):S24–31.

105. Thomas RK, Greulich H, Yuza Y, et al. Detection of oncogenic mutations in the EGFR gene in lung

adenocarcinoma with differential sensitivity to EGFR tyrosine kinase inhibitors. Cold Spring Harb Symp Quant Biol 2005;70:73–81.

106. Pao W, Wang TY, Riely GJ, et al. KRAS mutations and primary resistance of lung adenocarcinomas to gefitinib or erlotinib. PLoS Med 2005; 2(1):e17.

107. Pao W, Miller VA, Politi KA, et al. Acquired resistance of lung adenocarcinomas to gefitinib or erlotinib is associated with a second mutation in the EGFR kinase domain. PLoS Med 2005; 2(3):e73.

108. Bean J, Brennan C, Shih JY, et al. MET amplification occurs with or without T790M mutations in EGFR mutant lung tumors with acquired resistance to gefitinib or erlotinib. Proc Natl Acad Sci U S A 2007; 104(52):20932–7.

109. Engelman JA, Zejnullahu K, Mitsudomi T, et al. MET amplification leads to gefitinib resistance in lung cancer by activating ERBB3 signaling. Science 2007;316(5827):1039–43.

110. Gao SP, Mark KG, Leslie K, et al. Mutations in the EGFR kinase domain mediate STAT3 activation via IL-6 production in human lung adenocarcinomas. J Clin Invest 2007;117(12):3846–56.

111. Ishihara K, Hirano T. Molecular basis of the cell specificity of cytokine action. Biochim Biophys Acta 2002;1592(3):281–96.

112. Hong DS, Angelo LS, Kurzrock R. Interleukin-6 and its receptor in cancer: implications for translational therapeutics. Cancer 2007;110(9):1911–28.

113. Downward J. Targeting RAS signalling pathways in cancer therapy. Nat Rev Cancer 2003;3(1):11–22.

114. Karnoub AE, Weinberg RA. Ras oncogenes: split personalities. Nat Rev Mol Cell Biol 2008;9(7):517–31.

115. Rodenhuis S, Slebos RJ. Clinical significance of ras oncogene activation in human lung cancer. Cancer Res 1992;52(9 Suppl):2665s–9s.

116. Linardou H, Dahabreh IJ, Kanaloupiti D, et al. Assessment of somatic k-RAS mutations as a mechanism associated with resistance to EGFR-targeted agents: a systematic review and meta-analysis of studies in advanced non-small-cell lung cancer and metastatic colorectal cancer. Lancet Oncol 2008;9(10):962–72.

117. Riely GJ, Kris MG, Rosenbaum D, et al. Frequency and distinctive spectrum of KRAS mutations in never smokers with lung adenocarcinoma. Clin Cancer Res 2008;14(18):5731–4.

118. Adjei AA. K-ras as a target for lung cancer therapy. J Thorac Oncol 2008;3(6 Suppl 2):S160–3.

119. Ding L, Getz G, Wheeler DA, et al. Somatic mutations affect key pathways in lung adenocarcinoma. Nature 2008;455(7216):1069–75.

120. Davies H, Bignell GR, Cox C, et al. Mutations of the BRAF gene in human cancer. Nature 2002; 417(6892):949–54.

121. Naoki K, Chen TH, Richards WG, et al. Missense mutations of the BRAF gene in human lung adenocarcinoma. Cancer Res 2002;62(23):7001–3.

122. Sasaki H, Kawano O, Endo K, et al. Uncommon V599E BRAF mutations in Japanese patients with lung cancer. J Surg Res 2006;133(2):203–6.

123. Scholl C, Frohling S, Dunn IF, et al. Synthetic lethal interaction between oncogenic KRAS dependency and STK33 suppression in human cancer cells. Cell 2009;137(5):821–34.

124. Guo W, Wu S, Liu J, et al. Identification of a small molecule with synthetic lethality for K-ras and protein kinase C iota. Cancer Res 2008;68(18): 7403–8.

125. Luo J, Emanuele MJ, Li D, et al. A genome-wide RNAi screen identifies multiple synthetic lethal interactions with the Ras oncogene. Cell 2009; 137(5):835–48.

126. Singh A, Greninger P, Rhodes D, et al. A gene expression signature associated with "K-Ras addiction" reveals regulators of EMT and tumor cell survival. Cancer Cell 2009;15(6):489–500.

127. Sunaga N, Shames DS, Girard L, et al. Knockdown of oncogenic KRAS in non-small cell lung cancers suppresses tumor growth and sensitizes tumor cells to targeted therapy. Mol Cancer Ther 2011; 10(2):336–46.

128. Engelman JA, Chen L, Tan X, et al. Effective use of PI3K and MEK inhibitors to treat mutant Kras G12D and PIK3CA H1047R murine lung cancers. Nat Med 2008;14(12):1351–6.

129. Krystal G, Birrer M, Way J, et al. Multiple mechanisms for transcriptional regulation of the myc gene family in small-cell lung cancer. Mol Cell Biol 1988;8(8):3373–81.

130. Richardson GE, Johnson BE. The biology of lung cancer. Semin Oncol 1993;20(2):105–27.

131. Adhikary S, Eilers M. Transcriptional regulation and transformation by Myc proteins. Nat Rev Mol Cell Biol 2005;6(8):635–45.

132. Meyer N, Penn LZ. Reflecting on 25 years with MYC. Nat Rev Cancer 2008;8(12):976–90.

133. Nau MM, Brooks BJ Jr, Carney DN, et al. Human small-cell lung cancers show amplification and expression of the N-myc gene. Proc Natl Acad Sci U S A 1986;83(4):1092–6.

134. Broers JL, Viallet J, Jensen SM, et al. Expression of c-myc in progenitor cells of the bronchopulmonary epithelium and in a large number of non-small cell lung cancers. Am J Respir Cell Mol Biol 1993;9(1): 33–43.

135. Soda M, Choi YL, Enomoto M, et al. Identification of the transforming EML4-ALK fusion gene in non-small-cell lung cancer. Nature 2007;448(7153): 561–6.

136. Solomon B, Varella-Garcia M, Camidge DR. ALK gene rearrangements: a new therapeutic target in

a molecularly defined subset of non-small cell lung cancer. J Thorac Oncol 2009;4(12):1450–4.

137. Bertolini G, Roz L, Perego P, et al. Highly tumorigenic lung cancer CD133+ cells display stem-like features and are spared by cisplatin treatment. Proc Natl Acad Sci U S A 2009;106(38):16281–6.

138. De Francesco F, Tirino V, Desiderio V, et al. Human CD34/CD90 ASCs are capable of growing as sphere clusters, producing high levels of VEGF and forming capillaries. PLoS One 2009;4(8):e6537.

139. Tirino V, Camerlingo R, Franco R, et al. The role of CD133 in the identification and characterisation of tumour-initiating cells in non-small-cell lung cancer. Eur J Cardiothorac Surg 2009;36(3):446–53.

140. De Rosa A, De Francesco F, Tirino V, et al. A new method for the cryopreserving ASCs: an attractive and suitable large-scale and long-term cell banking technology. Tissue Eng Part C Methods 2009;15(4):659–67.

141. Costantino E, Maddalena F, Calise S, et al. TRAP1, a novel mitochondrial chaperone responsible for multi-drug resistance and protection from apoptosis in human colorectal carcinoma cells. Cancer Lett 2009;279(1):39–46.

142. Engelman JA, Luo J, Cantley LC. The evolution of phosphatidylinositol 3-kinases as regulators of growth and metabolism. Nat Rev Genet 2006;7(8):606–19.

143. Vivanco I, Sawyers CL. The phosphatidylinositol 3-kinase AKT pathway in human cancer. Nat Rev Cancer 2002;2(7):489–501.

144. West KA, Linnoila IR, Belinsky SA, et al. Tobacco carcinogen-induced cellular transformation increases activation of the phosphatidylinositol 3'-kinase/Akt pathway in vitro and in vivo. Cancer Res 2004;64(2):446–51.

145. Hay N. The Akt-mTOR tango and its relevance to cancer. Cancer Cell 2005;8(3):179–83.

146. Maulik G, Madhiwala P, Brooks S, et al. Activated c-Met signals through PI3K with dramatic effects on cytoskeletal functions in small cell lung cancer. J Cell Mol Med 2002;6(4):539–53.

147. Brognard J, Clark AS, Ni Y, et al. Akt/protein kinase B is constitutively active in non-small cell lung cancer cells and promotes cellular survival and resistance to chemotherapy and radiation. Cancer Res 2001;61(10):3986–97.

148. Tsurutani J, West KA, Sayyah J, et al. Inhibition of the phosphatidylinositol 3-kinase/Akt/mammalian target of rapamycin pathway but not the MEK/ERK pathway attenuates laminin-mediated small cell lung cancer cellular survival and resistance to imatinib mesylate or chemotherapy. Cancer Res 2005;65(18):8423–32.

149. Kendall J, Liu Q, Bakleh A, et al. Oncogenic cooperation and coamplification of developmental transcription factor genes in lung cancer. Proc Natl Acad Sci U S A 2007;104(42):16663–8.

150. Bingle CD. Thyroid transcription factor-1. Int J Biochem Cell Biol 1997;29(12):1471–3.

151. Ikeda K, Clark JC, Shaw-White JR, et al. Gene structure and expression of human thyroid transcription factor-1 in respiratory epithelial cells. J Biol Chem 1995;270(14):8108–14.

152. Tanaka H, Yanagisawa K, Shinjo K, et al. Lineage-specific dependency of lung adenocarcinomas on the lung development regulator TTF-1. Cancer Res 2007;67(13):6007–11.

153. Winslow MM, Dayton TL, Verhaak RG, et al. Suppression of lung adenocarcinoma progression by Nkx2-1. Nature 2011;473(7345):101–4.

154. Visakorpi T, Hyytinen E, Koivisto P, et al. In vivo amplification of the androgen receptor gene and progression of human prostate cancer. Nat Genet 1995;9(4):401–6.

155. Garraway LA, Widlund HR, Rubin MA, et al. Integrative genomic analyses identify MITF as a lineage survival oncogene amplified in malignant melanoma. Nature 2005;436(7047):117–22.

156. Holst F, Stahl PR, Ruiz C, et al. Estrogen receptor alpha (ESR1) gene amplification is frequent in breast cancer. Nat Genet 2007;39(5):655–60.

157. Garraway LA, Sellers WR. Lineage dependency and lineage-survival oncogenes in human cancer. Nat Rev Cancer 2006;6(8):593–602.

158. Knudson AG Jr. The ninth Gordon Hamilton-Fairley memorial lecture. Hereditary cancers: clues to mechanisms of carcinogenesis. Br J Cancer 1989;59(5):661–6.

159. Breuer RH, Postmus PE, Smit EF. Molecular pathology of non-small-cell lung cancer. Respiration 2005;72(3):313–30.

160. Takahashi T, Nau MM, Chiba I, et al. p53: a frequent target for genetic abnormalities in lung cancer. Science 1989;246(4929):491–4.

161. Hollstein M, Sidransky D, Vogelstein B, et al. p53 mutations in human cancers. Science 1991;253(5015):49–53.

162. Greenblatt MS, Bennett WP, Hollstein M, et al. Mutations in the p53 tumor suppressor gene: clues to cancer etiology and molecular pathogenesis. Cancer Res 1994;54(18):4855–78.

163. van Oijen MG, Slootweg PJ. Gain-of-function mutations in the tumor suppressor gene p53. Clin Cancer Res 2000;6(6):2138–45.

164. Ventura A, Kirsch DG, McLaughlin ME, et al. Restoration of p53 function leads to tumour regression in vivo. Nature 2007;445(7128):661–5.

165. Harbour JW, Lai SL, Whang-Peng J, et al. Abnormalities in structure and expression of the human retinoblastoma gene in SCLC. Science 1988;241(4863):353–7.

166. Yokota J, Mori N, Akiyama T, et al. Multiple genetic alterations in small-cell lung carcinoma. Princess Takamatsu Symp 1989;20:43–8.

167. Otterson GA, Kratzke RA, Coxon A, et al. Absence of p16INK4 protein is restricted to the subset of lung cancer lines that retains wildtype RB. Oncogene 1994;9(11):3375–8.

168. Wistuba II, Behrens C, Virmani AK, et al. High resolution chromosome 3p allelotyping of human lung cancer and preneoplastic/preinvasive bronchial epithelium reveals multiple, discontinuous sites of 3p allele loss and three regions of frequent breakpoints. Cancer Res 2000;60(7):1949–60.

169. Ito M, Ito G, Kondo M, et al. Frequent inactivation of RASSF1A, BLU, and SEMA3B on 3p21.3 by promoter hypermethylation and allele loss in non-small cell lung cancer. Cancer Lett 2005;225(1):131–9.

170. Kuroki T, Trapasso F, Yendamuri S, et al. Allelic loss on chromosome 3p21.3 and promoter hypermethylation of semaphorin 3B in non-small cell lung cancer. Cancer Res 2003;63(12):3352–5.

171. Feng Q, Hawes SE, Stern JE, et al. DNA methylation in tumor and matched normal tissues from non-small cell lung cancer patients. Cancer Epidemiol Biomarkers Prev 2008;17(3):645–54.

172. Wistuba II, Gazdar AF, Minna JD. Molecular genetics of small cell lung carcinoma. Semin Oncol 2001;28(2 Suppl 4):3–13.

173. Zochbauer-Muller S, Minna JD, Gazdar AF. Aberrant DNA methylation in lung cancer: biological and clinical implications. Oncologist 2002;7(5):451–7.

174. Siprashvili Z, Sozzi G, Barnes LD, et al. Replacement of Fhit in cancer cells suppresses tumorigenicity. Proc Natl Acad Sci U S A 1997;94(25):13771–6.

175. Agathanggelou A, Cooper WN, Latif F. Role of the Ras-association domain family 1 tumor suppressor gene in human cancers. Cancer Res 2005;65(9):3497–508.

176. Ji L, Roth JA. Tumor suppressor FUS1 signaling pathway. J Thorac Oncol 2008;3(4):327–30.

177. Deng WG, Kawashima H, Wu G, et al. Synergistic tumor suppression by coexpression of FUS1 and p53 is associated with down-regulation of murine double minute-2 and activation of the apoptotic protease-activating factor 1-dependent apoptotic pathway in human non-small cell lung cancer cells. Cancer Res 2007;67(2):709–17.

178. Tomizawa Y, Sekido Y, Kondo M, et al. Inhibition of lung cancer cell growth and induction of apoptosis after reexpression of 3p21.3 candidate tumor suppressor gene SEMA3B. Proc Natl Acad Sci U S A 2001;98(24):13954–9.

179. Ochi K, Mori T, Toyama Y, et al. Identification of semaphorin3B as a direct target of p53. Neoplasia 2002;4(1):82–7.

180. Castro-Rivera E, Ran S, Brekken RA, et al. Semaphorin 3B inhibits the phosphatidylinositol 3-kinase/Akt pathway through neuropilin-1 in lung and breast cancer cells. Cancer Res 2008;68(20):8295–303.

181. Brambilla E, Constantin B, Drabkin H, et al. Semaphorin SEMA3F localization in malignant human lung and cell lines: a suggested role in cell adhesion and cell migration. Am J Pathol 2000;156(3):939–50.

182. Kessler O, Shraga-Heled N, Lange T, et al. Semaphorin-3F is an inhibitor of tumor angiogenesis. Cancer Res 2004;64(3):1008–15.

183. Alessi DR, Sakamoto K, Bayascas JR. LKB1-dependent signaling pathways. Annu Rev Biochem 2006;75:137–63.

184. Hemminki A, Markie D, Tomlinson I, et al. A serine/threonine kinase gene defective in Peutz-Jeghers syndrome. Nature 1998;391(6663):184–7.

185. Sanchez-Cespedes M, Parrella P, Esteller M, et al. Inactivation of LKB1/STK11 is a common event in adenocarcinomas of the lung. Cancer Res 2002;62(13):3659–62.

186. Carretero J, Medina PP, Pio R, et al. Novel and natural knockout lung cancer cell lines for the LKB1/STK11 tumor suppressor gene. Oncogene 2004;23(22):4037–40.

187. Matsumoto S, Iwakawa R, Takahashi K, et al. Prevalence and specificity of LKB1 genetic alterations in lung cancers. Oncogene 2007;26(40):5911–8.

188. Shaw RJ, Bardeesy N, Manning BD, et al. The LKB1 tumor suppressor negatively regulates mTOR signaling. Cancer Cell 2004;6(1):91–9.

189. Onozato R, Kosaka T, Achiwa H, et al. LKB1 gene mutations in Japanese lung cancer patients. Cancer Sci 2007;98(11):1747–51.

190. Mahoney CL, Choudhury B, Davies H, et al. LKB1/KRAS mutant lung cancers constitute a genetic subset of NSCLC with increased sensitivity to MAPK and mTOR signalling inhibition. Br J Cancer 2009;100(2):370–5.

191. Reya T, Morrison SJ, Clarke MF, et al. Stem cells, cancer, and cancer stem cells. Nature 2001;414(6859):105–11.

192. Wang JC, Dick JE. Cancer stem cells: lessons from leukemia. Trends Cell Biol 2005;15(9):494–501.

193. Clarke MF, Dick JE, Dirks PB, et al. Cancer stem cells—perspectives on current status and future directions: AACR Workshop on cancer stem cells. Cancer Res 2006;66(19):9339–44.

194. Lapidot T, Sirard C, Vormoor J, et al. A cell initiating human acute myeloid leukaemia after transplantation into SCID mice. Nature 1994;367(6464):645–8.

195. Chen YC, Hsu HS, Chen YW, et al. Oct-4 expression maintained cancer stem-like properties in lung cancer-derived CD133-positive cells. PLoS One 2008;3(7):e2637.

196. Jiang F, Qiu Q, Khanna A, et al. Aldehyde dehydrogenase 1 is a tumor stem cell-associated marker in lung cancer. Mol Cancer Res 2009;7(3):330–8.

197. Kitamura H, Okudela K, Yazawa T, et al. Cancer stem cell: implications in cancer biology and therapy with special reference to lung cancer. Lung Cancer 2009;66(3):275–81.

198. Ho MM, Ng AV, Lam S, et al. Side population in human lung cancer cell lines and tumors is enriched with stem-like cancer cells. Cancer Res 2007;67(10):4827–33.

199. Eramo A, Lotti F, Sette G, et al. Identification and expansion of the tumorigenic lung cancer stem cell population. Cell Death Differ 2008;15(3):504–14.

200. Wicha MS, Liu S, Dontu G. Cancer stem cells: an old idea–a paradigm shift. Cancer Res 2006; 66(4):1883–90 [discussion: 1895–6].

201. Rubin LL, de Sauvage FJ. Targeting the Hedgehog pathway in cancer. Nat Rev Drug Discov 2006; 5(12):1026–33.

202. Riobo NA, Lu K, Emerson CP Jr. Hedgehog signal transduction: signal integration and cross talk in development and cancer. Cell Cycle 2006;5(15):1612–5.

203. Lauth M, Toftgard R. Non-canonical activation of GLI transcription factors: implications for targeted anti-cancer therapy. Cell Cycle 2007;6(20): 2458–63.

204. Watkins DN, Berman DM, Burkholder SG, et al. Hedgehog signalling within airway epithelial progenitors and in small-cell lung cancer. Nature 2003;422(6929):313–7.

205. Yuan Z, Goetz JA, Singh S, et al. Frequent requirement of hedgehog signaling in non-small cell lung carcinoma. Oncogene 2007;26(7):1046–55.

206. He B, You L, Uematsu K, et al. A monoclonal antibody against Wnt-1 induces apoptosis in human cancer cells. Neoplasia 2004;6(1):7–14.

207. You L, He B, Xu Z, et al. Inhibition of Wnt-2-mediated signaling induces programmed cell death in non-small-cell lung cancer cells. Oncogene 2004; 23(36):6170–4.

208. Winn RA, Van Scoyk M, Hammond M, et al. Antitumorigenic effect of Wnt 7a and Fzd 9 in non-small cell lung cancer cells is mediated through ERK-5-dependent activation of peroxisome proliferator-activated receptor gamma. J Biol Chem 2006; 281(37):26943–50.

209. Fukui T, Kondo M, Ito G, et al. Transcriptional silencing of secreted frizzled related protein 1 (SFRP 1) by promoter hypermethylation in non-small-cell lung cancer. Oncogene 2005;24(41): 6323–7.

210. Mazieres J, He B, You L, et al. Wnt inhibitory factor-1 is silenced by promoter hypermethylation in human lung cancer. Cancer Res 2004;64(14): 4717–20.

211. Uematsu K, He B, You L, et al. Activation of the Wnt pathway in non small cell lung cancer: evidence of dishevelled overexpression. Oncogene 2003; 22(46):7218–21.

212. Wissmann C, Wild PJ, Kaiser S, et al. WIF1, a component of the Wnt pathway, is down-regulated in prostate, breast, lung, and bladder cancer. J Pathol 2003;201(2):204–12.

213. Dang TP, Eichenberger S, Gonzalez A, et al. Constitutive activation of Notch3 inhibits terminal epithelial differentiation in lungs of transgenic mice. Oncogene 2003;22(13):1988–97.

214. Politi K, Feirt N, Kitajewski J. Notch in mammary gland development and breast cancer. Semin Cancer Biol 2004;14(5):341–7.

215. Parr C, Watkins G, Jiang WG. The possible correlation of Notch-1 and Notch-2 with clinical outcome and tumour clinicopathological parameters in human breast cancer. Int J Mol Med 2004;14(5): 779–86.

216. Hainaud P, Contreres JO, Villemain A, et al. The role of the vascular endothelial growth factor-Delta-like 4 ligand/Notch4-ephrin B2 cascade in tumor vessel remodeling and endothelial cell functions. Cancer Res 2006;66(17):8501–10.

217. Daniel VC, Peacock CD, Watkins DN. Developmental signalling pathways in lung cancer. Respirology 2006;11(3):234–40.

218. Olsen CL, Hsu PP, Glienke J, et al. Hedgehog-interacting protein is highly expressed in endothelial cells but down-regulated during angiogenesis and in several human tumors. BMC Cancer 2004; 4:43.

219. Nickoloff BJ, Osborne BA, Miele L. Notch signaling as a therapeutic target in cancer: a new approach to the development of cell fate modifying agents. Oncogene 2003;22(42):6598–608.

220. Hu T, Liu S, Breiter DR, et al. Octamer 4 small interfering RNA results in cancer stem cell-like cell apoptosis. Cancer Res 2008;68(16): 6533–40.

221. Von Hoff DD, LoRusso PM, Rudin CM, et al. Inhibition of the hedgehog pathway in advanced basal-cell carcinoma. N Engl J Med 2009;361(12): 1164–72.

222. Luistro L, He W, Smith M, et al. Preclinical profile of a potent gamma-secretase inhibitor targeting notch signaling with in vivo efficacy and pharmacodynamic properties. Cancer Res 2009;69(19): 7672–80.

223. Wei P, Walls M, Qiu M, et al. Evaluation of selective gamma-secretase inhibitor PF-03084014 for its antitumor efficacy and gastrointestinal safety to guide optimal clinical trial design. Mol Cancer Ther 2010;9(6):1618–28.

224. Sullivan JP, Spinola M, Dodge M, et al. Aldehyde dehydrogenase activity selects for lung adenocarcinoma stem cells dependent on notch signaling. Cancer Res 2010;70(23):9937–48.

225. Sholl LM, Barletta JA, Yeap BY, et al. Sox2 protein expression is an independent poor prognostic

indicator in stage I lung adenocarcinoma. Am J Surg Pathol 2010;34(8):1193–8.

226. Sholl LM, Long KB, Hornick JL. Sox2 expression in pulmonary non-small cell and neuroendocrine carcinomas. Appl Immunohistochem Mol Morphol 2010;18(1):55–61.

227. Korpanty G, Smyth E, Sullivan LA, et al. Antiangiogenic therapy in lung cancer: focus on vascular endothelial growth factor pathway. Exp Biol Med (Maywood) 2010;235(1):3–9.

228. Ferrara N. Vascular endothelial growth factor: basic science and clinical progress. Endocr Rev 2004; 25(4):581–611.

229. Stefanou D, Batistatou A, Arkoumani E, et al. Expression of vascular endothelial growth factor (VEGF) and association with microvessel density in small-cell and non-small-cell lung carcinomas. Histol Histopathol 2004;19(1):37–42.

230. Kaya A, Ciledag A, Gulbay BE, et al. The prognostic significance of vascular endothelial growth factor levels in sera of non-small cell lung cancer patients. Respir Med 2004;98(7):632–6.

231. Dudek AZ, Mahaseth H. Circulating angiogenic cytokines in patients with advanced non-small cell lung cancer: correlation with treatment response and survival. Cancer Invest 2005;23(3):193–200.

232. Jantus-Lewintre E, Sanmartin E, Sirera R, et al. Combined VEGF-A and VEGFR-2 concentrations in plasma: diagnostic and prognostic implications in patients with advanced NSCLC. Lung Cancer 2011. [Epub ahead of print].

233. Hasani A, Leighl NB. Targeting vascular endothelial growth factor in lung cancer. J Thorac Oncol 2010; 5(12 Suppl 6):S484–6.

234. Sandler A, Gray R, Perry MC, et al. Paclitaxel-carboplatin alone or with bevacizumab for non-small-cell lung cancer. N Engl J Med 2006;355(24): 2542–50.

235. Yang JC, Haworth L, Sherry RM, et al. A randomized trial of bevacizumab, an anti-vascular endothelial growth factor antibody, for metastatic renal cancer. N Engl J Med 2003;349(5):427–34.

236. Watson CJ, Webb NJ, Bottomley MJ, et al. Identification of polymorphisms within the vascular endothelial growth factor (VEGF) gene: correlation with variation in VEGF protein production. Cytokine 2000;12(8):1232–5.

237. Heist RS, Zhai R, Liu G, et al. VEGF polymorphisms and survival in early-stage non-small-cell lung cancer. J Clin Oncol 2008;26(6):856–62.

238. Schneider BP, Radovich M, Sledge GW, et al. Association of polymorphisms of angiogenesis genes with breast cancer. Breast Cancer Res Treat 2008;111(1):157–63.

239. Sautes-Fridman C, Cherfils-Vicini J, Damotte D, et al. Tumor microenvironment is multifaceted. Cancer Metastasis Rev 2011;30(1):13–25.

240. Paget S. The distribution of secondary growths in cancer of the breast. Lancet 1889;1:571–3.

241. Schwartz DL, Powis G, Thitai-Kumar A, et al. The selective hypoxia inducible factor-1 inhibitor PX-478 provides in vivo radiosensitization through tumor stromal effects. Mol Cancer Ther 2009;8(4): 947–58.

242. Williams KJ, Telfer BA, Shannon AM, et al. Combining radiotherapy with AZD2171, a potent inhibitor of vascular endothelial growth factor signaling: pathophysiologic effects and therapeutic benefit. Mol Cancer Ther 2007;6(2):599–606.

243. Thiery JP. Epithelial-mesenchymal transitions in tumour progression. Nat Rev Cancer 2002;2(6): 442–54.

244. Lee JM, Dedhar S, Kalluri R, et al. The epithelial-mesenchymal transition: new insights in signaling, development, and disease. J Cell Biol 2006; 172(7):973–81.

245. Thiery JP, Acloque H, Huang RY, et al. Epithelial-mesenchymal transitions in development and disease. Cell 2009;139(5):871–90.

246. Mani SA, Guo W, Liao MJ, et al. The epithelial-mesenchymal transition generates cells with properties of stem cells. Cell 2008;133(4):704–15.

247. Chiou SH, Wang ML, Chou YT, et al. Coexpression of Oct4 and Nanog enhances malignancy in lung adenocarcinoma by inducing cancer stem cell-like properties and epithelial-mesenchymal transdifferentiation. Cancer Res 2010;70(24):10433–44.

248. Wellner U, Schubert J, Burk UC, et al. The EMT-activator ZEB1 promotes tumorigenicity by repressing stemness-inhibiting microRNAs. Nat Cell Biol 2009;11(12):1487–95.

249. Hung JJ, Yang MH, Hsu HS, et al. Prognostic significance of hypoxia-inducible factor-1alpha, TWIST1 and Snail expression in resectable non-small cell lung cancer. Thorax 2009;64(12):1082–9.

250. Miura N, Yano T, Shoji F, et al. Clinicopathological significance of Sip1-associated epithelial mesenchymal transition in non-small cell lung cancer progression. Anticancer Res 2009;29(10):4099–106.

251. Soltermann A, Tischler V, Arbogast S, et al. Prognostic significance of epithelial-mesenchymal and mesenchymal-epithelial transition protein expression in non-small cell lung cancer. Clin Cancer Res 2008;14(22):7430–7.

252. Yauch RL, Januario T, Eberhard DA, et al. Epithelial versus mesenchymal phenotype determines in vitro sensitivity and predicts clinical activity of erlotinib in lung cancer patients. Clin Cancer Res 2005; 11(24 Pt 1):8686–98.

253. Thomson S, Buck E, Petti F, et al. Epithelial to mesenchymal transition is a determinant of sensitivity of non-small-cell lung carcinoma cell lines and xenografts to epidermal growth factor receptor inhibition. Cancer Res 2005;65(20):9455–62.

254. Roy BC, Kohno T, Iwakawa R, et al. Involvement of LKB1 in epithelial-mesenchymal transition (EMT) of human lung cancer cells. Lung Cancer 2010;70(2): 136–45.

255. Dohadwala M, Yang SC, Luo J, et al. Cyclooxygenase-2-dependent regulation of E-cadherin: prostaglandin E(2) induces transcriptional repressors ZEB1 and snail in non-small cell lung cancer. Cancer Res 2006;66(10):5338–45.

256. Krysan K, Lee JM, Dohadwala M, et al. Inflammation, epithelial to mesenchymal transition, and epidermal growth factor receptor tyrosine kinase inhibitor resistance. J Thorac Oncol 2008;3(2):107–10.

257. Park SM, Gaur AB, Lengyel E, et al. The miR-200 family determines the epithelial phenotype of cancer cells by targeting the E-cadherin repressors ZEB1 and ZEB2. Genes Dev 2008;22(7):894–907.

258. Gregory PA, Bert AG, Paterson EL, et al. The miR-200 family and miR-205 regulate epithelial to mesenchymal transition by targeting ZEB1 and SIP1. Nat Cell Biol 2008;10(5):593–601.

259. Gibbons DL, Lin W, Creighton CJ, et al. Contextual extracellular cues promote tumor cell EMT and metastasis by regulating miR-200 family expression. Genes Dev 2009;23(18):2140–51.

260. Tellez CS, Juri DE, Do K, et al. EMT and stem cell-like properties associated with miR-205 and miR-200 epigenetic silencing are early manifestations during carcinogen-induced transformation of human lung epithelial cells. Cancer Res 2011; 71(8):3087–97.

261. Albanell J, Lonardo F, Rusch V, et al. High telomerase activity in primary lung cancers: association with increased cell proliferation rates and advanced pathologic stage. J Natl Cancer Inst 1997;89(21): 1609–15.

262. Hiyama K, Hiyama E, Ishioka S, et al. Telomerase activity in small-cell and non-small-cell lung cancers. J Natl Cancer Inst 1995;87(12):895–902.

263. Frias C, Garcia-Aranda C, De Juan C, et al. Telomere shortening is associated with poor prognosis and telomerase activity correlates with DNA repair impairment in non-small cell lung cancer. Lung Cancer 2008;60(3):416–25.

264. Shay JW, Wright WE. Telomerase activity in human cancer. Curr Opin Oncol 1996;8(1):66–71.

265. Ouellette MM, Wright WE, Shay JW. Targeting telomerase-expressing cancer cells. J Cell Mol Med 2011;15(7):1433–42.

266. Molckovsky A, Siu LL. First-in-class, first-in-human phase I results of targeted agents: highlights of the 2008 American society of clinical oncology meeting. J Hematol Oncol 2008;1:20.

267. Vonderheide RH, Hahn WC, Schultze JL, et al. The telomerase catalytic subunit is a widely expressed tumor-associated antigen recognized by cytotoxic T lymphocytes. Immunity 1999;10(6):673–9.

268. Vonderheide RH. Telomerase as a universal tumor-associated antigen for cancer immunotherapy. Oncogene 2002;21(4):674–9.

269. Bird A. DNA methylation patterns and epigenetic memory. Genes Dev 2002;16(1):6–21.

270. Baylin SB, Esteller M, Rountree MR, et al. Aberrant patterns of DNA methylation, chromatin formation and gene expression in cancer. Hum Mol Genet 2001;10(7):687–92.

271. Kim H, Kwon YM, Kim JS, et al. Tumor-specific methylation in bronchial lavage for the early detection of non-small-cell lung cancer. J Clin Oncol 2004;22(12):2363–70.

272. Liu Y, Lan Q, Siegfried JM, et al. Aberrant promoter methylation of p16 and MGMT genes in lung tumors from smoking and never-smoking lung cancer patients. Neoplasia 2006;8(1):46–51.

273. Vaissiere T, Hung RJ, Zaridze D, et al. Quantitative analysis of DNA methylation profiles in lung cancer identifies aberrant DNA methylation of specific genes and its association with gender and cancer risk factors. Cancer Res 2009;69(1):243–52.

274. Buckingham L, Penfield Faber L, Kim A, et al. PTEN, RASSF1 and DAPK site-specific hypermethylation and outcome in surgically treated stage I and II nonsmall cell lung cancer patients. Int J Cancer 2010;126(7):1630–9.

275. Kaira K, Sunaga N, Tomizawa Y, et al. Epigenetic inactivation of the RAS-effector gene RASSF2 in lung cancers. Int J Oncol 2007;31(1):169–73.

276. Bibikova M, Lin Z, Zhou L, et al. High-throughput DNA methylation profiling using universal bead arrays. Genome Res 2006;16(3):383–93.

277. Christensen BC, Marsit CJ, Houseman EA, et al. Differentiation of lung adenocarcinoma, pleural mesothelioma, and nonmalignant pulmonary tissues using DNA methylation profiles. Cancer Res 2009;69(15):6315–21.

278. Rauch TA, Zhong X, Wu X, et al. High-resolution mapping of DNA hypermethylation and hypomethylation in lung cancer. Proc Natl Acad Sci U S A 2008;105(1):252–7.

279. Dai Z, Lakshmanan RR, Zhu WG, et al. Global methylation profiling of lung cancer identifies novel methylated genes. Neoplasia 2001;3(4):314–23.

280. Brena RM, Morrison C, Liyanarachchi S, et al. Aberrant DNA methylation of OLIG1, a novel prognostic factor in non-small cell lung cancer. PLoS Med 2007;4(3):e108.

281. Kim EH, Park AK, Dong SM, et al. Global analysis of CpG methylation reveals epigenetic control of the radiosensitivity in lung cancer cell lines. Oncogene 2010;29(33):4725–31.

282. Shames DS, Girard L, Gao B, et al. A genome-wide screen for promoter methylation in lung cancer identifies novel methylation markers for multiple malignancies. PLoS Med 2006;3(12):e486.

283. Zhong S, Fields CR, Su N, et al. Pharmacologic inhibition of epigenetic modifications, coupled with gene expression profiling, reveals novel targets of aberrant DNA methylation and histone deacetylation in lung cancer. Oncogene 2007;26(18): 2621–34.

284. Pfeifer GP, Rauch TA. DNA methylation patterns in lung carcinomas. Semin Cancer Biol 2009;19(3): 181–7.

285. Suzuki H, Gabrielson E, Chen W, et al. A genomic screen for genes upregulated by demethylation and histone deacetylase inhibition in human colorectal cancer. Nat Genet 2002;31(2):141–9.

286. Suzuki M, Yoshino I. Aberrant methylation in non-small cell lung cancer. Surg Today 2010;40(7): 602–7.

287. Heller G, Zielinski CC, Zochbauer-Muller S. Lung cancer: from single-gene methylation to methylome profiling. Cancer Metastasis Rev 2010;29(1): 95–107.

288. Kim DS, Kim MJ, Lee JY, et al. Aberrant methylation of E-cadherin and H-cadherin genes in nonsmall cell lung cancer and its relation to clinicopathologic features. Cancer 2007;110(12):2785–92.

289. Gu J, Berman D, Lu C, et al. Aberrant promoter methylation profile and association with survival in patients with non-small cell lung cancer. Clin Cancer Res 2006;12(24):7329–38.

290. Ota N, Kawakami K, Okuda T, et al. Prognostic significance of p16(INK4a) hypermethylation in non-small cell lung cancer is evident by quantitative DNA methylation analysis. Anticancer Res 2006;26(5B):3729–32.

291. Kim JS, Kim JW, Han J, et al. Cohypermethylation of p16 and FHIT promoters as a prognostic factor of recurrence in surgically resected stage I non-small cell lung cancer. Cancer Res 2006;66(8): 4049–54.

292. Wang J, Lee JJ, Wang L, et al. Value of p16INK4a and RASSF1A promoter hypermethylation in prognosis of patients with resectable non-small cell lung cancer. Clin Cancer Res 2004;10(18 Pt 1): 6119–25.

293. Maruyama R, Toyooka S, Toyooka KO, et al. Aberrant promoter methylation profile of bladder cancer and its relationship to clinicopathological features. Cancer Res 2001;61(24):8659–63.

294. Usadel H, Brabender J, Danenberg KD, et al. Quantitative adenomatous polyposis coli promoter methylation analysis in tumor tissue, serum, and plasma DNA of patients with lung cancer. Cancer Res 2002;62(2):371–5.

295. Brabender J, Usadel H, Danenberg KD, et al. Adenomatous polyposis coli gene promoter hypermethylation in non-small cell lung cancer is associated with survival. Oncogene 2001;20(27): 3528–32.

296. Kim DH, Nelson HH, Wiencke JK, et al. p16(INK4a) and histology-specific methylation of CpG islands by exposure to tobacco smoke in non-small cell lung cancer. Cancer Res 2001;61(8):3419–24.

297. Burbee DG, Forgacs E, Zochbauer-Muller S, et al. Epigenetic inactivation of RASSF1A in lung and breast cancers and malignant phenotype suppression. J Natl Cancer Inst 2001;93(9):691–9.

298. Tang X, Khuri FR, Lee JJ, et al. Hypermethylation of the death-associated protein (DAP) kinase promoter and aggressiveness in stage I non-small-cell lung cancer. J Natl Cancer Inst 2000; 92(18):1511–6.

299. Lu C, Soria JC, Tang X, et al. Prognostic factors in resected stage I non-small-cell lung cancer: a multivariate analysis of six molecular markers. J Clin Oncol 2004;22(22):4575–83.

300. Kim DH, Kim JS, Ji YI, et al. Hypermethylation of RASSF1A promoter is associated with the age at starting smoking and a poor prognosis in primary non-small cell lung cancer. Cancer Res 2003; 63(13):3743–6.

301. Tomizawa Y, Kohno T, Kondo H, et al. Clinicopathological significance of epigenetic inactivation of RASSF1A at 3p21.3 in stage I lung adenocarcinoma. Clin Cancer Res 2002;8(7):2362–8.

302. Toyooka S, Suzuki M, Maruyama R, et al. The relationship between aberrant methylation and survival in non-small-cell lung cancers. Br J Cancer 2004; 91(4):771–4.

303. Rhee I, Jair KW, Yen RW, et al. CpG methylation is maintained in human cancer cells lacking DNMT1. Nature 2000;404(6781):1003–7.

304. Ramalingam SS. Histone deacetylase, proteasome, and heat shock protein inhibitors for the treatment of lung cancer. J Thorac Oncol 2010; 5(12 Suppl 6):S458–60.

305. Mukhopadhyay NK, Weisberg E, Gilchrist D, et al. Effectiveness of trichostatin A as a potential candidate for anticancer therapy in non-small-cell lung cancer. Ann Thorac Surg 2006;81(3):1034–42.

306. Metzler M, Wilda M, Busch K, et al. High expression of precursor microRNA-155/BIC RNA in children with Burkitt lymphoma. Genes Chromosomes Cancer 2004;39(2):167–9.

307. Michael MZ, O' Connor SM, van Holst Pellekaan NG, et al. Reduced accumulation of specific microRNAs in colorectal neoplasia. Mol Cancer Res 2003;1(12): 882–91.

308. Calin GA, Dumitru CD, Shimizu M, et al. Frequent deletions and down-regulation of micro- RNA genes miR15 and miR16 at 13q14 in chronic lymphocytic leukemia. Proc Natl Acad Sci U S A 2002;99(24):15524–9.

309. Eis PS, Tam W, Sun L, et al. Accumulation of miR-155 and BIC RNA in human B cell lymphomas. Proc Natl Acad Sci U S A 2005;102(10):3627–32.

310. He L, Thomson JM, Hemann MT, et al. A microRNA polycistron as a potential human oncogene. Nature 2005;435(7043):828–33.

311. Ota A, Tagawa H, Karnan S, et al. Identification and characterization of a novel gene, C13orf25, as a target for 13q31-q32 amplification in malignant lymphoma. Cancer Res 2004;64(9):3087–95.

312. Voorhoeve PM, le Sage C, Schrier M, et al. A genetic screen implicates miRNA-372 and miR-NA-373 as oncogenes in testicular germ cell tumors. Cell 2006;124(6):1169–81.

313. Takamizawa J, Konishi H, Yanagisawa K, et al. Reduced expression of the let-7 microRNAs in human lung cancers in association with shortened postoperative survival. Cancer Res 2004;64(11): 3753–6.

314. Hayashita Y, Osada H, Tatematsu Y, et al. A polycistronic microRNA cluster, miR-17-92, is over-expressed in human lung cancers and enhances cell proliferation. Cancer Res 2005;65(21):9628–32.

315. O'Donnell KA, Wentzel EA, Zeller KI, et al. c-Myc-regulated microRNAs modulate E2F1 expression. Nature 2005;435(7043):839–43.

316. Esquela-Kerscher A, Slack FJ. Oncomirs—microRNAs with a role in cancer. Nat Rev Cancer 2006; 6(4):259–69.

317. Yu SL, Chen HY, Chang GC, et al. MicroRNA signature predicts survival and relapse in lung cancer. Cancer Cell 2008;13(1):48–57.

318. Yanaihara N, Caplen N, Bowman E, et al. Unique microRNA molecular profiles in lung cancer diagnosis and prognosis. Cancer Cell 2006;9(3):189–98.

319. Fabbri M, Garzon R, Cimmino A, et al. MicroRNA-29 family reverts aberrant methylation in lung cancer by targeting DNA methyltransferases 3A and 3B. Proc Natl Acad Sci U S A 2007;104(40): 15805–10.

320. Crawford M, Brawner E, Batte K, et al. MicroRNA-126 inhibits invasion in non-small cell lung carcinoma cell lines. Biochem Biophys Res Commun 2008;373(4):607–12.

321. Nasser MW, Datta J, Nuovo G, et al. Downregulation of microRNA-1 (miR-1) in lung cancer: suppression of tumorigenic property of lung cancer cells and their sensitization to doxorubicin induced apoptosis bymiR-1. J Biol Chem 2008;283(48): 33394–405.

322. Weiss GJ, Bemis LT, Nakajima E, et al. EGFR regulation by microRNA in lung cancer: correlation with clinical response and survival to gefitinib and EGFR expression in cell lines. Ann Oncol 2008; 19(6):1053–9.

323. Markou A, Tsaroucha EG, Kaklamanis L, et al. Prognostic value of mature microRNA-21 and MicroRNA-205 overexpression in non-small cell lung cancer by quantitative real-time RT-PCR. Clin Chem 2008;54(10):1696–704.

324. Garofalo M, Quintavalle C, Di Leva G, et al. MicroRNA signatures of TRAIL resistance in human non-small cell lung cancer. Oncogene 2008;27(27): 3845–55.

325. Volinia S, Calin GA, Liu CG, et al. A microRNA expression signature of human solid tumors defines cancer gene targets. Proc Natl Acad Sci U S A 2006;103(7):2257–61.

326. Raponi M, Dossey L, Jatkoe T, et al. MicroRNA classifiers for predicting prognosis of squamous cell lung cancer. Cancer Res 2009;69(14):5776–83.

327. Seike M, Goto A, Okano T, et al. MiR-21 is an EGFR-regulated anti-apoptotic factor in lung cancer in never-smokers. Proc Natl Acad Sci U S A 2009;106(29):12085–90.

328. Du L, Schageman JJ, Subauste MC, et al. miR-93, miR-98, and miR-197 regulate expression of tumor suppressor gene FUS1. Mol Cancer Res 2009;7(8): 1234–43.

329. Du L, Pertsemlidis A. microRNAs and lung cancer: tumors and 22-mers. Cancer Metastasis Rev 2010; 29(1):109–22.

330. Johnson SM, Grosshans H, Shingara J, et al. RAS is regulated by the let-7 microRNA family. Cell 2005;120(5):635–47.

331. Lee YS, Dutta A. The tumor suppressor microRNA let-7 represses the HMGA2 oncogene. Genes Dev 2007;21(9):1025–30.

332. Osada H, Takahashi T. let-7 and miR-17-92: small-sized major players in lung cancer development. Cancer Sci 2011;102(1):9–17.

333. Mayr C, Hemann MT, Bartel DP. Disrupting the pairing between let-7 and Hmga2 enhances oncogenic transformation. Science 2007;315(5818):1576–9.

334. Johnson CD, Esquela-Kerscher A, Stefani G, et al. The let-7 microRNA represses cell proliferation pathways in human cells. Cancer Res 2007; 67(16):7713–22.

335. Esquela-Kerscher A, Trang P, Wiggins JF, et al. The let-7 microRNA reduces tumor growth in mouse models of lung cancer. Cell Cycle 2008; 7(6):759–64.

336. Kumar MS, Erkeland SJ, Pester RE, et al. Suppression of non-small cell lung tumor development by the let-7 microRNA family. Proc Natl Acad Sci U S A 2008;105(10):3903–8.

337. Wang Z, Chen Z, Gao Y, et al. DNA hypermethylation of microRNA-34b/c has prognostic value for stage non-small cell lung cancer. Cancer Biol Ther 2011;11(5):490–6.

338. Gallardo E, Navarro A, Vinolas N, et al. miR-34a as a prognostic marker of relapse in surgically resected non-small-cell lung cancer. Carcinogenesis 2009;30(11):1903–9.

339. Donnem T, Eklo K, Berg T, et al. Prognostic impact of MiR-155 in non-small cell lung cancer evaluated by in situ hybridization. J Transl Med 2011;9:6.

340. Saito M, Schetter AJ, Mollerup S, et al. The association of microRNA expression with prognosis and progression in early-stage, non-small cell lung adenocarcinoma: a retrospective analysis of three cohorts. Clin Cancer Res 2011;17(7):1875–82.

341. Ma L, Reinhardt F, Pan E, et al. Therapeutic silencing of miR-10b inhibits metastasis in a mouse mammary tumor model. Nat Biotechnol 2010;28(4): 341–7.

342. Mercatelli N, Coppola V, Bonci D, et al. The inhibition of the highly expressed miR-221 and miR-222 impairs the growth of prostate carcinoma xenografts in mice. PLoS One 2008;3(12):e4029.

343. Felicetti F, Errico MC, Bottero L, et al. The promyelocytic leukemia zinc finger-microRNA-221/-222 pathway controls melanoma progression through multiple oncogenic mechanisms. Cancer Res 2008;68(8):2745–54.

344. Wickramasinghe NS, Manavalan TT, Dougherty SM, et al. Estradiol downregulates miR-21 expression and increases miR-21 target gene expression in MCF-7 breast cancer cells. Nucleic Acids Res 2009;37(8):2584–95.

345. Yang Y, Chaerkady R, Beer MA, et al. Identification of miR-21 targets in breast cancer cells using a quantitative proteomic approach. Proteomics 2009;9(5):1374–84.

346. Si ML, Zhu S, Wu H, et al. miR-21-mediated tumor growth. Oncogene 2007;26(19):2799–803.

347. Lebanony D, Benjamin H, Gilad S, et al. Diagnostic assay based on hsa-miR-205 expression distinguishes squamous from nonsquamous non-small-cell lung carcinoma. J Clin Oncol 2009;27(12):2030–7.

348. Liang Y. An expression meta-analysis of predicted microRNA targets identifies a diagnostic signature for lung cancer. BMC Med Genomics 2008;1:61.

349. Chen X, Hu Z, Wang W, et al. Identification of ten serum microRNAs from a genome-wide serum microRNA expression profile as novel non-invasive biomarkers for non-small cell lung cancer diagnosis. Int J Cancer 2011. [Epub ahead of print].

350. Wei J, Gao W, Zhu CJ, et al. Identification of plasma microRNA-21 as a biomarker for early detection and chemosensitivity of non-small cell lung cancer. Chin J Cancer 2011;30(6):407–14.

351. Yu L, Todd NW, Xing L, et al. Early detection of lung adenocarcinoma in sputum by a panel of microRNA markers. Int J Cancer 2010;127(12):2870–8.

352. Weidhaas JB, Babar I, Nallur SM, et al. MicroRNAs as potential agents to alter resistance to cytotoxic anticancer therapy. Cancer Res 2007;67(23): 11111–6.

353. Rupaimoole R, Han HD, Lopez-Berestein G, et al. MicroRNA therapeutics: principles, expectations, and challenges. Chin J Cancer 2011;30(6):368–70.

354. Nana-Sinkam SP, Croce CM. MicroRNA dysregulation in cancer: opportunities for the development of microRNA-based drugs. IDrugs 2010;13(12): 843–6.

355. Anguiano A, Nevins JR, Potti A. Toward the individualization of lung cancer therapy. Cancer 2008; 113(Suppl 7):1760–7.

356. Xie Y, Minna JD. Predicting the future for people with lung cancer. Nat Med 2008;14(8):812–3.

357. Sriram KB, Larsen JE, Yang IA, et al. Genomic medicine in non-small cell lung cancer: paving the path to personalized care. Respirology 2011; 16(2):257–63.

358. Shedden K, Taylor JM, Enkemann SA, et al. Gene expression-based survival prediction in lung adenocarcinoma: a multi-site, blinded validation study. Nat Med 2008;14(8):822–7.

359. Subramanian J, Simon R. Gene expression-based prognostic signatures in lung cancer: ready for clinical use? J Natl Cancer Inst 2010;102(7):464–74.

360. Jeong Y, Xie Y, Xiao G, et al. Nuclear receptor expression defines a set of prognostic biomarkers for lung cancer. PLoS Med 2010;7(12):e1000378.

361. Paik S, Shak S, Tang G, et al. A multigene assay to predict recurrence of tamoxifen-treated, node-negative breast cancer. N Engl J Med 2004; 351(27):2817–26.

362. Meyerson M, Gabriel S, Getz G. Advances in understanding cancer genomes through second-generation sequencing. Nat Rev Genet 2010; 11(10):685–96.

363. Kan Z, Jaiswal BS, Stinson J, et al. Diverse somatic mutation patterns and pathway alterations in human cancers. Nature 2010;466(7308):869–73.

364. Whitehurst AW, Bodemann BO, Cardenas J, et al. Synthetic lethal screen identification of chemosensitizer loci in cancer cells. Nature 2007;446(7137): 815–9.

365. Vicent S, Chen R, Sayles LC, et al. Wilms tumor 1 (WT1) regulates KRAS-driven oncogenesis and senescence in mouse and human models. J Clin Invest 2010;120(11):3940–52.

366. Duex JE, Sorkin A. RNA interference screen identifies Usp18 as a regulator of epidermal growth factor receptor synthesis. Mol Biol Cell 2009; 20(6):1833–44.

367. Yamanaka S, Gu Z, Sato M, et al. siRNA targeting against EGFR, a promising candidate for a novel therapeutic application to lung adenocarcinoma. Pathobiology 2008;75(1):2–8.

368. Lara R, Mauri FA, Taylor H, et al. An siRNA screen identifies RSK1 as a key modulator of lung cancer metastasis. Oncogene 2011;30(32):3513–21.

369. Lundberg AS, Randell SH, Stewart SA, et al. Immortalization and transformation of primary human airway epithelial cells by gene transfer. Oncogene 2002;21(29):4577–86.

370. Ramirez RD, Sheridan S, Girard L, et al. Immortalization of human bronchial epithelial cells in the

absence of viral oncoproteins. Cancer Res 2004; 64(24):9027–34.

371. Sato M, Vaughan MB, Girard L, et al. Multiple oncogenic changes (K-RAS(V12), p53 knockdown, mutant EGFRs, p16 bypass, telomerase) are not sufficient to confer a full malignant phenotype on human bronchial epithelial cells. Cancer Res 2006;66(4):2116–28.

372. Sasai K, Sukezane T, Yanagita E, et al. Oncogene-mediated human lung epithelial cell transformation produces adenocarcinoma phenotypes in vivo. Cancer Res 2011;71(7):2541–9.

373. Fisher GH, Wellen SL, Klimstra D, et al. Induction and apoptotic regression of lung adenocarcinomas by regulation of a K-Ras transgene in the presence and absence of tumor suppressor genes. Genes Dev 2001;15(24):3249–62.

374. Politi K, Pao W. How genetically engineered mouse tumor models provide insights into human cancers. J Clin Oncol 2011;29(16):2273–81.

375. Brough R, Frankum JR, Costa-Cabral S, et al. Searching for synthetic lethality in cancer. Curr Opin Genet Dev 2011;21(1):34–41.

376. Rehman FL, Lord CJ, Ashworth A. Synthetic lethal approaches to breast cancer therapy. Nat Rev Clin Oncol 2010;7(12):718–24.

377. Kobayashi S, Boggon TJ, Dayaram T, et al. EGFR mutation and resistance of non-small-cell lung cancer to gefitinib. N Engl J Med 2005;352(8): 786–92.

378. Balak MN, Gong Y, Riely GJ, et al. Novel D761Y and common secondary T790M mutations in epidermal growth factor receptor-mutant lung adenocarcinomas with acquired resistance to kinase inhibitors. Clin Cancer Res 2006;12(21): 6494–501.

379. Kosaka T, Yatabe Y, Endoh H, et al. Analysis of epidermal growth factor receptor gene mutation in patients with non-small cell lung cancer and acquired resistance to gefitinib. Clin Cancer Res 2006;12(19):5764–9.

380. Kwak EL, Sordella R, Bell DW, et al. Irreversible inhibitors of the EGF receptor may circumvent acquired resistance to gefitinib. Proc Natl Acad Sci U S A 2005;102(21):7665–70.

381. Kosaka T, Yatabe Y, Endoh H, et al. Mutations of the epidermal growth factor receptor gene in lung cancer: biological and clinical implications. Cancer Res 2004;64(24):8919–23.

382. Mascaux C, Iannino N, Martin B, et al. The role of RAS oncogene in survival of patients with lung cancer: a systematic review of the literature with meta-analysis. Br J Cancer 2005; 92(1):131–9.

383. Shields JM, Pruitt K, McFall A, et al. Understanding Ras: 'it ain't over 'til it's over'. Trends Cell Biol 2000; 10(4):147–54.

384. Kawano O, Sasaki H, Endo K, et al. PIK3CA mutation status in Japanese lung cancer patients. Lung Cancer 2006;54(2):209–15.

385. Yamamoto H, Shigematsu H, Nomura M, et al. PIK3CA mutations and copy number gains in human lung cancers. Cancer Res 2008;68(17): 6913–21.

386. Guertin DA, Sabatini DM. Defining the role of mTOR in cancer. Cancer Cell 2007;12(1):9–22.

387. Maehama T, Dixon JE. The tumor suppressor, PTEN/MMAC1, dephosphorylates the lipid second messenger, phosphatidylinositol 3,4,5-trisphosphate. J Biol Chem 1998;273(22):13375–8.

388. Soria JC, Lee HY, Lee JI, et al. Lack of PTEN expression in non-small cell lung cancer could be related to promoter methylation. Clin Cancer Res 2002;8(5):1178–84.

389. Marsit CJ, Zheng S, Aldape K, et al. PTEN expression in non-small-cell lung cancer: evaluating its relation to tumor characteristics, allelic loss, and epigenetic alteration. Hum Pathol 2005;36(7):768–76.

390. Higashiyama M, Doi O, Kodama K, et al. MDM2 gene amplification and expression in non-small-cell lung cancer: immunohistochemical expression of its protein is a favourable prognostic marker in patients without p53 protein accumulation. Br J Cancer 1997;75(9):1302–8.

391. Gazzeri S, Della Valle V, Chaussade L, et al. The human p19ARF protein encoded by the beta transcript of the p16INK4a gene is frequently lost in small cell lung cancer. Cancer Res 1998;58(17): 3926–31.

392. Vonlanthen S, Heighway J, Tschan MP, et al. Expression of p16INK4a/p16alpha and p19ARF/ p16beta is frequently altered in non-small cell lung cancer and correlates with p53 overexpression. Oncogene 1998;17(21):2779–85.

393. Ohtani N, Yamakoshi K, Takahashi A, et al. The p16INK4a-RB pathway: molecular link between cellular senescence and tumor suppression. J Med Invest 2004;51(3–4):146–53.

394. Reissmann PT, Koga H, Takahashi R, et al. Inactivation of the retinoblastoma susceptibility gene in non-small-cell lung cancer. The Lung Cancer Study Group. Oncogene 1993;8(7):1913–9.

395. Merlo A, Gabrielson E, Askin F, et al. Frequent loss of chromosome 9 in human primary non-small cell lung cancer. Cancer Res 1994;54(3):640–2.

396. Brambilla E, Moro D, Gazzeri S, et al. Alterations of expression of Rb, p16(INK4A) and cyclin D1 in non-small cell lung carcinoma and their clinical significance. J Pathol 1999;188(4):351–60.

397. Sato M, Takahashi K, Nagayama K, et al. Identification of chromosome arm 9p as the most frequent target of homozygous deletions in lung cancer. Genes Chromosomes Cancer 2005;44(4): 405–14.

398. Esteller M. Cancer epigenetics: DNA methylation and chromatin alterations in human cancer. Adv Exp Med Biol 2003;532:39–49.

399. Kotake Y, Cao R, Viatour P, et al. pRB family proteins are required for H3K27 trimethylation and Polycomb repression complexes binding to and silencing p16INK4alpha tumor suppressor gene. Genes Dev 2007;21(1):49–54.

400. Shigematsu H, Gazdar AF. Somatic mutations of epidermal growth factor receptor signaling pathway in lung cancers. Int J Cancer 2006; 118(2):257–62.

401. Yousem SA, Nikiforova M, Nikiforov Y. The histopathology of BRAF-V600E-mutated lung adenocarcinoma. Am J Surg Pathol 2008;32(9):1317–21.

402. Nakamura H, Saji H, Ogata A, et al. Correlation between encoded protein overexpression and copy number of the HER2 gene with survival in non-small cell lung cancer. Int J Cancer 2003; 103(1):61–6.

403. Hirashima N, Takahashi W, Yoshii S, et al. Protein overexpression and gene amplification of c-erb B-2 in pulmonary carcinomas: a comparative immunohistochemical and fluorescence in situ hybridization study. Mod Pathol 2001;14(6): 556–62.

404. Tatematsu A, Shimizu J, Murakami Y, et al. Epidermal growth factor receptor mutations in small cell lung cancer. Clin Cancer Res 2008; 14(19):6092–6.

405. Swanton C, Futreal A, Eisen T. Her2-targeted therapies in non-small cell lung cancer. Clin Cancer Res 2006;12(14 Pt 2):4377s–83s.

406. Rodenhuis S, van de Wetering ML, Mooi WJ, et al. Mutational activation of the K-ras oncogene. A possible pathogenetic factor in adenocarcinoma of the lung. N Engl J Med 1987;317(15):929–35.

407. De Biasi F, Del Sal G, Hand PH. Evidence of enhancement of the ras oncogene protein product (p21) in a spectrum of human tumors. Int J Cancer 1989;43(3):431–5.

408. Potiron VA, Roche J, Drabkin HA. Semaphorins and their receptors in lung cancer. Cancer Lett 2008; 273(1):1–14.

409. Lee JW, Soung YH, Kim SY, et al. PIK3CA gene is frequently mutated in breast carcinomas and hepatocellular carcinomas. Oncogene 2005;24(8): 1477–80.

410. Davies H, Hunter C, Smith R, et al. Somatic mutations of the protein kinase gene family in human lung cancer. Cancer Res 2005;65(17):7591–5.

411. Micke P, Hengstler JG, Ros R, et al. c-erbB-2 expression in small-cell lung cancer is associated with poor prognosis. Int J Cancer 2001;92(4): 474–9.

412. Potti A, Willardson J, Forseen C, et al. Predictive role of HER-2/neu overexpression and clinical features at initial presentation in patients with extensive stage small cell lung carcinoma. Lung Cancer 2002;36(3):257–61.

413. Dworakowska D, Jassem E, Jassem J, et al. MDM2 gene amplification: a new independent factor of adverse prognosis in non-small cell lung cancer (NSCLC). Lung Cancer 2004;43(3):285–95.

414. Cappuzzo F, Janne PA, Skokan M, et al. MET increased gene copy number and primary resistance to gefitinib therapy in non-small-cell lung cancer patients. Ann Oncol 2009;20(2):298–304.

415. Beau-Faller M, Ruppert AM, Voegeli AC, et al. MET gene copy number in non-small cell lung cancer: molecular analysis in a targeted tyrosine kinase inhibitor naive cohort. J Thorac Oncol 2008;3(4): 331–9.

416. Johnson BE, Russell E, Simmons AM, et al. MYC family DNA amplification in 126 tumor cell lines from patients with small cell lung cancer. J Cell Biochem Suppl 1996;24:210–7.

417. Ibson JM, Waters JJ, Twentyman PR, et al. Oncogene amplification and chromosomal abnormalities in small cell lung cancer. J Cell Biochem 1987; 33(4):267–88.

418. Shiraishi M, Noguchi M, Shimosato Y, et al. Amplification of protooncogenes in surgical specimens of human lung carcinomas. Cancer Res 1989; 49(23):6474–9.

419. Miller CT, Chen G, Gharib TG, et al. Increased C-CRK proto-oncogene expression is associated with an aggressive phenotype in lung adenocarcinomas. Oncogene 2003;22(39):7950–7.

420. Pezzella F, Turley H, Kuzu I, et al. bcl-2 protein in non-small-cell lung carcinoma. N Engl J Med 1993;329(10):690–4.

421. Kaiser U, Schilli M, Haag U, et al. Expression of bcl-2–protein in small cell lung cancer. Lung Cancer 1996;15(1):31–40.

422. Reissmann PT, Koga H, Figlin RA, et al. Amplification and overexpression of the cyclin D1 and epidermal growth factor receptor genes in non-small-cell lung cancer. Lung Cancer Study Group. J Cancer Res Clin Oncol 1999;125(2):61–70.

423. Eren B, Sar M, Oz B, et al. MMP-2, TIMP-2 and CD44v6 expression in non-small-cell lung carcinomas. Ann Acad Med Singapore 2008;37(1):32–9.

424. Junker K, Wiethege T, Muller KM. Pathology of small-cell lung cancer. J Cancer Res Clin Oncol 2000;126(7):361–8.

425. Micke P, Basrai M, Faldum A, et al. Characterization of c-kit expression in small cell lung cancer: prognostic and therapeutic implications. Clin Cancer Res 2003;9(1):188–94.

426. Cook RM, Miller YE, Bunn PA Jr. Small cell lung cancer: etiology, biology, clinical features, staging, and treatment. Curr Probl Cancer 1993;17(2): 69–141.

427. Araki K, Ishii G, Yokose T, et al. Frequent overexpression of the c-kit protein in large cell neuroendocrine carcinoma of the lung. Lung Cancer 2003; 40(2):173–80.

428. Rygaard K, Nakamura T, Spang-Thomsen M. Expression of the proto-oncogenes c-met and c-kit and their ligands, hepatocyte growth factor/scatter factor and stem cell factor, in SCLC cell lines and xenografts. Br J Cancer 1993;67(1):37–46.

429. Plummer H 3rd, Catlett J, Leftwich J, et al. c-myc expression correlates with suppression of c-kit protooncogene expression in small cell lung cancer cell lines. Cancer Res 1993;53(18):4337–42.

430. Hibi K, Takahashi T, Sekido Y, et al. Coexpression of the stem cell factor and the c-kit genes in small-cell lung cancer. Oncogene 1991;6(12): 2291–6.

431. Weiner DB, Nordberg J, Robinson R, et al. Expression of the neu gene-encoded protein (P185neu) in human non-small cell carcinomas of the lung. Cancer Res 1990;50(2):421–5.

432. Schneider PM, Hung MC, Chiocca SM, et al. Differential expression of the c-erbB-2 gene in human small cell and non-small cell lung cancer. Cancer Res 1989;49(18):4968–71.

433. Fernandes A, Hamburger AW, Gerwin BI. ErbB-2 kinase is required for constitutive stat 3 activation in malignant human lung epithelial cells. Int J Cancer 1999;83(4):564–70.

434. Rygaard K, Vindelov LL, Spang-Thomsen M. Expression of myc family oncoproteins in small-cell lung-cancer cell lines and xenografts. Int J Cancer 1993;54(1):144–52.

435. Takahashi T, Obata Y, Sekido Y, et al. Expression and amplification of myc gene family in small cell lung cancer and its relation to biological characteristics. Cancer Res 1989;49(10):2683–8.

436. Spencer CA, Groudine M. Control of c-myc regulation in normal and neoplastic cells. Adv Cancer Res 1991;56:1–48.

437. Zhang P, Gao WY, Turner S, et al. Gleevec (STI-571) inhibits lung cancer cell growth (A549) and potentiates the cisplatin effect in vitro. Mol Cancer 2003;2:1.

438. Rikova K, Guo A, Zeng Q, et al. Global survey of phosphotyrosine signaling identifies oncogenic kinases in lung cancer. Cell 2007;131(6): 1190–203.

439. Johnson FM, Krug LM, Tran HT, et al. Phase I studies of imatinib mesylate combined with cisplatin and irinotecan in patients with small cell lung carcinoma. Cancer 2006;106(2):366–74.

440. Rossi G, Cavazza A, Marchioni A, et al. Role of chemotherapy and the receptor tyrosine kinases KIT, PDGFRalpha, PDGFRbeta, and Met in large-cell neuroendocrine carcinoma of the lung. J Clin Oncol 2005;23(34):8774–85.

441. Ji H, Ramsey MR, Hayes DN, et al. LKB1 modulates lung cancer differentiation and metastasis. Nature 2007;448(7155):807–10.

442. Koivunen JP, Kim J, Lee J, et al. Mutations in the LKB1 tumour suppressor are frequently detected in tumours from Caucasian but not Asian lung cancer patients. Br J Cancer 2008;99(2): 245–52.

443. Carbone DP, Mitsudomi T, Chiba I, et al. p53 immunostaining positivity is associated with reduced survival and is imperfectly correlated with gene mutations in resected non-small cell lung cancer. A preliminary report of LCSG 871. Chest 1994; 106(Suppl 6):377S–81S.

444. Wistuba II, Berry J, Behrens C, et al. Molecular changes in the bronchial epithelium of patients with small cell lung cancer. Clin Cancer Res 2000;6(7):2604–10.

445. Chiba I, Takahashi T, Nau MM, et al. Mutations in the p53 gene are frequent in primary, resected non-small cell lung cancer. Lung Cancer Study Group. Oncogene 1990;5(10):1603–10.

446. Shimizu E, Zhao M, Shinohara A, et al. Differential expressions of cyclin A and the retinoblastoma gene product in histological subtypes of lung cancer cell lines. J Cancer Res Clin Oncol 1997; 123(10):533–8.

447. Salgia R, Skarin AT. Molecular abnormalities in lung cancer. J Clin Oncol 1998;16(3):1207–17.

448. Hensel CH, Hsieh CL, Gazdar AF, et al. Altered structure and expression of the human retinoblastoma susceptibility gene in small cell lung cancer. Cancer Res 1990;50(10):3067–72.

449. Girard L, Zochbauer-Muller S, Virmani AK, et al. Genome-wide allelotyping of lung cancer identifies new regions of allelic loss, differences between small cell lung cancer and non-small cell lung cancer, and loci clustering. Cancer Res 2000; 60(17):4894–906.

450. Thiberville L, Payne P, Vielkinds J, et al. Evidence of cumulative gene losses with progression of premalignant epithelial lesions to carcinoma of the bronchus. Cancer Res 1995;55(22):5133–9.

451. Sunaga N, Miyajima K, Suzuki M, et al. Different roles for caveolin-1 in the development of non-small cell lung cancer versus small cell lung cancer. Cancer Res 2004;64(12):4277–85.

452. Mori S, Ito G, Usami N, et al. p53 apoptotic pathway molecules are frequently and simultaneously altered in nonsmall cell lung carcinoma. Cancer 2004;100(8):1673–82.

453. Prudkin L, Behrens C, Liu DD, et al. Loss and reduction of FUS1 protein expression is a frequent phenomenon in the pathogenesis of lung cancer. Clin Cancer Res 2008;14(1):41–7.

454. Safar AM, Spencer H 3rd, Su X, et al. Methylation profiling of archived non-small cell lung cancer:

a promising prognostic system. Clin Cancer Res 2005;11(12):4400–5.

455. Toyooka S, Toyooka KO, Maruyama R, et al. DNA methylation profiles of lung tumors. Mol Cancer Ther 2001;1(1):61–7.

456. Shimamoto T, Ohyashiki JH, Hirano T, et al. Hyper-methylation of E-cadherin gene is frequent and independent of p16INK4A methylation in non-small cell lung cancer: potential prognostic implication. Oncol Rep 2004;12(2):389–95.

457. Jarmalaite S, Kannio A, Anttila S, et al. Aberrant p16 promoter methylation in smokers and former smokers with nonsmall cell lung cancer. Int J Cancer 2003;106(6):913–8.

458. Esteller M, Sanchez-Cespedes M, Rosell R, et al. Detection of aberrant promoter hypermethylation of tumor suppressor genes in serum DNA from non-small cell lung cancer patients. Cancer Res 1999;59(1):67–70.

459. Kim DS, Cha SI, Lee JH, et al. Aberrant DNA meth-ylation profiles of non-small cell lung cancers in a Korean population. Lung Cancer 2007;58(1):1–6.

460. Suh YA, Lee HY, Virmani A, et al. Loss of retinoic acid receptor beta gene expression is linked to aberrant histone H3 acetylation in lung cancer cell lines. Cancer Res 2002;62(14):3945–9.

461. Dammann R, Li C, Yoon JH, et al. Epigenetic inac-tivation of a RAS association domain family protein from the lung tumour suppressor locus 3p21.3. Nat Genet 2000;25(3):315–9.

462. Speicher MR, Gwyn Ballard S, Ward DC. Karyotyp-ing human chromosomes by combinatorial multi-fluor FISH. Nat Genet 1996;12(4):368–75.

463. Balsara BR, Testa JR. Chromosomal imbalances in human lung cancer. Oncogene 2002;21(45): 6877–83.

464. Luk C, Tsao MS, Bayani J, et al. Molecular cytoge-netic analysis of non-small cell lung carcinoma by spectral karyotyping and comparative genomic hybridization. Cancer Genet Cytogenet 2001; 125(2):87–99.

465. Petersen I, Bujard M, Petersen S, et al. Patterns of chromosomal imbalances in adenocarcinoma and squamous cell carcinoma of the lung. Cancer Res 1997;57(12):2331–5.

466. Petersen I, Langreck H, Wolf G, et al. Small-cell lung cancer is characterized by a high incidence of deletions on chromosomes 3p, 4q, 5q, 10q, 13q and 17p. Br J Cancer 1997;75(1):79–86.

467. Sung JM, Cho HJ, Yi H, et al. Characterization of a stem cell population in lung cancer A549 cells. Biochem Biophys Res Commun 2008;371(1): 163–7.

468. Levina V, Marrangoni AM, DeMarco R, et al. Drug-selected human lung cancer stem cells: cytokine network, tumorigenic and metastatic properties. PLoS One 2008;3(8):e3077.

469. Sullivan JP, Minna JD, Shay JW. Evidence for self-renewing lung cancer stem cells and their implications in tumor initiation, progression, and targeted therapy. Cancer Metastasis Rev 2010; 29(1):61–72.

470. Ucar D, Cogle CR, Zucali JR, et al. Aldehyde dehy-drogenase activity as a functional marker for lung cancer. Chem Biol Interact 2009;178(1–3):48–55.

471. Cui F, Wang J, Chen D, et al. CD133 is a temporary marker of cancer stem cells in small cell lung cancer, but not in non-small cell lung cancer. Oncol Rep 2011;25(3):701–8.

472. Gutova M, Najbauer J, Gevorgyan A, et al. Iden-tification of uPAR-positive chemoresistant cells in small cell lung cancer. PLoS One 2007;2(2): e243.

473. Wen J, Fu J, Zhang W, et al. Genetic and epige-netic changes in lung carcinoma and their clinical implications. Mod Pathol 2011;24(7):932–43.

474. Ji H, Wang Z, Perera SA, et al. Mutations in BRAF and KRAS converge on activation of the mitogen-activated protein kinase pathway in lung cancer mouse models. Cancer Res 2007;67(10):4933–9.

475. Ji H, Li D, Chen L, et al. The impact of human EGFR kinase domain mutations on lung tumorigenesis and in vivo sensitivity to EGFR-targeted therapies. Cancer Cell 2006;9(6):485–95.

476. Politi K, Zakowski MF, Fan PD, et al. Lung adeno-carcinomas induced in mice by mutant EGF recep-tors found in human lung cancers respond to a tyrosine kinase inhibitor or to down-regulation of the receptors. Genes Dev 2006;20(11):1496–510.

477. Regales L, Balak MN, Gong Y, et al. Development of new mouse lung tumor models expressing EGFR T790M mutants associated with clinical resistance to kinase inhibitors. PLoS One 2007; 2(8):e810.

478. Zhou W, Ercan D, Chen L, et al. Novel mutant-selective EGFR kinase inhibitors against EGFR T790M. Nature 2009;462(7276):1070–4.

479. Ji H, Zhao X, Yuza Y, et al. Epidermal growth factor receptor variant III mutations in lung tumorigenesis and sensitivity to tyrosine kinase inhibitors. Proc Natl Acad Sci U S A 2006;103(20):7817–22.

480. Chen Z, Sasaki T, Tan X, et al. Inhibition of ALK, PI3K/MEK, and HSP90 in murine lung adenocarci-noma induced by EML4-ALK fusion oncogene. Cancer Res 2010;70(23):9827–36.

481. Perera SA, Li D, Shimamura T, et al. HER2YVMA drives rapid development of adenosquamous lung tumors in mice that are sensitive to BIBW2992 and rapamycin combination therapy. Proc Natl Acad Sci U S A 2009;106(2):474–9.

482. Jackson EL, Willis N, Mercer K, et al. Analysis of lung tumor initiation and progression using condi-tional expression of oncogenic K-ras. Genes Dev 2001;15(24):3243–8.

483. Meuwissen R, Linn SC, van der Valk M, et al. Mouse model for lung tumorigenesis through Cre/lox controlled sporadic activation of the K-Ras oncogene. Oncogene 2001;20(45):6551–8.

484. Kim WY, Perera S, Zhou B, et al. HIF2alpha cooperates with RAS to promote lung tumorigenesis in mice. J Clin Invest 2009;119(8):2160–70.

485. Jackson EL, Olive KP, Tuveson DA, et al. The differential effects of mutant p53 alleles on advanced murine lung cancer. Cancer Res 2005;65(22): 10280–8.

486. Iwanaga K, Yang Y, Raso MG, et al. Pten inactivation accelerates oncogenic K-ras-initiated tumorigenesis in a mouse model of lung cancer. Cancer Res 2008;68(4):1119–27.

487. Olive KP, Tuveson DA, Ruhe ZC, et al. Mutant p53 gain of function in two mouse models of Li-Fraumeni syndrome. Cell 2004;119(6):847–60.

488. Meuwissen R, Linn SC, Linnoila RI, et al. Induction of small cell lung cancer by somatic inactivation of both Trp53 and Rb1 in a conditional mouse model. Cancer Cell 2003;4(3):181–9.

The Revised Stage Classification System for Primary Lung Cancer

Daniel J. Boffa, MD

KEYWORDS

• Stage classification • Primary lung cancer • Prognosis

The lung cancer stage classification system was revised for the seventh edition of the American Joint Committee on Cancer (AJCC) staging manual to reflect important changes in the understanding of prognostic significance of the tumor, node, metastasis (TNM) staging parameters. These advances were the direct result of a global staging project organized through the International Association for the Study of Lung Cancer (IASLC).[1] The revisions proposed by the IASLC were accepted by the Union Internationale Contre le Cancer (UICC) and AJCC and published in the seventh edition of the staging manual in 2009.[2] The revised staging parameters are listed in **Table 1** and all of the changes to the TNM staging parameters are listed in **Table 2**.

The revised stage classification system now applies the same TNM nomenclature to small cell lung cancer (replacing limited and extensive)[3]; however, the focus of this article is non–small cell lung cancer (NSCLC). In addition to the changes for each staging parameter, several important aspects of stage classification were clarified by the staging project and are outlined in the text. As with many advances, the considerable improvements have exposed/emphasized additional areas to be addressed in subsequent iterations of the staging project. Examples of such areas are also listed.

THE STAGING PROJECT

In 1999, the IASLC staging committees were organized to explore each of the TNM staging parameters. A global staging database was created containing 81,015 primary lung cancers diagnosed between 1990 and 2000. Submitted lung cancer cases originated in Europe (58%), North America (21%), Asia (14%), and Australia (7%), and were collected as part of case series (40%), registries (30%), and clinical trials (30%). The distribution of tumors included 16% small cell lung cancer (SCLC) and 84% NSCLC. The NSCLC treatment included surgery alone (41%), chemotherapy only (23%), radiotherapy (11%), and multimodality (25%).[1] Although all of the staging and survival data were validated, the treatment data were not and clinicians are cautioned against using the treatment data from the database to make clinical decisions.[4] In 2007, the results of the analysis were published in a series of articles outlining the proposed changes.[5–9] The key findings of the IASLC staging project were subsequently validated using data from the Surveillance, Epidemiology and End Results (SEER) database.[8]

T STAGE

The T staging parameter was evaluated using clinical M0, treatment-naive subsets of the IASLC staging database. Tumor size was explored using a learning set of 2284 completely resected pT1N0 and 2607 pT2N0 NSCLC tumors.[6] A log-rank statistical model identified 3 new size cut points (2, 5, and 7 cm) corresponding with significant differences in prognosis. As a result, the T parameter was reclassified as T1a (0–2 cm), T1b (>2–3 cm), T2a (>3–5 cm), T2b (>5–7 cm),

Thoracic Surgery, Yale University School of Medicine, 330 Cedar Street, BB205, 208062, New Haven, CT 06520, USA
E-mail address: daniel.boffa@yale.edu

Clin Chest Med 32 (2011) 741–748
doi:10.1016/j.ccm.2011.08.013
0272-5231/11/$ – see front matter © 2011 Elsevier Inc. All rights reserved.

chestmed.theclinics.com

Table 1
T staging parameters

Tumor and Subgroup[a]	Definition
T (primary tumor)	
T0	No primary tumor
T1	Tumor ≤3 cm,[b] surrounded by lung or visceral pleura, not more proximal than the lobar bronchus
T1a	Tumor ≤2 cm[b]
T1b	Tumor >2 but ≤3 cm[b]
T2	Tumor >3 but ≤7 cm[b] or tumor with any of the following[c]: invades visceral pleura, involves main bronchus ≥2 cm distal to the carina, atelectasis/obstructive pneumonia extending to hilum but not involving the entire lung
T2a	Tumor >3 cm but ≤5 cm[b]
T2b	Tumor >5 cm but ≤7 cm[b]
T3	
T3$_{>7}$	Tumor >7 cm[b]
T3$_{Inv}$	Directly invading chest wall, diaphragm, phrenic nerve, mediastinal pleura, parietal pericardium
T3$_{Centr}$	Tumor in the main bronchus <2 cm distal to the carina[d] or atelectasis/obstructive pneumonitis of entire lung
T3$_{Satell}$	Separate tumor nodule(s) in the same lobe
T4	
T4$_{Inv}$	Tumor of any size with invasion of heart, great vessels, trachea, recurrent laryngeal nerve, esophagus, vertebral body, or carina
T4$_{Ipsi\ Nod}$	Separate tumor nodule(s) in a different ipsilateral lobe
N (regional lymph nodes)	
N0	No region node metastasis
N1	Metastasis in ipsilateral peribronchial or perihilar lymph nodes and intrapulmonary nodes, including involvement by direct extension
N2	Metastasis in ipsilateral mediastinal or subcarinal lymph node(s)
N3	Metastasis in contralateral mediastinal, contralateral hilar, ipsilateral or contralateral scalene, or supraclavicular lymph node(s)
M (distant metastasis)	
M0	No distant metastasis
M1a	
M1 a$_{Contr\ Nod}$	Separate tumor nodule(s) in a contralateral lobe
M1 a$_{Pl\ Dissem}$	Tumor with pleural nodules or malignant pleural dissemination[e]
M1 b	Distant metastasis
Special situations	
TX, NX	T or N status not able to be assessed
T$_{is}$	Focus of in situ cancer
T1[d]	
T1$_{ss}$	Superficial spreading tumor of any size but confined to the wall of the trachea or mainstem bronchus

[a] These subgroup labels are not defined in the International Association for the study of Lung Cancer publications[1–4] but are added for clarity.
[b] In greatest dimension.
[c] T2 tumors with these features are classified as T2a if less than or equal to 5 cm.
[d] The uncommon, superficial spreading tumor in central airways is classified as T1.
[e] Pleural effusions that are cytologically negative, nonbloody, transudative, and clinically judged not to be caused by cancer are excluded.

From Detterbeck FC, Boffa DJ, Tanoue LT, et al. The new lung cancer staging system. Chest 2009;136:262; with permission.

Table 2
Summary of changes to TNM staging parameters

Previous (6th Edition)	Revised (7th Edition)
T1 (0–3 cm)	T1a (0–2 cm)
T2 (>3 cm)	T1b (>2–3 cm)
	T2a (3–5 cm)
	T2b (>5–7 cm)
	T3 (>7 cm)
T4 (multiple nodules in same lobe)	T3
T4 (malignant pleural effusion)	M1a
M1 (ipsilateral nodule in different lobe)	T4
M1 (systemic metastases)	M1a (separate nodules in contralateral lobe; malignant pleural dissemination)
	M1b (distant metastases)

and T3 (>7 cm) (**Fig. 1** and **Table 1**). This model was validated using 2589 pT1 and pT2N0M0 patients.

This staging project also reevaluated the prognostic impact of multiple ipsilateral tumor nodules. The number of cases was small (n = 363 for same-lobe nodules), forcing the committee to group together data from all resection types (complete and incomplete) and nodal statuses (N1, N2, N3). The analysis showed that multiple ipsilateral nodules in the same lobe or different lobes as the dominant tumor were associated with a better prognosis than their previous sixth edition staging cohorts (**Fig. 2**). Specifically, ipsilateral tumor

nodules occurring in the same lobe as the dominant tumor had a survival similar to the T3N0 staging category, and therefore were reclassified as T3 (previously T4) (see **Tables 1** and **2**). Similarly, the outcome with multiple nodules involving the different ipsilateral lobes more closely approximated T4N0 staging category, and as such are now classified as T4 (previously M1) (see **Fig. 2**).

There are several aspects to patients with multiple nodules that remain challenging. First, the additional tumor nodules must be derived from the dominant tumor nodule. The intention was not to include microscopic multicentricity, but grossly detectable separate nodules. However, the definition of gross is left to the pathologist and is subject to interpretation. Second is the need to distinguish between ipsilateral tumor nodules and multifocal lung cancer. Although concordance of histologic features supports a single tumor process (progeny of the dominant tumor), multifocal cancers may be similar histologically. Again, the onus for this determination is on the pathologist, which may impart a degree of variability. Multidisciplinary input is often critical to distinguish these processes. In addition, it must be a priority to clarify the cause of multiple nodules during the clinical staging evaluation. Thus far, the noninvasive and invasive staging recommendations have included interwoven considerations of the TNM staging variables with recommendations for studies targeting the TNM attributes based on cumulative probabilities and clinically important findings.[10,11] For example, the recommendation to perform invasive mediastinal staging reflects the pretest probability for mediastinal lymph node metastases as determined by considering T and M attributes. Invasive mediastinal staging is not recommended for peripheral T1a N0M0 lesions, but is recommended

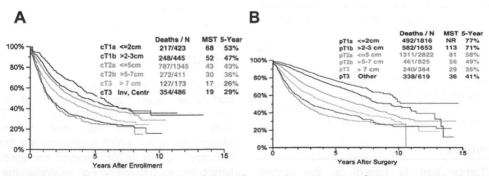

Fig. 1. Prognosis according to size category. (*A*) Overall survival by tumor size for patients with cT1 to 3N0M0 tumors using the IASLC classification. (*B*) Overall survival by tumor size for patients with pT1 to 3N0M0 R0 tumors using the IASLC classification. Centr, central; Inv, invasion; MST, median survival time (months); 5-year, 5-year overall survival. (*From* Rami-Porta R, Ball D, Crowley J, et al. The IASLC Lung Cancer Staging Project: proposals for revision of the T descriptors in the forthcoming (seventh) edition of the TNM classification of lung cancer. J Thorac Oncol 2007;2:593–602; with permission.)

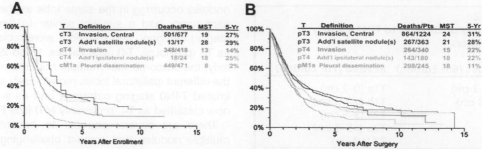

Fig. 2. Prognosis according to additional nodules, T4 invasion, and pleural dissemination. (*A*) Overall survival for patients with cT3,4/cM1a status because of additional tumor nodules using the IASLC classification (any cN), compared with other categories of T3 and T4. (*B*) Overall survival for patients with pT3,4/pM1a status because of additional tumor nodules using the IASLC classification (any pN, any R), compared with other categories of T3 and T4. (*From* Rami-Porta R, Ball D, Crowley J, et al. The IASLC Lung Cancer Staging Project: proposals for revision of the T descriptors in the forthcoming (seventh) edition of the TNM classification of lung cancer. J Thorac Oncol 2007;2:593–602, with permission.)

for T3N0M0 lesions that invade the chest wall because of an association of these tumors with mediastinal lymph node metastases. Less is known about the relationship between multiple pulmonary nodules and other N and M staging parameters, largely because most cases that have been studied did not appreciate the additional nodules during the clinical staging evaluation.[12–16] The IASLC analyses were based exclusively on pathologic data, because few cases were clinically staged as having multiple nodules.

There were insufficient data to evaluate the prognostic importance of visceral pleural invasion, so the staging committee left the designation as a T2 determinate (see **Table 1**).

The specific definitions of the T staging parameters are listed in **Table 1** and changes are summarized in **Table 2**. In addition to redefining the staging parameters, several important aspects of staging were clarified.[17]

Summary of Changes

- T1 and 2 separated into a and b by size
- Tumors greater than 7 cm become T3
- Multiple nodules in the same lobe become T3 (from T4)
- Multiple ipsilateral nodules in different lobes become T4 (from M1)
- Malignant pleural and pericardial dissemination moves from T4 to M1a

Clarifications

- Tumor size is based on the largest measurement by CT scanning
- T2 visceral pleural invasion considered invasion beyond elastic layer
- T3 includes invasion into, but not through, mediastinal pleura or parietal pericardium

- T4 includes invasion through mediastinal pleura, including recurrent nerve, superior vena cava, as well as intrapericardial pulmonary artery and veins
- Superior sulcus tumors (Pancoast) are T4 if they involve C8 nerve root, brachial plexus, subclavian vessels, vertebral bodies, or spinal canal
- Additional nodules must be grossly identifiable to be considered (as opposed to microscopic multicentricity)

Outstanding Issues

- Visceral pleural invasion prognosis not validated
- Unclear whether both invasive and lepidic tumor components to be considered in size determination for tumors with large ground-glass component and mixed histology
- Determining whether multiple nodules are metastases or separate primaries is left to pathologist
- Role of clinically detected multiple nodules

N STAGE

One of the first observations of the staging committee was the recognition of regional discrepancies in lymph node mapping. Specifically, the Japanese map and the map of Mountain-Dresler, which is used by the American Thoracic Society (ATS), handled the mediastinal lymph nodes differently. For example, the Japanese map tended to subdivide the lower paratracheal lymph nodes (ATS levels R4 and L4) into 2, 3, and 4. As a result, a significant advance has been the creation of an international consensus nodal map (**Fig. 3**). This map promotes greater

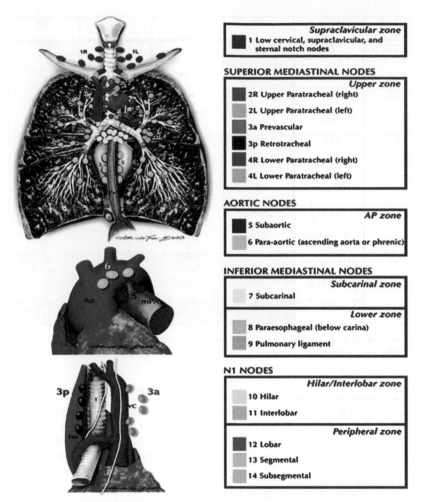

Fig. 3. The IASLC lymph node map, including the proposed grouping of lymph node stations into zones for prognostic analyses. (*From* Rusch VW, Asamura H, Watanabe H, et al. The IASLC Lung Cancer Staging Project: a proposal for a new international lymph node map in the forthcoming 7th edition of the TNM Classification for Lung Cancer. J Thorac Oncol 2009;4:574; with permission.)

consistency in future data collection. The N staging parameter explored 28,371 patients who were pathologically staged as M0 with complete nodal staging data.[7] This work confirmed the prognostic stratification associated with the N0, N1, N2, and N3 staging designations.

The committee also explored additional stratification by separating the hilar and mediastinal lymph node maps into zones. A total of 2876 tumors were staged with sufficient detail to analyze this strategy. Although multiple zone involvement seemed to portend a worse prognosis, the dataset was too small to justify changing the N staging parameter and there did seem to be questions with homogeneity (60% of the patients were submitted by Japan). This question will be explored in subsequent iterations of the stage classification system and may lead to a redefinition in the future.

Summary of Changes

- No changes

Clarifications

- A consensus nodal map was created
- Direct extension/invasion into a lymph node by the primary tumor is classified as nodal metastasis
- Nodal metastases invading adjacent structures are classified by the nodal station (N2 metastasis invading the trachea remains N2)
- Invasive mediastinal staging (mediastinoscopy, endobronchial ultrasound) considered clinical staging (clinical staging is defined as being before tumor resection)
- Micrometastases are considered positive nodes, but isolated tumors cells are not

T/M	Subgroups	N0	N1	N2	N3
T1	T1a	IA	IIA	IIIA	IIIB
	T1b	IA	IIA	IIIA	IIIB
T2	T2a	IB	IIA	IIIA	IIIB
	T2b	IIA	IIB	IIIA	IIIB
T3	T3 >7	IIB	IIIA	IIIA	IIIB
	T3 Inv	IIB	IIIA	IIIA	IIIB
	T3 Satell	IIB	IIIA	IIIA	IIIB
T4	T4 Inv	IIIA	IIIA	IIIB	IIIB
	T4 Ipsi Nod	IIIA	IIIA	IIIB	IIIB
M1	M1a Contr Nod	IV	IV	IV	IV
	M1a Pl Dissem	IV	IV	IV	IV
	M1b	IV	IV	IV	IV

Fig. 4. Stage groups according to TNM descriptor and subgroups. (*Reprinted from* Detterbeck FC, Boffa DJ, Tanoue LT, et al. The new lung cancer staging system. Chest 2009;136:267; with permission.)

Outstanding Issues

- Prognostic importance of multiple nodal zone involvement

M STAGE

The M stage was evaluated using 6596 cases represented by their best stage (pathologic rather than clinical, if both available).[9] The M staging parameter was separated into M1a and M1b. Malignant pleural dissemination was moved into M1a (previously T4) (see **Tables 1** and **2**). Contralateral pulmonary tumor nodules are considered M1a (previously M1). All other distant metastases are considered M1b. Patients with a single metatastic lesion (oligometastatic disease) were not found to have a better prognosis than patients with more widely disseminated disease, but the analysis was underpowered. Nonregional lymph nodes, such as intra-abdominal and axillary nodes, are considered M1b.

Summary of Changes

- M1 separated into a and b
- Malignant pleural and pericardial dissemination is M1a
- Contralateral pulmonary nodules are M1a
- Distant metastases are M1b

Clarifications

- Nonregional lymph node metastases are M1b[17]

Outstanding Issues

- Assess survival differences between oligometastatic, brain-limited oligometastatic and more widespread disease
- The importance in survival difference between M1a and M1b is unclear

Table 3
Types of staging assessments

Prefix	Name	Definition
c	Clinical	Before initiation of any treatment, using any and all information available (eg, including mediastinoscopy)
p	Pathologic	After resection, based on pathologic assessment
y	Restaging	After part or all of the treatment has been given
r	Recurrence	Stage at time of a recurrence
a	Autopsy	Stage as determined by autopsy

From Detterbeck FC, Boffa DJ, Tanoue LT, et al. The new lung cancer staging system. Chest 2009;136:261; with permission.

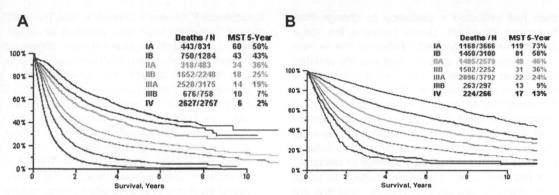

Fig. 5. Survival by stage groupings. (*A*) Overall survival by clinical stage for the proposed IASLC stage grouping. (*B*) Overall survival by pathologic stage for the proposed IASLC stage grouping. (*From* Goldstraw P, Crowley J, Chansky K, et al. The IASLC Lung Cancer Staging Project: proposals for the revision of the TNM stage groupings in the forthcoming (seventh) edition of the TNM Classification of malignant tumours. J Thorac Oncol 2007;2:706–14.)

STAGE GROUPINGS

For the most part, the changes in TNM staging parameters are clustered into the same stage groupings as the previous version of the stage classification system, with tumors moving in accordance with the revised parameters. The exceptions are T4N0M0 and T4N1M0, both of which were stage IIIB in the previous staging system but have become IIIA in the revised system. The new stage groupings are listed in **Fig. 4** and types of staging assessments in **Table 3**. The survival curves for clinically staged and pathologically staged patients are shown in **Fig. 5**.

STAGE SHIFTERS

As the seventh edition of the staging system was implemented, several tumors were assigned a staging designation in the revised version that differed from the previous version. These patients are referred to as the stage shifters, because of the apparent upstaging or downstaging by the change in staging nomenclature (**Table 4**). Between 10% and 15% of patients are be affected by this phenomenon.

It is not clear how these changes in staging nomenclature will affect treatment decisions. When lung cancer clinicians were surveyed, more

Table 4
The NSCLC stage shifters

	6th Edition Characteristics	Former Stage	New Stage	% IASLC Patients
Upstaged	T2$_{(>5\ but\ \leq7\ cm)}$ N0 M0	1B	2A	3.8
	T2$_{(>7\ cm)}$ N0 M0	1B	2B	1.7
	T2$_{(>7\ cm)}$ N0 M0	2B	3A	0.8
	Malignant pleural involvement	3B	4	2.5
Downstaged	T2$_{(\leq5\ cm)}$ N1	2B	2A	4.4
	Separate tumor nodules in same lobe, N0	3B	2B	0.6
	Separate tumor nodules in same lobe, N1, N2	3B	3A	0.7
	Separate tumor nodules in different ipsilateral lobe N0, N1	4	3A	0.4
	Separate tumor nodules in different ipsilateral lobe N2, 3	4	3B	0.3
	T4$_{(extension)}$ N0, N1	3B	3A	1.6

Abbreviations: IASLC, International Association for Study of Lung Cancer; NSCLC, non–small cell lung cancer.
From Boffa DJ, Detterbeck FC, Smith EJ, et al. Should the 7th edition of the lung cancer stage classification system change treatment algorithms in NSCLC? J Thorac Oncol 2010;5(11):1780; with permission.

than half indicated a tendency to change their treatment approach, simply because the stage designation had changed.[4] Although the revised stage classification system does provide updated prognostic information, prognosis alone does not define the best treatment. Other factors such as comorbidities, anatomic considerations, and local expertise all must be factored into a treatment plan. Furthermore, even if one wished to replicate the results observed in the staging database, because treatment data was defined or validated, it is not clear which treatment strategy to adopt and which to abandon. Therefore clinicians are encouraged to consider all aspects of a specific patient, and, whenever possible, apply randomized trial data that most closely approximate the tumor attributes of the patient in question.

SUMMARY

The revised NSCLC stage classification system has greatly improved the ability of clinicians to estimate prognosis based on specific TNM staging determinations. Several important questions have been addressed, although many remain and will likely fuel the discussion for subsequent revisions. Perhaps more than previous revisions, the current iteration may cause confusion because of the emphasis on stage-specific treatment recommendations. Clinicians are reminded that prognosis is only 1 of the factors in a multidisciplinary treatment plan, and they are encouraged to apply randomized trial data whenever possible. This global staging effort is testament to the progress that is possible through international collaboration.

REFERENCES

1. Goldstraw P, Crowley J. The International Association for the Study of Lung Cancer International Staging Project on Lung Cancer. J Thorac Oncol 2006;1(4):281–6.
2. AJCC, UICC. AJCC cancer staging manual. In: Edge S, Byrd DR, Compton CC, et al, editors. 7th edition. New York: Springer; 2009.
3. Shepherd F, Crowley J, Van Houtte P, et al. The International Association for the Study of Lung Cancer Lung Cancer Staging Project: proposals regarding the clinical staging of small cell lung cancer in the forthcoming (seventh) edition of the Tumor, Node, Metastasis Classification for Lung Cancer. J Thorac Oncol 2007;2(12):1067–77.
4. Boffa D, Detterbeck FC, Smith EJ, et al. Should the 7th edition of the Lung Cancer Stage Classification System change treatment algorithms in NSCLC? J Thorac Oncol 2010;5(11):1779–83.
5. Goldstraw P, Crowley J, Chansky K, et al. The IASLC Lung Cancer Staging Project: proposals for the revision of the TNM stage groupings in the forthcoming (seventh) edition of the TNM Classification of Malignant Tumours. J Thorac Oncol 2007;2(8):706–14.
6. Rami-Porta R, Ball D, Crowley J, et al. The IASLC Lung Cancer Staging Project: proposals for the revision of the T descriptors in the forthcoming (seventh) edition of the TNM Classification for Lung Cancer. J Thorac Oncol 2007;2(7):593–602.
7. Rusch VW, Crowley J, Giroux D, et al. The IASLC Lung Cancer Staging Project: proposals for the revision of the N descriptors in the forthcoming seventh edition of the TNM Classification for Lung Cancer. J Thorac Oncol 2007;2(7):603–12.
8. Groome PA, Bolejack V, Crowley J, et al. The IASLC Lung Cancer Staging Project: validation of the proposals for revision of the T, N, and M descriptors and consequent stage groupings in the forthcoming (seventh) edition of the TNM Classification of Malignant Tumours. J Thorac Oncol 2007;2(8):694–705.
9. Postmus PE, Brambilla E, Chansky K, et al. The IASLC Lung Cancer Staging Project: proposals for revision of the M descriptors in the forthcoming (seventh) edition of the TNM Classification of Lung Cancer. J Thorac Oncol 2007;2(8):686–93.
10. Detterbeck F, Jantz M, Wallace M, et al. Invasive mediastinal staging of lung cancer: An ACCP evidence based clinical practice guideline (2nd edition). Chest 2007;132(Suppl 3):202S–20S.
11. Silvestri G, Gould M, Margolis M, et al. Non-invasive staging of non-small cell lung cancer: ACCP evidenced-based clinical practice guidelines (2nd edition). Chest 2007;132(Suppl 3):178S–201S.
12. Trousse D, D'Journo X, Avaro J, et al. Multifocal T4 non-small cell lung cancer: a subset with improved prognosis. Eur J Cardiothorac Surg 2008;33(1):99–103.
13. Okada M, Tsubota N, Yoshimura M, et al. Evaluation of TMN classification for lung carcinoma with ipsilateral intrapulmonary metastasis. Ann Thorac Surg 1999;68(2):326–30.
14. Pennathur A, Lindeman B, Ferson P, et al. Surgical resection is justified in non-small cell lung cancer patients with node negative T4 satellite lesions. Ann Thorac Surg 2009;87(3):893–9.
15. Port JL, Korst R, Lee P, et al. Surgical resection for multifocal (T4) non-small cell lung cancer: is the T4 designation valid? Ann Thorac Surg 2007;83(2):397–400.
16. Rao J, Sayeed R, Tomaszek S, et al. Prognostic factors in resected satellite-nodule T4 non-small cell lung cancer. Ann Thorac Surg 2007;84(3):934–9.
17. Detterbeck FC, Boffa D, Tanoue L, et al. Details and difficulties regarding the new lung cancer staging system. Chest 2010;137(5):1172–80.

The Use and Misuse of Positron Emission Tomography in Lung Cancer Evaluation

Ching-Fei Chang, MD[a], Afshin Rashtian, MD[b],
Michael K. Gould, MD, MS[a,c],*

KEYWORDS

- Non–small-cell lung cancer • Positron emission tomography
- Pulmonary nodules • Mediastinum staging

Positron emission tomography (PET) has been studied for a variety of indications in patients with known or suspected non–small-cell lung cancer (NSCLC). This article discusses the potential benefits and limitations of PET for characterizing lung nodules, staging the mediastinum, identifying occult distant metastasis, determining prognosis and treatment response, guiding plans for radiation therapy, restaging during and after treatment, and selecting targets for tissue sampling (**Table 1**). Evidence from randomized, controlled trials supports the use of PET for initial staging in NSCLC, whereas lower quality evidence from studies of diagnostic accuracy and modeling studies supports the use of PET for characterizing lung nodules. For most other indications in NSCLC, additional studies are required to clarify the role of PET and determine who is most likely to benefit.

In many ways, the history of PET in lung cancer echoes the angst, introspection, and torment of Shakespeare's Hamlet, Prince of Denmark. Although the question "to PET or not to PET?" has been debated extensively, the more pressing concern is how to interpret PET results correctly in light of its performance in various situations.

To the uninitiated, a positive PET scan equals malignancy, and a negative PET scan rules it out, either in regard to the character of the primary lesion or the presence of mediastinal or distant metastasis—but these interpretations are often mistaken. Much like a Shakespearean play, the story of PET is complicated and multilayered, riddled with skeptics and converts, controversial and conflicting data, and shifting realities in which the hero morphs into a villain depending on the circumstances. Therefore, the real question faced by clinicians today is how to interpret the results and avoid misusing them to pursue or withhold potentially curative surgery. As Hamlet would have wisely advised us, "There is nothing either good or bad, but thinking makes it so."

This article presents the key findings from the medical literature regarding the capabilities and fallibilities of PET in lung cancer evaluation, including (but not limited to) characterization of pulmonary nodules and staging in patients with known or suspected NSCLC. The discussion is limited to PET imaging with fluorodeoxyglucose (FDG), recognizing that there is great interest in developing novel tracers for metabolic imaging.

Dr Gould receives grant support from NIH/NCI to study lung cancer diagnosis and staging. The authors have no other conflicts to disclose.

[a] Department of Medicine, Division of Pulmonary and Critical Care Medicine, Keck School of Medicine of USC, 2020 Zonal Avenue, IRD Room 723, Los Angeles, CA 90033, USA
[b] Department of Radiation Oncology, Keck School of Medicine of USC, Health Sciences Campus, Los Angeles, CA 90089, USA
[c] Department of Research and Evaluation, Kaiser Permanente Southern California, 100 South, Los Robles, Pasadena, CA 91101, USA
* Corresponding author.
E-mail address: michael.k.gould@kp.org

Clin Chest Med 32 (2011) 749–762
doi:10.1016/j.ccm.2011.08.012
0272-5231/11/$ – see front matter © 2011 Elsevier Inc. All rights reserved.

chestmed.theclinics.com

Table 1
Potential uses of PET imaging in lung cancer

CT Scan Finding:	How Pet May Be Helpful:
Clinical Stage IA (indeterminate pulmonary nodule):	1. Help characterize the nodule as benign or malignant (although a negative result may still require histologic confirmation unless the pretest probability for malignancy is low and active surveillance is acceptable) 2. Help rule out occult metastases to the mediastinum or extrathoracic sites, which may change plans from curative to palliative care 3. Help determine prognosis based on SUV intensity of the primary lesion and identify patients with more aggressive cell behavior who may benefit from adjuvant therapy after curative resection
Clinical Stage IB-IIB:	1. Help downstage or upstage the patient so that more accurate staging can lead to more appropriate care 2. Help assess early response to adjuvant therapy (after first cycle) so that second line or salvage therapy can be offered early without further waste of time, expense, and unnecessary toxicity
Clinical Stage IIIA-IIIB:	1. Help downstage or upstage the patient so that more accurate staging can lead to more appropriate care 2. Help assess response to induction chemotherapy (if surgical candidate) without the need and risk of re-mediastinoscopy to restage before curative resection 3. Help assess early response to definitive chemo/XRT (if nonsurgical candidate) so that the treatment plan can be changed without waste of time or unnecessary toxicity to the patient 4. Help tailor radiation therapy to provide maximum effect while minimizing toxicity to normal structures
Clinical Stage IV:	1. Potentially downstage the patient if contradictory data are found between CT and PET and a biopsy confirms benign pathologic condition at the M1 site.

The authors hope that the reader will carry away practical learning points that will positively affect their care of lung cancer patients in the future. The approach is skeptical as well as cautiously optimistic. As Shakespeare once said, "Modest doubt is the beacon of the wise," and this should guide the savvy PET-utilizing clinician.

INDICATIONS

In theory, PET can be useful in the evaluation of known or suspected lung cancer in several ways. The three most common indications for PET in lung cancer include

- Characterization of pulmonary nodules
- Staging the mediastinum and identification of occult distant metastasis
- Monitoring for recurrence after completion of treatment.

Over the last decade, there has been a surge of interest in PET scanning for novel indications, including

- Characterization of screening-detected lung nodules

- Assessing response to therapy early during the course of chemoradiation, so that ineffective and potentially toxic regimens can be modified
- Improving prognostication
- Identifying patients with resected NSCLC who are most likely to develop recurrence without additional therapy
- Restaging the mediastinum after neoadjuvant chemoradiation in patients with stage IIIA-N2 disease, to identify candidates who might benefit from surgery
- Confirming and restaging patients with suspected relapse so that aggressive salvage therapy can be planned
- Clarifying the boundaries between tumor and adjacent confounding processes (atelectasis, fibrosis, or postobstructive pneumonia) so that radiation therapy can be more precisely tailored and damage to surrounding structures can be minimized
- Providing a roadmap for high-yield biopsies in the mediastinum by endobronchial ultrasound (EBUS), endoscopic ultrasound (EUS), or mediastinoscopy to expedite staging.

Potentially, the role of PET in NSCLC spans the entire time from diagnosis to death. However, the high cost of PET suggests that its use should be limited to situations in which it is most likely to lead to improved outcomes. In some cases, use of PET may be particularly cost effective, especially if the information provided prevents patients from undergoing unnecessary mediastinoscopy or thoracotomy.[1-3] These indications are examined in turn.

HOW PET WORKS

PET is a functional imaging test that detects hypermetabolism in cells as a proxy for the presence of cancer. The tracer 18-FDG is a radio-labeled glucose analog that is selectively taken up by and then accumulates in metabolically active cells because it cannot pass through the complete glycolytic cycle. The trapped 18-fluorine isotope undergoes radioactive decay by releasing a positron, which subsequently collides with an electron to produce two high-energy photons in a so-called annihilation reaction. The photons travel in opposite directions and are detected by a ring scanner and registered when there is coincident detection of counts separated by 180 degrees. The resulting coincidence counts are processed by a computer for display. Modern PET scanners are typically mounted on a single gantry alongside a separate CT scanner, allowing for integration of functional data from PET with more precise anatomic information from CT.

The limitations of FDG-PET imaging primarily stem from the use of hypermetabolism as a proxy for the presence of cancer, although technical factors also play a role. Essentially, PET will miss slow-growing, relatively indolent cancers, and conversely it will detect many nonmalignant active infectious and noninfectious processes that involve recruitment of metabolically active inflammatory cells.

CHARACTERIZATION OF PULMONARY NODULES

Classically, the solitary pulmonary nodule is a well-circumscribed radiographic opacity that measures up to 3 cm in diameter in the lung periphery, without associated lymphadenopathy, atelectasis, or effusion.[4] The prevalence of malignancy varies widely, depending on the characteristics of the study sample. Before widespread availability of CT scans and PET, surgical resection was (and in some cases remains) the gold standard approach for simultaneous diagnosis and treatment.[5,6] These days, most nodules are incidentally detected by CT. In contrast to years past, nodules encountered today are smaller and few are solitary findings.[7,8] The availability of CT scans, PET, and an expanding menu of nonsurgical biopsy approaches improves the ability to discriminate between patients with benign and malignant nodules, enabling more selective use of surgery in patients with nodules that are most likely to be malignant.

Numerous studies have examined the accuracy of FDG-PET for characterization of focal pulmonary lesions and these studies have been summarized in multiple systematic reviews. In one such review of 40 studies of diagnostic accuracy, the pooled sensitivity and specificity of PET for identifying malignancy in focal pulmonary lesions of any size were 96.8% and 77.8%, respectively. The corresponding likelihood ratios were 4.4 for a positive PET result, and 0.04 for a negative result, suggesting that PET is more useful for excluding than confirming malignancy.[9] Diagnostic accuracy was similar when the analysis was limited to pulmonary nodules. In a subsequent review of seven prospective studies of diagnostic accuracy, sensitivity ranged from 79% to 100%, and specificity ranged from 40% to 90%, with variability in the latter stemming from study group differences in the prevalence of granulomatous disease, ground glass lesions, and nodules that measured less than 1 cm in diameter.[3] Another meta-analysis of 44 studies compared PET, CT, MRI, and single-photon emission computed tomography (SPECT) for identifying malignant lung nodules and found that diagnostic accuracy was similar for PET and SPECT,[10] with likelihood ratios of 5.4 and 0.06 for positive and negative findings, respectively. A prospective study of 344 veterans with newly identified lung nodules reported similar findings.[11] For the first time, this study confirmed that accuracy depended on the degree of FDG uptake, with likelihood ratios ranging from 0.03 for "definitely benign results" to 9.9 for "definitely malignant results," whereas the likelihood ratios were less definitive for "probably benign" (LR 0.15) and "probably malignant" (LR 3.2) results.

Studies of diagnostic accuracy may not capture all of the potential benefits of PET. First, even a false-positive PET result may have some value by alerting the clinician to another active process that requires additional investigation and treatment (eg, endemic mycoses, sarcoidosis). Second, there is some evidence that prognosis is relatively good in patients with false-negative PET results (ie, those with malignant nodules that are minimally or not hypermetabolic), even when surgery is delayed. For example, in one retrospective review of 192 patients with T1N0M0 (stage IA) lung cancer, prognosis was excellent among nine patients with non-hypermetabolic nodules, despite a mean delay of 27 months (range 3–120 months) until surgery.[12] However, these results were not confirmed in a post hoc analysis of data from a prospective study of diagnostic accuracy.[13] In this study, 204 patients had malignant nodules, including 10 patients with nodules that were non-hypermetabolic by PET. Differences in 2-year survival between those with hypermetabolic nodules (67%) and those with non-hypermetabolic nodules (80%) were neither confirmed nor excluded (relative risk 0.84, 95% CI 0.61–1.16).

Some proponents argue that PET may also help to identify occult metastasis in patients with nodules that are known or strongly suspected to be malignant, which may be seen in up to 6.3% of patients with clinical stage I tumors.[14] However, the 40% relapse rate in clinical stage I patients who undergo curative resection suggests that the reservoir of occult disease is even deeper, and that the negative predictive value of PET in these patients is limited.

Of note, no randomized, controlled trials have compared strategies for pulmonary nodule management with and without PET. However, several modeling studies have examined the cost-effectiveness of PET for lung nodule management. Two of these studies found that nonselective use of PET was cost-effective[15,16] while another demonstrated that PET-based strategies were most effective when the pretest probability of malignancy was low to moderate (≤50%).[17]

In summary, relatively low quality evidence, primarily from studies of diagnostic accuracy, supports using PET in many patients with lung nodules, and PET appears to be most useful (and most cost-effective) for identifying patients with non-hypermetabolic nodules who can be safely managed by active surveillance. However, there are several situations in which PET imaging is probably not indicated, including (1) patients with symptoms, signs, or imaging characteristics that suggest infection; (2) patients with larger (>3 cm) pulmonary mass lesions (of which 90% are malignant); (3) patients with small pulmonary nodules that measure less than 7 to 8 mm in diameter; (4) patients with nodular ground glass opacities; and (5) patients who are not candidates for curative treatment.

CHARACTERIZATION OF SCREENING-DETECTED NODULES

Preliminary results from the National Lung Screening Trial suggest that CT screening may be associated with a 20% reduction in lung cancer–specific mortality (Data Safety and Monitoring Board Statement Concerning the National Lung Screening Trial, October 28, 2010). If so, there will almost certainly be an explosion in the use of chest CT scans and a corresponding increase in the number of CT-detected pulmonary nodules, especially considering that roughly 25% to 50% of participants in uncontrolled trials of CT screening had one or more nodules detected on the baseline (prevalence) examination and data from the Lung Screening Study indicates that the cumulative probability of false-positive findings is 33% after two rounds of CT screening.[6,18,19] Given the large numbers of nodules detected by screening and the relatively low prevalence of malignancy in such nodules, the need for an accurate, noninvasive test to distinguish malignant from benign nodules is now even more relevant. Unfortunately, the imperfect ability of PET to characterize subcentimeter nodules potentially limits its utility for this indication.

However, in a recent study of 54 nodules detected by screening as part of the Danish Lung Cancer Screening Trial, the sensitivity and specificity of PET for identifying malignancy were 71% and 91%, respectively.[20] In this study, the prevalence of malignancy was 37%, and the mean was 13 mm, but separate results for patients with subcentimeter nodules were not provided. Nevertheless, this study suggests that PET may be helpful for characterizing screening-detected nodules, especially those measuring at least 7 to 8 mm in diameter.

INITIAL STAGING

Although many published studies of diagnostic accuracy have important limitations (eg, small samples, incomplete blinding, suboptimal reference standards), available data strongly suggest that PET is more sensitive than CT scanning for identifying mediastinal lymph node involvement in patients with known or suspected NSCLC. A systematic review and meta-analysis of 44 studies of diagnostic accuracy reported that the sensitivity and specificity of PET for this indication were 74% and 85%, respectively.[21,22] In the same review, CT scanning was noted to have similar specificity (86%) but substantially lower sensitivity (51%). Another meta-analysis demonstrated that the accuracy of PET depended on the CT findings in that PET results were more likely to be positive (either true-positive or false-positive) when lymph nodes were enlarged, and more likely to be negative (either true-negative or false-negative) when there was no lymph node enlargement.[23] Thus, PET seems to be less sensitive for identifying metastasis when lymph nodes are not enlarged and less specific when there is lymph node enlargement. The imperfect specificity of PET (especially in patients with enlarged lymph nodes) mandates confirmatory tissue sampling unless there is overwhelming evidence of tumor involvement with bulky, multistation adenopathy.

The availability of mediastinoscopy and newer, nonsurgical methods to sample mediastinal lymph nodes raises the question of if and when PET should be used for mediastinal staging. Indeed, there is a strong case to be made that enlarged nodes on CT should be sampled by invasive methods regardless of the PET results. If so, PET might still be indicated to identify occult distant metastasis, but this is controversial. One prospective study reported that the sensitivity and specificity of PET for identifying extrathoracic metastasis were 82% and 93%, respectively.[24] In light of these findings, proponents argue that the prevalence of occult extrathoracic metastasis is high in patients with clinical stage III disease by CT criteria, and that PET is reasonably sensitive for identifying these lesions. Others argue that the negative predictive value of a routine clinical evaluation is sufficiently high to obviate further testing.[25] However, there is little disagreement that, because of the test's imperfect specificity, positive extrathoracic findings on PET must be confirmed pathologically unless there is overwhelming evidence of metastasis, as is true in the mediastinum.

There is also disagreement about whether to use PET and/or invasive mediastinal staging in patients with no evidence of lymph node enlargement on CT. Although a full discussion of this debate is beyond the scope of this article, the authors believe that use of PET is reasonable in selected high-risk patients, including patients with primary tumors that are large, centrally-located, or adenocarcinoma by histology, as well as patients with hilar nodal enlargement.[26,27] However, because these are situations in which the likelihood of malignant mediastinal lymph node involvement is actually increased, many would argue that tissue sampling is mandatory in these patients and that PET is, therefore, superfluous except for the potential to more specifically direct mediastinal biopsies or evaluate for distant metastasis. Of note, EUS may be the preferred approach to identify occult involvement of posterior mediastinal nodes in patients with upper lobe primary tumors.[28,29]

Part of the reason for PET's limited sensitivity in the mediastinum may be related to micrometastatic foci in normal-sized lymph nodes. Nomori and colleagues[30] reported that PET loses its resolution for metastatic foci below 4 mm within mediastinal lymph nodes. Another group confirmed that the size of the lymph node affects PET sensitivity for malignancy: when the nodes were less than 1 cm, the sensitivity was a dismal 32.4%, but if the nodes were greater than 1 cm, the sensitivity jumped to 85.3%.[31] Of note, the prognostic significance of occult nodal micrometastasis is uncertain. It is also not clear whether preoperative detection (presumably followed by combined modality therapy) results in better outcomes in these patients, who would otherwise be treated with surgery followed by adjuvant chemotherapy.

Complementary to studies of diagnostic accuracy, several studies have demonstrated that use of PET often results in upstaging or downstaging, relative to CT or conventional staging. In one such prospective study of 105 consecutive patients with NSCLC who were referred for PET imaging (including only 59 patients who were referred for initial staging), PET altered management in 67% of participants by either upstaging to palliative care, downstaging to allow for potentially curative therapy, or changing radiation therapy plans.[32] The very high percentage of altered management observed in this study can probably be attributed to selection bias, at least in part. In another study of 153 consecutive patients with newly diagnosed NSCLC from the same group of Australian investigators, 33% of patients were upstaged by PET, 10% were downstaged, and management plans were meaningfully changed in 35%.[33]

The highest quality evidence regarding the use of PET for initial staging comes from randomized, controlled trials. No fewer than five randomized trials have examined PET for staging in NSCLC. A European multicenter trial compared conventional staging with conventional staging plus PET in 188 patients with known or suspected NSCLC that was potentially resectable. The primary outcome was the number of futile thoracotomies, defined as surgery for a benign lesion, intraoperative detection of N2, N3, or other stage IIIB disease; exploratory thoracotomy for some other reason; or tumor recurrence or death within 1 year. Similar numbers of patients in both groups underwent nonfutile thoracotomies, although the risk of futile thoracotomy was reduced from 41% in the conventional staging group to 21% in the PET group.[1]

These results were subsequently confirmed in two later studies, including a Danish study of 189 patients with NSCLC referred for preoperative staging, 60% of whom had clinical stage III disease. Compared with patients who underwent conventional staging, the risk of futile thoracotomy was reduced from 52% to 35% in those assigned to staging with integrated PET-CT.[34] Another trial performed in Canada enrolled 337 patients with potentially resectable, stage I-IIIA NSCLC and randomized participants to staging with integrated PET-CT or CT plus bone scan. In this study, PET-CT resulted in correct upstaging in 14% of participants, compared with 7% in the CT plus bone scan group, for an absolute reduction of 7% in the risk of unnecessary surgery.[35]

Two other trials reported less impressive results. In an Australian study of 184 patients with clinical stage I-II NSCLC who were randomized preoperatively to PET or no PET, 16% of patients in the PET group were either upstaged (8%) or downstaged (8%), but few thoracotomies were avoided in either group (4% vs 2%).[36] In another multicenter study, from the Netherlands, that compared "upfront" PET with conventional staging in 465 patients with a provisional diagnosis of lung cancer and no overt dissemination, there were fewer mediastinoscopies in the PET group, but the number of staging procedures was similar in the two groups.[37]

Some have also questioned the validity of recurrence or death within 1 year of surgery as an appropriate outcome in two of the three positive trials. If PET did not detect occult regional or distant metastatic disease in these patients, how can it be responsible for preventing recurrence or death? In addition, none of the studies reported improvements in survival or lung cancer mortality. Thus, the link between more accurate staging and survival has yet to be proved, and probably awaits the development of more effective stage-specific treatments.

Several studies have examined the cost effectiveness of PET for staging in NSCLC. One early study compared conventional staging with CT and mediastinoscopy to conventional staging plus PET and found that PET-based staging reduced costs by $1154 per patient and increased life expectancy by 3 days.[38] Another analysis reported that compared with CT followed by selective mediastinoscopy, a strategy of CT followed by mediastinoscopy (when CT showed enlarged lymph nodes) or PET (when there were no enlarged lymph nodes) cost approximately $25,000 per life-year gained.[39] Another modeling study compared mediastinoscopy alone with PET followed by selective mediastinoscopy and found that for every 100 patients treated, PET plus selective mediastinoscopy resulted in seven fewer futile thoracotomies and saved $212,800 Australian dollars.[40] An economic evaluation of data from a randomized, controlled trial of conventional staging versus conventional staging plus PET

reported that PET-based staging was less expensive by approximately €1,300.[2] However, a cost-minimization study that compared five approaches among patients with enlarged nodes on CT found that PET followed by selective mediastinoscopy was preferred only when the probability of lymph node metastasis was less than 25%. At higher probabilities, EUS-guided fine-needle aspiration (EUS-FNA) followed by negative mediastinoscopy was preferred, provided that the sensitivity of EUS-FNA was at least 75%.[41]

In summary, moderate-to-high quality evidence suggests that staging with PET is more accurate than CT, results in substantial upstaging and downstaging, and reduces the risk of futile thoracotomy. However, these benefits have not translated to improvements in survival. Economic evaluations suggest that several different PET-based strategies are either cost-saving or highly cost-effective.

PROGNOSIS

Several studies have confirmed that clinical TNM staging by PET is more strongly associated with prognosis than conventional staging with CT alone.[33,42] Given that PET is more accurate than CT for initial staging, this should come as no surprise.

Somewhat more controversial is the notion that the degree of FDG uptake in the primary tumor may be independently associated with prognosis. Although intuitively plausible, the correlations between hypermetabolism, growth, metastatic potential, and (ultimately) prognosis might be confounded by other factors, including tumor size and histology. A recent systematic review identified 21 studies that examined the association between primary tumor FDG uptake and survival in patients with NSCLC of any stage, and found that the hazard of death was twice as high when the standardized uptake value (SUV) was above the median value, although the investigators acknowledged that individual patient data would be needed to account for potential confounders.[43] Likewise, in another review limited to nine studies of patients with resected stage I NSCLC, higher degrees of FDG uptake in the primary tumor were associated with worse overall or disease-free survival, but differences were statistically significant in only five of the studies.[44] In a subsequent analysis of data from a prospective study of PET for lung nodule characterization, greater FDG uptake was independently associated with worse prognosis among patients with malignant nodules that were surgically resected, even after adjusting for age, tumor size, histology, and type of resection.[45]

Technical factors may explain differences in study results, at least in part. Published studies of prognosis used heterogeneous methods to perform examinations and measure FDG uptake. Standardization of protocols for acquisition and interpretation of PET images would greatly enhance both the validity and applicability of any results generated from future studies.[43,46,47]

PREDICTING TREATMENT RESPONSE

Although accurate prognostication is undeniably important to patients, predicting response to treatment is potentially even more valuable. Several studies have examined whether evidence of an early response to treatment by PET predicts longer term response. One such study reported that six of seven patients with advanced NSCLC and evidence of partial response on PET after one cycle of chemotherapy had a best overall response that was at least stable. In contrast, best overall response was stable in only 2 of 11 patients with evidence of progressive disease on early PET. In this study, PET response was not associated with survival.[48] However, a prospective study of 57 patients with advanced NSCLC found that early metabolic response (defined as a reduction in SUV mean of >20% after the first cycle of chemotherapy) was associated with a significantly longer time to disease progression and more frequent survival to 1 year (44% vs 10%).[49]

Other studies have examined the predictive value of PET following definitive treatment. In a study of 73 patients with NSCLC who underwent PET before and after completing radical radiotherapy or chemoradiotherapy, overall PET response was associated with survival before and after adjustment for performance status, stage, weight loss, and CT response.[50] Another study from the same group demonstrated that patients with a complete metabolic response had a longer median survival and were less subject to local failure and distant metastasis.[51]

Still other studies have used PET to assess response to induction chemotherapy before surgical resection. One study examined early response to induction chemotherapy by performing PET before and after chemotherapy cycles 1 and 3 in 47 patients with stage IIIA-N2 NSCLC.[52] In this study, both PET stage and various measures of FDG uptake were associated with survival. Another study of 56 patients with NSCLC who received neoadjuvant treatment with either chemoradiation or chemotherapy alone before surgical resection found that an 80% reduction in postinduction maximal SUV (SUVmax) was associated with a complete pathologic response.[53]

However, two other studies of patients with potentially resectable NSCLC who underwent neoadjuvant therapy found no association between FDG uptake and survival.[54,55]

One possible confounding factor in these studies is the timing of PET, especially in patients treated with radiation, which can be associated with false-positive findings. In a study of 109 patients treated with neoadjuvant chemoradiation, posttreatment PET was most accurate (compared with pathologic staging) in patients who underwent imaging between 21 and 30 days after the last dose of radiation.[56]

RESTAGING IN NSCLC

Because repeat mediastinoscopy is widely considered difficult and relatively low-yield, an accurate and less invasive option for restaging is highly desirable. Although there is great interest in using EBUS-guided and/or EUS-guided biopsy for this purpose,[57] these techniques are not yet widely available in community settings. The default method of restaging, until now, has always been CT.

At least in theory, PET has additional advantages over CT for restaging after neoadjuvant therapy or in patients with suspected relapse. Especially in cases in which radiation-induced fibrosis and distortion of intrathoracic structures makes assessment of the original target difficult,[50,58,59] or in cases of molecular targeted therapy in which the anatomic appearance of the tumor may not change at all,[60] physiologic assessment of disease activity might prove helpful.

Restaging Following Induction Therapy in Patients with Stage IIIA-N2 Disease

In light of accumulating data suggesting improved outcomes with combined multimodality treatment for patients with stage IIIA NSCLC and nonbulky N2 disease,[61–63] the accuracy of PET for identifying complete response following neoadjuvant therapy has been examined in several studies and summarized in two systematic reviews.[64,65] In one review, the sensitivity and specificity of PET for identifying residual N2 disease were only 64% and 85%, respectively,[64] suggesting that PET may have limited sensitivity for identifying residual disease in these circumstances.

However, another group reported that the accuracy of PET for restaging the mediastinum varied based on the location of involved lymph nodes, with excellent accuracy in anterior mediastinal nodes and relatively poor accuracy in posterior nodal stations.[66] This may have important implications for restaging in patients with upper lobe tumors, which often drain and metastasize to posterior nodes. In addition, the magnitude of reductions in FDG uptake following induction therapy may be more predictive than the categorical presence or absence of FDG uptake, for both the primary tumor and the involved lymph nodes. For example, in a prospective study of 93 patients with stage IIIA (N2) NSCLC who underwent pathologic staging following induction chemoradiotherapy, the sensitivity and specificity of an SUVmax greater than 2.5 for identifying residual N2 disease were 80% and 75%, respectively. Reductions in FDG uptake of at least 75% in the primary tumor and at least 50% in the involved lymph nodes were strongly associated with a "complete response" (and thus survival benefit with surgery).[57]

Restaging in Patients with Suspected Recurrence

Among patients who receive curative treatment for NSCLC, follow-up imaging often reveals suspicious nodules or masses in and outside the lung parenchyma. Although the early detection and treatment of relapses is of uncertain value, it seems that PET identifies relapse with a sensitivity and specificity of approximately 90%.[67,68] As is true for restaging following induction treatment, PET is often able to distinguish recurrent disease in areas of scarring and posttherapeutic change whereas CT cannot. In one study, PET correctly reclassified CT findings of recurrence in 24% of patients, thus sparing them the potential toxicity associated with unnecessary treatment.[68]

RADIOTHERAPY PLANNING

PET has been studied for several indications related to radiation therapy in patients with NSCLC, including selection of candidates for radical radiotherapy, delineation of radiation therapy volume, and determination of treatment response.[69]

Although many studies have examined the accuracy of PET for mediastinal and distant staging, relatively few studies have used PET stage to determine eligibility for curative radiation treatment. In one prospective study of 167 patients with clinical stage I-III NSCLC by CT scanning who were referred for radical radiation therapy, PET identified occult distant metastasis in 32 patients (19%), including 8% of those with stage I disease, 18% of those with stage II disease, and 24% of those with stage III disease by CT.[70] By upstaging these patients, PET changed the treatment plan from curative to palliative, possibly reducing treatment toxicity.

Accurate delineation of nodal metastasis is crucial for radiotherapy planning. Because the

negative predictive value of PET for lymph node staging is relatively high, radiation therapy can be designed to target positive nodes selectively. An extreme example of this approach was illustrated in a phase I-II trial of selective mediastinal irradiation based on FDG-PET scan results.[71] In this study, the addition of a PET scan changed nodal stage in 11 of the 44 patients, and only one out of 44 patients treated with the selective approach had an isolated nodal failure. In another study, PET led to an increase in planning target volume to incorporate positive nodal disease in 7 of 11 patients (64%), and the average increase was 19%.[72] In another study of 73 patients with NSCLC and positive lymph nodes on CT and/or PET who had lymph node metastasis confirmed pathologically, tumor coverage would have improved from 75% with CT to 89% if PET had been used.[73]

In some cases, radiation volumes determined by PET findings are smaller than those determined by CT, thus enabling delivery of lower doses to surrounding structures, such as the esophagus and heart. This enables the radiation oncologist to deliver a higher dose to the tumor without increasing side effects. Whether this will result in higher cure rates is a matter of ongoing research. In a small, theoretical study, PET results would have led to a reduction in the size or a change in shape of the portal in 12 of 34 patients, including eight patients with obstructive atelectasis that was distinguished from malignancy by PET.[74] In a subsequent prospective study of 24 patients with stages I-III NSCLC who had three-dimensional conformal radiation therapy, the addition of PET reduced gross tumor volume (GTV) in three patients (14%) and increased GTV in 11 patients.[75] More recently, GTV was modified by at least 25% in 10 of 19 patients who underwent planning with integrated PET-CT.[76]

Another area of interest is to use PET to monitor response and adjust treatment during the course of radiation therapy. In a small prospective study of 14 patients with stage I-III NSCLC who underwent integrated PET-CT before and midway through radiotherapy, the mean decrease in PET tumor volume was 44%, compared with 26% by CT.[77] This allowed for meaningful dose escalation and a reduction in the probability of complications. However, another similar study reported only modest dose escalation despite evidence of tumor shrinkage on integrated PET-CT.[78]

As outlined above, PET appears to have a role in designing the radiation field for the mediastinum, as well as distinguishing atelectasis from tumor at the primary site. However, most of the supporting studies were small and uncontrolled. In addition,

PET-defined radiotherapy fields can represent false-positive findings in up to 39% of patients.[79,80] Thus, positive findings on PET should be confirmed by histology whenever possible. In up to 70% of patients in whom PET scans indicate nodal metastasis, histologic confirmation can be obtained using EUS-FNA.[81] A combination of PET and EUS-FNA therefore holds potential as a minimally invasive approach for defining radiotherapy fields. This may allow for dose escalation to tumor and reduced dose to critical structures and, it is hoped, improved local control.

GUIDANCE FOR DIAGNOSTIC BIOPSY

A promising indication for PET in NSCLC is as a guide to high-yield diagnostic biopsies. By identifying potential intrathoracic and extrathoracic sites of metastatic involvement, PET can streamline the evaluation by helping to target the biopsy site that will establish the highest stage disease. Furthermore, by providing information about the location of potentially involved mediastinal lymph nodes, PET can help to guide the selection of a specific surgical or nonsurgical biopsy procedure. For example, a physician might choose EUS in a patient with hypermetabolic posterior subcarinal or paraesophageal nodes, whereas one would favor anterior mediastinotomy in a patient with isolated para-aortic lymph node involvement.

Systematic sampling of mediastinal nodes with combined EUS and EBUS is emerging as the potential gold standard for mediastinal staging.[82,83] However, this approach is time consuming and typically requires general anesthesia to keep the patient still and cough-free for a prolonged period of time. Although systematic staging is essential to completely exclude mediastinal involvement, targeted sampling of suspicious N2 or N3 nodes may be all that is necessary to confirm nonresectability in many patients. By identifying nodes that are the most hypermetabolic and/or most easily accessible, PET can facilitate planning for invasive staging.

Although several investigators have alluded to this potential indication for PET in NSCLC,[14,64,84,85] no data currently exist to confirm or refute whether PET-guided invasive staging is more efficient than systematic staging, making this a ripe target for investigation.

RECENT IMPROVEMENTS IN PET TECHNOLOGY

Integrated PET-CT allows for more precise localization of the specific anatomic structures responsible for FDG enhancement. Although of questionable value in the characterization of lung nodules, integration of PET and CT images seem to be potentially useful for evaluation of masses abutting the chest wall or mediastinum and for nodal staging. In one study, tumor stage was assigned correctly in 39 of 40 patients by integrated PET-CT, but only in 31 of 40 patients when results of dedicated PET and CT were visually correlated. Similarly, nodal stage was correctly assigned in 31 of 37 patients by integrated PET-CT, compared with 26 of 37 patients by visual correlation. Although widely cited, this small study was limited by incomplete blinding and failure to ascertain final stage in 30% of participants.[86] In a larger subsequent study of 129 consecutive patients with indeterminate solitary nodules or proven NSCLC, stage assignment by integrated PET-CT was more often correct than staging by dedicated PET alone, but integrated PET-CT was correct only 68% of the time and dedicated PET was correct less than 50% of the time.[85] It is also important to recognize that the CT portion of most integrated PET-CT scans has inferior image quality compared with that of a standard CT because it is primarily used as an attenuation correction tool and, thus, is subject to breathing and motion artifacts due to a lack of breath-holding.[87] Therefore, integrated PET-CT does not always obviate a dedicated CT of the chest.

Although integrated PET-CT has been widely adopted in clinical practice, other improvements have not yet been implemented, including standardization of protocols for image acquisition and interpretation so that there is a universally agreed-on fasting time, glucose threshold, delay time between injection of FDG and scanning, and a reproducible method of delineating a region of interest for the measurement of SUVmax. Another advance that has undergone preliminary study is dual-time scanning. With this technique, persistence of FDG uptake on a repeat scan helps, at least in theory, to distinguish malignancy from inflammation.[88,89]

In all likelihood, the most promising future advances will come from the development of novel tracers for metabolic imaging that are more sensitive or specific for identifying malignancy.

SUMMARY

In the last 2 decades, PET technology has become widely available and PET is now a standard part of the armamentarium for lung cancer diagnosis and staging. However, rational interpretation and use of PET requires careful consideration of the clinical context and the limitations of functional imaging with a tracer that uses metabolic activity as a proxy for the presence of cancer.

Above all else, it is important to re-emphasize that positive findings on PET, whether in the mediastinum or outside of the thorax, must be confirmed by biopsy before excluding a patient from potentially curative surgical resection, unless there is overwhelming evidence of malignancy. In some cases, absence of FDG uptake in the primary lesion or mediastinum may require confirmatory biopsy as well—especially if the PET-negative primary lesion is in a patient at high-risk for lung cancer, if the mediastinal lymph node size is only mildly enlarged (given that PET is less sensitive in smaller nodes), or if the radiographic presentation has any features that are associated with occult metastasis to the mediastinum (eg, centrally-located tumor, N1 hilar involvement, adenocarcinoma).

Areas of controversy include whether PET should be performed to identify occult metastasis in patients with suspected malignant small pulmonary nodules and whether PET is helpful or redundant for mediastinal staging in patients with clinical stage III disease. Likewise, it is unclear whether PET can identify high risk patients who are more likely to benefit from adjuvant chemotherapy following resection, or whether early detection of recurrence by PET is associated with better response to salvage treatment.

Although clinicians will always be faced with dilemmas of interpreting equivocal findings, PET can still be helpful in patients with known or suspected NSCLC if indications and results are not accepted at face value without additional deliberation. As Shakespeare eloquently put it, "Make not your thoughts your prisons." Given the rapid pace of technological innovation, the golden age of PET probably lies before us, and the indications will undoubtedly morph and reinvent themselves into clearer recommendations as additional studies are completed and experience accumulates.

REFERENCES

1. van Tinteren H, Hoekstra OS, Smit EF, et al. Effectiveness of positron emission tomography in the preoperative assessment of patients with suspected non-small-cell lung cancer: the PLUS multicentre randomised trial. Lancet 2002;359(9315):1388–92.

2. Verboom P, van Tinteren H, Hoekstra OS, et al. Cost-effectiveness of FDG-PET in staging non-small cell lung cancer: the PLUS study. Eur J Nucl Med Mol Imaging 2003;30(11):1444–9.

3. Ung YC, Maziak DE, Vanderveen JA, et al. 18Fluoro-deoxyglucose positron emission tomography in the diagnosis and staging of lung cancer: a systematic review. J Natl Cancer Inst 2007;99(23):1753–67.

4. Ost D, Fein AM, Feinsilver SH. Clinical practice. The solitary pulmonary nodule. N Engl J Med 2003; 348(25):2535–42.

5. Detterbeck FC. Seeking a home for a PET, part 1: defining the appropriate place for positron emission tomography imaging in the diagnosis of pulmonary nodules or masses. Chest 2004;125(6): 2294–9.

6. Wahidi MM, Govert JA, Goudar RK, et al. Evidence for the treatment of patients with pulmonary nodules: when is it lung cancer?: ACCP evidence-based clinical practice guidelines (2nd edition). Chest 2007; 132(Suppl 3):94S–107S.

7. Henschke CI, McCauley DI, Yankelevitz DF, et al. Early lung cancer action project: overall design and findings from baseline screening. Lancet 1999;354(9173):99–105.

8. Swensen SJ, Jett JR, Sloan JA, et al. Screening for lung cancer with low-dose spiral computed tomography. Am J Respir Crit Care Med 2002;165(4):508–13.

9. Gould MK, Jett JR, Sloan JA, et al. Accuracy of positron emission tomography for diagnosis of pulmonary nodules and mass lesions: a meta-analysis. JAMA 2001;285(7):914–24.

10. Cronin P, Dwamena BA, Kelly AM, et al. Solitary pulmonary nodules and masses: a meta-analysis of the diagnostic utility of alternative imaging tests. Eur Radiol 2008;18(9):1840–56.

11. Fletcher JW, Kymes SM, Gould M, et al. A comparison of the diagnostic accuracy of 18F-FDG PET and CT in the characterization of solitary pulmonary nodules. official publication, Society of Nuclear Medicine. J Nucl Med 2008;49(2):179–85.

12. Marom EM, Sarvis S, Herndon JE 2nd, et al. T1 lung cancers: sensitivity of diagnosis with fluorodeoxyglucose PET. Radiology 2002;223(2):453–9.

13. Barnett PG, Ananth L, Gould MK. Cost and outcomes of patients with solitary pulmonary nodules managed with PET scans. Chest 2010;137(1):53–9.

14. Reed CE, Harpole DH, Posther KE, et al. Results of the American College of Surgeons Oncology Group Z0050 trial: the utility of positron emission tomography in staging potentially operable non-small cell lung cancer. J Thorac Cardiovasc Surg 2003; 126(6):1943–51.

15. Gambhir SS, Shepherd JE, Shah BD, et al. Analytical decision model for the cost-effective management of solitary pulmonary nodules. official journal of the American Society of Clinical Oncology. J Clin Oncol 1998;16(6):2113–25.

16. Dietlein M, Weber K, Gandjour A, et al. Cost-effectiveness of FDG-PET for the management of solitary pulmonary nodules: a decision analysis based on cost reimbursement in Germany. Eur J Nucl Med 2000;27(10):1441–56.

17. Gould MK, Sanders GD, Barnett PG, et al. Cost-effectiveness of alternative management strategies

for patients with solitary pulmonary nodules. Ann Intern Med 2003;138(9):724–35.

18. Swensen SJ, Silverstein MD, Ilstrup DM, et al. The probability of malignancy in solitary pulmonary nodules. Application to small radiologically indeterminate nodules. Arch Intern Med 1997;157(8):849–55.

19. Croswell JM, Baker SG, Marcus PM, et al. Cumulative incidence of false-positive test results in lung cancer screening: a randomized trial. Ann Intern Med 2010;152(8):505–12, W176–80.

20. Ashraf H, Dirksen A, Loft A, et al. Combined use of positron emission tomography and volume doubling time in lung cancer screening with low-dose CT scanning. Thorax 2011;66(4):315–9.

21. Silvestri GA, Gould MK, Margolis ML, et al. Noninvasive staging of non-small cell lung cancer: ACCP evidenced-based clinical practice guidelines (2nd edition). Chest 2007;132(Suppl 3):178S–201S.

22. Toloza EM. Noninvasive staging of non-small cell lung cancer: a review of the current evidence. Chest 2003;123(90010):137S–46S.

23. Gould MK, Kuschner WG, Rydzak CE, et al. Test performance of positron emission tomography and computed tomography for mediastinal staging in patients with non-small-cell lung cancer: a meta-analysis. Ann Intern Med 2003;139(11):879–92.

24. Pieterman RM, van Putten JW, Meuzelaar JJ, et al. Preoperative staging of non-small-cell lung cancer with positron-emission tomography. N Engl J Med 2000;343(4):254–61.

25. Miller YE. Staging of non-small-cell lung cancer with positron-emission tomography. N Engl J Med 2000; 343(21):1571–2 [author reply: 1572–3].

26. Detterbeck FC. Seeking a home for a PET, Part 2: defining the appropriate place for positron emission tomography imaging in the staging of patients with suspected lung cancer. Chest 2004;125(6):2300–8.

27. Verhagen AF, Bootsma GP, Tjan-Heijnen VC, et al. FDG-PET in staging lung cancer: how does it change the algorithm? Lung Cancer 2004;44(2):175–81.

28. Cerfolio RJ, Bryant AS. Distribution and likelihood of lymph node metastasis based on the lobar location of nonsmall-cell lung cancer. Ann Thorac Surg 2006;81(6):1969–73 [discussion: 1973].

29. Cerfolio RJ, Bryant AS, Ojha B, et al. Improving the inaccuracies of clinical staging of patients with NSCLC: a prospective trial. Ann Thorac Surg 2005; 80(4):1207–13 [discussion: 1213–4].

30. Nomori H, Watanabe K, Ohtsuka T, et al. The size of metastatic foci and lymph nodes yielding false-negative and false-positive lymph node staging with positron emission tomography in patients with lung cancer. J Thorac Cardiovasc Surg 2004; 127(4):1087–92.

31. Bille A, Pelosi E, Skanjeti A, et al. Preoperative intrathoracic lymph node staging in patients with non-small-cell lung cancer: accuracy of integrated positron emission tomography and computed tomography. official journal of the European Association for Cardio-thoracic Surgery. Eur J Cardiothorac Surg 2009;36(3):440–5.

32. Kalff V, Hicks RJ, MacManus MP, et al. Clinical impact of (18)F fluorodeoxyglucose positron emission tomography in patients with non-small-cell lung cancer: a prospective study. official journal of the American Society of Clinical Oncology. J Clin Oncol 2001;19(1):111–8.

33. Hicks RJ, Kalff V, MacManus MP, et al. (18)F-FDG PET provides high-impact and powerful prognostic stratification in staging newly diagnosed non-small cell lung cancer. official publication, Society of Nuclear Medicine. J Nucl Med 2001;42(11):1596–604.

34. Fischer B, Lassen U, Mortensen J, et al. Preoperative staging of lung cancer with combined PET-CT. N Engl J Med 2009;361(1):32–9.

35. Maziak DE, Darling GE, Inculet RI, et al. Positron emission tomography in staging early lung cancer: a randomized trial. Ann Intern Med 2009;151(4): 221–8, W-48.

36. Viney RC, Boyer MJ, King MT, et al. Randomized controlled trial of the role of positron emission tomography in the management of stage I and II non-small-cell lung cancer. official journal of the American Society of Clinical Oncology. J Clin Oncol 2004;22(12):2357–62.

37. Herder GJ, Kramer H, Hoekstra OS, et al. Traditional versus up-front [18F] fluorodeoxyglucose-positron emission tomography staging of non-small-cell lung cancer: a Dutch cooperative randomized study. official journal of the American Society of Clinical Oncology. J Clin Oncol 2006;24(12):1800–6.

38. Gambhir SS, Hoh CK, Phelps ME, et al. Decision tree sensitivity analysis for cost-effectiveness of FDG-PET in the staging and management of non-small-cell lung carcinoma. official publication, Society of Nuclear Medicine. J Nucl Med 1996; 37(9):1428–36.

39. Scott WJ, Shepherd J, Gambhir SS. Cost-effectiveness of FDG-PET for staging non-small cell lung cancer: a decision analysis. Ann Thorac Surg 1998;66(6):1876–83 [discussion: 1883–5].

40. Yap KK, Yap KS, Byrne AJ, et al. Positron emission tomography with selected mediastinoscopy compared to routine mediastinoscopy offers cost and clinical outcome benefits for pre-operative staging of non-small cell lung cancer. Eur J Nucl Med Mol Imaging 2005;32(9):1033–40.

41. Harewood GC, Wiersema MJ, Edell ES, et al. Cost-minimization analysis of alternative diagnostic approaches in a modeled patient with non-small cell lung cancer and subcarinal lymphadenopathy. Mayo Clinic. Mayo Clin Proc 2002;77(2):155–64.

42. Dunagan D, Chin R Jr, McCain T, et al. Staging by positron emission tomography predicts survival in

patients with non-small cell lung cancer. Chest 2001; 119(2):333–9.

43. Paesmans M, Berghmans T, Dusart M, et al. Primary tumor standardized uptake value measured on fluorodeoxyglucose positron emission tomography is of prognostic value for survival in non-small cell lung cancer: update of a systematic review and meta-analysis by the European Lung Cancer Working Party for the International Association for the Study of Lung Cancer Staging Project. official publication of the International Association for the Study of Lung Cancer. J Thorac Oncol 2010;5(5):612–9.

44. Nair VS, Krupitskaya Y, Gould MK. Positron emission tomography 18F-fluorodeoxyglucose uptake and prognosis in patients with surgically treated, stage I non-small cell lung cancer: a systematic review. official publication of the International Association for the Study of Lung Cancer. J Thorac Oncol 2009;4(12):1473–9.

45. Nair VS, Barnett PG, Ananth L, et al. PET scan 18F-fluorodeoxyglucose uptake and prognosis in patients with resected clinical stage IA non-small cell lung cancer. Chest 2010;137(5):1150–6.

46. de Geus-Oei LF, van der Heijden HF, Corstens FH, et al. Predictive and prognostic value of FDG-PET in nonsmall-cell lung cancer: a systematic review. Cancer 2007;110(8):1654–64.

47. Vansteenkiste J, Fischer BM, Dooms C, et al. Positron-emission tomography in prognostic and therapeutic assessment of lung cancer: systematic review. Lancet Oncol 2004;5(9):531–40.

48. Lee DH, Kim SK, Lee HY, et al. Early prediction of response to first-line therapy using integrated 18F-FDG PET/CT for patients with advanced/metastatic non-small cell lung cancer. official publication of the International Association for the Study of Lung Cancer. J Thorac Oncol 2009;4(7):816–21.

49. Weber WA, Petersen V, Schmidt B, et al. Positron emission tomography in non-small-cell lung cancer: prediction of response to chemotherapy by quantitative assessment of glucose use. official journal of the American Society of Clinical Oncology. J Clin Oncol 2003;21(14):2651–7.

50. Mac Manus MP. Positron emission tomography is superior to computed tomography scanning for response-assessment after radical radiotherapy or chemoradiotherapy in patients with non-small-cell lung cancer. J Clin Oncol 2003;21(7):1285–92.

51. Mac Manus MP, Hicks RJ, Matthews JP, et al. Metabolic (FDG-PET) response after radical radiotherapy/chemoradiotherapy for non-small cell lung cancer correlates with patterns of failure. Lung Cancer 2005;49(1):95–108.

52. Hoekstra CJ, Stroobants SG, Smit EF, et al. Prognostic relevance of response evaluation using [18F]-2-fluoro-2-deoxy-D-glucose positron emission tomography in patients with locally advanced non-small-cell lung cancer. official journal of the American Society of Clinical Oncology. J Clin Oncol 2005;23(33):8362–70.

53. Cerfolio RJ, Bryant AS, Winokur TS, et al. Repeat FDG-PET after neoadjuvant therapy is a predictor of pathologic response in patients with non-small cell lung cancer. Ann Thorac Surg 2004;78(6): 1903–9 [discussion: 1909].

54. Tanvetyanon T, Eikman EA, Sommers E, et al. Computed tomography response, but not positron emission tomography scan response, predicts survival after neoadjuvant chemotherapy for resectable non-small-cell lung cancer. official journal of the American Society of Clinical Oncology. J Clin Oncol 2008;26(28):4610–6.

55. Pottgen C, Levegrün S, Theegarten D, et al. Value of 18F-fluoro-2-deoxy-D-glucose-positron emission tomography/computed tomography in non-small-cell lung cancer for prediction of pathologic response and times to relapse after neoadjuvant chemoradiotherapy. an official journal of the American Association for Cancer Research. Clin Cancer Res 2006;12(1):97–106.

56. Cerfolio RJ, Bryant AS. When is it best to repeat a 2-fluoro-2-deoxy-D-glucose positron emission tomography/computed tomography scan on patients with non-small cell lung cancer who have received neoadjuvant chemoradiotherapy? Ann Thorac Surg 2007;84(4):1092–7.

57. Cerfolio RJ, Bryant AS, Ojha B. Restaging patients with N2 (stage IIIa) non-small cell lung cancer after neoadjuvant chemoradiotherapy: a prospective study. J Thorac Cardiovasc Surg 2006;131(6):1229–35.

58. Port J. Positron emission tomography scanning poorly predicts response to preoperative chemotherapy in non-small cell lung cancer. Ann Thorac Surg 2004;77(1):254–9.

59. Xu X, Yu J, Sun X, et al. The prognostic value of 18F-fluorodeoxyglucose uptake by using serial positron emission tomography and computed tomography in patients with stage III nonsmall cell lung cancer. Am J Clin Oncol 2008;31(5):470–5.

60. de Langen AJ, van den Boogaart V, Lubberink M, et al. Monitoring response to antiangiogenic therapy in non-small cell lung cancer using imaging markers derived from PET and dynamic contrast-enhanced MRI. official publication, Society of Nuclear Medicine. J Nucl Med 2011;52(1):48–55.

61. Pisters KM, Kris MG, Gralla RJ, et al. Pathologic complete response in advanced non-small-cell lung cancer following preoperative chemotherapy: implications for the design of future non-small-cell lung cancer combined modality trials. official journal of the American Society of Clinical Oncology. J Clin Oncol 1993;11(9):1757–62.

62. Albain KS, Swann RS, Rusch VW, et al. Radiotherapy plus chemotherapy with or without surgical

resection for stage III non-small-cell lung cancer: a phase III randomised controlled trial. Lancet 2009;374(9687):379–86.

63. Paul S, Mirza F, Port JL, et al. Survival of patients with clinical stage IIIA non-small cell lung cancer after induction therapy: age, mediastinal downstaging, and extent of pulmonary resection as independent predictors. J Thorac Cardiovasc Surg 2011; 141(1):48–58.

64. Rebollo-Aguirre AC, Ramos-Font C, Villegas Portero R, et al. Is FDG-PET suitable for evaluating neoadjuvant therapy in non-small cell lung cancer? evidence with systematic review of the literature. J Surg Oncol 2010;101(6):486–94.

65. de Cabanyes Candela S, Detterbeck FC. A systematic review of restaging after induction therapy for stage IIIa lung cancer: prediction of pathologic stage. official publication of the International Association for the Study of Lung Cancer. J Thorac Oncol 2010;5(3):389–98.

66. Cerfolio RJ, Ojha B, Mukherjee S, et al. Positron emission tomography scanning with 2-fluoro-2-deoxy-d-glucose as a predictor of response of neoadjuvant treatment for non-small cell carcinoma. J Thorac Cardiovasc Surg 2003;125(4):938–44.

67. Hellwig D, Gröschel A, Graeter TP, et al. Diagnostic performance and prognostic impact of FDG-PET in suspected recurrence of surgically treated non-small cell lung cancer. Eur J Nucl Med Mol Imaging 2006;33(1):13–21.

68. Hicks RJ, Kalff V, MacManus MP, et al. The utility of (18)F-FDG PET for suspected recurrent non-small cell lung cancer after potentially curative therapy: impact on management and prognostic stratification. official publication, Society of Nuclear Medicine. J Nucl Med 2001;42(11):1605–13.

69. De Ruysscher D, Kirsch CM. PET scans in radiotherapy planning of lung cancer. journal of the European Society for Therapeutic Radiology and Oncology. Radiother Oncol 2010;96(3):335–8.

70. Mac Manus MP, Hicks RJ, Ball DL, et al. F-18 fluorodeoxyglucose positron emission tomography staging in radical radiotherapy candidates with nonsmall cell lung carcinoma: powerful correlation with survival and high impact on treatment. Cancer 2001;92(4): 886–95.

71. De Ruysscher D, Wanders S, van Haren E, et al. Selective mediastinal node irradiation based on FDG-PET scan data in patients with non-small-cell lung cancer: a prospective clinical study. Int J Radiat Oncol Biol Phys 2005;62(4):988–94.

72. Erdi YE, Rosenzweig K, Erdi AK, et al. Radiotherapy treatment planning for patients with non-small cell lung cancer using positron emission tomography (PET). journal of the European Society for Therapeutic Radiology and Oncology. Radiother Oncol 2002;62(1):51–60.

73. Vanuytsel LJ, Vansteenkiste JF, Stroobants SG, et al. The impact of (18)F-fluoro-2-deoxy-D-glucose positron emission tomography (FDG-PET) lymph node staging on the radiation treatment volumes in patients with non-small cell lung cancer. journal of the European Society for Therapeutic Radiology and Oncology. Radiother Oncol 2000;55(3):317–24.

74. Nestle U, Walter K, Schmidt S, et al. 18F-deoxyglucose positron emission tomography (FDG-PET) for the planning of radiotherapy in lung cancer: high impact in patients with atelectasis. Int J Radiat Oncol Biol Phys 1999;44(3):593–7.

75. Bradley J, Thorstad WL, Mutic S, et al. Impact of FDG-PET on radiation therapy volume delineation in non-small-cell lung cancer. Int J Radiat Oncol Biol Phys 2004;59(1):78–86.

76. Ashamalla H, Rafla S, Parikh K, et al. The contribution of integrated PET/CT to the evolving definition of treatment volumes in radiation treatment planning in lung cancer. Int J Radiat Oncol Biol Phys 2005;63(4): 1016–23.

77. Feng M, Kong FM, Gross M, et al. Using fluorodeoxyglucose positron emission tomography to assess tumor volume during radiotherapy for non-small-cell lung cancer and its potential impact on adaptive dose escalation and normal tissue sparing. Int J Radiat Oncol Biol Phys 2009;73(4):1228–34.

78. Gillham C, Zips D, Pönisch F, et al. Additional PET/CT in week 5-6 of radiotherapy for patients with stage III non-small cell lung cancer as a means of dose escalation planning? journal of the European Society for Therapeutic Radiology and Oncology. Radiother Oncol 2008;88(3):335–41.

79. Roberts PF, Follette DM, von Haag D, et al. Factors associated with false-positive staging of lung cancer by positron emission tomography. Ann Thorac Surg 2000;70(4):1154–9 [discussion: 1159–60].

80. Graeter TP, Hellwig D, Hoffmann K, et al. Mediastinal lymph node staging in suspected lung cancer: comparison of positron emission tomography with F-18-fluorodeoxyglucose and mediastinoscopy. Ann Thorac Surg 2003;75(1):231–5 [discussion: 235–6].

81. Annema JT, Hoekstra OS, Smit EF, et al. Towards a minimally invasive staging strategy in NSCLC: analysis of PET positive mediastinal lesions by EUS-FNA. Lung Cancer 2004;44(1):53–60.

82. Wallace MB, Pascual JM, Raimondo M, et al. Minimally invasive endoscopic staging of suspected lung cancer. the journal of the American Medical Association. JAMA 2008;299(5):540–6.

83. Wallace M, Pascual JM, Raimondo M, et al. Complete "medical mediastinoscopy" under conscious sedation: a prospective blinded comparison of endoscopic and endobronchial ultrasound to bronchoscopic fine needle aspiration for malignant mediastinal lymph nodes [abstract]. Gastrointest Endosc 2006;63:AB96.

84. Bryant AS, Cerfolio RJ, Klemm KM, et al. Maximum standard uptake value of mediastinal lymph nodes on integrated FDG-PET-CT predicts pathology in patients with non-small cell lung cancer. Ann Thorac Surg 2006;82(2):417–22 [discussion: 422–3].

85. Cerfolio RJ, Ojha B, Bryant AS, et al. The accuracy of integrated PET-CT compared with dedicated PET alone for the staging of patients with nonsmall cell lung cancer. Ann Thorac Surg 2004;78(3):1017–23 [discussion: 1017–23].

86. Lardinois D, Weder W, Hany TF, et al. Staging of non-small-cell lung cancer with integrated positron-emission tomography and computed tomography. N Engl J Med 2003;348(25):2500–7.

87. Kim SK, Allen-Auerbach M, Goldin J, et al. Accuracy of PET/CT in characterization of solitary pulmonary lesions. official publication, Society of Nuclear Medicine. J Nucl Med 2007;48(2):214–20.

88. Demura Y, Tsuchida T, Ishizaki T, et al. 18F-FDG accumulation with PET for differentiation between benign and malignant lesions in the thorax. official publication, Society of Nuclear Medicine. J Nucl Med 2003;44(4):540–8.

89. Uesaka D, Demura Y, Ishizaki T, et al. Evaluation of dual-time-point 18F-FDG PET for staging in patients with lung cancer. official publication, Society of Nuclear Medicine. J Nucl Med 2008;49(10):1606–12.

The Pulmonologist's Diagnostic and Therapeutic Interventions in Lung Cancer

Jonathan Puchalski, MD, MEd[a],*, David Feller-Kopman, MD[b]

KEYWORDS

- Bronchoscopy • Endobronchial ultrasound
- Electromagnetic navigation • Airway stents

Diagnostic and therapeutic strategies for lung cancer have improved with advancing technology and the acquisition of the necessary skills by bronchoscopists to fully use these advanced techniques. The diagnostic yield for lung cancer has significantly increased with the advent of technologies such as endobronchial ultrasound (EBUS), navigational systems, and improved imaging modalities. Similarly, the therapeutic benefit of bronchoscopy in advanced lung cancer has begun to be understood for its impact on quality and quantity of life. This article highlights the pulmonologists' diagnostic advances and therapeutic options, with an emphasis on outcomes.

DIAGNOSTIC BRONCHOSCOPY
Early Detection of Endobronchial Lung Cancer

Lung cancer is the leading cause of cancer death worldwide and accounted for approximately 157,300 deaths in the United States in 2010.[1] Although the potential benefits of lung cancer screening are eagerly anticipated,[2] unfortunately lung cancer is often detected in an advanced stage either incidentally or in patients with symptoms of late disease.

Lung cancer that is limited to the mucosa in the central airways is usually not detected with available imaging techniques. Imaging modalities such as autofluorescence, narrow band imaging, optical coherence tomography, confocal endomicroscopy, high magnification bronchoscopy, and multimodality fluorescein imaging are being investigated for the detection of early-stage lung cancer or carcinoma in situ.[3,4] Although many of these modalities have been found to have significantly higher sensitivity than white-light bronchoscopy for detecting high-grade dysplasia and carcinoma in situ, the primary limitation remains the poor specificity.[5] Miniaturized radial EBUS probes fitted with a catheter that carries a water-inflatable balloon at its tip (different from the peripheral and convex EBUS probes described later) improve bronchial wall contact to allow detailed images of the bronchial wall structure. EBUS images correlate extremely well with histologic specimens and are better than CT scans for determining airway invasion versus compression.[6] However, no gold standard currently exists for the bronchoscopic diagnosis of early-stage central-airway-limited lung cancer, and the efficacy of these techniques is less understood than EBUS, electromagnetic

This work was not supported by any grant.
The authors have nothing to disclose.
[a] Division of Pulmonary and Critical Care Medicine, Yale University School of Medicine, Boardman Building 205, 330 Cedar Street, New Haven, CT 06510, USA
[b] Bronchoscopy and Interventional Pulmonology, Division of Pulmonary and Critical Care Medicine, Johns Hopkins University, 1830 East Monument Street, Fifth Floor Baltimore, MD 21205, USA
* Corresponding author.
E-mail address: Jonathan.puchalski@yale.edu

Clin Chest Med 32 (2011) 763–771
doi:10.1016/j.ccm.2011.08.010
0272-5231/11/$ – see front matter © 2011 Elsevier Inc. All rights reserved.

navigation (EMN), and the techniques described in the following paragraphs for diagnosing mediastinal and hilar adenopathy and solitary pulmonary nodules and masses.

Endosonography for Adenopathy and Central Lesions

Esophageal ultrasound (EUS) and EBUS are highly accurate techniques for diagnosing and staging lung cancer. EUS was initially developed for gastrointestinal disease in the 1970s and is used during biopsy of lymph nodes for suspected lung cancer in stations 1L, 2L, 4L, 7, 8, and 9. It may also be the preferred technique for assessing metastases to the left adrenal gland. A recent meta-analysis described the ability of EUS to stage lung cancer, with a pooled sensitivity of 88% and specificity of 97% for patients with enlarged mediastinal lymph nodes. The sensitivity was 58% in the absence of mediastinal adenopathy.[7] The efficacy of EBUS advanced in the 1990s with miniaturization of the curvilinear ultrasound transducer. The convex probe EBUS bronchoscope allows real-time visualization of needle aspiration in stations 1, 2R, 2L, 4R, 4L, 7, 10R, 10L, 11R, and 11L. A meta-analysis of EBUS for these lesions reported a 93% sensitivity, with a 9% false-negative rate.[8]

EUS and EBUS are complementary techniques that, when used together, further increase the diagnostic yield. Although the two different scopes with different practitioners may be used, the EBUS scope may be passed into the esophagus, enabling both procedures to be accomplished by one operator in the same setting. This approach has been shown to increase the diagnostic accuracy and the number of lymph node stations that can be biopsied.[9,10]

Although mediastinoscopy has long been considered the gold standard for mediastinal lymph node staging, the technique is used in fewer than 30% of patients undergoing lung resection, and when performed, lymph node tissue is obtained in fewer than 50%.[11] Additionally, EBUS has been shown to have a higher diagnostic yield compared with mediastinoscopy, especially at station 7.[12] The yield of endoscopic evaluation (EUS/EBUS) plus mediastinoscopy is higher than either modality alone.[13] Therefore, the need for mediastinoscopy has decreased in most institutions that routinely use EUS and EBUS.

The Assessment of Peripheral Lesions

Nonmalignant lesions are found in up to 55% of patients undergoing resection for suspicious pulmonary opacities.[14] CT-guided biopsy has a high diagnostic yield but is associated with a pneumothorax rate of 20% to 25%, higher than the 5% to

10% quoted for bronchoscopic biopsies.[15] Although the historical yield for bronchoscopy in diagnosing peripheral lesions has been low, new techniques have significantly improved bronchoscopists' ability to obtain the correct diagnosis.

Peripheral EBUS (pEBUS) uses a 20-MHz radial-type probe and may be used with or without a guide sheath. The typical "snowstorm" seen in the parenchyma will convert to a more homogenous image when the lesion in question is approached. A recent meta-analysis reviewed 16 studies that included 1420 patients and found a point sensitivity of 0.73 for the detection of lung cancer, with a positive likelihood ratio of 26.84 and a negative likelihood ratio of 0.28. The sensitivity for diagnosing malignant lesions smaller than 2 cm is increased with the use of peripheral EBUS.[16] The addition of transbronchial needle aspiration to conventional techniques such as biopsy forceps, cytology brushing, and bronchoalveolar lavage increased the yield when using pEBUS.[17] Prototype bronchoscopes that are smaller and can navigate further into the periphery are currently under investigation.

Electromagnetic navigation (EMN) combines real-time three-dimensional CT images with virtual bronchoscopy and uses a locatable guide that has active steering capability to guide more readily and accurately to peripheral lung lesions. The steps of the process have been well summarized and include planning, mapping, navigation, and then the biopsies.[18] Its use has increased since 2003 and the overall diagnostic yield has ranged from 59% to 77%. The efficacy of the technique is not necessarily impacted by the size of the lesion, with several studies showing a similar diagnostic accuracy for lesions smaller or larger than 2 cm.[13] Lesions in which a bronchus leads to the abnormality in question ("bronchus sign") have a significantly higher yield than those without a visible airway to the lesion.[19] Combining EMN with pEBUS in a randomized controlled trial improved the diagnostic yield to 88% compared with pEBUS (69%) and EMN (59%) alone.[20] New technologies using both virtual bronchoscopic navigation and combined virtual bronchoscopic and electromagnetic navigation are being developed and actively investigated. Images from these advanced endoscopic techniques are shown in **Fig. 1** and diagnostic procedures are summarized in **Table 1**.

Therapeutics

Interventional procedures for lung cancer are often palliative in nature, although early-stage lung cancers may also be treated definitively. This section focuses on topical endobronchial modalities, airway stenting, and palliative pleural

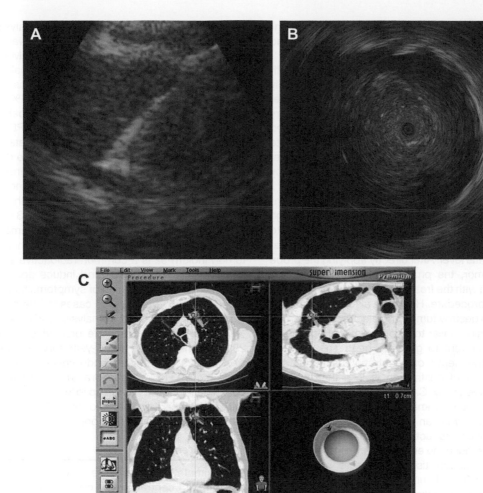

Fig. 1. Advanced diagnostic tools include the convex probe EBUS (*A*), peripheral EBUS (*B*), and EMN (*C*). The lesion is biopsied in real-time (*A*), and identified with advanced techniques before biopsy (*B, C*).

procedures aimed at improving dyspnea. It highlights not only the technical success of the procedures but also what is known regarding the outcomes related to dyspnea and quality of life stemming from these procedures.

Topical Therapies

Various forms of topical therapy may be applied to the tracheobronchial tree through a bronchoscope. These techniques include mechanical debulking and the use of thermal and nonthermal modalities,

Table 1
The pulmonologist's advanced tools for diagnosing malignancy[a]

Convex EBUS	Meta-analysis: sensitivity 0.88–0.93 for mediastinal staging in patients with lung cancer[43,44]
Peripheral EBUS	Meta-analysis: Sensitivity 0.73 for detection of lung cancer[16]
EMN	May increase diagnostic accuracy when added to peripheral EBUS[20]
Ultrasound-guided thoracentesis	Ultrasound improves safety of thoracentesis[45]; the yield of thoracentesis for malignant effusions is 62%–90% and increases with multiple fluid collections[46]
Pleuroscopy	Diagnostic sensitivity for malignant effusions is 93%–95%[41]

[a] Newer technologies have improved the diagnostic yield for common bronchoscopic and pleural procedures.

such as laser, electrocautery, argon plasma coagulation (APC), cryotherapy, brachytherapy, and photodynamic therapy (PDT).

Mechanical debulking is often accomplished with the rigid bronchoscope itself. Tumors may be easily cored out, achieving airway patency within a matter of minutes. The microdebrider is a tool with a rotary blade and continuous suction capability. It is used with the rigid bronchoscope to rapidly recanalize the airway.[21] Both of these techniques are faster and more efficacious than flexible bronchoscopy with biopsy forceps.

Various forms of thermal energy can be used endobronchially. Cryotherapy uses a probe through the working channel of a flexible bronchoscope to freeze exophytic airway lesions down to the lobar or segmental level. After directly applying the probe to the tumor, the probe and bronchoscope are withdrawn with the frozen pieces of tumor in a rapid and safe procedure. Heat may also be used in the airways to destroy tumor. The electrocautery probe is technically similar to cryotherapy but applies an electrical current to generate heat. The operator controls the depth of penetration, although the visual extent of destruction is less than what is seen pathologically. Cautery may also be delivered through a snare or knife. APC uses ionized argon gas charged with an electric current to achieve thermal tissue destruction. It does not require direct contact because the energized argon gas finds the nearest grounded tissue to create necrosis to a depth of 3 to 4 mm. A unique risk of APC is systemic gas embolization.[21] The most common laser used in the tracheobronchial tree is the neodymium:yttrium-aluminum-garnet (Nd:YAG), although carbon dioxide may also used in the airway. Tissue vaporization is immediate and the depth of penetration can be up to 10 mm with the Nd:YAG. With all therapies that use heat, the patient's fraction of inspired oxygen requirements must be 40% or less to prevent airway fires. The immediate response rate ranges from 69% to 100%.[22] Most of these techniques are used together as a combined approach to endobronchial therapy.

PDT uses systemic injection of light-activated chemical compounds that cause cell death. It is used for centrally located early-stage or inoperable cancers, although its use in the periphery has also been described. Light of a specific wavelength (nonthermal laser) is used to activate the drug, and tumor destruction results from the generation of cytotoxic singlet oxygen species. The effects of PDT are delayed and thus it is indicated predominantly for patients who are nonoperable and not candidates for external-beam radiation therapy, or as palliative treatment in the absence of acute

dyspnea.[22] In a recent retrospective analysis of 529 cases in 133 patients, the distal airway was opened in 81% of patients, the Modified Medical Research Council (MMRC) dyspnea scale improved in 74% of patients, morbidity was 15%, and the median 5-year survival was 43%. The authors commented on equal efficacy between PDT and laser therapy but preferred PDT for patients with bloody tumors, such as metastatic renal cell carcinoma and melanoma.[23] One disadvantage is that patients remain photosensitized for 4 to 6 weeks after the procedure and thus must avoid sunlight; another is the cost of the Photofrin, which is currently approximately $13,000.

Brachytherapy involves the direct placement of radioactive seeds into or in proximity to an airway tumor. Iridium-92 is a common radioactive source and is used to alter DNA and induce apoptosis. Improvement and palliation of symptoms has been reported in 65% to 95% of cases.[22] The median survival in a retrospective analysis of 226 patients who received high-dose rate brachytherapy was 28.6 months, with 2- and 5-year survival rates of 57% and 29%. Complete endobronchial response was seen in 93.6% of patients at 3 months, although complications were seen in up to 30%.[24] High-dose rate brachytherapy followed by PDT has been described in a small patient population.[25]

Airway Stenting

Approximately 30% of patients with lung cancer present with central airway obstruction.[26] Airway stenting is often useful in addition to the ablative techniques described earlier and is the only endoscopic modality that can treat airway obstruction caused by external compression. Stents are made of metal, silicone, or a hybrid combination of the two, and are available from different manufacturers. They are available in tubular, Y, L, or T configurations. Silicone stents require rigid bronchoscopy for insertion, whereas metal stents may be placed via flexible bronchoscopy. Silicone stents, however, can be much easier to remove, because tumor ingrowth and epithelization occur less frequently than with metal stents. Other complications include migration, mucus plugging, granuloma formation, and infection.[26] Examples of therapeutic bronchoscopic procedures are shown in **Fig. 2** and a summary of these procedures is shown in **Table 2**.

Therapeutic Outcomes for Airway Disease

The aforementioned airway interventions require specialized training and have their associated risks. A recent prospective analysis of 554 therapeutic procedures performed in four hospitals showed

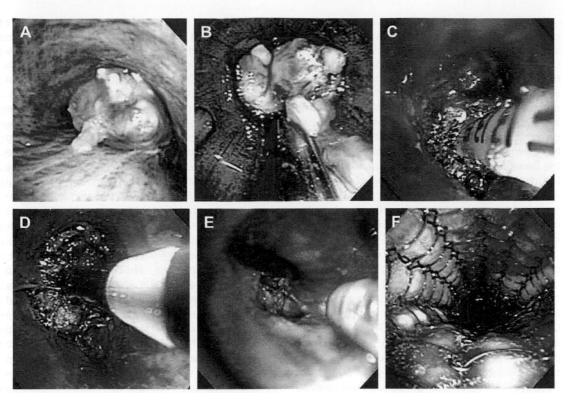

Fig. 2. Therapeutic bronchoscopy. Rigid bronchoscopy can debulk large central tumors (A, B). Heat modalities, including APC (C), electrocautery (D), and laser (E) may be used to topically ablate endobronchial tumor. Prolonged therapy may result from stent placement (F).

that complications were common (19.8%) and that the 30-day mortality was 7.8%. Patients with malignant indications who had the highest rate of complications included current smokers and patients with hypertension, diabetes, and endobronchial disease. Of the deaths at 30 days, only one was procedure-related, whereas the others were related to the progression of underlying disease. Patients with an American Society of Anesthesiologists score of greater than two and higher Zubrod scores were at the greatest risk for complications.[27]

Table 2
The pulmonologist's therapeutic tools for treating malignancy[a]

Laser resection	Success rate for symptoms, radiographic or endoscopic findings approaches 93%[47]
Electrocautery	Success rate is similar to laser, although the cost is less[47]
Argon plasma coagulation	Success rate is similar to laser, although the cost is less[47]
Brachytherapy	Low-dose and high-dose brachytherapy response rates may approach 89%–94%[47]
Photodynamic therapy	Efficacy similar to laser[23]
Airway stenting	Relief of symptoms in up to 90% of patients[48]
Rigid bronchoscopy	Combined with flexible bronchoscopy to core-out central airway obstruction; all of these techniques are often used in conjunction as multimodality therapy
Tunneled pleural catheter	Symptomatic improvement in 96% of patients[37]
Pleurodesis	Talc poudrage via pleuroscopy is successful in up to 90% of patients[41]

[a] Common techniques used by pulmonologists for symptomatic relief in patients with lung cancer.

Many studies show the immediate value of reopening a large central airway that has been obstructed by tumor. The techniques are usually combinations of debulking, heat or cold destruction, and stenting. The greatest benefit is seen when the obstruction is in the trachea, right or left mainstem, or bronchus intermedius (eg, the central airways). Lobar obstruction may be relieved when disease is proximal and the resultant atelectasis has been present for less than 1 month, although the benefits may not be as pronounced as when the central airways are reestablished. The technical success of achieving patency is high. More recent studies have begun to define the benefits of therapeutic airway procedures beyond the immediate postprocedural period.

In 2008, Amjadi, and colleagues[28] performed one of the first studies evaluating quality of life in patients receiving interventional airway procedures. They used the validated European Organisation for Research and Treatment of Cancer Quality of Life Questionnaire (EORTC QLQ-C30) and included 20 patients over 6 months. These patients were nonoperable and did not undergo chemotherapy or radiation therapy during the first 30 days of the study. Therapeutic procedures included mechanical debulking and dilation, Nd:YAG laser, cryotherapy, or stents. More than 80% of the airway caliber was restored in 80% of patients, and 85% of patients showed improved dyspnea scores within 24 hours that extended to 30 days, and most went from a severe category to slight. Significant variability was seen in overall quality of life changes after the procedure. Patients with the best and worst preprocedure quality of life scores seemed to benefit the least, whereas those with an intermediate quality of life benefited the most. The investigators hypothesized that improved dyspnea led to improvements in quality of life but that other factors were also important in overall quality of life assessments.

A recent prospective cohort study of 37 patients with high-grade symptomatic central airway obstruction were evaluated for exercise capacity, lung function, and quality of life. Most (91.9%) had restoration of airway patency (>50% of airway lumen restored). Statistically significant improvements in the 6-minute walk test were noted at days 30, 90, and 180 compared with baseline. The dyspnea scores, resting Borg, forced expiratory volume in 1 second, and forced vital capacity were also improved at day 30. An improvement in overall quality of life was seen in 43% of patients. The median survival was 166 days (23.7 weeks) and the 6-month survival was 46%.[29]

Some emerging reports show potential survival benefits related to interventional pulmonary procedures. A retrospective study of 50 patients who underwent stenting for central airway obstruction suggested that symptoms were effectively palliated as measured by the Medical Research Council (MRC) dyspnea score and Eastern Cooperative Oncology Group performance status. Compared with historical controls, patients in the intermediate performance status group experienced a significant survival advantage. This finding was not seen in patients with a poor performance status. The median survival was 117 days and the 6-month survival was 40%. A median survival of approximately 8 months was seen in patients who underwent airway stenting, compared with 3 months in patients with a high MRC score or poor performance status and 1 to 2 months in historical untreated patients with central airway obstruction.[30] In contrast, a retrospective study of 65 patients showed no survival benefit with airway stenting. Although 98% of patients experienced immediate relief of the airway obstruction, the 1-year survival was 25.2% and the median survival was 6.2 months. A 4-month increase in median survival was seen in patients who received stenting plus adjuvant chemotherapy, but overall survival was not changed.[31] Despite terminal central airway obstruction, other studies have shown the overall benefit of providing palliative care for these patients. In a study of 14 patients with imminent airway obstruction who could choose euthanasia, all patients undergoing stent placement experienced immediate improvement in symptoms.[32] In another study consisting of patients requiring intensive care, 62.5% of the 32 patients could be transferred to a lower level of care immediately after emergency intervention. Benefits also included withdrawal from mechanical ventilation, relief of symptoms, and extended survival.[33] Compared with patients without central airway obstruction receiving therapy for advanced non–small cell lung cancer, those who were treated for central airway obstruction did not have a worsened overall survival.[34] Additional studies report the value of therapeutic bronchoscopy as a combined approach before surgery for curative intent, noting that this may permit parenchyma-sparing surgery in patients with lung cancer.[35]

Diagnostic and Therapeutic Approaches for Malignant Pleural Disease

Of the 150,000 patients per year who develop malignant pleural effusions, lung cancer and breast cancer account for up to 75%.[36] The median survival for patients with a malignant pleural effusion is 4 months.[37] Dyspnea results from loss of functional lung tissue caused by atelectasis, mediastinal shift, and, most importantly, reduced compliance of the chest wall. The diagnosis may be established through routine thoracentesis in up to 80% of cases, although more than one thoracentesis is often necessary. Pleural biopsy may be required for cytologically negative effusions. Once diagnosed, the options for management include treatment of the underlying malignancy, repeated thoracentesis, chest tube placement with pleurodesis, thoracoscopy with pleurodesis, or placement of pleural catheters. Pleurectomy and pleuroperitoneal shunts are rarely performed.[38] Given that the life expectancy is poor, early and aggressive pleural palliation may be the best option for some patients.

Thoracentesis may be performed and several liters of fluid can be removed. For recurrent effusions, however, repeated thoracentesis subjects patients to the risks of the procedure in addition to the uncertainty that revolves around how quickly the effusion will reaccumulate and contribute to respiratory distress. Therefore, most patients should undergo a more definitive therapy. Chest tube placement with instillation of a sclerosing agent requires inpatient hospitalization to enable ongoing drainage of the effusion and adhesion of the pleural surfaces. Smaller chest tubes (10–14 French) work as well as larger chest tubes.

Doxycycline has a reported pleurodesis rate of 76% compared with talc (95%).[38] Controversy exists as to whether talc slurry is as efficacious as aerosolized talc (via thoracoscopy).[36] The two techniques are likely equally effective, although talc poudrage may be preferred in patients with malignant effusions from lung or breast cancer.[39] In a recent phase III prospective study of 482 patients, no overall difference in pleurodesis was seen between talc slurry and insufflation, although the rate was higher with insufflation in patients with lung cancer.[40]

The concern with using talc is the risk for lung injury and acute respiratory distress syndrome (ARDS), possibly related to particle size. None of the patients in a recent prospective study of 558 patients developed ARDS with the use of large talc particles.[36]

Thoracoscopic pleurodesis can be achieved either through video-assisted thoracoscopic surgery or medical pleuroscopy. The latter may be performed with a rigid scope or a flexi-rigid scope. Medical pleuroscopy can be performed outside of the operating room without general anesthesia or single lung ventilation. Talc poudrage performed thoracoscopically has a pleurodesis rate of at least 90%.[41] Discharge from the hospital may be accomplished sooner through placing a tunneled

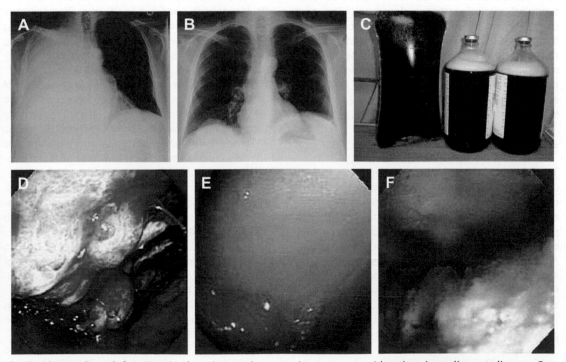

Fig. 3. Diagnostic and therapeutic pleural procedures are important considerations in malignant disease. One-time (thoracentesis) and recurrent drainage of effusions (tunneled catheters) may improve dyspnea (A, B, C). Pleuroscopy may be used to biopsy pleural lesions (D) and then pleurodese with agents such as talc (E, F).

pleural catheter at the same time as thoracoscopic pleurodesis.[42]

The tunneled pleural catheter system (PleurX, CareFusion, Waukwgan, IL USA) is a 15.5-French catheter that may be placed in an outpatient setting. Drainage is typically performed daily or every other day by the patient, family members, or visiting health care professionals. Spontaneous pleurodesis occurs in 46% of patients at 29 to 56 days postplacement of the catheter, although rates from 21% to 58% have been reported. Symptomatic improvement occurs in 81% to 100% of patients,[38] with a recent review of 1370 patients showing a 95.6% improvement in symptoms.[37] Quality of life measurements are infrequently reported, but 46 of 46 patients showed improvement.[37] Additional systems exist but have not been well-studied. Complications are generally considered to be low, but range from 5% to 27%[38] and are absent in 87.5% of cases.[37] The major complications include empyemas (2.8%), other infection (2%), and pneumothorax (5.9%).[37] Survival after placement of tunneled pleural catheter is a mean of 87 days and median of 59.5 to 144 days.[37] Because these catheters may be placed on an outpatient basis without general anesthesia, costs seem to be less than for tube thoracostomy and thoracoscopy.[36] A more recent study suggested that talc pleurodesis may be less expensive than tunneled pleural catheter placement. The cost of the drainage bottles significantly contributes to the price, and thus patients surviving longer may incur this larger expense.[37] Combining pleurodesis with placement of a tunneled catheter may provide a minimal hospital stay (1.7 days) and short catheter duration (7 days).[42] **Fig. 3** shows examples of these procedures.

SUMMARY

The diagnostic bronchoscopic approach to lung cancer has changed significantly with the advent of new technology and appropriate training. Therapeutic strategies have also developed that provide an improvement in symptoms and quality of life for patients with advanced lung cancer. Aggressive palliation of pleural disease provides similar benefits. These improvements are likely foreshadowing of future advances as technology continues to expand.

REFERENCES

1. Cataldo VD, Gibbons DL, Perez-Soler R, et al. Treatment of non-small-cell lung cancer with erlotinib or gefitinib. N Engl J Med 2011;364(10):947–55.

2. Aberle DR, Berg CD, Black WC, et al. The National Lung Screening Trial: overview and study design. Radiology 2011;258(1):243–53.

3. Yarmus L, Feller-Kopman D. Bronchoscopes of the twenty-first century. Clin Chest Med 2010;31(1):19–27.

4. Colt HG, Murgu SD. Interventional bronchoscopy from bench to bedside: new techniques for early lung cancer detection. Clin Chest Med 2010;31(1):29–37.

5. Haussinger K, Becker H, Stanzel F, et al. Autofluorescence bronchoscopy with white light bronchoscopy compared with white light bronchoscopy alone for the detection of precancerous lesions: a European randomised controlled multicentre trial. Thorax 2005;60(6):496–503.

6. Yasufuku K. Early diagnosis of lung cancer. Clin Chest Med 2010;31(1):39–47.

7. Micames CG, McCrory DC, Pavey DA, et al. Endoscopic ultrasound-guided fine-needle aspiration for non-small cell lung cancer staging: a systematic review and metaanalysis. Chest 2007;131(2):539–48.

8. Gomez M, Silvestri GA. Endobronchial ultrasound for the diagnosis and staging of lung cancer. Proc Am Thorac Soc 2009;6(2):180–6.

9. Herth FJ, Krasnik M, Kahn N, et al. Combined endoscopic-endobronchial ultrasound-guided fine-needle aspiration of mediastinal lymph nodes through a single bronchoscope in 150 patients with suspected lung cancer. Chest 2010;138(4):790–4.

10. Hwangbo B, Lee GK, Lee HS, et al. Transbronchial and transesophageal fine-needle aspiration using an ultrasound bronchoscope in mediastinal staging of potentially operable lung cancer. Chest 2010; 138(4):795–802.

11. Little AG, Rusch VW, Bonner JA, et al. Patterns of surgical care of lung cancer patients. Ann Thorac Surg 2005;80(6):2051–6.

12. Ernst A, Anantham D, Eberhardt R, et al. Diagnosis of mediastinal adenopathy-real-time endobronchial ultrasound guided needle aspiration versus mediastinoscopy. J Thorac Oncol 2008;3(6):577–82.

13. Annema JT, van Meerbeeck JP, Rintoul RC, et al. Mediastinoscopy vs endosonography for mediastinal nodal staging of lung cancer: a randomized trial. JAMA 2010;304(20):2245–52.

14. Isbell JM, Deppen S, Putnam JB Jr, et al. Existing general population models inaccurately predict lung cancer risk in patients referred for surgical evaluation. Ann Thorac Surg 2011;91(1):227–33.

15. Hergott CA, Tremblay A. Role of bronchoscopy in the evaluation of solitary pulmonary nodules. Clin Chest Med 2010;31(1):49–63.

16. Steinfort DP, Khor YH, Manser RL, et al. Radial probe endobronchial ultrasound for the diagnosis of peripheral lung cancer: systematic review and meta-analysis. Eur Respir J 2011;37(4):902–10.

17. Chao TY, Chien MT, Lie CH, et al. Endobronchial ultrasonography-guided transbronchial needle aspiration increases the diagnostic yield of peripheral pulmonary lesions: a randomized trial. Chest 2009; 136(1):229–36.

18. Schwarz Y. Electromagnetic navigation. Clin Chest Med 2010;31(1):65–73.

19. Seijo LM, de Torres JP, Lozano MD, et al. Diagnostic yield of electromagnetic navigation bronchoscopy is highly dependent on the presence of a Bronchus sign on CT imaging: results from a prospective study. Chest 2010;138(6):1316–21.

20. Eberhardt R, Anantham D, Ernst A, et al. Multimodality bronchoscopic diagnosis of peripheral lung lesions: a randomized controlled trial. Am J Respir Crit Care Med 2007;176(1):36–41.

21. Gorden JA, Ernst A. Endoscopic management of central airway obstruction. Semin Thorac Cardiovasc Surg 2009;21(3):263–73.

22. Folch E, Mehta AC. Airway interventions in the tracheobronchial tree. Semin Respir Crit Care Med 2008;29(4):441–52.

23. Minnich DJ, Bryant AS, Dooley A, et al. Photodynamic laser therapy for lesions in the airway. Ann Thorac Surg 2010;89(6):1744–8.

24. Aumont-le Guilcher M, Prevost B, Sunyach MP, et al. High-dose-rate brachytherapy for non-small-cell lung carcinoma: a retrospective study of 226 patients. Int J Radiat Oncol Biol Phys 2011;79(4): 1112–6.

25. Weinberg BD, Allison RR, Sibata C, et al. Results of combined photodynamic therapy (PDT) and high dose rate brachytherapy (HDR) in treatment of obstructive endobronchial non-small cell lung cancer (NSCLC). Photodiagnosis Photodyn Ther 2010;7(1):50–8.

26. Lee P, Kupeli E, Mehta AC. Airway stents. Clin Chest Med 2010;31(1):141–50.

27. Ernst A, Simoff M, Ost D, et al. Prospective risk-adjusted morbidity and mortality outcome analysis after therapeutic bronchoscopic procedures: results of a multi-institutional outcomes database. Chest 2008;134(3):514–9.

28. Amjadi K, Voduc N, Cruysberghs Y, et al. Impact of interventional bronchoscopy on quality of life in malignant airway obstruction. Respiration 2008; 76(4):421–8.

29. Oviatt PL, Stather DR, Michaud G, et al. Exercise capacity, lung function, and quality of life after interventional bronchoscopy. J Thorac Oncol 2011;6(1):38–42.

30. Razi SS, Lebovics RS, Schwartz G, et al. Timely airway stenting improves survival in patients with malignant central airway obstruction. Ann Thorac Surg 2010;90(4):1088–93.

31. Saji H, Furukawa K, Tsutsui H, et al. Outcomes of airway stenting for advanced lung cancer with central airway obstruction. Interact Cardiovasc Thorac Surg 2010;11(4):425–8.

32. Vonk-Noordegraaf A, Postmus PE, Sutedja TG. Tracheobronchial stenting in the terminal care of cancer patients with central airways obstruction. Chest 2001;120(6):1811–4.

33. Colt HG, Harrell JH. Therapeutic rigid bronchoscopy allows level of care changes in patients with acute respiratory failure from central airways obstruction. Chest 1997;112(1):202–6.

34. Chhajed PN, Baty F, Pless M, et al. Outcome of treated advanced non-small cell lung cancer with and without central airway obstruction. Chest 2006; 130(6):1803–7.

35. Chhajed PN, Eberhardt R, Dienemann H, et al. Therapeutic bronchoscopy interventions before surgical resection of lung cancer. Ann Thorac Surg 2006; 81(5):1839–43.

36. Musani AI. Treatment options for malignant pleural effusion. Curr Opin Pulm Med 2009;15(4):380–7.

37. Van Meter ME, McKee KY, Kohlwes RJ. Efficacy and safety of tunneled pleural catheters in adults with malignant pleural effusions: a systematic review. J Gen Intern Med 2011;26(1):70–6.

38. Spector M, Pollak JS. Management of malignant pleural effusions. Semin Respir Crit Care Med 2008;29(4):405–13.

39. Dresler CM, Olak J, Herndon JE II, et al. Phase III intergroup study of talc poudrage vs talc slurry sclerosis for malignant pleural effusion. Chest 2005; 127(3):909–15.

40. Chen H, Brahmer J. Management of malignant pleural effusion. Curr Oncol Rep 2008;10(4):287–93.

41. Michaud G, Berkowitz DM, Ernst A. Pleuroscopy for diagnosis and therapy for pleural effusions. Chest 2010;138(5):1242–6.

42. Reddy C, Ernst A, Lamb C, et al. Rapid pleurodesis for malignant pleural effusions: a pilot study. Chest 2011;139(6):1419–23.

43. Adams K, Shah PL, Edmonds L, et al. Test performance of endobronchial ultrasound and transbronchial needle aspiration biopsy for mediastinal staging in patients with lung cancer: systematic review and meta-analysis. Thorax 2009;64(9):757–62.

44. Gu P, Zhao YZ, Jiang LY, et al. Endobronchial ultrasound-guided transbronchial needle aspiration for staging of lung cancer: a systematic review and meta-analysis. Eur J Cancer 2009;45(8):1389–96.

45. Gordon CE, Feller-Kopman D, Balk EM, et al. Pneumothorax following thoracentesis: a systematic review and meta-analysis. Arch Intern Med 2010;170(4):332–9.

46. Heffner JE. Diagnosis and management of malignant pleural effusions. Respirology 2008;13(1):5–20.

47. Lee P, Tamm M, Chhajed PN. Advances in bronchoscopy–therapeutic bronchoscopy. J Assoc Physicians India 2004;52:905–14.

48. Theodore PR. Emergent management of malignancy-related acute airway obstruction. Emerg Med Clin North Am 2009;27(2):231–41.

Functional Evaluation before Lung Resection

Florian von Groote-Bidlingmaier, MD,
Coenraad F.N. Koegelenberg, MD, Chris T. Bolliger, MD, PhD*

KEYWORDS

- Lung resection • Operability • Preoperative evaluation
- Regional lung function • Cardiopulmonary exercise test

Lung cancer is the leading cause of cancer-related death worldwide, accounting for approximately 160,000 deaths in the United States in 2010.[1] Lung resection remains the only curative approach to lung cancer, despite continuous advances in chemotherapy and radiotherapy.[2,3] In the Western world, lung cancer is one of the main indications for lung resection, despite only 15% to 25% of all lung cancers being operable at the time of presentation. In developing countries, this figure is even lower: recent data from South Africa suggest that only 6% of all patient with lung cancer were operable at the time of presentation.[4] However, post-tuberculous bronchiectasis, complicated by hemoptysis or recurrent lower respiratory tract infections, remains the most common indication for lung resection.[5]

In most cases of operable lung cancer, a substantial part of functional lung tissue has to be resected, which leads to a permanent loss of pulmonary function. An estimated 90% of all patients with lung cancer have underlying chronic obstructive pulmonary disease (COPD) and cardiovascular disorders in varying degrees caused by the shared risk factor from tobacco smoking, making lung resection in those patients a procedure associated with a higher risk of intraoperative and postoperative complications.[2,3] Resection in patients with insufficient pulmonary reserves can result in permanent respiratory disability. The assumption that there is a level of respiratory impairment beyond which resection bears a high risk and is prohibitive drives the ongoing search for the ideal test to predict postoperative lung function and identify the patients at high risk.

This article reviews the current standards of preoperative assessment, including tests for measurement of preoperative pulmonary function and gas exchange, calculation of predicted postoperative (ppo) function, exercise testing, and assessment of regional lung function.

PARAMETERS OF FUNCTIONAL OPERABILITY

The main parameters of functional operability are age, general health and performance status, cardiac function, pulmonary mechanics, diffusion capacity, exercise capacity, and extent of resection. All functional parameters must be measured in optimal therapy to achieve the best possible results. Patients' COPD treatment therefore needs to be optimized, smoking cessation should be encouraged, and even short term physiotherapy and rehabilitation need to be considered. The lack of chest physiotherapy has been shown to be an independent risk factor for postoperative complications.[6] In patients who have lung cancer, the potential period for functional improvement is only 4 to 6 weeks, because further delays necessitate reevaluation of tumor staging given the often rapid progression of disease.

Age, General Health, Performance Status

Although age greater than 70 years has been associated with a higher risk of complications,[7,8] it is the comorbidities associated with advanced age rather than age itself that are responsible for this observation.[9] Patients more than 70 years of age with good performance status and preserved

The authors have nothing to disclose.
Division of Pulmonology, Department of Medicine, University of Stellenbosch, PO Box 19063, Tygerberg 7505, Cape Town, South Africa
* Corresponding author.
E-mail address: ctb@sun.ac.za

Clin Chest Med 32 (2011) 773–782
doi:10.1016/j.ccm.2011.08.001
0272-5231/11/$ – see front matter © 2011 Elsevier Inc. All rights reserved.

cardiopulmonary reserves have a long-term survival comparable with younger patients.[10] Newer surgical techniques, such as video-assisted thoracic surgery (VATS),[11] and limited resections for stage Ia lung cancers may also negate some of the effects of comorbidity in elderly patients. Surgery should therefore not be withheld from any patient based on age alone.[2]

COPD is the most frequently identified risk factor for pulmonary complications among patients undergoing any form of surgery, and overt COPD has a relative risk of 4.7 of developing postoperative complications following thoracic surgery.[9] Moreover, both the presence of abnormalities on physical examination and the degree of obstruction correlate with complications. There is currently no prospective evidence to estimate the risk of postoperative complications in patients with restrictive ventilatory impairment.[12] Well-controlled asthma is not associated with postoperative complications, and neither is a short course of oral corticosteroids.[12]

The American Society of Anesthesiologists' (ASA) classification has been shown to predict postoperative complications. The odds ratio for postoperative complications in patients with ASA class III or higher is 2.6 compared with patients with ASA class I and II.[12] Partial and total dependence are major risk factors for postoperative complications.[13] Patients who are dependent are unlikely to be candidates for major pulmonary resection. Metabolic disturbances contribute to postoperative complications. Malnutrition (albumin <30 g/L) reduces ventilatory drive to hypoxia and hypercapnia, contributes to respiratory muscle dysfunction, alters lung elasticity, and impairs immunity. However, nutritional intervention before surgery has not been shown to attenuate the risk. Renal impairment (blood urea >30 mg/dL [10.7 mmol/L]) carries an odds ratio of 2.3 for postoperative complications.[12,13]

Cigarette smoking increases the risk of postoperative pulmonary complications irrespective of the presence of COPD.[9] A significant reduction of this risk is only noted after 8 weeks of cessation.[10] It had previously been suggested that quitting less than 8 weeks before surgery might even increase the risk for complications.[14,15] Recent meta-analyses confirm that smoking cessation before surgery does not increase the risk for postoperative complications. The data indicate that stopping smoking before surgery might lower the risk of complications, with a growing effect with longer duration of smoking cessation.[16,17] Therefore, smokers should be encouraged to quit smoking and should be supported with appropriate treatment.

Cardiac Risk Assessment

Patients with lung cancer and underlying COPD often suffer from cardiovascular disease as well, because smoking is a risk factor for both lung and heart disease. Those patients are at higher risk for postoperative complications than patients without underlying lung and cardiovascular disease. As far back as 1961, Mittman[18] showed that an abnormal resting electrocardiogram (ECG) was associated with an increased risk of intraoperative or postoperative cardiac complications. In the late 1970s, a multifactorial cardiac risk index was published,[19] was revised in 1999.[20] It contains 6 independent variables that correlate with postoperative cardiac complications (**Box 1**). Two or more variables indicate a high risk and are associated with a postoperative cardiac complication rate of greater than 10%. Lung resection represents high-risk surgery (ie, 1 positive variable), and any patient with another positive variable needs evaluation and potential intervention by a cardiologist.

Box 1
Revised Goldman Cardiac Risk Index: the number of positive variables correlates with the risk for postoperative cardiac complications (no risk factors, 0.4%; 1 risk factor, 0.9%; 2 risk factors, 7%; 3 and more risk factors, 11%)

1. High-risk type of surgery

2. History of ischemic heart disease

    a. History of myocardial infarction (within 6 months)

    b. Positive exercise test

    c. Current complaint of ischemic chest pain

    d. Use of nitrate therapy

    e. Pathologic Q waves on ECG

(Not included: prior coronary revascularization procedure unless one of the other criteria for ischemic heart disease is present)

3. History of cardiac failure

4. History of cerebrovascular disease

5. Diabetes mellitus requiring treatment with insulin

6. Preoperative serum creatinine >2.0 mg/dL (177 μmol/L)

From Lee TH, Marcantonio ER, Mangione CM, et al. Derivation and prospective validation of a simple index for prediction of cardiac risk of major noncardiac surgery. Circulation 1999;100(10):1043–9; with permission.

Coronary stenting can be performed before lung resection, although it has not been shown to influence cardiac risk.[3] Coronary artery bypass surgery before lung surgery, as suggested previously, might delay curative resection, which is problematic because of the time constraints in the management of lung cancer. Combining lung cancer surgery and conventional bypass surgery increases the risk of morbidity and mortality.[21,22] Minimally invasive (off-pump) direct coronary artery bypass surgery simultaneous with lung resection has comparable complications with lung resection alone.[23]

Spirometry

Many parameters of pulmonary mechanics have been recommended for preoperative assessment, but only forced expiratory volume in 1 second (FEV_1), suggested in the early 1970s,[24,25] has stood the test of time. It correlates well with the degree of respiratory impairment and provides an indirect measure of pulmonary reserves. Most studies that have reported on FEV_1 have used absolute values. Early recommendations of FEV_1 values for safe resections were more than 2 L for pneumonectomy[26,27] and more than 1.5 L for lobectomy.[27,28] However, the use of absolute values has never been universally accepted, because they do not take gender, height, weight, and age into consideration, nor do they consider the functional contribution of the tissue to be removed . Three investigators suggested cutoffs for FEV_1 in percentage predicted: Mittman[18] suggested greater than 70%, whereas Nagasaki[8] and, more recently, Pate[29] suggested greater than 40%. None of the 3 studies mentioned the extent of resection possible with these values.

The concept of so-called predicted postoperative (ppo) values has recently been introduced. These values are ideally expressed as percent of ppo (%ppo). Thresholds prohibiting resections of various extents have been validated. Patients with preoperative FEV_1 greater than 80% of predicted (in combination with a carbon monoxide diffusion capacity [DL_{CO}] >80% of predicted) are generally considered at low risk for resection up to pneumonectomy. Markos and colleagues,[30] Wahi and colleagues,[31] and Bolliger and colleagues[32] all found mortality rates of approximately 50% in patients with %FEV_1-ppo less than 40%. Nakahara and colleagues[33] found an even higher mortality (60%) in patients with %FEV_1-ppo less than 30%. Technical aspects regarding ppo calculations are discussed later in this article.

DL_{CO}

The DL_{CO} is a proxy measurement of alveolar oxygen exchange.[34] As early as 1963, Cander[35]

suggested that a value of less than 50% of predicted precluded pulmonary resections. Ferguson and colleagues[36] showed that the DL_{CO} was an independent predictor of morbidity and mortality after pulmonary resection. They identified a DL_{CO} of less than 60% of predicted as a cutoff value for major pulmonary resection. Similar findings were reported by Markos and colleagues.[30] The predicted postoperative DL_{CO} (ppo-DL_{CO}) is currently used, rather than the actual value, particularly in patients with impaired pulmonary reserves.[34] A ppo-DL_{CO} value of less than 40% identifies high-risk patients.[37] The ppo-DL_{CO} values derived from various methods tend to overestimate immediate postoperative values, but there is a significant correlation between actual values 1 month after resection and ppo-DL_{CO} values.[34] Despite being included in current guidelines, the European Thoracic Surgery Database recently showed that DL_{CO} values were only measured in approximately 25% of patients before pulmonary resection.[38]

Formal Cardiopulmonary Exercise Testing

Formal cardiopulmonary exercise testing (CPET) is a comprehensive investigation that assesses integrated cardiopulmonary reserves. The testing is performed in a controlled environment and has the advantage of good reproducibility. Measured values are dependent on pulmonary function, cardiovascular function, and oxygen use by peripheral tissues, thus assessing the overall fitness of a patient.[2] CPET is well validated, but requires expertise and is not universally available. The most widely used exercise tests are maximal or symptom-limited incremental exercise tests on treadmill or bicycle. Various parameters, including cardiac ischemia, can be assessed with good reproducibility. The most important measurement in CPET is the level of work achieved, measured as maximum oxygen consumption (Vo_2max). Vo_2max is measured either directly in a noninvasive fashion or can be calculated. Invasive hemodynamic measurements have been shown to add little useful additional information.[39] An early study reported no mortality versus 75% mortality at greater than and less than a threshold of 1 L/min. Expressing Vo_2max as mL/kg/min takes the patient's body mass into account and should therefore be used. Until recently, a Vo_2max of greater than 20 mL/kg/min or greater than 75% of predicted was considered sufficient to undergo pneumonectomy, whereas a Vo_2max of less than 10 mL/kg/min or less than 40% of predicted would preclude any resection.[25,40] Most recently, the Vo_2max value precluding any resection was lowered to

35% of predicted.[41] A cutoff of 15 mL/kg/min is considered to be sufficient for lobectomy.[42–44]

Low-Cost Alternatives

The lack of access to sophisticated exercise equipment and expertise often necessitates the use of other forms of exercise testing. Low-technology alternatives have been proposed to evaluate patients before lung resection, stair climbing tests being the most widely used and validated form. The advantages of stair climbing are availability, low cost, and familiarity of patients with this kind of exercise, and it has been reported that stair climbing yields greater values for Vo_2max than cycle ergometry.[45–47] The largest prospective study reports on 160 patients who underwent stair climbing testing before pulmonary resection.[48] It was shown that patients with no complications climbed to a significantly greater height than patients with complications. A cutoff of 20 m was suggested, although the extent of resection was not taken into consideration. The same group investigated the correlation between the height reached and directly measured Vo_2max in 109 patients. They concluded that patients who reached 22 m or more can proceed directly to surgery because they generated high values of Vo_2max.[49] In another recent study, the speed of ascent, rather than the height alone, showed a linear correlation with Vo_2max measured by cycle ergometry.[5] Compared with the oxygen consumption values, a speed of ascent of 15 m/min correlated with a Vo_2max of 20 mL/kg/min, and a speed of 12 m/min correlated with a Vo_2max of 15 mL/kg/min, suggesting potential cutoffs for pneumonectomy and lobectomy, respectively. The use of shuttle walking tests cannot be recommended, because prospective studies failed to validate the tests.[50,51]

ASSESSMENT OF REGIONAL LUNG FUNCTION AND CALCULATING THE EXTENT OF RESECTION
Anatomic Calculations

Anatomic calculations are an old, tested, and simple method of assessing regional lung function. With the advent of pulmonary perfusion scintigraphy, they were abandoned to a degree, but were revived in the 1990s and have now been re-established as reliable predictors of postoperative lung function.[52] Anatomic calculations are based on the number of segments to be resected (ie, the ppo value is a fraction of remaining segments or subsegments). The simplest formula to calculate (eg, ppo-FEV_1) is preoperative $FEV_1 \times$ [19 - patent segments to be removed/19]. Nineteen

represents the number of total lung segments. ppo-DL_{CO} and ppo-Vo_2max are calculated in a similar fashion. Anatomic calculations overestimate the extent of functional loss, because destroyed or collapsed lung parenchyma might be resected with little loss of function.[52] Subanalysis of one prospective study showed that anatomic calculations were less accurate than lobectomy at predicting postresectional lung function following pneumonectomy.[53]

Radionucleotide Ventilation/Perfusion Scanning

The usefulness of radionucleotide perfusion scanning was established in the 1970s by a study showing accurate prediction of functional loss 3 months after pneumonectomy by perfusion scanning using intravenous technetium-99 macroaggregates.[54] The feasibility of this method to estimate ventilatory function was subsequently confirmed. Patients are scanned in 4 projections and images obtained by a γ camera (single-photon emission computed tomography [SPECT]). The technetium particles are trapped in the capillary bed of the lungs and emit γ rays proportional to regional pulmonary perfusion. Quantification of regional perfusion is performed by a system-integrated program (**Fig. 1**). A prospective study in 44 patients who had lung resection showed that estimates based on perfusion scanning had the highest correlations with postoperatively measured values for FEV_1, FVC, DL_{CO} and Vo_2max. Perfusion scanning outperformed calculations based on quantitative dynamic computed tomography (CT) scanning anatomic calculations for the range of functional parameters.[53]

Quantitative CT Scanning

Quantitative CT scanning is a simple, universally available method of assessing regional lung function. It has gained in popularity, because almost every lung resection candidate has a staging CT scan. It should be performed at inspiration and viewed with a standard-spatial-frequency reconstruction algorithm. The total functional lung volume (TFLV) is identified by semiautomated analyses. Using a cursor, the lung parenchyma is outlined and 3 quantitative segments are generated according to Hounsfield units (HU) (**Fig. 2**). The part of the lung to be resected is calculated as the regional functional lung volume (RFLV). Values for ppo are calculated as follows (eg, ppo-FEV_1): ppo-FEV_1 = preoperative $FEV_1 \times$ (1-(RFLV/TFLV)).

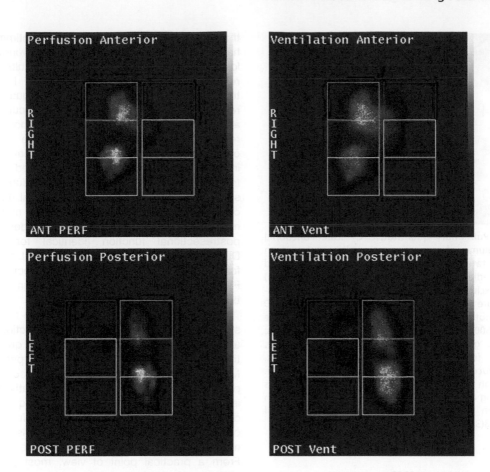

	Perfusion% Geometric Mean		Ventilation% Geometric Mean	
	Right	Left	Right	Left
Upper	28.0	4.5	24.6	8.8
Middle	33.5	7.1	31.0	10.0
Lower	25.6	1.4	23.6	2.0
Total	87.0	13.0	79.2	20.8

Fig. 1. Radionucleotide perfusion ventilation scan. An example of a radionucleotide ventilation perfusion scan performed on a patient with almost completely destroyed left lung and only 13% of total perfusion left on that side. Quantification is performed according to zones and evaluation of anterior and posterior views. (*Courtesy of* Prof J. Warwick, Medical Imaging and Clinical Oncology, Stellenbosch University and Tygerberg Hospital, Cape Town, South Africa.)

This method has been shown to be accurate in predicting postoperative FEV$_1$ and FVC.[55–57] One prospective study reported on the correlation of prediction based on quantitative CT scanning for DL$_{CO}$ and Vo$_2$max. Predictions for DL$_{CO}$ correlated well, whereas, for Vo$_2$max, CT-derived estimates were outperformed by radionucleotide scanning.[53]

Dynamic Contrast-Enhanced Perfusion Magnetic Resonance Imaging

The most recently established standard method is perfusion magnetic resonance imaging (MRI), using contrast-enhanced MRI calculating the regional pulmonary blood volume. This technique requires some expertise as well as appropriate software, but has been shown to reliably predict

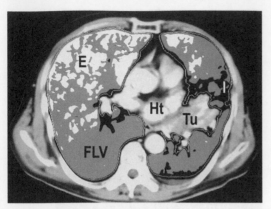

Fig. 2. Pulmonary quantitative CT scan. Functional lung volume of a representative slice is shown on a quantitative CT map. Lung parenchyma is outlined from mediastinum and chest wall with tumor (Tu) being excluded. Then 3 segments in the lung parenchyma are generated. The white area, less than −910 HU, denotes emphysema (E); the black area, more than −500 HU, denotes infiltration and atelectasis; and the gray area, between −500 and −910 HU, denotes functional lung volume (FLV). Ht, heart. (*Reproduced from* Wu MT, Pan HB, Chiang AA, et al. Prediction of postoperative lung function in patients with lung cancer: comparison of quantitative CT with perfusion scintigraphy. AJR Am J Roentgenol 2002;178(3):668; with permission.)

than other techniques. Anatomic estimations have been shown to overestimate the functional loss, because minimal loss often results after resection of destroyed or collapsed lung or tumor-bearing tissue. Many patients qualify for resection based on these simple calculations, and more sophisticated methods should be reserved for borderline patients.[52] The number of functional segments (segments patent on imagery or bronchoscopy) to be resected is subtracted from the total number of functional segments and then divided by the total number of functional segments. This fraction must be multiplied by preoperative values to determine postresectional function (identical for FEV_1, DL_{CO}, and Vo_2max. Thus the general formula for the ppo function (F) is: F-ppo = preoperative $F \times (19 - $ the number of functional segments to be resected/19).

Radionucleotide scanning used to be the gold standard in assessing regional lung function, but advances in radiological technology (ie, quantitative CT and dynamic contrast-enhanced perfusion MRI) have been shown to be at least as accurate in predicting certain parameters. Postoperative FEV_1 is predicted well by the different techniques, but direct comparison regarding other functional parameters is difficult because protocols, equipment, and expertise vary throughout the studies. From a practical point of view, most patients undergo staging CT scanning, and only additional software and expertise is needed to predict postoperative lung function using quantitative CT.

In general, anatomic calculations should be performed on all patients who require estimation of postoperative lung function. For patients who require further evaluation, availability, cost, and local expertise usually determine the choice of method.

postoperative values.[56,58] Dynamic perfusion MRI studies are performed with a phased array coil and images acquired with a three-dimensional radiofrequency-spoiled gradient-echo sequence (**Fig. 3**). Gadolinium is used as a contrast agent. Regional pulmonary blood volume is calculated from the signal intensity-time course curve. ppo-FEV_1 = preoperative $FEV_1 \times [1 - (\%$ perfusion of resected lobe or lung/100)].[56,58]

A large prospective study compared the performance of perfusion MRI and SPECT in predicting postoperative FEV_1 and showed that MRI is superior to SPECT.[58] Other parameters of lung function (ie, DL_{CO} and Vo_2max) were not assessed in that study.

APPROACH TO ASSESSMENT OF REGIONAL LUNG FUNCTION

Values of ppo for FEV_1, DL_{CO}, and Vo_2max have to be calculated in every patient who does not qualify for lung resection based on basic lung function (ie, FEV_1 or DL_{CO} <80%) or exercise testing (Vo_2max<20 mL/kg/min or <75%). Calculating ppo lung function based on anatomic values is the simplest way of predicting postoperative function, although it is less accurate

ALGORITHM FOR THE ASSESSMENT OF THE LUNG RESECTION CANDIDATE

Patients undergoing lung resection surgery should be assessed regarding their fitness for surgery, focusing on cardiovascular and respiratory function. A stepwise approach is useful in assessing patients before pulmonary resection. A widely used algorithm initially proposed by Bolliger and Perruchoud[59] in 1998 has recently been revised by an ERS/ESTS task force and cutoff values have been lowered, because previous thresholds have been shown to be conservative and err on the side of safety (**Fig. 4**).[41,59,60]

Every patient should have a resting ECG and cardiac disease needs to be identified and managed. Ventilatory impairment should be optimized

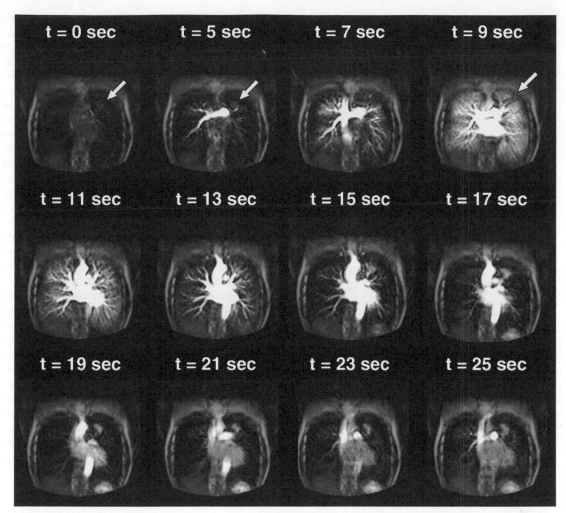

Fig. 3. Dynamic perfusion MRI. A dynamic perfusion MRI of a patient with a left upper lobe adenocarcinoma. The images show heterogeneous, but well-enhanced, pulmonary parenchyma at 5 and 13 seconds in portions of lungs not affected by the cancer (*arrows*). The adenocarcinoma also is enhanced after 13 seconds. (*Reproduced from Ohno Y, Koyama H, Nogami M, et al. Postoperative lung function in lung cancer patients: comparative analysis of predictive capability of MRI, CT, and SPECT. AJR Am J Roentgenol 2007;189(2):404; with permission.*)

before functional evaluation. The first step in assessing pulmonary function should include spirometry (FEV_1) and DL_{CO}. An uncomplicated postoperative course can be assumed in patients with FEV_1 and DL_{CO} values greater than 80% of predicted. Should either of these values be less than 80% of predicted, formal exercise testing with measurement of maximum oxygen consumption is recommended. Thus, for example, a poor FEV_1 can be compensated for by a preserved Vo_2max, making the algorithm inclusive rather than exclusive. A Vo_2max of greater than 20 mL/kg/min or greater than 75% of predicted allows for surgery up to pneumonectomy. In further steps for patients who do not qualify for

a resection up to a pneumonectomy based on the tests mentioned earlier, split functions must be calculated considering the extent of resection. This extent of resection used in the estimation must always be considered when a patient is deemed operable based on split functions.

This and other algorithms not mentioned in this article can only serve as guides but, in general, patients should be considered functionally inoperable if regarded as high risk by any algorithm. Exceptions can be made on an individual basis, provided patients are informed of the significant increased risk of morbidity and mortality. Recent advances in surgical techniques and the advent of minimally invasive surgery

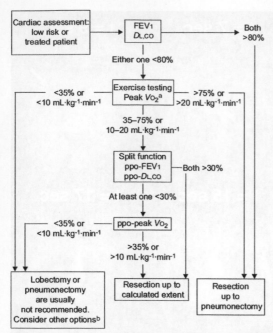

Fig. 4. Revised algorithm for the assessment of cardiorespiratory reserve and operability before pulmonary resection. Patients undergo a stepwise evaluation until they either qualify for varying extent of resection or are deemed inoperable. All percentages refer to percent of predicted value. FEV_1, forced expiratory volume in 1 second; DL_{CO}, carbon monoxide diffusion capacity; Vo_2, maximal oxygen consumption; ppo, predicted postoperative. [a]If peak Vo_2 is not available, cardiopulmonary exercise testing can be replaced by stair climbing. [b]See sections entitled Surgical techniques in lung cancer (p. 27) and Chemo-radiotherapy in lung cancer (p. 28) in original publication. (*Reproduced from* Brunelli A, Charloux A, Bolliger CT, et al. ERS/ESTS clinical guidelines on fitness for radical therapy in lung cancer patients (surgery and chemo-radiotherapy). Eur Respir J 2009;34(1):22; with permission.)

(eg, VATS) have, to an extent, also challenged the current thresholds.

SUMMARY

Lung resection remains a high-risk procedure because many candidates suffer from concomitant obstructive lung disease or cardiovascular disease. For lung cancer, resection represents the only potentially curative treatment. Every pulmonary resection candidate should therefore undergo a careful and structured evaluation while on optimal treatment. This assessment should take cardiac, pulmonary, and general fitness into consideration. Cardiac evaluation should identify patients

with cardiovascular disease at the beginning of a stepwise approach. The initial pulmonary function parameters to be obtained are FEV_1 and DL_{CO}. Patients with values greater than 80% of predicted for both parameters have been shown to have an uncomplicated surgical course and can proceed directly to resection up to pneumonectomy. All other patients warrant further evaluation by formal cardiopulmonary exercise testing. Vo_2max greater than 20 mL/kg/min or greater than 75% of predicted allows resection up to pneumonectomy, whereas a Vo_2max less than 10 mL/kg/min or less than 35% of predicted is usually prohibitive for any resection. Patients who are between those thresholds require assessment of their regional lung function by various methods and calculation of ppo lung function. ppo-FEV_1 and ppo-DL_{CO} greater than 30% and a ppo-Vo_2max of 10 mL/kg/min or greater than 35% allow surgery up to the calculated extent. In case sophisticated exercise testing equipment is not available, low-cost alternatives can be used, stair climbing being the most validated test. Lung volume reduction surgery combined with pulmonary resection may improve postoperative lung function in selected patients and thus allow surgery in patients otherwise deemed inoperable. Ongoing developments in surgical and anesthetic techniques, together with the trend for tissue-sparing resections for very small tumors, will lower the minimal required limits of functional reserves in the future.[61]

REFERENCES

1. Jemal A, Siegel R, Xu J, et al. Cancer statistics, 2010. CA Cancer J Clin 2010;60(5):277–300.
2. Bolliger CT. Evaluation of operability before lung resection. Curr Opin Pulm Med 2003;9(4):321–6.
3. Bolliger CT, Koegelenberg CF, Kendal R. Preoperative assessment for lung cancer surgery. Curr Opin Pulm Med 2005;11(4):301–6.
4. Nanguzgambo AB, Aubeelack K, von Groote-Bidlingmaier F, et al. Radiologic features, staging, and operability of primary lung cancer in the Western Cape, South Africa: a 1-year retrospective study. J Thorac Oncol 2011;6(2):343–50.
5. Koegelenberg CF, Diacon AH, Irani S, et al. Stair climbing in the functional assessment of lung resection candidates. Respiration 2008;75(4):374–9.
6. Algar FJ, Alvarez A, Salvatierra A, et al. Predicting pulmonary complications after pneumonectomy for lung cancer. Eur J Cardiothorac Surg 2003;23(2):201–8.
7. Didolkar MS, Moore RH, Takita H. Evaluation of the risk in pulmonary resection for bronchogenic carcinoma. Am J Surg 1974;127(6):700–3.

8. Nagasaki F, Flehinger BJ, Martini N. Complications of surgery in the treatment of carcinoma of the lung. Chest 1982;82(1):25–9.

9. Smetana GW. Preoperative pulmonary evaluation. N Engl J Med 1999;340(12):937–44.

10. Conti B, Brega Massone PP, Lequaglie C, et al. Major surgery in lung cancer in elderly patients? Risk factors analysis and long-term results. Minerva Chir 2002;57(3):317–21.

11. Koizumi K, Haraguchi S, Hirata T, et al. Lobectomy by video-assisted thoracic surgery for lung cancer patients aged 80 years or more. Ann Thorac Cardiovasc Surg 2003;9(1):14–21.

12. Smetana GW, Lawrence VA, Cornell JE. Preoperative pulmonary risk stratification for noncardiothoracic surgery: systematic review for the American College of Physicians. Ann Intern Med 2006;144(8):581–95.

13. Arozullah AM, Khuri SF, Henderson WG, et al. Development and validation of a multifactorial risk index for predicting postoperative pneumonia after major noncardiac surgery. Ann Intern Med 2001;135(10):847–57.

14. Warner MA, Offord KP, Warner ME, et al. Role of preoperative cessation of smoking and other factors in postoperative pulmonary complications: a blinded prospective study of coronary artery bypass patients. Mayo Clin Proc 1989;64(6):609–16.

15. Bluman LG, Mosca L, Newman N, et al. Preoperative smoking habits and postoperative pulmonary complications. Chest 1998;113(4):883–9.

16. Mills E, Eyawo O, Lockhart I, et al. Smoking cessation reduces postoperative complications: a systematic review and meta-analysis. Am J Med 2011;124(2):144.e8–54.e8.

17. Myers K, Hajek P, Hinds C, et al. Stopping smoking shortly before surgery and postoperative complications: a systematic review and meta-analysis. Arch Intern Med 2011;171(11):983–9.

18. Mittman C. Assessment of operative risk in thoracic surgery. Am Rev Respir Dis 1961;84:197–207.

19. Goldman L, Caldera DL, Nussbaum SR, et al. Multifactorial index of cardiac risk in noncardiac surgical procedures. N Engl J Med 1977;297(16):845–50.

20. Lee TH, Marcantonio ER, Mangione CM, et al. Derivation and prospective validation of a simple index for prediction of cardiac risk of major noncardiac surgery. Circulation 1999;100(10):1043–9.

21. Johnson JA, Landreneau RJ, Boley TM, et al. Should pulmonary lesions be resected at the time of open heart surgery? Am Surg 1996;62(4):300–3.

22. Miller DL, Orszulak TA, Pairolero PC, et al. Combined operation for lung cancer and cardiac disease. Ann Thorac Surg 1994;58(4):989–93 [discussion: 993–4].

23. Dyszkiewicz W, Jemielity MM, Piwkowski CT, et al. Simultaneous lung resection for cancer and myocardial revascularization without cardiopulmonary bypass (off-pump coronary artery bypass grafting). Ann Thorac Surg 2004;77(3):1023–7.

24. Burke JR, Duarte IG, Thourani VH, et al. Preoperative risk assessment for marginal patients requiring pulmonary resection. Ann Thorac Surg 2003;76(5):1767–73.

25. Datta D, Lahiri B. Preoperative evaluation of patients undergoing lung resection surgery. Chest 2003;123(6):2096–103.

26. Peters RM, Clausen JL, Tisi GM. Extending resectability for carcinoma of the lung in patients with impaired pulmonary function. Ann Thorac Surg 1978;26(3):250–60.

27. Boushy SF, Billig DM, North LB, et al. Clinical course related to preoperative and postoperative pulmonary function in patients with bronchogenic carcinoma. Chest 1971;59(4):383–91.

28. Perruchoud A, Meili U, Kopp C, et al. Presurgical determination of lung function in patients with bronchogenic carcinoma. Schweiz Med Wochenschr 1979;109(22):832–5 [in German].

29. Pate P, Tenholder MF, Griffin JP, et al. Preoperative assessment of the high-risk patient for lung resection. Ann Thorac Surg 1996;61(5):1494–500.

30. Markos J, Mullan BP, Hillman DR, et al. Preoperative assessment as a predictor of mortality and morbidity after lung resection. Am Rev Respir Dis 1989;139(4):902–10.

31. Wahi R, McMurtrey MJ, DeCaro LF, et al. Determinants of perioperative morbidity and mortality after pneumonectomy. Ann Thorac Surg 1989;48(1):33–7.

32. Bolliger CT, Wyser C, Roser H, et al. Lung scanning and exercise testing for the prediction of postoperative performance in lung resection candidates at increased risk for complications. Chest 1995;108(2):341–8.

33. Nakahara K, Ohno K, Hashimoto J, et al. Prediction of postoperative respiratory failure in patients undergoing lung resection for lung cancer. Ann Thorac Surg 1988;46(5):549–52.

34. Ferguson MK, Lehman AG, Bolliger CT, et al. The role of diffusing capacity and exercise tests. Thorac Surg Clin 2008;18(1):9–17, v.

35. Cander L. Physiologic assessment and management of the preoperative patient with pulmonary emphysema. Am J Cardiol 1963;12:324–6.

36. Ferguson MK, Little L, Rizzo L, et al. Diffusing capacity predicts morbidity and mortality after pulmonary resection. J Thorac Cardiovasc Surg 1988;96(6):894–900.

37. Ferguson MK, Reeder LB, Mick R. Optimizing selection of patients for major lung resection. J Thorac Cardiovasc Surg 1995;109(2):275–81 [discussion: 281–3].

38. Berrisford R, Brunelli A, Rocco G, et al. The European Thoracic Surgery Database project: modelling

the risk of in-hospital death following lung resection. Eur J Cardiothorac Surg 2005;28(2):306–11.

39. Ribas J, Diaz O, Barbera JA, et al. Invasive exercise testing in the evaluation of patients at high-risk for lung resection. Eur Respir J 1998;12(6):1429–35.

40. Bolliger CT, Jordan P, Soler M, et al. Exercise capacity as a predictor of postoperative complications in lung resection candidates. Am J Respir Crit Care Med 1995;151(5):1472–80.

41. Brunelli A, Charloux A, Bolliger CT, et al. ERS/ESTS clinical guidelines on fitness for radical therapy in lung cancer patients (surgery and chemo-radiotherapy). Eur Respir J 2009;34(1):17–41.

42. Morice RC, Peters EJ, Ryan MB, et al. Exercise testing in the evaluation of patients at high risk for complications from lung resection. Chest 1992; 101(2):356–61.

43. Smith TP, Kinasewitz GT, Tucker WY, et al. Exercise capacity as a predictor of post-thoracotomy morbidity. Am Rev Respir Dis 1984;129(5):730–4.

44. Wang JS, Abboud RT, Evans KG, et al. Role of CO diffusing capacity during exercise in the preoperative evaluation for lung resection. Am J Respir Crit Care Med 2000;162(4 Pt 1):1435–44.

45. Pollock M, Roa J, Benditt J, et al. Estimation of ventilatory reserve by stair climbing. A study in patients with chronic airflow obstruction. Chest 1993;104(5): 1378–83.

46. Holden DA, Rice TW, Stelmach K, et al. Exercise testing, 6-min walk, and stair climb in the evaluation of patients at high risk for pulmonary resection. Chest 1992;102(6):1774–9.

47. Swinburn CR, Wakefield JM, Jones PW. Performance, ventilation, and oxygen consumption in three different types of exercise test in patients with chronic obstructive lung disease. Thorax 1985;40(8):581–6.

48. Brunelli A, Al Refai M, Monteverde M, et al. Stair climbing test predicts cardiopulmonary complications after lung resection. Chest 2002;121(4):1106–10.

49. Brunelli A, Xiume F, Refai M, et al. Peak oxygen consumption measured during the stair-climbing test in lung resection candidates. Respiration 2010;80(3):207–11.

50. Win T, Jackson A, Groves AM, et al. Relationship of shuttle walk test and lung cancer surgical outcome. Eur J Cardiothorac Surg 2004;26(6):1216–9.

51. Win T, Jackson A, Groves AM, et al. Comparison of shuttle walk with measured peak oxygen consumption in patients with operable lung cancer. Thorax 2006; 61(1):57–60.

52. Koegelenberg CF, Bolliger CT. Assessing regional lung function. Thorac Surg Clin 2008;18(1):19–29, v–vi.

53. Bolliger CT, Guckel C, Engel H, et al. Prediction of functional reserves after lung resection: comparison between quantitative computed tomography, scintigraphy, and anatomy. Respiration 2002;69(6):482–9.

54. Olsen GN, Block AJ, Tobias JA. Prediction of post-pneumonectomy pulmonary function using quantitative macroaggregate lung scanning. Chest 1974; 66(1):13–6.

55. Wu MT, Chang JM, Chiang AA, et al. Use of quantitative CT to predict postoperative lung function in patients with lung cancer. Radiology 1994;191(1): 257–62.

56. Ohno Y, Koyama H, Nogami M, et al. Postoperative lung function in lung cancer patients: comparative analysis of predictive capability of MRI, CT, and SPECT. AJR Am J Roentgenol 2007;189(2):400–8.

57. Wu MT, Pan HB, Chiang AA, et al. Prediction of postoperative lung function in patients with lung cancer: comparison of quantitative CT with perfusion scintigraphy. AJR Am J Roentgenol 2002;178(3):667–72.

58. Ohno Y, Hatabu H, Higashino T, et al. Dynamic perfusion MRI versus perfusion scintigraphy: prediction of postoperative lung function in patients with lung cancer. AJR Am J Roentgenol 2004; 182(1):73–8.

59. Bolliger CT, Perruchoud AP. Functional evaluation of the lung resection candidate. Eur Respir J 1998; 11(1):198–212.

60. Wyser C, Stulz P, Soler M, et al. Prospective evaluation of an algorithm for the functional assessment of lung resection candidates. Am J Respir Crit Care Med 1999;159(5 Pt 1):1450–6.

61. Bolliger CT. Functional reserve before lung resection: how low can we go? Respiration 2009;78(1):20–2.

Evaluation and Treatment of High-Risk Patients with Early-Stage Lung Cancer

Hiren J. Mehta, MD[a], Christopher Ross, MD[b], Gerard A. Silvestri, MD, MS[a,*], Roy H. Decker, MD, PhD[b]

KEYWORDS

- Lung cancer • Elderly • Wedge resection • Segmentectomy
- Preoperative assessment • Stereotactic body radiotherapy

Although lung cancer is the most common cancer worldwide, only 25% to 30% of cases are diagnosed at an early stage. Standard therapy for early-stage non–small cell lung cancer (NSCLC) is lobectomy for patients who are able to tolerate such surgery. However, the risk of postoperative morbidity is not trivial, with a 30% to 40% incidence of postoperative complications and a 1% to 5% incidence of operative mortality.[1] Despite the intention to consider all patients with stage I/II disease for surgery, there are those who, although technically resectable, refuse surgery or are considered medically inoperable because of insufficient respiratory reserve, cardiovascular disease, or general frailty. This group is considered either "high risk" or "medically inoperable."[2,3] Approximately 20% of patients with early-stage NSCLC are considered medically inoperable.[4,5]

APPROACH TO DECISION MAKING IN HIGH-RISK PATIENTS WITH EARLY-STAGE LUNG CANCER
Physiologic Tests

A general assessment of a patient's ability to tolerate major lung resection includes a careful history and physical examination. Physiologic factors indicative of increased operative risk include advanced age (but not alone), poor performance status, altered mental status, diabetes, hypertension, cerebrovascular disease, and end-organ dysfunction from renal or hepatic insufficiency. Cardiovascular status is important to assess, as operative morbidity and mortality are increased in patients with coronary artery disease, severe valve dysfunction, congestive heart failure, ventricular dysrhythmia, and moderate to severe pulmonary hypertension. Other factors that have an impact on perioperative outcomes include the patient's smoking status, hospital volume for the procedure, the training of the surgeon, and the approach used for lung resection.[6–11]

Since the first pneumonectomy in 1933[12] there have been wide-ranging efforts to identify the best predictive tests and to define the threshold values necessary for minimizing surgical risk.[13] Tests that are commonly considered include preoperative pulmonary function (mainly forced expiratory volume in 1 second [FEV_1] and diffusion capacity of carbon monoxide [DLCO]), prediction of postoperative pulmonary function, exercise testing, and cardiovascular evaluation.[14] While certain values are proposed as cutoffs to identify those at increased risk, there are no absolute criteria. The decision to operate should be based

The authors have nothing to disclose.
a Division of Pulmonary and Critical Care Medicine, Medical University of South Carolina, 171 Ashley Avenue, Charleston, SC 29425, USA
b Department of Therapeutic Radiology, Yale University School of Medicine, PO Box 20804, New Haven, CT 06520-8040, USA
* Corresponding author.
E-mail address: silvestr@musc.edu

Clin Chest Med 32 (2011) 783–797
doi:10.1016/j.ccm.2011.08.011
0272-5231/11/$ – see front matter © 2011 Elsevier Inc. All rights reserved.

on individual evaluation of risk and patient preference. This evaluation is discussed in detail in the article entitled "Functional Evaluation Before Lung Resection" elsewhere in this issue, and is presented briefly here.

Spirometric evaluation of FEV_1 provides an indirect measure of pulmonary reserve. Some studies have suggested that DLCO and predicted postoperative DLCO are the most important predictors of mortality and postoperative morbidity.[15,16] DLCO is an independent prognostic factor for long-term survival after curative lung resection for cancer.[17] Preoperative DLCO also predicts quality of life at 6 months following lobectomy.[18] Patients with preoperative results for FEV_1 and DLCO that are both greater than 80% predicted do not need further physiologic testing.[19]

Patients who do not meet the aforementioned FEV_1 and DLCO criteria should undergo further testing to allow calculation of predicted postoperative lung function. A variety of techniques is currently in use to assess regional function, including the function segment method, radionuclide scanning, and quantitative computed tomography (CT). Each method permits reasonable estimation of postoperative values, especially in patients undergoing lobectomy, although radionuclide scanning is superior to the segment method in patients in whom endobronchial obstruction is present, who require pneumonectomy, or when there is substantial functional heterogeneity.[20–26] The correlation between predicted postoperative lung function and observed postoperative lung function is particularly good (and stable over time) following pneumonectomy. However, following lobectomy, there is a disproportionate early loss in observed function (compared with the predicted loss), followed by significant functional improvement over time.[24] Patients with predicted postoperative values for either FEV_1 or DLCO less than 40 are at increased risk for lung resection.[19] Preoperative exercise testing is recommended for patients with either of these criteria to further assess surgical risk. Preoperative exercise testing includes a spectrum of tests from stair climbing to complete cardiopulmonary exercise testing.

Various tests including stair climbing, shuttle walking, exercise oximetry, and the 6-minute walk have all been variably shown to predict increased morbidity and mortality associated with lung resection.[27–29] Multiple studies have suggested different cutoffs for each of these methods. Patients with lung cancer being considered for surgery who walk less than 25 shuttles on two shuttle walks or less than one flight of stairs are at increased risk for postoperative death and cardiopulmonary complications with standard lung resection. The American College of Chest Physicians (ACCP)

recommends that these patients be counseled about nonstandard surgery and nonoperative treatment options for their lung cancer.[19]

Peak VO_2 measured by formal cardiopulmonary exercise testing is often used to determine whether individuals with unacceptable lung function by other metrics might still be able to tolerate resection. Measurement of peak VO_2 does not add to risk stratification if the preoperative FEV_1 and DLCO are greater than 80% predicted. In several studies of patients with predicted postoperative FEV_1 and DLCO of less than 40% of predicted, major resection was well tolerated if peak VO_2 was greater than 10 mL/kg/min.[30–32] An algorithm to risk-stratify patients for lung resection used at the authors' institution is shown in **Fig. 1**. An alternative algorithm is also discussed in the article by von Groote-Bedlingmaier and colleagues elsewhere in this issue.

Both the ACCP and the European Respiratory Society/European Society of Thoracic Surgeons (ERS/ESTS) have produced clinical practice guidelines to assess risk in patients being considered for lung resection.[19,32] While both provide a framework to help guide physicians they are different in their approaches, suggesting there is there is no "one size fits all" approach. The take-home message is that each case must be dealt with on an individualized basis, with the goal of providing each patient with optimal treatment.

TREATMENT OPTIONS FOR HIGH-RISK PATIENTS WITH EARLY-STAGE LUNG CANCER
Surgery

Surgery is the treatment of choice in patients with early-stage NSCLC.[33] Lobectomy is generally accepted as the optimal procedure because of its ability to preserve pulmonary function.[34] For proximal tumors that cannot be readily resected by lobectomy, sleeve resection is preferred over pneumonectomy, based on the fact that comparatively it results in fewer complications, equivalent oncologic efficacy, and better preservation of lung function.[35] However, lobectomy is frequently not a surgical option in high-risk patients with low FEV_1 and DLCO. For patients considered to be at high risk for lobectomy, lesser resections could be considered.

Sublobar resection
Sublobar resection for lung cancer can be performed with a simple wedge resection technique, with appropriate attention being paid to obtaining an adequate surgical margin, or anatomic segmental resection (segmentectomy), which achieves a detailed anatomic bronchial

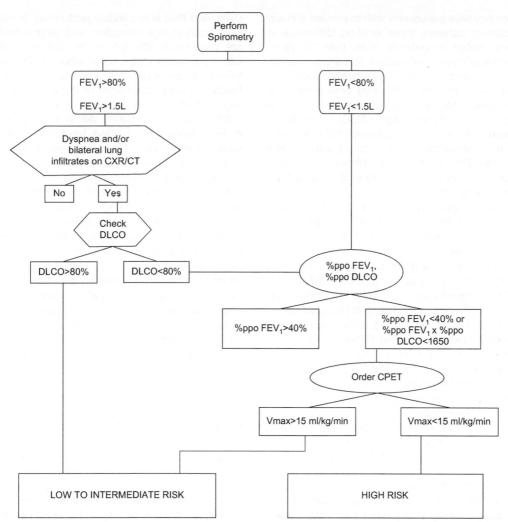

Fig. 1. Preoperative risk stratification for patients with early-stage lung cancer considered for lung resection. CPET, cardiopulmonary exercise testing; DLCO, diffusion capacity of carbon monoxide; FEV$_1$, forced expiratory volume in the first second; PPO, predicted postoperative; Vmax, maximal oxygen consumption.

and vascular dissection, with selective division of these structures. Extended segmentectomy ensures the complete removal of the targeted anatomic segment with its vascular and lymphatic distribution.

Jensik and colleagues[36] were among the first to report that an anatomic segmental resection might represent an adequate operation for stage I NSCLC. Sublobar resection is currently viewed as a "compromised" procedure, only to be performed in patients with significant comorbidities or impairment in cardiopulmonary function. Data regarding the relative efficacy of limited resection in comparison with lobectomy are scarce. Lung Cancer Study Group Trial 801 is the only prospective randomized controlled trial comparing lobectomy with sublobar resection; 276 patients with peripheral T1N0 (stage IA) NSCLC were randomly assigned to either lobectomy or a more limited procedure (ie, wedge resection, segmentectomy). The study showed a threefold increase in local recurrence (17.2% vs 6.4%) and a significant trend toward a 30% increase in mortality in patients who had sublobar resection.[34] Nonetheless, sublobar resection still has some distinct advantages over lobectomy. Sublobar resections achieve comparable perioperative morbidity and reduced operative mortality.[37,38] In addition, sublobar resection has been associated with preservation of pulmonary function compared with lobectomy, and may represent the only feasible surgical option in high-risk patients with compromised cardiopulmonary function.[39,40]

In a study using the Surveillance, Epidemiology, and End Results database, 14,555 patients underwent anatomic lung resection for NSCLC. Though lobectomy was associated with improved survival in younger patients, there was no difference in survival noted in patients older than 75 years undergoing either a lobectomy or sublobar resection.[41] Kilic and colleagues[42] compared outcomes of patients older than 75 years who underwent either lobectomy (n = 106) or anatomic segmentectomy (n = 78) for stage I NSCLC. Anatomic segmentectomy was associated with reduced operative morbidity (29.5% vs 50%) and mortality (1.3% vs 4.7%). There was no difference in locoregional recurrence (6% vs 4%) or overall survival (49.8% vs 45.5%).

Sublobar resection appears to be equivalent to lobectomy in the treatment of small peripheral tumors. Okada and colleagues[43] found no statistical difference in the 5-year disease-free survival in lobectomy or segmentectomy patients with tumors 2 cm or less in diameter (87.4% vs 84.6%, respectively). Similarly, El-Sherif and colleagues[44] compared lobar and sublobar resections for T1 tumors less than 2 cm and found there was no difference in survival. Other reports examining sublobar resection in the setting of subcentimeter tumors document no difference in local recurrence or survival.[40,44] A prospective, randomized, multi-institutional study is currently under way (CALGB 140503) evaluating the outcomes of sublobar resection compared with those of lobectomy for small tumors (<2 cm).[45,46] Tumor histology may be helpful in making a decision about lobar versus sublobar resection. Sublobar resection of a dominant lesion suspected or known to be adenocarcinoma in situ (bronchioloalveolar carcinoma) in a patient with other radiographic areas of ground-glass abnormalities suggestive of premalignancy or early malignancy allows complete excision of the suspect lesion, while preserving pulmonary parenchyma against the possibility of a need for future resections.[47]

Several studies have shown that anatomic segmentectomy may represent the ideal approach to minimize recurrence in situations where parenchyma-sparing techniques may be beneficial. The LCSG trial, comparing wedge resection with anatomic segmentectomy in high-risk patients with early-stage lung cancer, showed that recurrence rates for segmentectomy were similar to lobectomy and significantly lower than simple wedge resection.[34] El-Sherif and colleagues[44] evaluated 81 patients with stage I NSCLC treated by either wedge resection (n = 55) or anatomic segmentectomy (n = 26), and found a significantly higher risk of locoregional recurrence with the former (14/55, 25.5% compared with 1/26, 3.8%). Segmentectomy, despite its advantages, is a prolonged procedure and requires more advanced surgical skills, and thus is not widely performed. In conclusion, both wedge resection and segmentectomy are reasonable alternatives in high-risk patients with early-stage lung cancer who cannot tolerate lobectomy because of a significant loss of lung function, though the weight of the evidence favors segmentectomy over wedge resection.

Although most patients will lose some degree of lung function and effort tolerance even with sublobar resections, there is a specific subgroup of lung cancer patients, mainly those with heterogeneous upper lobe emphysema, who may have improved lung function and quality of life after surgery by the simultaneous performance of lung volume reduction surgery (LVRS) and lung cancer resection. In multiple studies, patients with an FEV_1 of less than 40% predicted and emphysema in the lobe containing the lung cancer tolerate lobectomy well.[48] Patient selection for the combined surgery is important. Several centers have proposed various selection criteria, including FEV_1 less than 40% predicted, a technically resectable tumor, and the target lobe demonstrating emphysema and contributing less than 10% of overall perfusion. The national emphysema treatment trial (NETT) showed that patients benefited most from LVRS if they had predominantly upper lobe emphysema and had poor functional capacity.[49] LVRS in well-selected patients with severe emphysema results in postoperative improvement of symptoms and measured pulmonary function.[50] Combined LVRS and nodule resection has been shown to improve postoperative FEV_1, functional capacity measured by 6-minute walk, and quality of life, as well as reduce chronic obstructive pulmonary disease (COPD) exacerbations at 1 year after surgery. Cancer-free survival and recurrence rates have been similar to other non-COPD lung cancer patients at 1, 3, and 5 years.[51] In conclusion, the combination of lung cancer resection with LVRS offers carefully selected patients, who by traditional criteria would be considered unsuitable surgical candidates because of limited pulmonary reserve, the opportunity to undergo resection of their cancer with physiologic improvement rather than further reduction in their pulmonary function.

Newer minimally invasive methods for lung resection have become available, which might provide high-risk patients with procedures that can make recovery and quality of life better. Video-assisted thoracoscopic surgery (VATS) is associated with a reduction in surgical morbidity, including perioperative pain, and appears particularly useful for those with significant medical comorbidities.[52] It has been demonstrated that VATS and conventional surgery are both efficacious for early-stage NSCLC, with similar perioperative mortality.[53] In addition, the completeness of lymph node dissection, 5-year survival, and local recurrence rates are similar between the two approaches.[54,55] There has been substantial evidence showing that VATS lobectomy is an appropriate alternative to open lobectomy if performed in experienced hands.[54,55] To date there have been no studies comparing VATS with open thoracotomy in high-risk patients, but existing evidence suggests that VATS might be particularly beneficial to this group of patients in decreasing perioperative morbidity.

Therapeutic Radiation

Despite the best efforts to offer some form of surgery for high-risk early-stage lung cancer, there are times when patients prefer not to have surgery or when physicians believe that patients are not suitable surgical candidates. Radiation therapy is a well-studied, reasonable, and frequently used alternative therapy in these cases.

Radiofrequency ablation

Radiofrequency ablation (RFA) is a minimally invasive procedure typically performed under conscious sedation, which involves inserting a radiofrequency probe percutaneously into a lung tumor under image guidance. The tumor is then heated to a target temperature of 50°C to 100°C to induce coagulative necrosis[56] using an alternating electric current with a frequency in the range of radio waves (460–500 kHz).[57] As the internal tumor temperature exceeds 50°C cellular proteins begin to denature, damaging cellular membranes and causing coagulation. If temperatures are allowed to exceed 100°C charring and cavitation occurs, which limits current flow, thereby reducing the effectiveness of thermal ablation.[58]

The use of RFA to treat lung tumors in humans was first reported in 2000.[59] Since that time many of the published prospective and retrospective series of RFA for lung tumors have focused on the treatment of lung metastases, but a recent review by Chan and colleagues[60] identified 479 cases of primary NSCLC treated with RFA among 33 studies reported in the literature. Eleven of these studies[61–71] included more than one patient with NSCLC treated with RFA alone with a median follow-up of at least 12 months (**Table 1**). From this series the 1- to 2-year local control rates range from 60% to 88% and 1- to 2-year overall survival rates range from 46% to 95%. Long-term results are lacking, with the only 5-year outcomes for RFA treatment of early-stage NSCLC reported in a retrospective study by Simon and colleagues[62] examining the long-term safety and efficacy of 153 patients treated with pulmonary RFA. Of the 75 patients with stage I NSCLC lesions, the 5-year overall survival rate was 27%. The 5-year local control rates, reported based on tumor size

Table 1
Summary of published studies using radiofrequency ablation alone to treat non–small cell lung cancer with at least 12 months of follow-up

Study	No. of Patients[a]	Follow-Up (months)	Local Control (%)		Overall Survival (%)	
			1 Year	2 Years	1 Year	2 Years
Lencioni et al[61] (RAPTURE Study)	33[b]	12–24	87.5	—	70	48
Simon et al[62]	75 (80)	20.5	—	—	78	57
Fernando et al[63]	18 (21)[b]	14	62		83	
Jin et al[64]	10	19	—	70[c]	—	50
Lee et al[65]	10	13.5	60[c]	—	80	—
Hiraki et al[66]	24 (25)	12	72	60	—	—
de Baère et al[67]	9	18	—	88	85	61
Pennathur et al[68]	19	29	58		95	68
Hiraki et al[69]	20	21.8	72	63	90	84
Choe et al[70]	65 (76)[b]	20.8	—	—	67	46
Lanuti et al[71]	31 (34)	17	—	68	85	78

[a] Number in parentheses represents the number of treated lesions.
[b] Included early-stage as well as advanced-stage NSCLC patients.
[c] Reported as "complete ablation" or "complete necrosis" at the given time point.

as opposed to tumor status as a primary lung cancer or a metastasis, were 47% for tumors 3 cm or smaller and 25% for tumors larger than 3 cm. This trend toward improved outcomes with T1 lesions in comparison with T2 lesions was also observed in several other trials.[65,69–71]

The largest prospective multicenter intention-to-treat trial of RFA for lung tumors is the RAPTURE study.[61] This European trial enrolled 106 patients with 183 lung tumors consisting of primary NSCLC (33 patients) and metastatic lesions (73 patients) who were considered unsuitable for surgery and unfit for standard radiotherapy or chemotherapy. Patients were treated with RFA and followed for up to 2 years. Technical success, defined as correct placement of the device in the target with completion of the planned treatment, was achieved in 99% of the patients. Overall survival and cancer-specific survival at 2 years for patients with stage I NSCLC (n = 13) were 75% and 92%, respectively. A confirmed complete response lasting at least 1 year was observed in 87.5% of NSCLC patients.

In the reported studies of pulmonary RFA the most prevalent adverse effects include pneumothorax (28% minor, 14% requiring chest drain), pleural effusion (15%), and pain (14%).[60] Less common side effects (<5% each) include hemoptysis, fever, pneumonia, bronchopleural fistula, abscess, and subcutaneous emphysema.[60] Procedure-related mortality ranged from 0% to 5.6%, with an overall rate of 0.2% in the reported literature.[60] There appears to be no significant worsening of pulmonary function following treatment with RFA.[61]

Stereotactic body radiotherapy

Stereotactic body radiotherapy (SBRT) is a method of delivering a highly conformal dose of radiation to a tumor using multiple converging static beams or a rotational arc technique. Typical treatment regimens include 1 to 5 treatments delivered over 1 to 2 weeks. With SBRT, the treatment volume is limited by using precise targeting and conformal treatment delivery to provide an ablative dose of radiation to the tumor while minimizing radiation to adjacent normal tissues. This process allows a much higher biologically equivalent dose (BED) of radiation to be delivered to the tumor than with conventional fractionated radiotherapy. SBRT can be performed on a variety of platforms, including a modified linear accelerator or a dedicated SBRT device. SBRT treatment requires careful patient immobilization, precise tumor localization, the ability to account for tumor motion, and a radiation oncologist with the appropriate expertise.

The growing interest in SBRT can in part be attributed to recent advances in imaging techniques and treatment planning, which allow for greater treatment precision.[72] In particular, the inability to precisely localize lung tumors and account for their motion during treatment can result in geographic misses when tight margins around the tumor volume are used. The contribution of tumor motion to geographic errors in the treatment of lung cancer was first formally evaluated in 1990.[73] Since that time significant improvements have been made in imaging techniques, which enable much better target delineation. This mode requires accounting for tumor motion, which can be accomplished by a variety of methods. One common approach involves the use of 4-dimensional CT scans, incorporating the element of time to allow visualization of tumor movement during the respiratory cycle.[74] Abdominal compression is also widely used, which limits diaphragmatic excursion, thereby limiting tumor motion. Accurate localization must occur during each of the 3 to 5 treatment fractions, which historically was accomplished via tight immobilization in a rigid body frame with an external stereotactic coordinate system. Modern SBRT more commonly relies on image guidance, either by fluoroscopic tracking of an internal, radiographically visible fiducial marker, or with treatment units that have integrated imaging capabilities, allowing for a CT scan to be acquired before treatment delivery, thereby ensuring proper patient positioning and tumor localization.[75] Taken together, these advances permit the use of a smaller treatment margin around the tumor, such that a much higher dose of radiation can be delivered safely. For example, the recently published Radiation Therapy Oncology Group (RTOG) 0236 trial delivered 54 Gy in 3 fractions, which is biologically equivalent to 126 Gy delivered using conventional 2-Gy fractions—nearly twice the 66 Gy total dose historically used with conventional fractionation.

As a result of increasing the BED delivered to the tumor, SBRT has resulted in excellent local control rates[76–86] compared with conventional radiotherapy, ranging from 80% to 96% at 3 years. The largest retrospective experience is a Japanese multi-institutional study that evaluated 257 patients with stage I NSCLC. All patients were treated with SBRT to a total dose of 18 to 74 Gy in 1 to 22 fractions.[87] The results demonstrated a significant improvement in local control for patients treated with a fractionation scheme that delivered a BED of 100 Gy or more (calculated using a linear-quadratic model and assuming $\alpha/\beta = 10$), with a local recurrence rate of 8% compared with 43% for a BED less than 100 Gy.

While there remains some controversy as to the optimal fractionation scheme for SBRT, a BED of 100 Gy or greater is a commonly accepted standard.

Several prospective trials of SBRT for early-stage NSCLC have now been completed and reported. A phase I dose-escalation trial was performed at Indiana University to determine the maximum tolerated radiation dose. Stage IA and IB NSCLC patients were treated with escalating doses starting at 3 fractions of 8 Gy to a total dose of 24 Gy.[88,89] The maximum tolerated dose was 72 Gy for tumors larger than 5 cm (T2b lesions), but was not reached for T1 lesions (maximum dose = 60 Gy). In this cohort of 37 patients there were 10 local recurrences, but only 1 in patients who were treated with a fraction size 18 Gy or more (total dose ≥54 Gy, BED >120 Gy). This trial confirmed that SBRT doses can be safely achieved, even for large tumors, and the dose fractionation scheme of 54 Gy in 3 fractions served as the basis for future studies conducted by the RTOG.

The largest multi-institutional SBRT trial performed in the United States for surgically ineligible patients with early-stage NSCLC is the RTOG 0236 trial.[77] Fifty-five patients were treated with SBRT consisting of 54 Gy in 3 fractions, which most closely reflects current practice for peripherally located tumors. With a median follow-up of 34 months there was only one primary tumor failure, yielding a 3-year tumor control rate of 98%.

Three-year local control, including primary tumor control and involved lobe control, was 91%. Overall survival at 3 years was 56%.

Table 2 summarizes studies examining outcomes of SBRT in stage I NSCLC; these studies all limited enrollment to patients with biopsy-proven NSCLC, and used an SBRT dose with a BED of 100 Gy or greater. The 3-year overall survival rates for this patient population treated with SBRT ranged from 43% to 91%.[76–86] Five-year survival rates were reported in 3 of the trials, and ranged from 26% to 80%.[79,81,82] The majority of these patients were not medically eligible for surgery, due to comorbid medical illness or poor pulmonary function at baseline, and not unexpectedly many of the patients treated on these trials died of causes other than lung cancer. The reported 3-year cancer-specific survival ranged from 66% to 88%,[76,79,81,84,85] which is a dramatic improvement compared with historical 3-year cancer-specific survival rates of 22% to 42% with the use of conventionally fractionated radiotherapy.[90–92]

There has been growing interest in comparing SBRT with sublobar resection in patients who are deemed ineligible for lobectomy. It is important to recognize that local control and survival rates determined from cohorts of medically inoperable patients may not be generalizable to a younger, healthier population. Several retrospective analyses address this. A Japanese study evaluated local control and overall survival in 87 medically

Table 2
Summary of stereotactic body radiotherapy trials for the treatment of stage I non–small cell lung cancer

Study	No. of Patients	Follow-Up Duration (months)	Fractionation	Local Control at 3 Years (%)	Overall Survival at 3 Years (%)
Fakiris et al[76,86]	70	50	20–22 Gy × 3	88	43
Timmerman et al[77] (RTOG 0236)	55	34	18 Gy × 3	91	56
Zimmerman et al[78]	30	18	12.5 Gy × 3[a]	87[b]	44
Nyman et al[79]	45	43	15 Gy × 3	80	55
Fritz et al[80]	33	18	30 Gy × 1	83[c]	53
Baumann et al[81]	138	33	15 Gy × 3[d]	85	52
Nagata et al[82]	45	30	12 Gy × 4	94	80
Xia et al[83]	25	27	5 Gy × 10	96	91
Ricardi et al[84]	62	28	15 Gy × 3	88	57
Baumann et al[85]	57	35	15 Gy × 3	92	60

[a] Most patients received 12.5 Gy × 3, but total dose ranged from 24 to 40 Gy.
[b] 2-Year local control rate.
[c] 4-Year local control rate.
[d] Most patients received 15 Gy × 3, but total dose ranged from 30 to 48 Gy.

operable patients with stage IA and IB NSCLC who were treated with SBRT after refusing surgery.[93] The results demonstrated 5-year local control rates of 92% and 73% for T1 and T2 lesions, respectively, and 5-year overall survival rates of 72% and 62%, respectively. These survival rates are similar to those seen after lobectomy for clinically staged T1 and T2 lesions reported in series from the United States[94] and Japan.[95,96] To further compare SBRT with sublobar resection, a study by Grills and colleagues[97] evaluated 124 patients with stage I NSCLC treated with wedge resection or SBRT. All patients were ineligible for anatomic lobectomy, and 95% of the SBRT patients were considered medically inoperable. With a median follow-up of 2.5 years SBRT was associated with a 4% risk for local recurrence compared with 20% with wedge resection ($P = .07$). When excluding synchronous primaries and tumors lacking biopsy confirmation, there was a statistically significant reduction in local recurrence (5% vs 24%) and locoregional recurrence (5% vs 29%) with the use of SBRT. Overall survival was lower with SBRT, as expected, but cancer-specific survival was identical.

SBRT for surgical candidates is being evaluated in two ongoing phase 2 trials, RTOG 0618 and JCOG 0403. Early results from JCOG 0403 with a median follow-up of 45 months were recently presented with a 3-year reported overall survival of 76%.[98] There are also two ongoing phase 3 trials randomizing surgically eligible patients to surgery or SBRT.[99]

A comprehensive study of lung SBRT toxicity identified 15 studies including 683 patients that were treated for primary NSCLC or lung metastases.[100] Overall Grade 3 to 5 toxicity was reported in up to 15% of patients, with a treatment-related mortality rate of 0.3%. More common toxicities occurring in 5% to 40% of patients include fatigue, cough, dyspnea, chest pain, and dermatitis.[85] Evidence of radiographic pneumonitis following treatment is extremely common[101]; however, these findings are often asymptomatic, with rates of clinically apparent pneumonitis less than 20%.[85] In a comprehensive evaluation of pulmonary function test (PFT) changes following SBRT, there appears to be no significant overall change in PFT values, including FEV_1 and DLCO.[102] There also appears to be no significant difference in survival or posttreatment-related PFT values between patients in the lowest quartile of pretreatment FEV_1 and those patients in the upper 3 quartiles.[76] These data suggest that SBRT is safe and well tolerated, even for patients with significant COPD.

Severe SBRT toxicity appears to be rare, but a phase 2 trial performed at Indiana Univeristy[76,86]

suggests that significant toxicity may be more common in the treatment of central tumors, defined as within 2 cm of the proximal bronchial tree. In this study, which included both peripheral and central tumors, a total of 12 patients (17%) experienced Grade 3 to 5 toxicities that were reported as possibly treatment related, including apnea, pneumonia, pleural effusion, decline in PFT values, anxiety, and erythema. Five deaths (7%) were reported as possibly treatment related, due to pneumonia (n = 3), hemoptysis (n = 1), and respiratory failure (n = 1). When stratified by proximity to the central bronchi, the mature results from this study showed a 10.4% risk for Grade 3 to 5 toxicities for peripheral lesions, compared with 27.3% for centrally located lesions.[76] This difference did not reach statistical significance, likely because of the low total number of severe toxicities; however, these data have promoted caution in the use of SBRT for centrally located tumors. In the RTOG 0236, which included only peripheral tumors, Grade 3 or greater adverse events were noted in 9 of 59 patients, and there were no treatment-related deaths. The delivery of lower doses or the use of more fractionated schemes does seem safe and well tolerated for patients with central tumors, based on retrospective studies.[103–105] A prospective RTOG trial (RTOG 0813) is currently under way for patients with centrally located tumors to determine the maximum tolerated dose using 5 fractions.[99]

Following treatment, patients typically undergo serial CT imaging to monitor treatment response. Evaluation of these images following SBRT can be difficult, due to persistent radiographic changes at the site of the tumor including fibrosis and ground-glass opacities, which occur in the majority of patients.[101] Positron emission tomography (PET) and/or biopsy can be used to further evaluate suspicious CT findings, but PET can continue to show persistent hypermetabolic activity at the treatment site in the absence of disease for up to 22 to 26 months following treatment,[106] and can result in unnecessary diagnostic interventions.[107]

MULTIDISCIPLINARY TUMOR BOARDS

Several guideline panels suggest that a multidisciplinary approach is optimal in assessing the patient with high-risk, early-stage lung cancer, including discussion at a thoracic oncology tumor board. Tumor boards provide a treatment-planning approach in which several clinicians in different specialties review and discuss the medical condition and treatment options of a patient. Based on a survey published in 1989,

90% of hospitals with greater than 100 beds have a tumor board, with approximately 50 physician hours per month spent in preparation or conducting their tumor conference.[108] Tumor boards can positively affect clinical decision making and thereby directly influence patient care in an array of clinical settings. These boards function not only as mechanisms for improving patient care but also as educational forums. Tumor boards give every patient the full spectrum of management strategies, some of which might be overlooked by a single consultation or sequential consultations. The multidisciplinary approach is an important patient-centered strategy that provides patients with evaluation and second opinion in one visit in one location.[109] A review at tumor board can lead to change in management decisions in up to 30% to 45% of the patients presented.[110,111] Tumor board discussions have been shown to independently predict adherence to clinical practice guidelines and prompt the creation of treatment algorithms to achieve greater quality and consistency for commonly treated disease entities. Emphasizing a multidisciplinary approach to the management plan can help overcome the potential bias of the treating or diagnosing physician.[112,113] Consultations result in positive patient outcomes in terms of diagnosis and/or treatment planning.[114] Tumor board recommendations improve overall survival in complex cancer patients, patient satisfaction, and clinician satisfaction.[115,116] Tumor boards are essential for generating coordinated treatment plans, and improve timely access to care.[117] Recommendations made at tumor conferences are generally implemented. Multidisciplinary tumor boards also provide a significant educational opportunity for postgraduate trainees.[118,119] The American College of Surgeons Commission on Cancer, a national medical accreditation body, recognizes tumor boards as an essential component of excellence in cancer care. All high-risk early-stage lung cancers should ideally be discussed within multidisciplinary tumor boards for consideration of management options.

PATIENT PREFERENCES

Patient preferences should be respected as physicians consider treatment options. It is essential to educate patients about the advantages and disadvantages of available treatment. A broad spectrum of individual patient choices regarding active therapy versus best supportive care should be offered irrespective of age, gender, or educational background. Individual preferences are based not only on potential survival benefits but also reflect patient attitudes regarding the chances of treatment success, toxicities related to therapy, and short-term and long-term effects on overall quality of life.[120,121] Patients' assessments of their own survival play an important role in their choices regarding treatment.[122] Approximately 61% of patients with early-stage lung cancer receive recommended therapy. Older age, race, and marital status contribute significantly to patients not receiving recommended therapy.[123] Several factors play a role in decision making by patients in complying with recommended therapy. There is a marginally higher refusal rate for surgery by black patients than white patients, with proposed driving factors including cultural beliefs, distrust, and limited access to subspecialty care.[124–126] Patients' negative perceptions about the communication process and misperceptions of quality of life and prognosis 1 year after lung cancer diagnosis also relate to lower surgical rates. Other factors that affect patient preferences for accepting recommended therapy include patient's age, the presence of comorbidities, religious beliefs, lower socioeconomic status, and emotional adjustment to the diagnosis of cancer.[127,128]

EVALUATION AND TREATMENT OF EARLY-STAGE LUNG CANCER IN THE ELDERLY

Approximately 80% of all the lung cancers diagnosed in 2010 falls into the category of NSCLC.[129] The median age of diagnosis of lung cancer in the United States is 69 years in men and 67 years in women, with as many as 50% of the patients being diagnosed when older than 65 years.[130] Thirty percent of all lung cancers are diagnosed in patients older than 70 and 14% in patients older than 80 years.[131] The question still remains as regards the age cutoff used to define "elderly." In the United States and Europe, age greater than 70 is accepted as "elderly."[132] Some investigators define elderly patients in geriatric oncology as "old" when their health status begins to interfere with oncologic decision making.[133] Regardless of definition, the elderly population is grossly underrepresented in the clinical trials, with only 25% of clinical trials historically opening enrollment to patients older than 65 years.[134] Extrapolation of the clinical data in management of elderly patients is a clinical dilemma.

With regard to the diagnosis of lung cancer, elderly patients obtain lower histologic confirmation rates and less accurate staging.[135,136] However, several studies have shown that fiberoptic bronchoscopy and/or CT-guided needle biopsy commonly used for histologic diagnosis and staging of lung cancer are safe and very well tolerated by most patients irrespective of age, and should be routinely used to diagnose and stage elderly patients.[137,138] Surgery is the treatment of choice for early-stage lung cancer provided that it can be performed with acceptable risk. Elderly patients traditionally are considered to be at an increased operative risk for early-stage lung cancer irrespective of comorbidities or functional status. In one study of approximately 1600 patients, 37% of all patients younger than 65 years underwent surgery, compared with only 15% of patients older than 75. In addition, postoperative mortality was significantly higher (42% vs 58%) in the elderly population than in younger patients.[139] However, the elderly population had significantly higher comorbidity and the risk was not adjusted. Over the last decade, with the introduction of minimally invasive surgical techniques, advances in anesthesia, and better surgical risk stratification, there has been a significant decline in postoperative mortality and improvement in long-term survival. Given that average life expectancy in octogenarians can be as long as 5 to 9 years, and that without any intervention the survival in early-stage lung cancer is less than 2 years, treatment should be considered for every elderly patient.[140] Elderly patients should undergo preoperative evaluation similar to any other patient with early-stage lung cancer, and should be considered for surgery if they are deemed fit and prefer a surgical over a nonsurgical approach.

Lobectomy is the surgical procedure of choice even for elderly patients, because of higher rates of local recurrences with lesser surgeries.[39] In patients who cannot tolerate lobectomy, wedge resection and segmentectomies are reasonable alternatives. Although some older studies done in the late 1980s show decreased survival in the elderly population undergoing lung cancer surgery, this finding did not reach statistical significance.[141,142] Most recent studies, however, show similar survival between the two groups, as summarized in **Table 3**.

While surgery remains the treatment of choice for early-stage lung cancer in elderly patients, a significant proportion of these subjects remain unsuitable for such an approach because of the presence of comorbidities or patient refusal. Standard external beam radiation and SBRT are reasonable alternative management strategies in high-risk elderly patients with early-stage lung cancer. A retrospective review by Gauden and Tripcony[146] on 347 patients treated with a standard technique involving external beam radiation therapy to a dose of 50 Gy minimum tumor dose in 20 fractions over 4 weeks for early-stage NSCLC showed no difference in 5-year overall

Table 3 Surgery outcomes based on age in patients with early-stage non–small cell lung cancer				
Author	Year	Patients (n)	Age (y)	% Survival at 5 years
Morandi et al[143]	1997	130	<70	28
		85	>70	35
Kamiyoshihara et al[144]	2000	123	<70	50.8
		37	>70	35.1
Palma et al[145]	2010	63	<75	65
		247	>75	69

survival (22% vs 32%) or recurrence-free survival (18% vs 30%) between patients younger than 70 years and patients 70 years and older. The incidence of both acute and late Grade 3/4 toxicities was similar among all ages. A further discussion of SBRT is offered in the article by Paoletti and colleagues elsewhere in this issue.

SUMMARY

Much work has been done to identify and stratify high-risk patients with early-stage NSCLC. Surgery remains the treatment of choice, and surgical techniques have improved dramatically so to mitigate the risk for marginal patients. When surgery is not possible, SBRT appears to be the best therapy, while RFA is a promising alternative when SBRT is not available. As the population ages, the median age of those diagnosed with lung cancer will increase. Though special attention should be paid to the elderly, age alone should not be used as a criterion for treatment options. Multidisciplinary tumor board recommendations and incorporation of patient preferences in management decisions are important aspects of the evaluation and treatment of high-risk lung cancer patients.

REFERENCES

1. Myrdal G, Gustafsson G, Lambe M, et al. Outcome after lung cancer surgery. Factors predicting early mortality and major morbidity. Eur J Cardiothorac Surg 2001;20(4):694–9.
2. Mountain CF. Revisions in the international system for staging lung cancer. Chest 1997;111(6):1710–7.
3. Boffa DJ, Allen MS, Grab JD, et al. Data from The Society of Thoracic Surgeons General Thoracic Surgery database: the surgical management of primary lung tumors. J Thorac Cardiovasc Surg 2008;135(2):247–54.

4. Scott WJ, Howington J, Feigenberg S, et al. Treatment of non-small cell lung cancer stage I and stage II: ACCP evidence-based clinical practice guidelines (2nd edition). Chest 2007;132(Suppl 3):234S–42S.

5. Williams DE, Pairolero PC, Davis CS, et al. Survival of patients surgically treated for stage I lung cancer. J Thorac Cardiovasc Surg 1981;82(1):70–6.

6. Cheung MC, Hamilton K, Sherman R, et al. Impact of teaching facility status and high-volume centers on outcomes for lung cancer resection: an examination of 13,469 surgical patients. Ann Surg Oncol 2009;16(1):3–13.

7. Meguid RA, Brooke BS, Chang DC, et al. Are surgical outcomes for lung cancer resections improved at teaching hospitals? Ann Thorac Surg 2008;85(3):1015–24 [discussion: 1024–5].

8. Berry MF, Villamizar-Ortiz NR, Tong BC, et al. Pulmonary function tests do not predict pulmonary complications after thoracoscopic lobectomy. Ann Thorac Surg 2010;89(4):1044–51 [discussion: 1051–2].

9. Goodney PP, Lucas FL, Stukel TA, et al. Surgeon specialty and operative mortality with lung resection. Ann Surg 2005;241(1):179–84.

10. Mason DP, Subramanian S, Nowicki ER, et al. Impact of smoking cessation before resection of lung cancer: a Society of Thoracic Surgeons General Thoracic Surgery Database study. Ann Thorac Surg 2009;88(2):362–70 [discussion: 370–1].

11. Silvestri GA, Handy J, Lackland D, et al. Specialists achieve better outcomes than generalists for lung cancer surgery. Chest 1998;114(3):675–80.

12. Graham EA, Berck M. Principles versus details in the treatment of acute empyema. Ann Surg 1933;98(4):520–7.

13. Bolliger CT, Koegelenberg CF, Kendal R. Preoperative assessment for lung cancer surgery. Curr Opin Pulm Med 2005;11(4):301–6.

14. Datta D, Lahiri B. Preoperative evaluation of patients undergoing lung resection surgery. Chest 2003;123(6):2096–103.

15. Ferguson MK, Little L, Rizzo L, et al. Diffusing capacity predicts morbidity and mortality after pulmonary resection. J Thorac Cardiovasc Surg 1988;96(6):894–900.

16. Ferguson MK, Vigneswaran WT. Diffusing capacity predicts morbidity after lung resection in patients without obstructive lung disease. Ann Thorac Surg 2008;85(4):1158–64 [discussion: 1164–5].

17. Liptay MJ, Basu S, Hoaglin MC, et al. Diffusion lung capacity for carbon monoxide (DLCO) is an independent prognostic factor for long-term survival after curative lung resection for cancer. J Surg Oncol 2009;100(8):703–7.

18. Handy JR Jr, Asaph JW, Skokan L, et al. What happens to patients undergoing lung cancer surgery? Outcomes and quality of life before and after surgery. Chest 2002;122(1):21–30.

19. Colice GL, Shafazand S, Griffin JP, et al. Physiologic evaluation of the patient with lung cancer being considered for resectional surgery: ACCP evidenced-based clinical practice guidelines (2nd edition). Chest 2007;132(Suppl 3):161S–77S.

20. Bolliger CT, Guckel C, Engel H, et al. Prediction of functional reserves after lung resection: comparison between quantitative computed tomography, scintigraphy, and anatomy. Respiration 2002;69(6):482–9.

21. Smulders SA, Smeenk FW, Janssen-Heijnen ML, et al. Actual and predicted postoperative changes in lung function after pneumonectomy: a retrospective analysis. Chest 2004;125(5):1735–41.

22. Giordano A, Calcagni ML, Meduri G, et al. Perfusion lung scintigraphy for the prediction of postlobectomy residual pulmonary function. Chest 1997;111(6):1542–7.

23. Zeiher BG, Gross TJ, Kern JA, et al. Predicting postoperative pulmonary function in patients undergoing lung resection. Chest 1995;108(1):68–72.

24. Ali MK, Mountain CF, Ewer MS, et al. Predicting loss of pulmonary function after pulmonary resection for bronchogenic carcinoma. Chest 1980;77(3):337–42.

25. Bria WF, Kanarek DJ, Kazemi H. Prediction of postoperative pulmonary function following thoracic operations. Value of ventilation-perfusion scanning. J Thorac Cardiovasc Surg 1983;86(2):186–92.

26. Corris PA, Ellis DA, Hawkins T, et al. Use of radionuclide scanning in the preoperative estimation of pulmonary function after pneumonectomy. Thorax 1987;42(4):285–91.

27. Holden DA, Rice TW, Stelmach K, et al. Exercise testing, 6-min walk, and stair climb in the evaluation of patients at high risk for pulmonary resection. Chest 1992;102(6):1774–9.

28. Ninan M, Sommers KE, Landreneau RJ, et al. Standardized exercise oximetry predicts postpneumonectomy outcome. Ann Thorac Surg 1997;64(2):328–32 [discussion: 332–3].

29. Olsen GN, Bolton JW, Weiman DS, et al. Stair climbing as an exercise test to predict the postoperative complications of lung resection. Two years' experience. Chest 1991;99(3):587–90.

30. Morice RC, Peters EJ, Ryan MB, et al. Exercise testing in the evaluation of patients at high risk for complications from lung resection. Chest 1992;101(2):356–61.

31. Pate P, Tenholder MF, Griffin JP, et al. Preoperative assessment of the high-risk patient for lung resection. Ann Thorac Surg 1996;61(5):1494–500.

32. Brunelli A, Belardinelli R, Refai M, et al. Peak oxygen consumption during cardiopulmonary exercise test improves risk stratification in candidates to major lung resection. Chest 2009;135(5):1260–7.

33. Raz DJ, Zell JA, Ou SH, et al. Natural history of stage I non-small cell lung cancer: implications for early detection. Chest 2007;132(1):193–9.

34. Ginsberg RJ, Rubinstein LV. Randomized trial of lobectomy versus limited resection for T1 N0 non-small cell lung cancer. Lung Cancer Study Group. Ann Thorac Surg 1995;60(3):615–22.

35. Ferguson MK, Lehman AG. Sleeve lobectomy or pneumonectomy: optimal management strategy using decision analysis techniques. Ann Thorac Surg 2003;76(6):1782–8.

36. Jensik RJ, Faber LP, Milloy FJ, et al. Segmental resection for lung cancer. A fifteen-year experience. J Thorac Cardiovasc Surg 1973;66(4):563–72.

37. Ginsberg RJ, Hill LD, Eagan RT, et al. Modern thirty-day operative mortality for surgical resections in lung cancer. J Thorac Cardiovasc Surg 1983; 86(5):654–8.

38. Wada H, Nakamura T, Nakamoto K, et al. Thirty-day operative mortality for thoracotomy in lung cancer. J Thorac Cardiovasc Surg 1998;115(1):70–3.

39. Keenan RJ, Landreneau RJ, Maley RH Jr, et al. Segmental resection spares pulmonary function in patients with stage I lung cancer. Ann Thorac Surg 2004;78(1):228–33 [discussion: 228–33].

40. Harada H, Okada M, Sakamoto T, et al. Functional advantage after radical segmentectomy versus lobectomy for lung cancer. Ann Thorac Surg 2005;80(6):2041–5.

41. Mery CM, Pappas AN, Bueno R, et al. Similar long-term survival of elderly patients with non-small cell lung cancer treated with lobectomy or wedge resection within the surveillance, epidemiology, and end results database. Chest 2005;128(1): 237–45.

42. Kilic A, Schuchert MJ, Pettiford BL, et al. Anatomic segmentectomy for stage I non-small cell lung cancer in the elderly. Ann Thorac Surg 2009; 87(6):1662–6 [discussion: 1667–8].

43. Okada M, Nishio W, Sakamoto T, et al. Effect of tumor size on prognosis in patients with non-small cell lung cancer: the role of segmentectomy as a type of lesser resection. J Thorac Cardiovasc Surg 2005;129(1):87–93.

44. El-Sherif A, Fernando HC, Santos R, et al. Margin and local recurrence after sublobar resection of non-small cell lung cancer. Ann Surg Oncol 2007; 14(8):2400–5.

45. Ketchedjian A, Daly B, Landreneau R, et al. Sublobar resection for the subcentimeter pulmonary nodule. Semin Thorac Cardiovasc Surg 2005; 17(2):128–33.

46. Martin-Ucar AE, Nakas A, Pilling JE, et al. A case-matched study of anatomical segmentectomy versus lobectomy for stage I lung cancer in high-risk patients. Eur J Cardiothorac Surg 2005;27(4): 675–9.

47. Owens JM, Roberts DB, Myers JN. The role of postoperative adjuvant radiation therapy in the treatment of mucosal melanomas of the head and neck region. Arch Otolaryngol Head Neck Surg 2003;129(8):864–8.

48. Edwards JG, Duthie DJ, Waller DA. Lobar volume reduction surgery: a method of increasing the lung cancer resection rate in patients with emphysema. Thorax 2001;56(10):791–5.

49. Fishman A, Martinez F, Naunheim K, et al. A randomized trial comparing lung-volume-reduction surgery with medical therapy for severe emphysema. N Engl J Med 2003;348(21):2059–73.

50. Cooper JD, Patterson GA, Sundaresan RS, et al. Results of 150 consecutive bilateral lung volume reduction procedures in patients with severe emphysema. J Thorac Cardiovasc Surg 1996; 112(5):1319–29 [discussion: 1329–30].

51. Choong CK, Meyers BF, Battafarano RJ, et al. Lung cancer resection combined with lung volume reduction in patients with severe emphysema. J Thorac Cardiovasc Surg 2004;127(5):1323–31.

52. Flores RM, Alam N. Video-assisted thoracic surgery lobectomy (VATS), open thoracotomy, and the robot for lung cancer. Ann Thorac Surg 2008;85(2):S710–5.

53. Farjah F, Wood DE, Mulligan MS, et al. Safety and efficacy of video-assisted versus conventional lung resection for lung cancer. J Thorac Cardiovasc Surg 2009;137(6):1415–21.

54. Onaitis MW, Petersen RP, Balderson SS, et al. Thoracoscopic lobectomy is a safe and versatile procedure: experience with 500 consecutive patients. Ann Surg 2006;244(3):420–5.

55. McKenna RJ Jr, Houck W, Fuller CB. Video-assisted thoracic surgery lobectomy: experience with 1,100 cases. Ann Thorac Surg 2006;81(2):421–5 [discussion: 425–6].

56. Hiraki T, Gobara H, Mimura H, et al. Percutaneous radiofrequency ablation of lung cancer. Lancet Oncol 2008;9(7):604–5.

57. Gazelle GS, Goldberg SN, Solbiati L, et al. Tumor ablation with radio-frequency energy. Radiology 2000;217(3):633–46.

58. Nahum Goldberg S, Dupuy DE. Image-guided radiofrequency tumor ablation: challenges and opportunities–part I. J Vasc Interv Radiol 2001; 12(9):1021–32.

59. Dupuy DE, Zagoria RJ, Akerley W, et al. Percutaneous radiofrequency ablation of malignancies in the lung. AJR Am J Roentgenol 2000;174(1):57–9.

60. Chan VO, McDermott S, Malone DE, et al. Percutaneous radiofrequency ablation of lung tumors: evaluation of the literature using evidence-based techniques. J Thorac Imaging 2011;26(1):18–26.

61. Lencioni R, Crocetti L, Cioni R, et al. Response to radiofrequency ablation of pulmonary tumours:

a prospective, intention-to-treat, multicentre clinical trial (the RAPTURE study). Lancet Oncol 2008;9(7):621–8.

62. Simon CJ, Dupuy DE, DiPetrillo TA, et al. Pulmonary radiofrequency ablation: long-term safety and efficacy in 153 patients. Radiology 2007;243(1):268–75.

63. Fernando HC, De Hoyos A, Landreneau RJ, et al. Radiofrequency ablation for the treatment of non-small cell lung cancer in marginal surgical candidates. J Thorac Cardiovasc Surg 2005;129(3):639–44.

64. Jin GY, Lee JM, Lee YC, et al. Primary and secondary lung malignancies treated with percutaneous radiofrequency ablation: evaluation with follow-up helical CT. AJR Am J Roentgenol 2004;183(4):1013–20.

65. Lee JM, Jin GY, Goldberg SN, et al. Percutaneous radiofrequency ablation for inoperable non-small cell lung cancer and metastases: preliminary report. Radiology 2004;230(1):125–34.

66. Hiraki T, Sakurai J, Tsuda T, et al. Risk factors for local progression after percutaneous radiofrequency ablation of lung tumors: evaluation based on a preliminary review of 342 tumors. Cancer 2006;107(12):2873–80.

67. de Baère T, Palussière J, Aupérin A, et al. Midterm local efficacy and survival after radiofrequency ablation of lung tumors with minimum follow-up of 1 year: prospective evaluation. Radiology 2006;240(2):587–96.

68. Pennathur A, Luketich JD, Abbas G, et al. Radiofrequency ablation for the treatment of stage I non-small cell lung cancer in high-risk patients. J Thorac Cardiovasc Surg 2007;134(4):857–64.

69. Hiraki T, Gobara H, Iishi T, et al. Percutaneous radiofrequency ablation for clinical stage I non-small cell lung cancer: results in 20 nonsurgical candidates. J Thorac Cardiovasc Surg 2007;134(5):1306–12.

70. Choe YH, Kim SR, Lee KS, et al. The use of PTC and RFA as treatment alternatives with low procedural morbidity in non-small cell lung cancer. Eur J Cancer 2009;45(10):1773–9.

71. Lanuti M, Sharma A, Digumarthy SR, et al. Radiofrequency ablation for treatment of medically inoperable stage I non-small cell lung cancer. J Thorac Cardiovasc Surg 2009;137(1):160–6.

72. Haasbeek CJ, Slotman BJ, Senan S. Radiotherapy for lung cancer: clinical impact of recent technical advances. Lung Cancer 2009;64(1):1–8.

73. Ross CS, Hussey DH, Pennington EC, et al. Analysis of movement of intrathoracic neoplasms using ultrafast computerized tomography. Int J Radiat Oncol Biol Phys 1990;18(3):671–7.

74. Keall P. 4-Dimensional computed tomography imaging and treatment planning. Semin Radiat Oncol 2004;14(1):81–90.

75. Grills IS, Hugo G, Kestin LL, et al. Image-guided radiotherapy via daily online cone-beam CT substantially reduces margin requirements for stereotactic lung radiotherapy. Int J Radiat Oncol Biol Phys 2008;70(4):1045–56.

76. Fakiris AJ, McGarry RC, Yiannoutsos CT, et al. Stereotactic body radiation therapy for early-stage non-small-cell lung carcinoma: four-year results of a prospective phase II study. Int J Radiat Oncol Biol Phys 2009;75(3):677–82.

77. Timmerman R, Paulus R, Galvin J, et al. Stereotactic body radiation therapy for inoperable early stage lung cancer. JAMA 2010;303(11):1070–6.

78. Zimmermann FB, Geinitz H, Schill S, et al. Stereotactic hypofractionated radiation therapy for stage I non-small cell lung cancer. Lung Cancer 2005;48(1):107–14.

79. Nyman J, Johansson KA, Hultén U. Stereotactic hypofractionated radiotherapy for stage I non-small cell lung cancer–mature results for medically inoperable patients. Lung Cancer 2006;51(1):97–103.

80. Fritz P, Kraus HJ, Mühlnickel W, et al. Stereotactic, single-dose irradiation of stage I non-small cell lung cancer and lung metastases. Radiat Oncol 2006;1:30.

81. Baumann P, Nyman J, Lax I, et al. Factors important for efficacy of stereotactic body radiotherapy of medically inoperable stage I lung cancer. A retrospective analysis of patients treated in the Nordic countries. Acta Oncol 2006;45(7):787–95.

82. Nagata Y, Takayama K, Matsuo Y, et al. Clinical outcomes of a phase I/II study of 48 Gy of stereotactic body radiotherapy in 4 fractions for primary lung cancer using a stereotactic body frame. Int J Radiat Oncol Biol Phys 2005;63(5):1427–31.

83. Xia T, Li H, Sun Q, et al. Promising clinical outcome of stereotactic body radiation therapy for patients with inoperable Stage I/II non-small-cell lung cancer. Int J Radiat Oncol Biol Phys 2006;66(1):117–25.

84. Ricardi U, Filippi AR, Guarneri A, et al. Stereotactic body radiation therapy for early stage non-small cell lung cancer: results of a prospective trial. Lung Cancer 2010;68(1):72–7.

85. Baumann P, Nyman J, Hoyer M, et al. Outcome in a prospective phase II trial of medically inoperable stage I non-small-cell lung cancer patients treated with stereotactic body radiotherapy. J Clin Oncol 2009;27(20):3290–6.

86. Timmerman R, McGarry R, Yiannoutsos C, et al. Excessive toxicity when treating central tumors in a phase II study of stereotactic body radiation therapy for medically inoperable early-stage lung cancer. J Clin Oncol 2006;24(30):4833–9.

87. Onishi H, Shirato H, Nagata Y, et al. Hypofractionated stereotactic radiotherapy (HypoFXSRT) for stage I non-small cell lung cancer: updated results

of 257 patients in a Japanese multi-institutional study. J Thorac Oncol 2007;2(7 Suppl 3):S94–100.

88. Timmerman R, Papiez L, McGarry R, et al. Extracranial stereotactic radioablation: results of a phase I study in medically inoperable stage I non-small cell lung cancer. Chest 2003;124(5):1946–55.

89. McGarry RC, Papiez L, Williams M, et al. Stereotactic body radiation therapy of early-stage non-small-cell lung carcinoma: phase I study. Int J Radiat Oncol Biol Phys 2005;63(4):1010–5.

90. Krol AD, Aussems P, Noordijk EM, et al. Local irradiation alone for peripheral stage I lung cancer: could we omit the elective regional nodal irradiation? Int J Radiat Oncol Biol Phys 1996;34(2): 297–302.

91. Sandler HM, Curran WJ, Turrisi AT. The influence of tumor size and pre-treatment staging on outcome following radiation therapy alone for stage I non-small cell lung cancer. Int J Radiat Oncol Biol Phys 1990;19(1):9–13.

92. Kaskowitz L, Graham MV, Emami B, et al. Radiation therapy alone for stage I non-small cell lung cancer. Int J Radiat Oncol Biol Phys 1993;27(3): 517–23.

93. Onishi H, Shirato H, Nagata Y, et al. Stereotactic body radiotherapy (SBRT) for operable stage I non-small-cell lung cancer: can SBRT be comparable to surgery? Int J Radiat Oncol Biol Phys 2010. [Epub ahead of print].

94. Mountain CF. The international system for staging lung cancer. Semin Surg Oncol 2000;18(2):106–15.

95. Asamura H, Goya T, Koshiishi Y, et al. A Japanese lung cancer registry study: prognosis of 13,010 resected lung cancers. J Thorac Oncol 2008;3(1): 46–52.

96. Naruke T, Tsuchiya R, Kondo H, et al. Prognosis and survival after resection for bronchogenic carcinoma based on the 1997 TNM-staging classification: the Japanese experience. Ann Thorac Surg 2001;71(6):1759–64.

97. Grills IS, Mangona VS, Welsh R, et al. Outcomes after stereotactic lung radiotherapy or wedge resection for stage I non-small-cell lung cancer. J Clin Oncol 2010;28(6):928–35.

98. Nagata Y, Hiraoka M, Shibata T, et al. A phase II trial of stereotactic body radiation therapy for operable T1N0M0 non-small cell lung cancer: Japan Clinical Oncology Group (JCOG0403). Int J Radiat Oncol Biol Phys 2010;78:S27–8.

99. NIH Clinical Trials database. Available at: http://www.clinicaltrials.gov. Accessed March 13, 2011.

100. Carey Sampson M, Katz A, Constine LS. Stereotactic body radiation therapy for extracranial oligometastases: does the sword have a double edge? Semin Radiat Oncol 2006;16(2):67–76.

101. Trovo M, Linda A, El Naqa I, et al. Early and late lung radiographic injury following stereotactic body radiation therapy (SBRT). Lung Cancer 2010;69(1):77–85.

102. Stephans KL, Djemil T, Reddy CA, et al. Comprehensive analysis of pulmonary function test (PFT) changes after stereotactic body radiotherapy (SBRT) for stage I lung cancer in medically inoperable patients. J Thorac Oncol 2009;4(7):838–44.

103. Lagerwaard FJ, Haasbeek CJ, Smit EF, et al. Outcomes of risk-adapted fractionated stereotactic radiotherapy for stage I non-small-cell lung cancer. Int J Radiat Oncol Biol Phys 2008;70(3):685–92.

104. Senan S, Haasbeek NJ, Smit EF, et al. Stereotactic radiotherapy for centrally located early-stage lung tumors. J Clin Oncol 2007;25(4):464 [author reply: 465].

105. Guckenberger M, Heilman K, Wulf J, et al. Pulmonary injury and tumor response after stereotactic body radiotherapy (SBRT): results of a serial follow-up CT study. Radiother Oncol 2007;85(3): 435–42.

106. Hoopes DJ, Tann M, Fletcher JW, et al. FDG-PET and stereotactic body radiotherapy (SBRT) for stage I non-small-cell lung cancer. Lung Cancer 2007;56(2):229–34.

107. Takeda A, Kunieda E, Takeda T, et al. Possible misinterpretation of demarcated solid patterns of radiation fibrosis on CT scans as tumor recurrence in patients receiving hypofractionated stereotactic radiotherapy for lung cancer. Int J Radiat Oncol Biol Phys 2008;70(4):1057–65.

108. Fleming ID. Multidisciplinary treatment planning. Tumor boards. Cancer 1989;64(Suppl 1):279–81 [discussion: 282–4].

109. Chang JH, Vines E, Bertsch H, et al. The impact of a multidisciplinary breast cancer center on recommendations for patient management: the University of Pennsylvania experience. Cancer 2001;91(7): 1231–7.

110. Burton S, Brown G, Daniels IR, et al. MRI directed multidisciplinary team preoperative treatment strategy: the way to eliminate positive circumferential margins? Br J Cancer 2006;94(3):351–7.

111. Newman EA, Guest AB, Helvie MA, et al. Changes in surgical management resulting from case review at a breast cancer multidisciplinary tumor board. Cancer 2006;107(10):2346–51.

112. Abraham NS, Gossey JT, Davila JA, et al. Receipt of recommended therapy by patients with advanced colorectal cancer. Am J Gastroenterol 2006;101(6):1320–8.

113. Lutterbach J, Pagenstecher A, Spreer J, et al. The brain tumor board: lessons to be learned from an interdisciplinary conference. Onkologie 2005; 28(1):22–6.

114. Zorbas H, Barraclough B, Rainbird K, et al. Multidisciplinary care for women with early breast cancer in the Australian context: what does it mean? Med J Aust 2003;179(10):528–31.

115. Junor EJ, Hole DJ, Gillis CR. Management of ovarian cancer: referral to a multidisciplinary team matters. Br J Cancer 1994;70(2):363–70.

116. Sainsbury R, Haward B, Rider L, et al. Influence of clinician workload and patterns of treatment on survival from breast cancer. Lancet 1995; 345(8960):1265–70.

117. Gabel M, Hilton NE, Nathanson SD. Multidisciplinary breast cancer clinics. Do they work? Cancer 1997;79(12):2380–4.

118. Petty JK, Vetto JT. Beyond doughnuts: tumor board recommendations influence patient care. J Cancer Educ 2002;17(2):97–100.

119. Gatcliffe TA, Coleman RL. Tumor board: more than treatment planning—a 1-year prospective survey. J Cancer Educ 2008;23(4):235–7.

120. Silvestri G, Pritchard R, Welch HG. Preferences for chemotherapy in patients with advanced non-small cell lung cancer: descriptive study based on scripted interviews. BMJ 1998;317(7161):771–5.

121. Brundage MD, Feldman-Stewart D, Cosby R, et al. Cancer patients' attitudes toward treatment options for advanced non-small cell lung cancer: implications for patient education and decision support. Patient Educ Couns 2001;45(2):149–57.

122. Weeks JC, Cook EF, O'Day SJ, et al. Relationship between cancer patients' predictions of prognosis and their treatment preferences. JAMA 1998; 279(21):1709–14.

123. Potosky AL, Saxman S, Wallace RB, et al. Population variations in the initial treatment of non-small-cell lung cancer. J Clin Oncol 2004;22(16):3261–8.

124. McCann J, Artinian V, Duhaime L, et al. Evaluation of the causes for racial disparity in surgical treatment of early stage lung cancer. Chest 2005; 128(5):3440–6.

125. Farjah F, Wood DE, Yanez ND 3rd, et al. Racial disparities among patients with lung cancer who were recommended operative therapy. Arch Surg 2009;144(1):14–8.

126. Margolis ML, Christie JD, Silvestri GA, et al. Racial differences pertaining to a belief about lung cancer surgery: results of a multicenter survey. Ann Intern Med 2003;139(7):558–63.

127. Cykert S, Dilworth-Anderson P, Monroe MH, et al. Factors associated with decisions to undergo surgery among patients with newly diagnosed early-stage lung cancer. JAMA 2010;303(23): 2368–76.

128. Clever SL, Edwards KA, Feudtner C, et al. Ethics and communication: does students' comfort addressing: ethical issues vary by specialty team? J Gen Intern Med 2001;16(8):559–63.

129. Jemal A, Siegel R, Ward E, et al. Cancer statistics, 2009. CA Cancer J Clin 2009;59(4):225–49.

130. Havlik RJ, Yancik R, Long S, et al. The National Institute on Aging and the National Cancer Institute

SEER collaborative study on comorbidity and early diagnosis of cancer in the elderly. Cancer 1994; 74(Suppl 7):2101–6.

131. Owonikoko TK, Ragin CC, Belani CP, et al. Lung cancer in elderly patients: an analysis of the surveillance, epidemiology, and end results database. J Clin Oncol 2007;25(35):5570–7.

132. Balducci L. Geriatric oncology: challenges for the new century. Eur J Cancer 2000;36(14):1741–54.

133. Extermann M. Measuring comorbidity in older cancer patients. Eur J Cancer 2000;36(4):453–71.

134. Hutchins LF, Unger JM, Crowley JJ, et al. Underrepresentation of patients 65 years of age or older in cancer-treatment trials. N Engl J Med 1999; 341(27):2061–7.

135. Brown JS, Eraut D, Trask C, et al. Age and the treatment of lung cancer. Thorax 1996;51(6):564–8.

136. Janssen-Heijnen ML, Schipper RM, Razenberg PP, et al. Prevalence of co-morbidity in lung cancer patients and its relationship with treatment: a population-based study. Lung Cancer 1998;21(2): 105–13.

137. Hehn B, Haponik EF. Flexible bronchoscopy in the elderly. Clin Chest Med 2001;22(2):301–9, viii.

138. Brown TS, Kanthapillai P. Transthoracic needle biopsy for suspected thoracic malignancy in elderly patients using CT guidance. Clin Radiol 1998;53(2):116–9.

139. Peake MD, Thompson S, Lowe D, et al. Ageism in the management of lung cancer. Age Ageing 2003;32(2):171–7.

140. Anderson RN. United States life tables, 1997. Natl Vital Stat Rep 1999;47(28):1–37.

141. Sherman S, Guidot CE. The feasibility of thoracotomy for lung cancer in the elderly. JAMA 1987;258(7):927–30.

142. Ishida T, Yokoyama H, Kaneko S, et al. Long-term results of operation for non-small cell lung cancer in the elderly. Ann Thorac Surg 1990; 50(6):919–22.

143. Morandi U, Stefani A, Golinelli M, et al. Results of surgical resection in patients over the age of 70 years with non small-cell lung cancer. Eur J Cardiothorac Surg 1997;11(3):432–9.

144. Kamiyoshihara M, Kawashima O, Ishikawa S, et al. Long-term results after pulmonary resection in elderly patients with non-small cell lung cancer. J Cardiovasc Surg (Torino) 2000;41(3):483–6.

145. Palma DA, Tyldesley S, Sheehan F, et al. Stage I non-small cell lung cancer (NSCLC) in patients aged 75 years and older: does age determine survival after radical treatment? J Thorac Oncol 2010;5(6):818–24.

146. Gauden SJ, Tripcony L. The curative treatment by radiation therapy alone of Stage I non-small cell lung cancer in a geriatric population. Lung Cancer 2001;32(1):71–9.

Approach to the Ground-Glass Nodule

Frank C. Detterbeck, MD[a],*, Robert J. Homer, MD, PhD[b]

KEYWORDS

- Ground-glass opacity • Chest CT • Lung cancer
- Lung nodule • CT scan

Patients are increasingly being identified with a ground-glass lesion on a chest computed tomography (CT) scan. It is not clear whether this is because of an increased incidence, increased awareness (ie, recognition of an abnormality as opposed to considering it an inconsequential finding), or increased identification because of an increasing prevalence of CT imaging. Whatever the reason, how to approach these patients is an issue that increasingly confronts clinicians. This article reviews the available data and proposes management recommendations for these patients.

A ground-glass opacity (GGO) is defined as a hazy increased lung opacity (on CT) with preservation of bronchial and vascular markings.[1] However, this definition requires clarification because such densities are seen in many different contexts. This article discusses abnormalities that are seen in the absence of another disease process, such as a pneumonia (including a viral pneumonia) or interstitial lung disease. It discusses only persistent (not transient) GGOs, and excludes diffuse GGO throughout the lung, or infiltrates that are geographic and not focal (these are generally associated with an underlying disease process). This article is concerned only about a focal GGO in patients who are middle aged or older. Although a GGO may have a solid component, this article primarily focuses on the approach to a pure GGO, or lesion with a solid component but that is still more than 50% GGO. These are usually found incidentally on a CT scan (and generally not visible on a chest radiograph). Examples of GGOs according to the Suzuki classification are shown in

Fig. 1.[2] This article addresses only types 1 to 4 in this classification.

This article discusses the range of possible entities, whether there are identifiable risk factors or characteristics that help make a presumptive clinical diagnosis, how often and for how long these should be observed, when and how a biopsy should be done, how these lesions should be treated (ie, lobectomy, segmentectomy, wedge resection, stereotactic body radiotherapy [SBRT], or radiofrequency ablation [RFA]), and how multifocal GGOs should be approached.

PATHOLOGIC ENTITIES

A GGO that is not related to another pulmonary or systemic process is most likely to be either a nonspecific benign process or an entity in the adenocarcinoma (AC) spectrum. These entities are predominantly characterized by growth at least in part along preexisting alveolar structures. This pattern of growth is also known as lepidic growth (named after butterflies, Order Lepidoptera, alighting on a branch but not disturbing it). The entities currently recognized in this spectrum include atypical adenomatous hyperplasia (AAH; defined as a lesion <0.5 cm, with mild to moderate nuclear atypia, without stromal invasion), AC in situ (AIS; <3 cm, with moderate to severe nuclear atypia, without stromal invasion), minimally invasive AC (stromal invasion present but overall tumor size <3 cm with <0.5 cm of invasion), lepidic pattern AC (extent of invasion >0.5 cm but predominantly lepidic pattern of growth), and

The authors have nothing to disclose.
[a] Yale Thoracic Surgery, Yale School of Medicine, 330 Cedar Street, PO Box 208062, New Haven, CT 06520-8062, USA
[b] Department of Pathology, Yale School of Medicine, 310 Cedar Street, New Haven, CT 06510-3218, USA
* Corresponding author.
E-mail address: frank.detterbeck@yale.edu

Clin Chest Med 32 (2011) 799–810
doi:10.1016/j.ccm.2011.08.002
0272-5231/11/$ – see front matter © 2011 Elsevier Inc. All rights reserved.

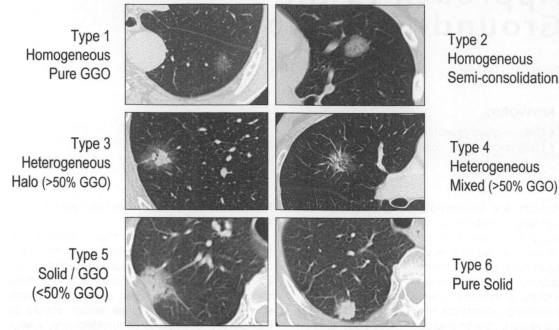

Type 1
Homogeneous
Pure GGO

Type 2
Homogeneous
Semi-consolidation

Type 3
Heterogeneous
Halo (>50% GGO)

Type 4
Heterogeneous
Mixed (>50% GGO)

Type 5
Solid / GGO
(<50% GGO)

Type 6
Pure Solid

Fig. 1. Suzuki classification of GGOs. Radiographic classification of lung nodules according to the ground-glass component by Suzuki and colleagues.[2] (*Data from* Suzuki K, Kusumoto M, Watanabe S, et al. Radiologic classification of small adenocarcinoma of the lung: radiologic-pathologic correlation and its prognostic impact. Ann Thorac Surg 2006;81:413–9.)

conventional acinar and papillary AC with minor lepidic growth around the periphery of the tumor.[3] The key concept in this progression is the presence and relative extent of invasion. Historically (since the 1999 World Health Organization [WHO] classification), the presence of invasion has separated AAH and bronchioloalveolar carcinoma (BAC) from invasive AC, but the extent of invasion was not a key criterion. A critical supporting concept is that the entire tumor needs to be examined (not just a biopsy) to pathologically exclude invasion. Thus any reported series of BAC based on biopsy only is inappropriately classified. Similarly, multicentric tumors or pneumonic tumors commonly show noninvasive components on biopsy despite obvious radiologic evidence for invasion.[4] Widespread lack of awareness of the need to examine the entire (resected) tumor to appropriately classify these tumors has led to the recommendation to abandon the term BAC[3]; however, the concept of complete assessment also applies to the new terminology (AAH, AIS, AC.[3] These entities are discussed further in the article by Travis elsewhere in this issue.

In most cases, stromal invasion leads to dense scarring that is apparent as a solid density radiographically. This dense scar is the basis of the Suzuki system described earlier. The exceptions are that of papillary and micropapillary AC, which are

recent additions to the spectrum of pulmonary AC. In some cases, the papillary AC component had been confused with the BAC pattern, which is a consideration in analysis of the existing literature. The significance is that papillary ACs are believed to have a similar prognosis as conventional invasive ACs, whereas micropapillary ACs are generally considered to have a worse prognosis. Most lung ACs are mixtures of different patterns, thus pure papillary or micropapillary ACs are rare.

If AAH and AIS are considered precursor lesions to more aggressive, invasive AC, there should be similar but increased genetic complexity in the invasive portion of the AC component in comparison with the noninvasive portion of the same tumor. This prediction has been shown to be true in at least some tumors.[5,6] AAH clearly has a lower level of complexity than AIS,[7] but the rate of progression of AAH and AIS to more clinically significant lesions is hard to estimate. Specifically, because AAH is generally an incidental finding in a lobe resected for another purpose, it is not possible to estimate its rate of progression.

APPROACH TO MANAGEMENT
Clinical Diagnosis

The first step in approaching a patient is to make a presumptive clinical diagnosis, along with an estimate of how reliable this is. The risk of malignant disease, namely AC in situ and invasive AC, must be estimated. The best treatment of AIS is debatable, but there is no substantial experience with observation as a strategy, and a diagnosis of AIS is assumed to be an indication for treatment.

Among GGOs that were resected, most were AIS or AC (**Fig. 2**A, B). The rate of AC is increased if there is a solid component. Because all of these patients were resected, these data probably do not apply to all patients with a GGO, of whom many are believed to be more appropriately observed, presumably because their risk of cancer is believed to be low.

The influence of size in pure and semisolid GGOs is shown in **Fig. 3**A, B among studies involving a period of follow-up (or biopsy). For pure GGO that are less than or equal to 10 mm in size, the chance of invasive AC seems to be minimal, although there is about a 25% chance of AIS. Pure GGOs greater than 10 mm in size have a higher risk of AIS (~40%) and a small risk of AC (~20%). The presence of a solid portion seems to be more significant; even if the lesion is less than or equal to 10 mm, about 50% have AIS and about 25% have AC. Most semisolid lesions greater than 10 mm have AIS or AC. However, the number of studies is limited, and the data in part come from a skewed patient population in which the suspicion of malignancy was high enough to justify surgical removal of the lesion.

There are few data regarding other patient or lesion characteristics that can influence the risk of cancer. There is some evidence that GGOs have little relationship to smoking,[8,9] although this has not been clearly addressed. Whether a prior history of lung cancer affects the incidence of malignancy in a GGO is unclear.[10,11] Other factors, such as age or geographic location, have not been studied. All the studies to date have come from Asia, with 1 exception.[12]

Observation: When and How?

This article focuses on GGOs that are persistent, but being exact about this definition is difficult. No standard criteria have been established, but we propose that the lesion appears unchanged during a period of approximately 2 to 3 months. CT screening shows that about 30% of GGOs on baseline scan disappear after 2 months, as do about 50% of new GGO lesions detected on repeat screening evaluations.[13] Most of the GGO lesions that disappear are believed to be related to infection. In particular, lesions with radiographic features that suggest infection (ie, lesions that are less focal, often with borders that fade gradually and with a more irregular shape) should be treated with antibiotics and a follow-up scan to show that they have resolved. Data show that most (~95%) lesions that disappear do so within the first 3 months.[14,15]

What happens in time to a persistent GGO? Data from several studies are shown in **Fig. 4**. The length of follow-up ranged from 9 to 40 months. The reported outcomes vary, probably because the patients included, and the nature of the endpoints and follow-up, have varied. Most lesions either remained the same or decreased in size. About 10% to 20% increased in size, although the proportion was higher (~50%) in 2 studies.[16,17] One of these studies[16] only reported on patients who were selected for resection; no reason is apparent why

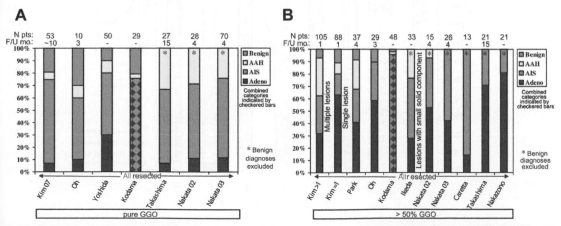

Fig. 2. Findings at resection of a GGO. Distribution of diagnoses of resected lesions for (*A*) pure GGO and (*B*) semisolid GGO lesions. AAH, atypical adenomatous hyperplasia; Adeno, adenocarcinoma; AIS, adenocarcinoma in situ; F/U mo, follow-up period (in months); N pts, number of patients. (Part (*A*) *Data from* Refs.[15,26,44,46,73–75]; and (*B*) *Data from* Refs.[12,15,26,46,59,60,74–77])

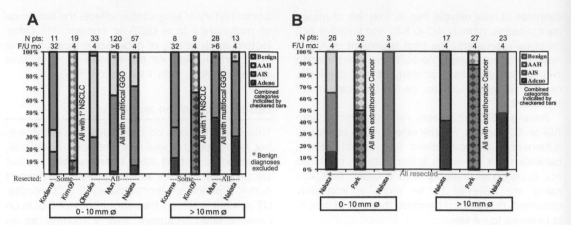

Fig. 3. Diagnosis according to size. Diagnosis according to size for (A) pure GGO and (B) semisolid GGO. AAH, atypical adenomatous hyperplasia; Adeno, adenocarcinoma; AIS, adenocarcinoma in situ; F/U mo, follow-up period (in months); N pts, number of patients; NSCLC, non–small cell lung carcinoma. (Part (A) *Data from* Refs.[17,46,58,60,78]; and (B) *Data from* Refs.[46,59,75])

the incidence of an increase in size was so high in the other.[17] The incidence of development of a solid component seems to be low. Whether the lesion is a pure GGO or semisolid seems to have little influence in predicting subsequent changes,[10] but the data are limited.

A study of 125 GGOs (after documented stability for 3 months) found that, by multivariate analysis, the initial lesion size, and perhaps a prior history of lung cancer, were the only factors affecting the risk of growth over time.[10] The risk of growth at 5 years was 66% for lesions greater than 10 mm versus 14% if less than or equal to 10 mm initially.[10]

There was no sign of a plateau that could support termination of follow-up after a certain point.[10]

It is difficult to measure a GGO. The difference between the lesion and the underlying lung is subtle, often the borders are indistinct, and the lesion may change in size with breathing. Even for the more usual (ie, solid) cl tumors, data show false-positive and false-negative (FN) assessments of growth of 10% to 50%, using different measurement methods (maximal length, diameter, volume),[18] and poor interobserver and intraobserver consistency for size differences of less than 1.5 to 2 mm.[19,20] Volumetric programs that

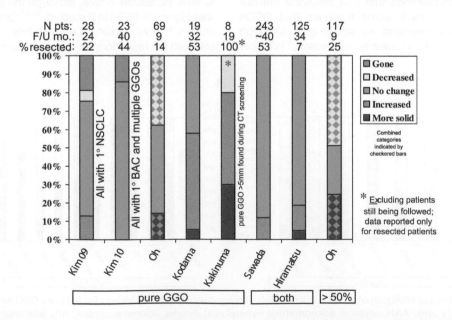

Fig. 4. Outcomes during observation. Outcomes of GGO lesions after a period of observation. BAC, bronchioloalveolar carcinoma; F/U mo, follow-up period (in months); N pts, number of patients. (*Data from* Refs.[10,15–17,57,60,79])

work well with solid lesions do not seem to function with GGOs,[21] although recent programs show intraobserver and interobserver differences for volume measurements of approximately plus or minus 15% to 20% for GGOs greater than or equal to 8 mm and plus or minus 30% to 40% if less than 8 mm.[22]

In addition, a decrease in size cannot be taken as an indication that a lesion is benign. Several studies observed a decrease in size during an observation period in approximately 20% (range 14%–25%) of resected ACs that appeared as a GGO.[16,23–26] This may be a select group, because they were chosen for resection despite the decrease in size. A decrease in size may be associated with the development of a solid component (but not always). There is also a suggestion that a period of decrease in size may be an expected occurrence during the progression of a GGO into an invasive cancer.[27]

The traditional approach of putting a great deal of importance on the growth of a lesion is problematic. Studies of screening CT have shown that the growth rate of malignant nodules is often not as consistent as expected.[14,23,27,28] The difficulty in determining the size of a lesion seems to account for only part of this variation.

Among lesions that were observed, approximately 5% were eventually found to be AC, and approximately 10% to 30% were AIS (Fig. 5). The incidence of AC may be slightly higher in patients with semisolid lesions or in patients with a history of non–small cell lung carcinoma

(NSCLC).[11,15] The rest of the lesions were either benign or are still being followed. It is possible that some of the followed lesions are malignancies (ie, indolent). It is also likely that a proportion of the lesions still being followed would be diagnosed as AAH if they were biopsied.

A significant amount of data show that, on average, cancers arising from GGO lesions exhibit slow rates of growth (volume doubling times [VDT] of ~500 and ~750 days for semisolid and pure GGO lesions).[29–32] Among pure GGO lesions, 50% to 90% of patients have tumors with a VDT of greater than 400 days, and this was greater than 800 days in 20% to 50%.[29–32] For semisolid lesions, about 50% have a VDT of greater than 400 days, but, in at least 1 study, a small proportion has a short VDT of less than 100 days. These data come from studies involving CT screening, which may be skewed toward more indolent tumors.[32] Furthermore, some variability exists in the growth patterns observed among GGO lesions that were followed and eventually shown to be NSCLC.[23]

Given the variability of results and limited number of studies, an initial interval between scans of 6 months for pure GGO and 3 months for a semisolid lesion seems reasonable. If stability is shown, subsequently increasing the interval to 12 and 6 months, respectively, seems to be justified.

Confirmatory Tests

Positron emission tomography (PET) imaging has no usefulness for GGO lesions.[11,33,34] A study of

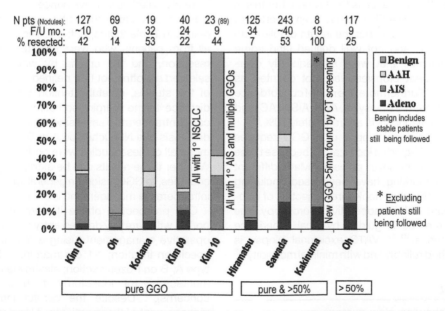

Fig. 5. Diagnoses during observation. Diagnoses made during observation. AAH, atypical adenomatous hyperplasia; Adeno, adenocarcinoma; AIS, adenocarcinoma in situ; F/U mo, follow-up period (in months); N pts, number of patients. (Data from Refs.[10,15–17,57,60,73,79])

GGOs 1 to 3 cm in size reported a sensitivity of 10% and a FN rate of 90%.[33] For lesions that have a solid component, the usefulness of PET is limited because of the size. The amount of PET uptake decreases almost linearly for solid lesions less than 2 cm; particularly for lesions less than 10 mm, the sensitivity is low and the FN rate is high.[33–35]

Methods of biopsy include bronchoscopic biopsy, transthoracic needle, or surgical (excisional) biopsy, typically via video-assisted thoracic surgery (VATS). Bronchoscopy for peripheral lesions has a low yield (~30%),[36] and a GGO that cannot be visualized with fluoroscopy is even more difficult. Electromagnetic navigation can guide a biopsy, but confirmation of being in the right place (ie, with peripheral ultrasound) may not be possible. No data have been reported regarding the yield of such techniques specifically for GGO lesions.

Specific potential issues with CT-guided transthoracic needle biopsy include that GGO lesions are small and, by definition, not very cellular, and bleeding can obscure the lesion and make a second pass difficult. The sensitivity has been reported to be about 50% to 90%, but, with inclusion of indeterminate results, it is about 50% to 75%.[37–39] The sensitivity is slightly worse in smaller lesions (35%–67% for lesions ≤10 mm vs 75%–80% for lesions >15–20 mm).[37,39] The sensitivity also seems slightly worse for pure GGO lesions than for lesions that are greater than 50% GGO (50% vs 80%).[39] CT fluoroscopy may yield slightly better results.[39]

However, the real issue is the FN rate, but this is not well defined. The FN rate has been reported to be about 20% to 30%, but the length of follow-up has been short and not well defined (and some negative biopsies that were subsequently overturned by repeat biopsies were not counted as negative).[38,39] Furthermore, the rate of concordance between the needle biopsy (ie, AAH, AIS of AC) and the resection diagnosis is approximately 70%.[38]

A VATS excisional biopsy of a GGO requires preoperative CT-guided localization, because these lesions are almost never palpable. Many different methods of marking have been used, including technetium, blue dye, hook wires, injection of lipiodol or barium with intraoperative fluoroscopy. The choice of method is guided by local experience and preference.[40–42] VATS excisional biopsy is accomplished reliably and with minimal morbidity.[42]

Treatment

The data showing slow average growth rates of malignant GGO lesions prompt the question of whether a less aggressive treatment than lobectomy is warranted. One way to assess this is to examine the incidence of nodal involvement among resected malignant GGOs (Table 1). The incidence of nodal involvement seems to be consistently low for lesions that are greater than 50% GGO, with only 1 exception.[43] This study was not limited to patients who were at clinical stage I; it is possible that inclusion of patients who were at cII and cIIIa accounted for the high incidence of nodal involvement. However, for cI GGO lesions of less than 2 cm, the surrogate endpoint of nodal involvement suggests that sublobar resection may be reasonable. These results are true even for GGO lesions that were classified as invasive cancer.

Outcomes of patients with greater than 50% GGO tumors who underwent primarily sublobar resection are consistently excellent, as shown in Table 2. This finding is true for both retrospective analyses as well as prospective studies.[44–48] It is not possible to compare lobectomy, segmentectomy, and wedge resection in these studies, but there does not seem to be any trend toward worse outcomes in studies with a large proportion of wedge resections. However, overall and disease-free survival may not be optimal endpoints in this case (because patients may survive despite recurrence of an indolent tumor, unrelated deaths with no evidence of recurrence are counted as an event, and new primary lung cancers are counted as an event). The best treatment outcome measure is recurrence, which is uniformly zero after sublobar resection. Again, these excellent results for GGO lesions are true even for tumors that were classified as invasive cancer.

However, caution should be used in applying the results in Table 2 prospectively. These results were all from patients who were selected for sublobar resection, and the criteria by which they were selected are often not fully defined. In at least some of the studies, careful attention was paid to the distance to the margin, sometimes with sophisticated intraoperative assessment, or a frozen section diagnosis of a Noguchi type A or B tumor. Furthermore, all of these studies were performed in Japan. Whether these results can be extrapolated to other countries, to GGO lesions in general, or without strict intraoperative management, is uncertain.

One prospective phase II study has been reported with carefully defined entry criteria and intraoperative management (using a modified stapler; specimen inflation; ≥1 cm margin; only Noguchi type A, B on frozen section; elastin stain; and segmentectomy or lobectomy if there were any concerns).[44] Despite the careful intraoperative management of these patients, 3 local recurrences at the staple line were reported in this study.[49] The final results of this study have not yet been released.

Table 1
Incidence of nodal involvement of resected malignant GGO lesions

Study	Total n	Histologic Size			% GGO	% N1	N2
		Stage	Type	Size (cm)			
Park et al,[61] 2009	58	—	—	—	Pure	0	0
Seki et al,[8] 2008	38	cIa	—	—	Pure	0	0
Mun and Kohno,[58] 2007	27	—	—	—	Pure	0	0
Suzuki et al,[63] 2002	24	cI	—	—	Pure	0	0
Suzuki et al,[2] 2006	22	cIa	Ad	≤2	Pure	0	0
Nomori et al,[64] 2003	18	cIa	Ad	—	Pure	0	0
Takamochi et al,[43] 2001	156	cI-IIIa	Ad	—	>50[a]	20	
Hashizume et al,[62] 2008	152	cIa	Ad	≤2	>50	0	0
Suzuki et al,[2] 2006	116	cIa	Ad	≤2	>50	1	0
Okada et al,[65] 2003	88	—	Ad	≤3	>50[a]	1	
Kondo et al,[66] 2002	66	—	—	<2	>50	2	
Ichiki et al,[67] 2011	62	cIa	Ad	1–2	>50	0	0
Kodama et al,[68] 2001	52	—	—	≤2	>50	0	0
Ikeda et al,[69] 2004	44	—	—	≤2	>50	0	0
Yamato et al,[45] 2001	42	cIa	Ad	≤2	>50	0	0
Suzuki et al,[63] 2002	33	cI	—	—	>50	0	0
Matsuguma et al,[70] 2004	31	cIa	—	—	>50	0	0
Nomori et al,[64] 2003	28	cIa	Ad	—	Mixed	0	4
Nakata et al,[46] 2003	28	—	—	≤2	>50	0	0
Seki et al,[8] 2008	27	cI	—	—	>50	4	—
Matsuguma et al,[71] 2002	26	cIa	—	—	>50	0	0
Zhou et al,[52] 2010	24	cI	—	≤1	>50	0	0

Inclusion criteria: studies of resection of >50% GGO lesions in >20 patients, with node assessment in >80%.
Abbreviation: Ad, adenocarcinoma.
[a] By tumor disappearance ratio (the ratio of lesion size on lung and mediastinal windows).

Some investigators have advocated limited resection of AIS (ie, BAC), noting that, in general, a GGO lesion is more likely to be AIS. These investigators reported 94% to 100% reliability of a frozen section to correctly diagnose AIS.[44,45,47,48,50] These data are from studies that used sophisticated and stringent criteria for how the frozen section was performed; applying this more broadly may not yield the same result.

The lack of nodal involvement with a GGO is in contrast with that for solid cI lesions, for which several studies have shown that, even for solid nodules less than or equal to 1 cm, there is a worrisome incidence of nodal involvement (average 22%, range 7%–54%).[51–55]

MANAGEMENT OF MULTIFOCAL GGO

A particular problem is how to manage patients with multiple GGOs, which we call multifocal disease. It is probably best not to think of this mechanistically as hematogenous (or aerogenous) dissemination, but as a manifestation of cancer development at multiple sites (ie, field cancerization and multiple primary tumors), given consistent survival results that are dramatically different than other forms of distant dissemination (even to solitary sites, with 23% 1-year survival in the staging revision database).[56] Multiple (vs single) GGOs do not seem to be more ominous for risk of invasive cancer, either in general or with a dominant lesion that is AIS or AC.[10,11,57–60]

The risk of cancer being present in a GGO seems to be similarly influenced by the size and presence of a solid component, whether there are multiple GGOs or a single GGO.[58–60] During a median follow-up period of 46 months, new lesions developed in 26% in a study of 27 patients with 91 GGOs.[58] All new lesions were pure GGOs of less than 10 mm (most were simply observed and not resected because they showed no signs of being invasive cancers). No new lesions were noted in

Table 2
Outcomes with sublobar resection of malignant GGO lesions

Study	n	Stage	Size (cm)	GGO Criteria	% Wedge	% Segment	% Lobectomy	% 5-y Survival OS	% 5-y Survival DFS	% Recurrence Local	% Recurrence Any
Yoshida et al,[44] 2005[a]	50	cI	<2	Pure	60	12	28	100	100	0	0
Yamada et al,[50] 2004	39	—	<2	Pure	72	10	18	—	—	0	0
Nakata et al,[46] 2003[a]	33	cIa	≤1	Pure	100	0	0	—	—	0	0
Nakamura et al,[72] 2004	27	—	—	Pure	97[b]	3[b]	0[b]	94	—	0	0
Mun and Kohno,[58] 2007	27	—	—	Pure	88[c]	2[c]	10[c]	100	(70)[d]	0	0
Okada et al,[65] 2003	88	—	≤3	>50%[e]	11[b]	50[b]	39[b]	99	—	—	—
Kondo et al,[66] 2002	66	—	<2	>50%	0	52	48	100	100	0	0
Kodama et al,[68] 2001 #3765	52	—	≤2	>50%	40	31	29	—	(100)[f]	0	0
Ikeda et al,[69] 2004	44	—	<2	>50%	70[b]	13[b]	17[b]	100	—	0	0
Yamato et al,[45] 2001[a]	42	cIa	<2	>50%	81	5	14	100	—	0	0
Watanabe et al,[48] 2005[a]	34	cIa	<2	>50%	41	59	0	—	—	0	3
Ichiki et al,[67] 2011	33	cIa	<2	>50%	46	54	0	100	100	0	0
Matsuguma et al,[70] 2004	31	cIa	≤3	>50%	—	—	—	100	100	0	0
Koike et al,[47] 2009[a]	20	cI	—	>50%	96	4	0	93	93	0	0

Inclusion criteria: studies involving mostly sublobar resection of >50% GGO lesions.
Abbreviations: DFS, disease free survival; n, number of patients undergoing sublobar resection; OS, overall survival.
[a] Prospective study.
[b] Data for whole cohort; not for a specific subgroup.
[c] Data reported per lesion (150 GGO lesions in 27 multifocal patients).
[d] New primary cancers were counted as a recurrence.
[e] By tumor disappearance ratio (between lung and mediastinal windows).
[f] Two-year survival.

another study of 58 patients (14 with multiple GGOs) with a median follow-up of 24 months.[61]

Thus the management of patients with multiple GGOs should be determined primarily by the size of the lesion and the presence of a solid component. The management is not different for multiple lesions; the nature of the lesions themselves does not seem to be changed if there are many or only 1.

SUMMARY OF MANAGEMENT RECOMMENDATIONS

Lesions that appear inflammatory in nature (eg, irregular, nonfocal, indistinct borders) should undergo a follow-up CT scan in 6 to 12 weeks. Antibiotics can be given if there is a strong suspicion of a bacterial infection. A lesion that is persistent with little change after 3 months is unlikely to disappear later, so a definitive management plan should be defined at this time.

A pure GGO less than or equal to 10 mm has approximately a 25% chance of being AIS and less than a 5% chance of being AC; for a pure GGO of greater than 10 mm, the chances of AIS and AC are approximately 40% and 20%. A semisolid (>50%) GGO has approximately a 50% chance of being AIS and a 25% chance of being AC if less than or equal to 10 mm and a 50% chance of being AC if greater than 10 mm.

The documented low rate of growth of pure GGOs less than or equal to 10 mm[10] and the typically indolent growth of AIS justify observation of such lesions. It may be reasonable to observe very small semisolid GGO or those with a very small solid component, but this has not been addressed in studies to date. Given the uncertainties of growth rates, initial intervals between scans of 6 months for pure GGO and 3 months for a semisolid lesion seems reasonable. If stability is shown, subsequently increasing the interval to 12 and 6 months, respectively, seems to be justified. The data currently available suggest that follow-up should be continued indefinitely, although perhaps eventually at extended (eg, 2 year) intervals if prolonged stability has already been shown.

The chance of progression of a GGO during observation seems to be about 20% to 30% over several years, although few are eventually found to be AC (most are AIS). The risk seems to be substantial for larger pure GGO lesions (>10 mm) and is also higher for semisolid lesions. A decrease in size does not indicate that further imaging is unnecessary, unless the decrease is dramatic and serially observed in multiple scans. The imprecision of all current methods (including volumetric) must be kept in mind when interpreting small changes in size.[18–22] The appearance of a solid component in a lesion is an indication for intervention.

A pure GGO greater than 10 mm or one with a solid component, in general, requires intervention. PET imaging has no role. Some physicians prefer to use a positive result of a needle biopsy to plan therapy, but a negative result warrants further intervention given the FN rates of 20% to 30% reported so far.[38,39] A VATS excisional biopsy is definitive, but generally requires some form of preoperative localization.

The data from both retrospective and prospective studies in Asia are consistent that a cT1aN0M0 tumor that is either a pure GGO or greater than 50% GGO can be effectively managed with a sublobar resection. This seems to be true regardless of whether the final histologic diagnosis is AIS or invasive AC.[62] However, it has not been shown that these results apply in other parts of the world, and, in general, they have involved careful attention to many details (eg margin status, distance to margin). Sublobar resection can reasonably be recommended for patients with a cIa greater than 50% GGO lesion of less than 2 cm in the context of a careful preoperatively planned protocol. Although the incidence of node involvement has been low, systematic N1 and N2 node sampling should be done until further data are available. Other forms of local therapy (eg, SBRT or RFA) that lack the histologic confirmation, careful attention to margin status, or invasive nodal staging can only be recommended in the context of a clinical trial.

SUMMARY

The detection of GGO is increasingly common. Sufficient data have been accumulated for recommendations for observation, intervention, and treatment modalities to be made. However, an understanding of many nuances and uncertainties in the available data is needed to avoid making management errors.

REFERENCES

1. Hansell DM, Bankier AA, MacMahon H, et al. Fleischner society: glossary of terms for thoracic imaging. Radiology 2008;246:697–722.
2. Suzuki K, Kusumoto M, Watanabe S, et al. Radiologic classification of small adenocarcinoma of the lung: radiologic-pathologic correlation and its prognostic impact. Ann Thorac Surg 2006;81:413–9.
3. Travis WD, Brambilla E, Noguchi M, et al. International Association for the Study of Lung Cancer/American Thoracic Society/European Respiratory Society International Multidisciplinary Classification

of Lung Adenocarcinoma. J Thorac Oncol 2011;6: 244–85.

4. Travis WD, Garg K, Franklin WA, et al. Evolving concepts in the pathology and computed tomography imaging of lung adenocarcinoma and bronchioloalveolar carcinoma. J Clin Oncol 2005;23: 3279–87.

5. Yoshikawal T, Aoyagi Y, Kodama K, et al. Topographical distribution of allelic loss in individual lung adenocarcinomas with lymph node metastases. Mod Pathol 2004;17:204–13.

6. Iijima H, Tomizawa Y, Dobashi K, et al. Allelic losses on chromosome 3p are accumulated in relation to morphological changes of lung adenocarcinoma. Br J Cancer 2004;91:1143–8.

7. Kerr KM. Pulmonary preinvasive neoplasia. J Clin Pathol 2001;54:257–71.

8. Seki N, Sawada S, Nakata M, et al. Lung cancer with localized ground-glass attenuation represents early-stage adenocarcinoma in nonsmokers. J Thorac Oncol 2008;3(5):483–90.

9. Okada M, Tauchi S, Iwanaga K, et al. Associations among bronchioloalveolar carcinoma components, positron emission tomographic and computed tomographic findings, and malignant behavior in small lung adenocarcinomas. J Thorac Cardiovasc Surg 2007;133:1448–54.

10. Hiramatsu M, Inagaki T, Inagaki T, et al. Pulmonary ground-glass opacity (GGO) lesions-large size and a history of lung cancer are risk factors for growth. J Thorac Oncol 2008;3:1245–50.

11. Kim H, Choi Y, Kim K, et al. Management of ground-glass opacity lesions detected in patients with otherwise operable non-small cell lung cancer. J Thorac Oncol 2009;4:1242–6.

12. Carretta A, Ciriaco P, Melloni G, et al. Surgical treatment of multiple primary adenocarcinomas of the lung. Thorac Cardiovasc Surg 2009;57:30–4.

13. Libby DM, Wu N, Lee IJ, et al. CT screening for lung cancer: the value of short-term CT follow-up. Chest 2006;129:1039–42.

14. Kaneda H, Sakaida N, Saito T, et al. Appearance of bronchioloalveolar carcinoma and the rapid progression into invasive papillary adenocarcinoma. Gen Thorac Cardiovasc Surg 2009;57:224–7.

15. Oh JY, Kwon SY, Yoon HI, et al. Clinical significance of a solitary ground-glass opacity (GGO) lesion of the lung detected by chest CT. Lung Cancer 2007; 55:67–73.

16. Kakinuma R, Ohmatsu H, Kaneko M, et al. Progression of focal pure ground-glass opacity detected by low-dose helical computed tomography screening for lung cancer. J Comput Assist Tomogr 2004;28:17–23.

17. Kodama K, Higashiyama M, Yokouchi H, et al. Natural history of pure ground-glass opacity after long-term follow-up of more than 2 years. Ann Thorac Surg 2002;73:386–93.

18. Jennings SG, Winer-Muram HT, Tarver RD, et al. Lung tumor growth: assessment with CT–comparison of diameter and cross-sectional area with volume measurements. Radiology 2004;231:866–71.

19. Nietert PJ, Ravenel JG, Leue WM, et al. Imprecision in automated volume measurements of pulmonary nodules and its effect on the level of uncertainty in volume doubling time estimation. Chest 2009;135: 1580–7.

20. Revel MP, Bissery A, Bienvenu M, et al. Are two-dimensional CT measurements of small noncalcified pulmonary nodules reliable? Radiology 2004;231: 453–8.

21. Ko JP, Rusinek H, Jacobs EL, et al. Small pulmonary nodules: volume measurement at chest CT–phantom study. Radiology 2003;228:864–70.

22. Oda S, Awai K, Murao K, et al. Computer-aided volumetry of pulmonary nodules exhibiting ground-glass opacity at MDCT. AJR Am J Roentgenol 2010;194: 398–406.

23. Lindell RM, Hartman TE, Swensen SJ, et al. 5-year lung cancer screening experience. Chest 2009; 136:1586–95.

24. Jennings SG, Winer-Muram HT, Tann M, et al. Distribution of stage I lung cancer growth rates determined with serial volumetric CT measurements. Radiology 2006;241:554–63.

25. Winer-Muram HT, Jennings SG, Tarver RD, et al. Volumetric growth rate of stage I lung cancer prior to treatment: serial CT scanning. Radiology 2002; 223:798–805.

26. Takashima S, Maruyama Y, Hasegawa M, et al. CT findings and progression of small peripheral lung neoplasms having a replacement growth pattern. AJR Am J Roentgenol 2003;180:817–26.

27. Min JH, Lee HY, Lee KS, et al. Stepwise evolution from a focal pure pulmonary ground-glass opacity nodule into an invasive lung adenocarcinoma: an observation for more than 10 years. Lung Cancer 2010;69:123–6.

28. Nakamura H, Kawasaki N, Taguchi M, et al. A minute small-cell lung cancer showing a latent phase early in growth. Ann Thorac Cardiovasc Surg 2007;13: 254–7.

29. Hasegawa M, Sone S, Takashima S, et al. Growth rate of small lung cancers detected on mass CT screening. Br J Radiol 2000;73:1252–9.

30. Lindell RM, Hartman TE, Swensen SJ, et al. Five-year lung cancer screening experience: CT appearance, growth rate, location, and histologic features of 61 lung cancers. Radiology 2007;242:555–62.

31. Sone S, Nakayama T, Honda T, et al. CT findings of early-stage small cell lung cancer in a low-dose CT screening programme. Lung Cancer 2007;56:207–15.

32. Detterbeck F, Gibson C. Turning gray: the natural history of lung cancer over time. J Thorac Oncol 2008;3:781–92.

33. Nomori H, Watanabe K, Ohtsuka T, et al. Evaluation of F-18 fluorodeoxyglucose (FDG) PET scanning for pulmonary nodules less than 3 cm in diameter, with special reference to the CT images. Lung Cancer 2004;45:19–27.

34. Detterbeck F, Khandani AH. The role of PET imaging in solitary pulmonary nodules. Clin Pulm Med 2009; 16:81–8.

35. Herder GJ, Golding RP, Hoekstra OS, et al. The performance of 18F-fluorodeoxyglucose positron emission tomography in small solitary pulmonary nodules. Eur J Nucl Med Mol Imaging 2004;31: 1231–6.

36. Rivera MP, Mehta AC. Initial diagnosis of lung cancer: ACCP evidence-based clinical practice guidelines (2nd edition). Chest 2007;132:131S–48S.

37. Shimizu K, Ikeda N, Tsuboi M, et al. Percutaneous CT-guided fine needle aspiration for lung cancer smaller than 2 cm and revealed by ground-glass opacity at CT. Lung Cancer 2006;51:173–9.

38. Kim TJ, Lee JH, Lee CT, et al. Diagnostic accuracy of CT-guided core biopsy of ground-glass opacity pulmonary lesions. AJR Am J Roentgenol 2008;190:234–9.

39. Hur J, Lee HJ, Nam JE, et al. Diagnostic accuracy of CT fluoroscopy-guided needle aspiration biopsy of ground-glass opacity pulmonary lesions. AJR Am J Roentgenol 2009;192:629–34.

40. Daniel T, Altes T, Rehm P, et al. A novel technique for localization and excisional biopsy of small or ill-defined pulmonary lesions. Ann Thorac Surg 2004; 77:1756–62 [discussion: 1762].

41. Kondo R, Yoshida K, Hamanaka K, et al. Intraoperative ultrasonographic localization of pulmonary ground-glass opacities. J Thorac Cardiovasc Surg 2009;138:837–42.

42. Sortini D, Feo C, Maravegias K, et al. Intrathoracoscopic localization techniques. Surg Endosc 2006; 20:1341–7.

43. Takamochi K, Nagai K, Yoshida J, et al. Pathologic N0 status in pulmonary adenocarcinoma is predictable by combining serum carcinoembryonic antigen level and computed tomographic findings. J Thorac Cardiovasc Surg 2001;122:325–30.

44. Yoshida J, Nagai K, Yokose T, et al. Limited resection trial for pulmonary ground-glass opacity nodules: fifty-case experience. J Thorac Cardiovasc Surg 2005;129:991–6.

45. Yamato Y, Tsuchida M, Watanabe T, et al. Early results of a prospective study of limited resection for bronchioloalveolar adenocarcinoma of the lung. Ann Thorac Surg 2001;71:971–4.

46. Nakata M, Sawada S, Saeki H, et al. Prospective study of thoracoscopic limited resection for ground-glass opacity selected by computed tomography. Ann Thorac Surg 2003;75:1601–6.

47. Koike T, Togashi KI, Shirato T, et al. Limited resection for noninvasive bronchioloalveolar carcinoma diagnosed by intraoperative pathologic examination. Ann Thorac Surg 2009;88:1106–11.

48. Watanabe T, Okada A, Imakiire T, et al. Intentional limited resection for small peripheral lung cancer based on intraoperative pathologic exploration. Jpn J Thorac Cardiovasc Surg 2005;53:29–35.

49. Yoshida J, Ishii G, Yokose T, et al. Possible delayed cut-end recurrence after limited resection for ground-glass opacity adenocarcinoma, intraoperatively diagnosed as Noguchi type B, in three patients. J Thorac Oncol 2010;5:546–50.

50. Yamada S, Kohno T. Video-assisted thoracic surgery for pure ground-glass opacities 2 cm or less in diameter. Ann Thorac Surg 2004;77:1911–5.

51. Moriya Y, Iyoda A, Hiroshima K, et al. Clinicopathological analysis of clinical N0 peripheral lung cancers with a diameter of 1 cm or less. Thorac Cardiovasc Surg 2004;52:196–9.

52. Zhou Q, Suzuki K, Anami YI, et al. Clinicopathologic features in resected subcentimeter lung cancer - status of lymph node metastases. Interact Cardiovasc Thorac Surg 2010;10:53–7.

53. Miller DL, Rowland CM, Deschamps C, et al. Surgical treatment of non-small cell lung cancer 1 cm or less in diameter. Ann Thorac Surg 2002;73:1545–51.

54. Yoshida J, Nagai K, Yokose T, et al. Primary peripheral lung carcinoma smaller than 1 cm in diameter. Chest 1998;114:710–2.

55. Lee P, Korst R, Port J, et al. Long-term survival and recurrence in patients with resected non-small cell lung cancer 1 cm or less in size. J Thorac Cardiovasc Surg 2006;132:1382–8.

56. Postmus P, Brambilla E, Chansky K, et al. The IASLC Lung Cancer Staging Project: proposals for revision of the M descriptors in the forthcoming (seventh) edition of the TNM classification of lung cancer. J Thorac Oncol 2007;2:686–93.

57. Kim H, Choi Y, Kim J, et al. Management of multiple pure ground-glass opacity lesions in patients with bronchioloalveolar carcinoma. J Thorac Oncol 2010;5:206–10.

58. Mun M, Kohno T. Efficacy of thoracoscopic resection for multifocal bronchioloalveolar carcinoma showing pure ground-glass opacities of 20 mm or less in diameter. J Thorac Cardiovasc Surg 2007;134:877–82.

59. Park CM, Goo JM, Kim TJ, et al. Pulmonary nodular ground-glass opacities in patients with extrapulmonary cancers: what is their clinical significance and how can we determine whether they are malignant or benign lesions? Chest 2008;133:1402–9.

60. Kim TJ, Goo JM, Lee KW, et al. Clinical, pathological and thin-section CT features of persistent multiple ground-glass opacity nodules: comparison with solitary ground-glass opacity nodule. Lung Cancer 2009;64:171–8.

61. Park JH, Lee KS, Kim JH, et al. Malignant pure pulmonary ground-glass opacity nodules: prognostic implications. Korean J Radiol 2009;10:12–20.

62. Hashizume T, Yamada K, Okamoto N, et al. Prognostic significance of thin-section CT scan findings in small-sized lung adenocarcinoma. Chest 2008; 133:441–7.

63. Suzuki K, Asamura H, Kusumoto M, et al. "Early" peripheral lung cancer: prognostic significance of ground glass opacity on thin-section computed tomographic scan. Ann Thorac Surg 2002;74:1635–9.

64. Nomori H, Ohtsuka T, Naruke T, et al. Histogram analysis of computed tomography numbers of clinical T1 N0 M0 lung adenocarcinoma, with special reference to lymph node metastasis and tumor invasiveness. J Thorac Cardiovasc Surg 2003;126:1584–9.

65. Okada M, Nishio W, Sakamoto T, et al. Discrepancy of computed tomographic image between lung and mediastinal windows as a prognostic implication in small lung adenocarcinoma. Ann Thorac Surg 2003;76:1828–32 [discussion: 1832].

66. Kondo T, Yamada K, Noda K, et al. Radiologic-prognostic correlation in patients with small pulmonary adenocarcinomas. Lung Cancer 2002;36:49–57.

67. Ichiki Y, Hanagiri T, Baba T, et al. Limited pulmonary resection for peripheral small-sized adenocarcinoma of the lung. Int J Surg 2011;9:155–9.

68. Kodama K, Higashiyama M, Yokouchi H, et al. Prognostic value of ground-glass opacity found in small lung adenocarcinoma on high-resolution CT scanning. Lung Cancer 2001;33:17–25.

69. Ikeda N, Maeda J, Yashima K, et al. A clinicopathological study of resected adenocarcinoma 2 cm or less in diameter. Ann Thorac Surg 2004;78: 1011–6.

70. Matsuguma H, Nakahara R, Anraku M, et al. Objective definition and measurement method of ground-glass opacity for planning limited resection in patients with clinical stage IA adenocarcinoma of the lung. Eur J Cardiothorac Surg 2004;25:1102–6.

71. Matsuguma H, Yokoi K, Anraku M, et al. Proportion of ground-glass opacity on high-resolution computed tomography in clinical T1 N0 M0 adenocarcinoma of the lung: a predictor of lymph node metastasis. J Thorac Cardiovasc Surg 2002;124: 278–84.

72. Nakamura H, Saji H, Ogata A, et al. Lung cancer patients showing pure ground-glass opacity on computed tomography are good candidates for wedge resection. Lung Cancer 2004;44:61–8.

73. Kim H, Shim Y, Lee K, et al. Persistent pulmonary nodular ground-glass opacity at thin-section CT: histopathologic comparisons. Radiology 2007;245: 267–75.

74. Kodama K, Higashiyama M, Takami K, et al. Treatment strategy for patients with small peripheral lung lesion(s): intermediate-term results of prospective study. Eur J Cardiothorac Surg 2008;34: 1068–74.

75. Nakata M, Saeki H, Takata I, et al. Focal ground-glass opacity detected by low-dose helical CT. Chest 2002;121:1464–7.

76. Ikeda K, Awai K, Mori T, et al. Differential diagnosis of ground-glass opacity nodules: CT number analysis by three-dimensional computerized quantification. Chest 2007;132:984–90.

77. Nakazono T, Sakao Y, Yamaguchi K, et al. Subtypes of peripheral adenocarcinoma of the lung: differentiation by thin-section CT. Eur Radiol 2005;15:1563–8.

78. Ohtsuka T, Watanabe KI, Kaji M, et al. A clinicopathological study of resected pulmonary nodules with focal pure ground-glass opacity. Eur J Cardiothorac Surg 2006;30:160–3.

79. Sawada S, Komori E, Nogami N, et al. Evaluation of lesions corresponding to ground-glass opacities that were resected after computed tomography follow-up examination. Lung Cancer 2009;65:176–9.

Additional Pulmonary Nodules in the Patient with Lung Cancer: Controversies and Challenges

Anthony W. Kim, MD[a,*], David T. Cooke, MD[b]

KEYWORDS
• Cancer • Lung • Pulmonary nodule • Staging

The optimal management of an additional pulmonary nodule in a patient with a known primary lung cancer is unclear. The literature on the additional pulmonary nodule is equivocal largely because additional pulmonary nodules are often identified during pathologic evaluation after resection of a primary tumor rather than before surgery. Although correlating these pathologic data with preoperative information can be useful, their applicability to management and decision making is often limited.

This article assumes that the additional nodule is another malignant lesion. It focuses on the malignant additional pulmonary nodule in the same lobe as the known primary tumor (T3 nodule) (**Fig. 1**), in a different lobe in the same lung as the known primary tumor (T4 nodule) (**Fig. 2**), and in a different lobe in the contralateral lung (**Fig. 3**). (The article elsewhere in this issue by Boffa and colleagues describes in detail the TNM staging nomenclature.) The additional pulmonary nodule may be either a metastatic lesion of the initial primary tumor or a synchronous primary lung cancer. However, for nodules in the contralateral lung, the presence of an M1a lesion is not discussed. Also, although some studies considered in this article included tumors previously classified as bronchoalveolar carcinoma, this tumor type is

not discussed because its management differs from that of other types of non–small cell lung cancer (NSCLC) and is discussed elsewhere (see the article by Detterbeck and colleagues elsewhere in this issue).

THE ADDITIONAL PULMONARY NODULE DETECTED ON IMAGING

The most important preintervention information for managing an additional pulmonary nodule in a patient with NSCLC is whether or not the nodule is malignant. However, this information is not always available. Additional solid, noncalcified pulmonary nodules occur in approximately 15% of patients with a potentially resectable lung cancer.[1] Most such additional lesions are found to be benign.[1–3] Computed tomography (CT) screening for lung cancer has also shown that most such lesions, especially those smaller than 8 mm in diameter, are benign.[4,5] There is also evidence that observation is appropriate for additional foci of ground-glass opacity that are smaller than 8 mm.[6–8]

For a suspicious pulmonary nodule (eg, one with growth characteristics consistent with cancer on CT imaging, or fluorodeoxyglucose positron emission tomography [FDG-PET] avidity consistent

The authors have nothing to disclose.
a Section of Thoracic Surgery, Department of Surgery, Yale School of Medicine, 330 Cedar Street, BB 205, New Haven, CT 06520, USA
b Division of Cardiothoracic Surgery, The University of California, Davis Medical Center, 2221 Stockton Boulevard, Room 2117, Sacramento, CA 95817-2214, USA
* Corresponding author.
E-mail address: anthony.kim@yale.edu

Clin Chest Med 32 (2011) 811–825
doi:10.1016/j.ccm.2011.08.007
0272-5231/11/$ – see front matter © 2011 Elsevier Inc. All rights reserved.

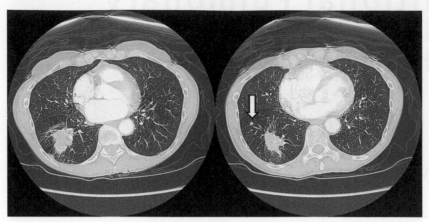

Fig. 1. The T3 additional pulmonary nodule (*arrow*) in the same lobe (right lower lobe).

with malignancy), decision making requires evaluation of the nature of the lesion and its biologic behavior. However, histologic evaluation is problematic because it requires that tissue be obtained, and needle biopsy misidentifies the histologic subtype in 30% of tumors.[9] Therefore, the biologic nature and potential clinical behavior of additional nodules is largely speculative.[10–12] As a result, the principles used to evaluate solitary pulmonary nodules are often used to evaluate the additional pulmonary nodule in a patient with an existing lung cancer.

CHALLENGES IN NOMENCLATURE

The term additional pulmonary nodule has not been used consistently in the literature. The term satellite nodule was originally designated to describe additional small nodules occurring in the same lobe as an existing lung cancer but that are anatomically distinct and grossly recognizable.[13,14] The term satellite nodule has also been used to describe the additional nodule in a different lobe in the ipsilateral or contralateral lung.[15,16] As a result of the confusion, the American Joint

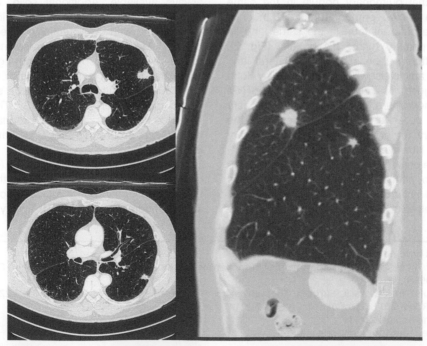

Fig. 2. The T4 additional pulmonary nodule in a different lobe in the ipsilateral lung (left lung).

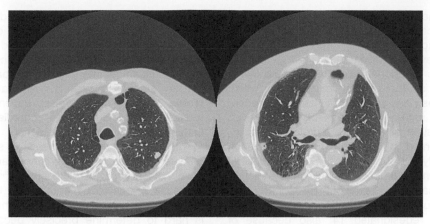

Fig. 3. The additional pulmonary nodule in a different lobe in the contralateral lung.

Committee on Cancer (AJCC) has recommended replacing the term satellite nodule with the term additional tumor nodule.[13,17]

In 1975, Martini and Melamed[17] proposed a classification system to categorize additional malignant pulmonary nodules (**Table 1**). Detterbeck and colleagues[14,18] proposed a similar classification system (**Box 1**). In both systems, the designation synchronous primary lung cancer refers to additional pulmonary nodules in a different lobe with either the same or different histology and without involvement of mediastinal lymph nodes; there is no distinction between lesions occurring in the ipsilateral or the contralateral lung. Synchronous

primary lung cancers may be distinguished from metastatic lesions when there is an absence of mediastinal lymph node involvement and other distant disease. In both systems, intrapulmonary metastases to a different lobe in the ipsilateral

---

Table 1
Martini and Melamed[17] criteria for synchronous primary lung tumors

Synchronous Lung Tumors		
Anatomic Location	**Identical Histology**	**Different Histology**
Same segment	Metastasis	Synchronous primary
Different Segment	Metastasis: cancer in shared lymph basin or systemic metastasis or no CIS	Synchronous primary
	Synchronous primary: no cancer in shared lymph basin and no systemic metastasis and CIS	Synchronous primary

Abbreviation: CIS, carcinoma in situ.
Data from Martini N, Melamed MR. Multiple primary lung cancers. J Thorac Cardiovasc Surg 1975;70:606–12.

Box 1
Alternative categorization scheme of satellite nodules, multiple primary lung cancers, and pulmonary metastases

Satellite nodules

- Satellite nodules from primary tumor

  ○ Same histology and same lobe as primary cancer and no systemic metastasis

Multiple primary lung cancers

- Same histology, anatomically separated

  ○ Cancers in different lobes and no N2,3 involvement and no systematic metastases

- Same histology, temporally separated

  ○ ≥4-y interval between cancers and no systemic metastases from either cancer

- Different histology

  ○ Different histologic type or different molecular genetic characteristics or arising separately from foci of carcinoma in situ

Hematogenously spread pulmonary metastases

- Same histology and multiple systemic metastases

- Same histology, in different lobes, and presence of N2,3 involvement, or <2-y interval

From Detterbeck FC, Jones DR, Kernstine KH, et al. Special treatment issues. Chest 2003;123(1):248s; with permission.

chest without lymph node involvement are not specifically distinguished from synchronous primary tumors.[18]

In the seventh edition of the AJCC staging system, the additional pulmonary nodule in the same lobe as the primary lung cancer, which was previously designated a T4 lesion, was redesignated T3, primarily because of the improved survival in such patients after surgical resection, as documented in the International Association for the Study of Lung Cancer (IASLC) database.[19] The additional pulmonary nodule in a separate lobe of the same lung as the primary cancer, which was previously designated M1 (distant metastasis), was redesignated T4, also because of improved survival compared with other M1 tumors.[13,19] The additional pulmonary nodule in a separate lobe of the contralateral lung retains its M1 status, except when it is confirmed to be a synchronous primary cancer.[13,19]

The current understanding of the additional pulmonary nodule does not allow for a consistently reliable algorithm to distinguishing a metastatic additional pulmonary nodule from a synchronous primary cancer. Therefore, the simple designation of additional pulmonary nodule is likely to be sufficient for describing the outcomes associated with this entity.

The Additional Pulmonary Nodule in the Same Lobe (T3 Nodule)

The approach to patients with a suspected additional focus of cancer in the same lobe as a primary NSCLC, according to the American College of Chest Physicians (ACCP) lung cancer guidelines, is to proceed in the same manner as for a primary lung cancer alone.[3] No additional biopsy is recommended, and the staging evaluation (eg, PET or invasive mediastinal staging) is the same as if the additional nodule were not present. This recommendation is based on the good outcomes of patients who are managed in this manner; however, the evidence is considered poor to moderate.[3]

The incidence of an additional pulmonary nodule in the same lobe as a primary cancer ranges from 3% to 7%.[14,20,21] **Table 2** shows survival data for patients with an additional pulmonary nodule in the same lobe as the known lung cancer (T3 lesion). An additional pulmonary nodule is detected before surgery in approximately 17% of patients with known lung cancer. The 5-year survival rate for patients with an additional pulmonary nodule in the same lobe is approximately 40% (range 20%–46%). Smaller studies have shown similar or higher 5-year survival rates for

such patients.[22,23] These smaller studies notwithstanding, the 5-year survival rates observed in the larger studies are corroborated by results from population-based registries and large regional, national, or international databases reporting an average 5-year survival rate of 27% **(Table 3)**. This figure involves patients primarily treated by surgical resection, regardless of nodal status or completeness of resection.

There is a moderate decrease in survival rate between cohorts with and without an additional pulmonary nodule for each stage.[16,20,24–28] This decrease seems to be about 10% to 15% per stage. However, the magnitude of the difference is hard to determine precisely because of the limited number of studies, the long time periods involved, the variability in survival results potentially stemming from small cohorts when divided by stage, and the different stage classification systems used. A recent study reported a 5-year survival rate for stage I, II, and III disease (ignoring the additional nodule in the stage classification) of 64%, 31%, and 0, respectively.[24]

The Additional Pulmonary Nodule in a Different Lobe of the Ipsilateral Lung (T4 Nodule)

Presumed metastasis

There is little information specifically on the presumed metastatic additional pulmonary nodule in a different lobe of the ipsilateral lung.[25,29–32] Most of the literature in the past 2 decades has focused on second primary lung cancers rather than metastatic disease, perhaps because intrapulmonary metastases are rare. Alternatively, the incidence of such metastatic disease may be low because these tumors are classified as synchronous primary cancers by the different criteria used by various investigators.

The average 5-year survival rate for presumed metastatic pulmonary nodules in a different lobe of the ipsilateral lung is only 17% **(Table 4)**. Many of the reports of these additional nodules have come from outside the United States, mostly from Asia[22,23,25,29,30] and Europe,[31,32] possibly suggesting a different cause of the tumors and different biologic behavior. It could also be because of an increased prevalence of CT screening. However, no differences in outcomes are apparent between continents. Also, based on limited data, it seems that only a minority of these additional nodules (an average of 21%) are detected on preoperative imaging. It does not seem to be the case that the survival rate is poor because intraoperative detection of the nodule in a different lobe results in a more limited resection.[14]

Table 2
Survival associated with T3 additional pulmonary nodule(s) with same or similar histology

Study Reference	N	% Detected Before Surgery	% R0 Resection[a]	% Adjuvant Therapy	% 5-y Survival
Battafarano et al[78]	27	—	100	—	66[3y]
Finley et al[34]	27	—	100	—	64[b]
Bryant et al[63]	26	—	100	73	57[c]
Rao et al[50]	35	51	100	—	57[c]
Trousse et al[79]	35	0	100	—	52
Fukuse et al[29]	20	—	100	45	49[3y]
Port et al[24]	53	15	100	—	48
Terzi et al[21]	32	25	100	0	42[c]
Shimizu et al[20]	37	—	100	—	41[2y]
Yano et al[26]	39	—	100	—	36
Okumura et al[25]	152	9	69	—	34
Rostad et al[32]	44	7	100	—	34[c]
Okada et al[30]	51	0	100	—	30
Riquet et al[80]	25	—	100	—	29
Osaki et al[49]	36	3[d]	92	42[e,f]	27
Pennathur et al[54]	51	47	100	—	26
Oliaro et al[31]	39	—	100	—	20
Average	—	17	—	—	40

Inclusion criteria: studies of 20 or more patients with T3 additional pulmonary nodules reporting 5-year survival from January 1990 to December 2010.

Abbreviations: 2y, 2-year survival; 3y, 3-year survival.

[a] R0 resection is complete resection, and this is presumed to be 100% in the context of publications describing surgical series unless otherwise stated.

[b] Estimated from survival curves and/or tables provided.

[c] Included minority with bronchoalveolar carcinomas.

[d] Based on administration of neoadjuvant therapy.

[e] Different modalities of adjuvant therapy administered including chemotherapy alone, radiation therapy alone, or combined chemoradiation therapy.

[f] Included non-R0 resections.

Data from Detterbeck FC, Jones DR, Kernstine KH, Naunheim KS. Special treatment issues. Chest 2003;123(1):244S–58S.

Synchronous primary lung cancer

The incidence of additional pulmonary nodules that are presumed to be synchronous primary lung cancers has been estimated to be approximately 1% of all lung cancer cases.[33] Synchronous tumors are readily distinguished when they are of different histologic types (or subtypes) from the initial tumor, but only a minority of tumors differs histologically from the known tumor. It has been estimated that more than half of synchronous primary NSCLCs are of the same histologic type as the initial cancer and that most of these tumors are squamous cell carcinomas.[14] The empiric criteria of Martini and Melamed[17] (see **Table 1**) have been most commonly used to define synchronous primary cancers, but a modification that considers morphologic tumor subtyping is gaining recognition.[8,34] Synchronous primary cancers account for approximately one-third of all multiple primary

lung cancers, and approximately one-third of these are detected incidentally during resection.[14]

The long-term survival rate of patients with synchronous primary cancers in a different lobe (whether of the same or different histologic type from the initial cancer) is highly variable and consistent with the difficulty of reliably classifying these tumors.[3,14] This specific survival rate is difficult to ascertain because it is often aggregated with data from patients with additional nodules in the same lobe.[14] However, careful analysis of the existing data can reveal long-term survival associated with additional pulmonary nodules in different lobes (**Table 5**). The average 5-year survival rate for patients with the T4 additional pulmonary nodule is 40%. This figure is similar to the survival rate observed among patients with the T3 additional nodule in the same lobe, but remains greater than the survival rate associated with those

Table 3
Survival associated with the T3 additional pulmonary nodule(s) in the same lobe among national or international database or registry studies

Database	Time Period	N	% 5-y Survival
SEER[81]	1999–2003	633	35
IASLC[27]	1990–2000	363	28
JJCLCR[35]	2001	317	27
SEER[28]	1998–2003	2285	24
CCR[82]	1999–2003	422	23
Average	—	—	27

Inclusion criteria: national or international database or registry studies of patients with an additional nodule in the same lobe as the dominant primary lung cancer from January 1990 to December 2010.
Abbreviations: CCR, California Cancer Registry; JJCLCR, Japanese Joint Committee of Lung Cancer Registry; SEER, Surveillance, Epidemiology, End-Results registry.

patients with lesions believed to be intrapulmonary metastases. In addition, population-based registries and large regional, national, and international databases that have included most patients undergoing surgical resection for T4 additional nodules have shown similar 5-year survival rates to patients undergoing surgical resection for T3 additional nodules.[27,35] When those with unresected T4 additional nodules are included, then the 5-year survival rate is less than that observed following resection (**Table 6**).

These findings, combined with the data mostly arising from surgically resected tumors, suggest that there is a different pathophysiology occurring with synchronous primary lung cancers than with same-lobe metastasis, suggesting a field defect rather than disease spread, which may portend a better outcome. The 5-year survival rate for all patients ranges from 0 to 70%, and the survival rate of patients in whom both tumors are classified as stage I ranges from 0 to 79%.[3,14] The wide range underscores what little is known about presumed synchronous primary cancers.

Managing the patient with an additional pulmonary nodule in a different lobe

Determining whether an additional pulmonary nodule is a metastasis or a synchronous primary cancer is frequently not possible. However, ruling out distant disease through imaging and invasive mediastinal staging is prudent. If no other sites of disease are found, resection of both lesions is reasonable when possible, although the outcomes are not good.

The Additional Pulmonary Nodule in the Contralateral Lung

There are only a few series in which most patients have the additional pulmonary nodule in the contralateral lung.[36–38]

In their study of 37 patients who had a contralateral nodule exclusively, De Leyn and colleagues[36] found that the 5-year survival rate was 38%. Other studies with a predominance of additional nodules in the contralateral lung have reported 5-year survival rates ranging from 20% to 34%.[37,39] By virtue of N2 mediastinal lymph node involvement, surgical resection with curative intent is not offered, but there are some survival data on such patients who have had surgical therapy (see **Table 5**). These limited data show that the 5-year survival rate is reasonable considering that an

Table 4
Survival associated with the T4 additional pulmonary nodule(s) believed to be an intrapulmonary metastasis (same or similar histology)

Study Reference	N	% Detected Before Surgery	% R0 Resection[a]	% Adjuvant Therapy	% 5-y Survival
Fukuse et al[29]	21	—	100	33	21[3y]
Rostad et al[32]	41	15	100	—	24[b]
Okada et al[30]	38	10	100	—	23
Okumura et al[25]	48	39	37	—	11
Oliaro et al[31]	35	—	100	—	10
Average	—	21	—	—	17

Inclusion criteria: studies of 20 or more patients with an additional nodule in a different lobe as the primary lung cancer and also considered to be a pulmonary metastasis within the ipsilateral lung from January 1990 to December 2010.
Abbreviation: 3y, 3-year survival.
[a] Unless stated explicitly, presumed to be 100% in the context of publications describing surgical series.
[b] Included minority with bronchoalveolar carcinomas.

Table 5
Survival associated with additional pulmonary nodule(s) in different lobes

| Study Reference | Nodule | | | | % Resection | % Resection of Malignancy | % Same Histology | % 5-y Survival | T4 Specific % 5-y Survival |
	N	T3	T4 Specific	Contralateral					
Kushibe et al[48]	32	19		24	73	30[a]	86	83[b]	—
Battafarano et al[78]	44	27	17		100	100	68	65[c,d,e,3y]	—
Voltolini et al[39]	50	0	15	35	86	100	60	34	34
Vansteenkiste et al[47]	54	16	22	10	89	65[a]	—	33	—
Watanabe et al[46]	49	—	—	—	—	—	—	14	—
Subtotal	—	—	—	—	—	—	—	27	—
Okada et al[43]	28	21	7	7	100	100	71	70	70
Finley et al[34]	175	27	78	70	100	100	4	64[3y]	52[e]
Jung et al[40]	32	8	15	9	100	100	44	61[c]	60
Rosengart et al[42]	33	36	39	24	91	100	48	44[c]	—
De Leyn et al[36]	57	0	0	57	74	86	50	38	38
Chang et al[83]	92	55	26	11	100	100	97	35[c]	—
Trousse et al[53]	125	63	28	34	100	100	83	34	34[e]
Riquet et al[80]	118	57	51	10	100	100	51	26	16
Pommier et al[44]	27	—	—	—	37	100	55	24[c,f] [45]	—
Van Rens et al[37]	85	16	26	43	100	100	68	19	16
Deschamps et al[41]	36	31		14	100	100	33	16[c]	—
Antakli et al[84]	26	—	—	—	84	100	50[d]	5[c,f] [12]	—
Ribet and Dambron[45]	24	9	—	15	62	100	58[d]	0	—
Subtotal	—	—	—	—	—	—	—	31	—
Average	—	—	—	—	—	—	—	30	40

Inclusion criteria: studies of 20 or more patients with heterogeneous groups of additional pulmonary nodules reporting % 5-year survival according to lymph node status from January 1990 to December 2010. Number of patients with different-lobe additional pulmonary nodules must have been 50% or greater in studies incorporating same-lobe additional pulmonary nodules, unless a specific subgroup of different-lobe data is provided. Studies above the subtotal are those that included a mixture of patients who may have had intrapulmonary metastasis or synchronous primary lung cancers. Studies below the subtotal are those that explicitly reported on synchronous primary lung cancers. The numbers in square brackets reflect the completely resected patients from the entire cohort.

Abbreviation: 3y, 3-year survival.

[a] Based on denominator that included patients who did not undergo resection.
[b] Includes patients with and without lung cancer.
[c] Includes minority with bronchoalveolar carcinoma.
[d] Based on whole cohort in study.
[e] Estimated from survival curves and/or tables provided.
[f] Includes patients in whom resection was not performed.

Table 6
Survival associated with the T4 additional pulmonary nodule(s) among registry or database studies

Database	Time Period	N	%5-y Survival
JJCLCR[35]	2001	128	22
IASLC[27]	1990–2000	180	22
CCR[82]	1999–2003	745	9[a]
SEER[28]	1998–2003	3019	8[a]
SEER[81]	1999–2003	3010	7[a]
Average	—	—	14

Inclusion criteria: national or international database or registry studies including patients with an additional nodule in a different ipsilateral lobe from the dominant primary lung cancer independent of lymph node status from January 1990 to December 2010.

Abbreviations: CCR, California Cancer Registry; JJCLCR, Japanese Joint Committee of Lung Cancer Registry; SEER, Surveillance, Epidemiology, End-Results registry.

[a] Most patients did not undergo resection.

additional pulmonary nodule in the presence of N2 lymph node may represent M1a or stage IV disease.

According to the currently used nomenclature schemes, an additional pulmonary nodule in the contralateral lung should be considered a metastasis when there is mediastinal lymph node involvement and its presence suggests spread via the mediastinum. The additional pulmonary nodule in the contralateral lung without lymph node involvement detected on mediastinal staging may reasonably be presumed to be a synchronous primary cancer.

CHALLENGES ASSOCIATED WITH LYMPH NODE STAGING
Lymph Node Involvement

Lymph node status is a strong determinant of long-term outcome after pulmonary resection for malignancy. In a T3 or T4 lesion, the presence of positive mediastinal lymph nodes indicates locally advanced disease. It has been argued that N2 lymph node involvement by mediastinal staging indicates that lesions considered to be synchronous primary cancers in the contralateral lung may be metastatic lesions. If lesions in the contralateral lung are confirmed on pathologic analysis to be a different histologic type than the initial lung cancer, then positive mediastinal lymph nodes suggest the coexistence of an early-stage cancer and a locally advanced cancer. However, this may be more unlikely than the presence of metastatic disease. Also, having pathologic

confirmation before definitive treatment of the lesions is not common.

Because most of the data on lymph node status were obtained from patients who had undergone surgical resection, it is likely that such patients were believed to have had early-stage disease. This assumption is supported by most patients with additional pulmonary nodules having stage I or II disease. However, several studies included patients with known stage III disease by virtue of mediastinal lymph node involvement.[20,24,34,37,40–50] The use of neoadjuvant therapy or definitive chemoradiation therapy is now widely accepted in such patients; therefore, it is unclear why surgery was the initial therapy in these patient with stage III disease. It is possible that a belief in the efficacy of adjuvant therapy in lymph node–positive mediastinal disease may have been the motivation behind pursuing surgery as the primary mode of therapy. Nevertheless, mediastinal lymph node involvement should raise concerns of metastases rather than a locally advanced synchronous primary cancer. The mediastinal lymph node–positive subsets described in the literature may represent surprise N2 disease.[51]

The Additional Pulmonary Nodule in the Same Lobe (T3N2) with N2 Lymph Nodes

The incidence of lymph node–negative disease in patients with an additional pulmonary nodule in the same lobe as the initial cancer is approximately 42% (**Table 7**). This finding suggests that most patients have lymph node involvement. The 42% figure is largely based on surgical series that did not all routinely use invasive mediastinal staging, suggesting that the patients in the study were most likely not believed to have N2 involvement before resection.

The 5-year survival rate for patients who are lymph node negative on average is 53% and ranges from 37% to 67% (see **Table 7**). Therefore, the survival rate is slightly less than expected for patients with early-stage lung cancer without an additional pulmonary nodule.

Determining the average 5-year survival rate for patients with lymph node–positive disease is more difficult because survival rate is not often broken down by node distribution. It seems that patients with N1 disease have a 5-year survival rate that ranges from 40% to 61%, which is similar to that of patients with N1 disease and no additional pulmonary nodule (see **Table 7**). Similarly, the 5-year survival rate for patients with N2 disease seems to range from 0 to 47%, which also is similar to that of patients without an additional pulmonary nodule. This finding suggests that the

Table 7
Survival associated with same-lobe additional pulmonary nodule (T3N2)

Study Reference	N	% Positive				% 5-y Survival				
		N0	N1	N1	N3	N0	N1	N2	N3	All
Rao et al[50]	35	51	49			64	47			57
Port et al[24]	53	68	25	7	—	58	36		—	48
Shimizu et al[20]	37	46	18	36	—	$(51)^{3y}$	$(22)^{3y}$	$(0)^{3y}$	—	41^{2y}
Yano et al[26]	39	25	31	44	—	—	—	—	—	36
Okumura et al[25]	105	32	22	49	2	37	40	24	—	34
Okada et al[30]	48	—	—	—	—	67	61	0	—	30
Riquet et al[80]	25	32	20	48	—	—	—	—	—	29
Osaki et al[49]	36	44	20	36	—	—	—	—	—	27
Pennathur et al[54]	51	67	20	14	—	40	0		—	26
Oliaro et al[31]	39	17	6	16	—	$(33)^{4y}$	—	—	—	20
Average	—	42	23	33		53	—	—	—	34

Inclusion criteria: studies of 20 or more patients with T3 additional pulmonary nodules reporting either distribution of pathologic lymph node status or % 5-year survival according to lymph node status from January 1990 to December 2010, numbers in parentheses ( ) are not 5-year survival figures.
Abbreviations: 2y, 2-year survival; 3y, 3-year survival.

presence of an additional pulmonary nodule confers a worse prognosis in patients with lymph node–negative disease but plays only a secondary role in patients with lymph node–positive disease.

The Additional Pulmonary Nodule in a Different Lobe in the Ipsilateral Lung with N2 Lymph Nodes (T4N2)

Patients with an additional pulmonary nodule in a different lobe of the ipsilateral lung with N2 involvement are considered to have stage IIIb disease in the new lung cancer stage classification system.[52] In the past 2 decades, several studies of more than 20 patients each have evaluated outcomes for such patients (**Table 8**), but only 2 have reported specifically on patients with an additional nodule in a different lobe of the ipsilateral lung.[31,35] Both of these studies, one of which was a registry study, found that any node involvement (N1 or N2) is associated with worse long-term survival than that in patients who are node negative.[31,35]

A study that evaluated the Surveillance, Epidemiology, End-Results (SEER) registry database from 1998 to 2003 found that 66% of cases of additional pulmonary nodules in a different lobe were associated with positive mediastinal lymph nodes.[28] Of this cohort, the 5-year survival rate was 2%, which was markedly less than the rate that was observed among smaller institutional studies, and may have been caused by N3 lymph nodes being included in the analysis, and most of the patients did not undergo resection.[28] In

the only other significant database study, Nagai and colleagues[35] identified 128 patients in the Japanese Joint Committee on Lung Cancer Registry who had additional pulmonary nodules in a different lobe with positive mediastinal lymph nodes. The 5-year survival rate for this cohort was 10%, which was similar to the rate that is averaged from individual institution reports and most likely reflects this cohort consisting of patients who had undergone resection of their additional pulmonary nodule.

Predicting the Need for Invasive Mediastinal Staging

The high incidence of mediastinal lymph node involvement in the patients with T3 or T4 additional pulmonary nodules who underwent surgical resection (approximately one-third) suggests that mediastinoscopy is warranted before consideration of surgical therapy (see **Tables 7** and **8**). This approach is further supported by the survival rates in lymph node–negative disease among the T3 and T4 subsets being respectable (see **Tables 7** and **8**). The long-term survival for patients with mediastinal lymph node involvement is less clear and is variable, but generally seems to be similar to survival in the typical patient with mediastinal lymph node involvement.[13] In these cases, mediastinal staging is recommended and, therefore, this recommendation should also apply to patients with an additional pulmonary nodule.

The use of PET scanning in the evaluation of the additional pulmonary nodule has increased in

Table 8
Survival associated with lymph node involvement among same-lobe additional pulmonary nodules including both intrapulmonary metastasis and synchronous primary lung cancers

Study Reference	N	% Positive				% 5-y Survival				
		N0	N1	N2	N3	N0	N1	N2	N3	All
Okada et al[43]	28	39	61			79		41		70
Finley et al[34]	175	73	14	13	—	(69)[3y]	(49)[3y]	(51)[3y]	—	64[3y]
Jung et al[40]	32	78	16	6	—	64	54		—	61
Rosengart et al[42]	33	—	—	—	—	—	—	—	—	44
De Leyn et al[36]	36	67	31	3	—	—	—	—	—	38
Trousse et al[53]	125	44	54			51	15			34
Voltolini et al[39]	43	58	21	21	—	57	0		—	34
Fukuse et al[29]	41	44	10	44	2	30[a]	100[a]	13[a]	0	26
Riquet et al[80]	118	46	14	40	—	38	—	—	—	26
Pommier et al[44]	27	44	54			38		0		24 [45]
Van Rens et al[37]	73	55	45			23	—	13		19
Deschamps et al[41]	36[b]	67	19	11	—	24	—	—	—	16
Oliaro et al[31]	35	54	20	26		16	—	—	—	10
Antakli et al[84]	26	—	—	—	—	—	—	—	—	5 [12]
Ribet and Dambron[45]	24	63	29	8	—	—	—	—	—	0
Average	—	54	30	31	—	34	—	—	—	28

Inclusion criteria: studies of 20 or more patients with an additional nodule in a different lobe as the primary lung cancer reporting either distribution of pathologic lymph node status or % 5-year survival according to lymph node status from January 1990 to December 2010. Among studies with fewer than 20 patients with an additional pulmonary nodule in a different lobe, the number of patients with same-lobe additional pulmonary nodules must have been 50% or greater in studies incorporating same-lobe additional pulmonary nodules, unless a specific subgroup of same-lobe data was provided. The numbers in square brackets reflect the completely resected patients from the entire cohort.
[a] Estimated from survival curves provided.
[b] Includes minority with unknown lymph node (N) status.

recent series.[21,31,39,40,53,54] This increase may reflect the increased use of PET scans in general. It may also reflect their use either in guiding invasive staging, or in lieu of invasive staging, or in evaluating for distant disease. However, there does not seem to be additional benefit in staging the mediastinum with PET scanning in patients with an additional pulmonary nodule, although its use has been advocated.[39,53] Therefore, the importance of invasive mediastinal lymph node staging techniques, such as mediastinoscopy, in these patients cannot be overemphasized. PET scanning may be responsible for the increased detection of additional pulmonary nodules that may be synchronous primary cancers.[36]

THERAPEUTIC OPTIONS FOR THE ADDITIONAL PULMONARY NODULE

Lobectomy should be performed when possible in the fit patient with a T3 additional pulmonary nodule because the synchronous nodule is in the same lobe. However, treatment algorithms for T4 additional pulmonary nodules and synchronous primary cancers in the contralateral lobe are more complex, especially because lung parenchyma must be preserved in patients with limited pulmonary reserve. Lobectomy for the synchronous T4 nodule may not be practical and might require segmentectomy or sublobar wedge resection for local control in addition to lobectomy for the primary lesion. For solitary lung cancers, sublobar resection has historically been considered inferior to anatomic lobectomy for local recurrence.[55] However, recent studies suggest that sublobar resection for peripheral lung tumors smaller than 2 cm in diameter results in local control similar to that of lobectomy, with favorable local recurrence rates.[56,57] In the study by Finley and colleagues[34] of 102 patients who had a single-stage operation for synchronous primary cancers, 66% underwent lobectomy or bilobectomy and 31% sublobar resection. In the patients who underwent staged resections, 14%

underwent bilateral lobectomy and 56% lobectomy plus sublobar resection. Hospital morbidity and mortality were 33% and only 1.2%, respectively.[34]

Some clinicians, including the authors of this review, increasingly use hybrid approaches in patients with limited pulmonary reserve who cannot tolerate more than 1 lobectomy. Such hybrid approaches involve lobar or sublobar resection of the primary tumor, and, if the additional nodule is not amenable to sublobar resection and the patient has poor pulmonary reserve, radiofrequency ablation or stereotactic body radiotherapy to the additional pulmonary nodule in a staged setting. Radiofrequency ablation and stereotactic body radiotherapy have resulted in favorable local control of small tumors in poor surgical candidates.[58,59] This approach requires multidisciplinary collaboration with interventional radiologists or radiation oncologists and is an ideal candidate for a multi-institution clinical trial.

An experimental treatment algorithm consists of video-assisted thoracoscopic surgery or open resection of the primary lung cancer, with intraoperative radiofrequency ablation of an unresectable T4 additional pulmonary nodule in the ipsilateral lung. By palpating the additional nodule, the surgeon can guide needle placement, at the same time avoiding and protecting adjacent vascular and bronchial structures. Small, single-institution studies suggest that this approach is feasible.[60–62] Its limitations include accurately judging an appropriate tumor ablation radius. Studies using intraoperative CT scanning or ultrasound are needed to determine the extent of this limitation.

ROLE OF ADJUVANT THERAPIES

There is no solid evidence to support the use of adjuvant chemotherapy or chemoradiation therapy in the node-negative patient, even though the presence of the additional nodule makes the cancer greater than stage I. In the T3 additional pulmonary nodule, it is unknown whether adjuvant therapy is used. Among the 4 studies that specifically discussed the use of adjuvant therapies in this population, 2 studies addressed its use in the context of lymph node–negative disease. One study explicitly reported not using adjuvant therapy,[21] whereas another reported its use in 73% of their patients.[63] Two other studies reported using adjuvant therapy in 42% and 45% of their patients, respectively, but these studies reported lymph node involvement in 55% and 56% of their patients, respectively.[29,49]

The additional pulmonary nodule in a different lobe of the ipsilateral lung is designated T4 and therefore is at least stage IIIA. The use of adjuvant therapy would likely be more common in such cases. However, adjuvant therapy is not routinely used in patients with NSCLC and intrapulmonary metastasis.[29]

Platinum-based adjuvant chemotherapy is reserved for node-positive stage II and III disease. Multiple clinical trials have evaluated the role of adjuvant chemotherapy for resected primary lung cancer. A meta-analysis of clinical trials after 1965, including adjuvant trials, found a total 5-year survival benefit of 4%, with a survival advantage for patients with stage II and III disease.[64] The use of adjuvant chemotherapy in lymph node–positive disease in patients with an additional pulmonary nodule should be consistent with its use in patients without an additional nodule.

Numerous clinical trials are evaluating adjuvant chemotherapy and immunomodulator therapy for early-stage lung cancer. The Eastern Cooperative Oncology Group study 1505 is a phase III trial of adjuvant platinum-based chemotherapy with or without the vascular endothelial growth factor (VEGF) angiogenesis inhibitor bevacizumab for patients with resected stage IB (tumor greater than 4 cm in diameter) to IIIA NSCLC.[65] The Southwest Oncology Group study 0720 is a phase II adjuvant therapy trial of the DNA excision repair protein ERCC1 and the ribonucleoside diphosphate reductase large subunit (RRM1) in patients with stage I NSCLC.[66] Patients whose tumors show low expression of ERCC1 and RRM1 are sensitive to platinum-based therapy.[67] The GlaxoSmithKline study 109493 is a phase III study that assesses the efficacy of RecMAGE-A3 plus AS15 (an antigen-specific cancer immunotherapeutic agent) as adjuvant therapy in patients with MAGE-A3–positive NSCLC.[68] However, patients with synchronous primary tumors are not eligible for these clinical trials. Most current clinical trials are based on the sixth edition of the AJCC TNM lung cancer staging system, in which synchronous tumors are stage IIIB (same lobe) or higher; however, in the current, seventh edition, these tumors have been downstaged. As more adjuvant early-stage NSCLC trials are developed, it will be important that they include patients with additional pulmonary nodules.

ROLE OF HISTOLOGIC AND MOLECULAR PROFILING

The Martini and Melamed[17] criteria were developed in 1979 from a study that consisted primarily of metachronous tumors and tumors designated simply as adenocarcinoma, squamous cell carcinoma, and carcinoma in situ. Most synchronous primary cancers defined by the Martini and Mel-amed[17] criteria (see **Table 1**) have the same histo-logic type (eg, adenocarcinoma or squamous cell carcinoma.)[3,14,36,69] This approach is logical, because the cause of both of these types is likely the same (ie, genetics and environmental expo-sures). However, histology is beneficial in defining a relationship between additional foci of cancer in only a minority of cases involving additional pulmonary nodules. Other available modalities to differentiate synchronous primary cancer from pulmonary metastasis include molecular profiling and histologic analysis of tumor subtype by light microscopy.

Evaluating multiple primary lung cancers by molecular profiling has produced conflicting results.[70–74] However, there is some promise. Microdissection and DNA extraction of tumors, followed by polymerase chain reaction amplifica-tion of tumor DNA polymorphisms, such as *p53*, can identify patterns of loss of heterozygosity of chromosome loci and genes.[72] Clonal metastatic lesions would have similar loss of heterozygosity, and synchronous primary tumors would have disparate gene patterns, despite similar simple histology. Comparison of somatic point mutations of other genes has been shown to augment Martini and Melamed's[17] overall model (**Box 2**).[75] The advantage of genotype profiling is its diagnostic accuracy. The disadvantage is the expense as well as the access to the technology, especially for small medical centers.

Assessment of tumor histologic subtypes by light microscopy can be effective in differentiating synchronous primary cancer from metastasis.[76,77] Girard and colleagues[76] showed that comprehen-sive analysis by light microscopy of histologic subtypes, including grade; stroma characteristics; necrosis; and clear cell, basaloid, and sarcoma-tous components, not only were comparable with Martini and Melamed's[17] criteria, but were consistent with concurrent molecular determi-nants of synchronous primary cancers versus metastasis in 91% of specimens. Histologic sub-typing by light microscopy is advantageous because it is inexpensive and may be more suit-able to medical centers with limited resources.

SUMMARY

Management of the patient with an additional pulmonary nodule and a known primary lung cancer is a challenge. The evidence used to manage these patients is largely biased by the postoperative pathologic nature of the data. Therefore, in a sense, a leap of faith has been taken in assuming that the rules of those resected apply to those who are about to undergo resection or an alternative form of therapy. In defense of this strategy, there is little other evidence to guide decision making. Therefore, recommendations are made with the best available information, although largely based on surgical data.

The presence of an additional pulmonary nodule in a patient with a suspected or known malignancy does not always indicate the presence of a metas-tasis or a synchronous primary lung cancer. The long-term survival rate associated with the addi-tional pulmonary nodule in the same or a different lobe is respectable but varies slightly depending on how these lesions are classified. The findings of this review suggest that, irrespective of the loca-tion of the additional pulmonary nodule, invasive mediastinal staging should be performed because lymph node–positive disease is detected in the re-sected specimens in approximately one-third of patients.

Lobectomy is the gold standard for the local treatment of the additional pulmonary nodule, particularly for T3 lesions. Although lobectomy is desirable for the T4 lesion or synchronous primary lung cancers, it is not always feasible. In these clinical situations, limited resection or hybrid approaches may be reasonable alternatives for the additional pulmonary nodules and may become more common as more data about their efficacy

---

Box 2
Genes that have been used to identify patterns of loss of heterozygosity of synchronous tumors

Gene

AKT1 = RAC-α serine/threonine-protein kinase

BRAF = Serine/threonine-protein kinase B-Raf

EGFR = Epidermal growth factor receptor

ERBB2 (HER2/neu) = Human epidermal growth factor receptor 2

KRAS = V-Ki-ras2 Kirsten rat sarcoma viral onco-gene homolog

MEK1 = Dual-specificity mitogen-activated protein kinase 1

p53 = Protein 53

Data from Huang J, Behrens C, Wistuba I, et al. Molec-ular analysis of synchronous and metachronous tumors of the lung: Impact on management and prog-nosis. Ann Diagn Pathol 2001;5(6):321–9; and Girard N, Ostrovnaya I, Lau C, et al. Genomic and mutational profiling to assess clonal relationships between multiple non–small cell lung cancers. Clin Cancer Res 2009;15(16):5184–90.

accumulate. The role of adjuvant therapy in lymph node–negative disease is also a promising area for investigation because little is known about its benefit. In addition, advances in molecular profiling and histologic subtyping may improve characterization of the clinical and biologic behavior of the additional pulmonary nodules. Continued investigation in this area may improve management of the additional pulmonary nodule by determining which patients may respond to a specific type of therapy.

REFERENCES

1. Keogan MT, Tung KT, Kaplan DK, et al. The significance of pulmonary nodules detected on CT staging for lung cancer. Clin Radiol 1993;48:94–6.

2. Kunitoh H, Eguchi K, Yamada K, et al. Intrapulmonary sublesions detected before surgery in patients with lung cancer. Cancer 1992;70:1876–9.

3. Shen KR, Meyers BF, Larner JM, et al. Special treatment issues in lung cancer: ACCP evidence-based clinical practice guidelines (2nd edition). Chest 2007;132(Suppl 3):290S–305S.

4. Swensen SJ, Jett JR, Hartman TE, et al. CT screening for lung cancer: five-year prospective experience. Radiology 2005;235(1):259–65.

5. Pastorino U, Bellomi M, Landoni C, et al. Early lung-cancer detection with spiral CT and positron emission tomography in heavy smokers: 2-year results. Lancet 2003;362(9384):593–7.

6. Kim H, Choi Y, Kim J, et al. Management of multiple pure ground-glass opacity lesions in patients with bronchioloalveolar carcinoma. J Thorac Oncol 2010;5(2):206–10.

7. Kim H, Choi Y, Kim K, et al. Management of ground-glass opacity lesions detected in patients with otherwise operable non-small cell lung cancer. J Thorac Oncol 2009;4(10):1242–6.

8. Detterbeck FC. Synchronous, separate, and similar. J Thorac Oncol 2010;5(2):150–2.

9. Rivera MP, Detterbeck FC, Loomis DP. Epidemiology and classification of lung cancer. In: Detterbeck FC, Rivera MP, Socinski MA, et al, editors. Diagnosis and treatment of lung cancer: an evidence-based guide for the practicing clinician. Philadelphia: WB Saunders; 2001. p. 25–44.

10. Lindell RM, Hartman TE, Swensen SJ, et al. 5-year lung cancer screening experience. Chest 2009; 136(6):1586–95.

11. Detterbeck F, Boffa DJ, Tanoue L, et al. Details, difficulties and dilemmas regarding the new lung cancer staging system. Chest 2010;137(5):1172–80.

12. Detterbeck F, Tanoue L, Boffa D. Anatomy, biology and concepts pertaining to lung cancer stage classification. J Thorac Oncol 2009;4(4):437–43.

13. AJCC, UICC. AJCC cancer staging manual. 7th edition. New York: Springer; 2009.

14. Detterbeck FC, Jones DR, Funkhouser WK Jr. Satellite nodules and multiple primary cancers. In: Detterbeck FC, Rivera MP, Socinski MA, et al, editors. Diagnosis and treatment of lung cancer: an evidence-based guide for the practicing clinician. Philadelphia: WB Saunders; 2001. p. 437–49.

15. Urschel JD, Urschel DM, Anderson TM, et al. Prognostic implications of pulmonary satellite nodules: are the 1997 staging revisions appropriate? Lung Cancer 1998;21:83–7.

16. Deslauriers J, Brisson J, Cartier R, et al. Carcinoma of the lung: evaluation of satellite nodules as a factor influencing prognosis after resection. J Thorac Cardiovasc Surg 1989;97:504–12.

17. Martini N, Melamed MR. Multiple primary lung cancers. J Thorac Cardiovasc Surg 1975;70:606–12.

18. Detterbeck FC, Jones DR, Kernstine KH, et al. Special treatment issues. Chest 2003;123(1):244S–58S.

19. Groome PA, Bolejack V, Crowley J, et al. The IASLC Lung Cancer Staging Project: validation of the proposals for revision of the T, N, and M descriptors and consequent stage groupings in the forthcoming (seventh) edition of the TNM classification of malignant tumours. J Thorac Oncol 2007;2(8): 694–705.

20. Shimizu N, Ando A, Date H, et al. Prognosis of undetected intrapulmonary metastases in resected lung cancer. Cancer 1993;71:3868–72.

21. Terzi A, Falezza G, Benato C, et al. Survival following complete resection of multifocal T4 node-negative NSCLC: a retrospective study. Thorac Cardiovasc Surg 2007;55(1):44–7.

22. Okubo K, Bando T, Miyahara R, et al. Resection of pulmonary metastasis of non-small cell lung cancer. J Thorac Oncol 2009;4(2):203–7.

23. Yoshino I, Nakanishi R, Osaki T, et al. Postoperative prognosis in patients with non-small cell lung cancer with synchronous ipsilateral intrapulmonary metastasis. Ann Thorac Surg 1997;64:809–13.

24. Port JL, Korst RJ, Lee PC, et al. Surgical resection for multifocal (T4) non-small cell lung cancer: is the T4 designation valid? Ann Thorac Surg 2007;83(2): 397–400.

25. Okumura T, Asamura H, Suzuki K, et al. Intrapulmonary metastasis of non-small cell lung cancer: a prognostic assessment. J Thorac Cardiovasc Surg 2001; 122(1):24–8.

26. Yano M, Arai T, Inagaki K, et al. Intrapulmonary satellite nodule of lung cancer as a T factor. Chest 1998; 114:1305–8.

27. Rami-Porta R, Ball D, Crowley J, et al. The IASLC Lung Cancer Staging Project: proposals for revision of the T descriptors in the forthcoming (7th) edition of the TNM classification of lung cancer. J Thorac Oncol 2007;2(7):593–602.

28. Williams W Jr, Lin H, Lee J, et al. Revisiting stage IIIB and IV non-small cell lung cancer. Chest 2009; 136(3):701–9.

29. Fukuse T, Hirata T, Tanaka F, et al. Prognosis of ipsilateral intrapulmonary metastases in resected non-small cell lung cancer. Eur J Cardiothorac Surg 1997;12:218–23.

30. Okada M, Tsubota N, Yoshimura M, et al. Evaluation of TMN classification for lung carcinoma with ipsilateral intrapulmonary metastasis. Ann Thorac Surg 1999;68(2):326–31.

31. Oliaro A, Filosso PL, Cavallo A, et al. The significance of intrapulmonary metastasis in non-small cell lung cancer: upstaging or downstaging? A re-appraisal for the next TNM staging system. Eur J Cardiothorac Surg 2008;34(2):438–43 [discussion: 43].

32. Rostad H, Strand TE, Naalsund A, et al. Resected synchronous primary malignant lung tumors: a population-based study. Ann Thorac Surg 2008;85(1): 204–9.

33. Ferguson MK. Synchronous primary lung cancers. Chest 1993;103:398S–400S.

34. Finley D, Yoshizawa A, Travis W, et al. Predictors of outcomes after surgical treatment of synchronous primary lung cancers. J Thorac Oncol 2010;5: 197–205.

35. Nagai K, Sohara Y, Tsuchiya R, et al. Prognosis of resected non-small cell lung cancer patients with intrapulmonary metastases. J Thorac Oncol 2007;2(4): 282–6.

36. De Leyn P, Moons J, Vansteenkiste J, et al. Survival after resection of synchronous bilateral lung cancer. Eur J Cardiothorac Surg 2008;34(6):1215–22.

37. van Rens MT, Zanen P, Brutel de la Rivière A, et al. Survival in synchronous vs single lung cancer. Chest 2000;118(4):952–8.

38. Vogt-Moykopf I, Krysa S, Bulzebruck H, et al. Surgery for pulmonary metastases: the Heidelberg experience. Chest Surg Clin N Am 1994;4:85–112.

39. Voltolini L, Rapicetta C, Luzzi L, et al. Surgical treatment of synchronous multiple lung cancer located in a different lobe or lung: high survival in node-negative subgroup. Eur J Cardiothorac Surg 2010; 37(5):1198–204.

40. Jung EJ, Lee JH, Jeon K, et al. Treatment outcomes for patients with synchronous multiple primary non-small cell lung cancer. Lung Cancer 2011;73(2): 237–42.

41. Deschamps C, Pairolero PC, Trastek VF, et al. Multiple primary lung cancers: results of surgical treatment. J Thorac Cardiovasc Surg 1990;99:769–78.

42. Rosengart TK, Martini N, Ghosn P, et al. Multiple primary lung carcinomas: prognosis and treatment. Ann Thorac Surg 1991;52:273–9.

43. Okada M, Tsubota N, Yoshimura M, et al. Operative approach for multiple primary lung carcinomas. J Thorac Cardiovasc Surg 1998;115:836–40.

44. Pommier RF, Vetto JT, Lee JT, et al. Synchronous non-small cell lung cancers. Am J Surg 1996; 171(5):521–4.

45. Ribet M, Dambron P. Multiple primary lung cancers. Eur J Cardiothorac Surg 1995;9:231–6.

46. Watanabe Y, Shimizu J, Oda M, et al. Proposals regarding some deficiencies in the new international staging system for non-small cell lung cancer. Jpn J Clin Oncol 1991;21(3):160–8.

47. Vansteenkiste JF, De Belie B, Deneffe GJ, et al. Practical approach to patients presenting with multiple synchronous suspect lung lesions: a reflection on the current TNM classification based on 54 cases with complete follow-up. Lung Cancer 2001; 34(2):169–75.

48. Kushibe K, Kawaguchi T, Nishimoto Y, et al. Operative indications for lung cancer with satellite lesions. Asian Cardiovasc Thorac Ann 2006;14(4):316–20.

49. Osaki T, Sugio K, Hanagiri T, et al. Survival and prognostic factors of surgically resected T4 non-small cell lung cancer. Ann Thorac Surg 2003;75(6): 1745–51 [discussion: 1751].

50. Rao J, Sayeed RA, Tomaszek S, et al. Prognostic factors in resected satellite-nodule T4 non-small cell lung cancer. Ann Thorac Surg 2007;84(3):934–9.

51. Detterbeck F. What to do with surprise N2: intraoperative management of patients with non-small cell lung cancer. J Thorac Oncol 2008;3(3):289–302.

52. Detterbeck F, Tanoue L, Boffa DJ. The new lung cancer staging system. Chest 2009;136:260–71.

53. Trousse D, Barlesi F, Loundou A, et al. Synchronous multiple primary lung cancer: an increasing clinical occurrence requiring multidisciplinary management. J Thorac Cardiovasc Surg 2007;133(5):1193–200.

54. Pennathur A, Lindeman B, Ferson P, et al. Surgical resection is justified in non-small cell lung cancer patients with node negative T4 satellite lesions. Ann Thorac Surg 2009;87(3):893–9.

55. Ginsberg RJ, Rubinstein LV. Randomized trial of lobectomy versus limited resection for T1 N0 non-small cell lung cancer. Lung Cancer Study Group. Ann Thorac Surg 1995;60:615–23.

56. Okada M, Nishio W, Sakamoto T, et al. Effect of tumor size on prognosis in patients with non-small cell lung cancer: the role of segmentectomy as a type of lesser resection. J Thorac Cardiovasc Surg 2005;129(1):87–93.

57. Fernando HC, Santos RS, Benfield JR, et al. Lobar and sublobar resection with and without brachytherapy for small stage IA non-small cell lung cancer. J Thorac Cardiovasc Surg 2005;129(2):261–7.

58. Grills IS, Mangona VS, Welsh R, et al. Outcomes after stereotactic lung radiotherapy or wedge resection for stage I non–small-cell lung cancer. J Clin Oncol 2010;28(6):928–35.

59. Healey TT, Dupuy DE. Radiofrequency ablation: a safe and effective treatment in nonoperative

patients with early-stage lung cancer. Cancer J 2011;17(1):33–7.

60. Pennathur A, Abbas G, Qureshi I, et al. Radiofrequency ablation for the treatment of pulmonary metastases. Ann Thorac Surg 2009;87(4):1030–9.

61. Schneider T, Warth A, Herpel E, et al. Intraoperative radiofrequency ablation of lung metastases and histologic evaluation. Ann Thorac Surg 2009;87(2): 379–84.

62. Linden PA, Wee JO, Jaklitsch MT, et al. Extending indications for radiofrequency ablation of lung tumors through an intraoperative approach. Ann Thorac Surg 2008;85(2):420–3.

63. Bryant AS, Pereira SJ, Miller DL, et al. Satellite pulmonary nodule in the same lobe (T4N0) should not be staged as IIIB non-small cell lung cancer. Ann Thorac Surg 2006;82(5):1808–14.

64. Arriagada R, Auperin A, et al, NSCLC Meta-analyses Collaborative Group. Adjuvant chemotherapy, with or without postoperative radiotherapy, in operable non-small-cell lung cancer: two meta-analyses of individual patient data. Lancet 2010;375(9722):1267–77.

65. Eastern Cooperative Oncology Group (ECOG) Physician and patient education materials for E1505. Available at: http://ecog.dfci.harvard.edu/general/E1505info.html. Accessed June 3, 2011.

66. Southwestern Oncology Group (SWOG) Protocol abstract: S0720. Available at: http://swog.org/Visitors/ViewProtocolDetails.asp?ProtocolNumber=S0720. Accessed June 3, 2011.

67. Simon G, Sharma A, Li X, et al. Feasibility and efficacy of molecular analysis-directed individualized therapy in advanced non-small-cell lung cancer. J Clin Oncol 2007;25(19):2741–6.

68. Glaxo Smith Kline (GSK) Protocol summary for 109493. Available at: http://www.gsk-clinicalstudyregister.com/protocol_detail.jsp;jsessionid=D7BE392270D24AA9D34CDE273823D0DC?protocolId=109493&compound=GSK1572932. Accessed June 3, 2011.

69. Lee JG, Lee CY, Kim DJ, et al. Non-small cell lung cancer with ipsilateral pulmonary metastases: prognosis analysis and staging assessment. Eur J Cardiothorac Surg 2008;33(3):480–4.

70. Wang X, Wang M, MacLennan GT, et al. Evidence for common clonal origin of multifocal lung cancers. J Natl Cancer Inst 2009;101(8):560–70.

71. Hiroshima K, Toyozaki T, Kohno H, et al. Synchronous and metachronous lung carcinomas: molecular evidence for multicentricity. Pathol Int 1998; 48(11):869.

72. Huang J, Behrens C, Wistuba I, et al. Molecular analysis of synchronous and metachronous tumors of the lung: impact on management and prognosis. Ann Diagn Pathol 2001;5(6):321–9.

73. Dacic SM, Ionescu DN, Finkelstein SM, et al. Patterns of allelic loss of synchronous adenocarcinomas of the lung. Am J Surg Pathol 2005;29(7): 897–902.

74. Chang YL, Wu CT, Lin SC, et al. Clonality and prognostic implications of p53 and epidermal growth factor receptor somatic aberrations in multiple primary lung cancers. Clin Cancer Res 2007;13(1):52–8.

75. Girard N, Ostrovnaya I, Lau C, et al. Genomic and mutational profiling to assess clonal relationships between multiple non–small cell lung cancers. Clin Cancer Res 2009;15(16):5184–90.

76. Girard ND, Lau C, Finley D, et al. Comprehensive histologic assessment helps to differentiate multiple lung primary non-small cell carcinomas from metastases. Am J Surg Pathol 2009;33(12):1752–64.

77. Motoi N, Szoke J, Riely GJ, et al. Lung adenocarcinoma: modification of the 2004 WHO mixed subtype to include the major histologic subtype suggests correlations between papillary and micropapillary adenocarcinoma subtypes, EGFR mutations and gene expression analysis. Am J Surg Pathol 2008; 32(6):810–27.

78. Battafarano RJ, Meyers BF, Guthrie TJ, et al. Surgical resection of multifocal non-small cell lung cancer is associated with prolonged survival. Ann Thorac Surg 2002;74(4):988–94.

79. Trousse D, D'Journo XB, Avaro JP, et al. Multifocal T4 non-small cell lung cancer: a subset with improved prognosis. Eur J Cardiothorac Surg 2008;33(1):99–103.

80. Riquet M, Cazes A, Pfeuty K, et al. Multiple lung cancers prognosis: what about histology? Ann Thorac Surg 2008;86(3):921–6.

81. Zell J, Ignatius Ou SH, Ziogas A, et al. Survival improvements for advanced stage nonbronchioloalveolar carcinoma-type nonsmall cell lung cancer cases with ipsilateral intrapulmonary nodules. Cancer 2008;112(1):136–43.

82. Ou SHI, Zell JA. Validation study of the proposed IASLC staging revisions of the T4 and M non-small cell lung cancer descriptors using data from 23,583 patients in the California Cancer Registry. J Thorac Oncol 2008;3(3):216–27.

83. Chang YL, Wu CT, Lee YC. Surgical treatment of synchronous multiple primary lung cancers: experience of 92 patients. J Thorac Cardiovasc Surg 2007;134(3):630–7.

84. Antakli T, Schaefer RF, Rutherford JE, et al. Second primary lung cancer. Ann Thorac Surg 1995;59:863–7.

A Decade of Advances in Treatment of Early-Stage Lung Cancer

Luca Paoletti, MD[a], Nicholas J. Pastis, MD[a],
Chadrick E. Denlinger, MD[b], Gerard A. Silvestri, MD, MS[a,*]

KEYWORDS

• Lung cancer • Treatment • Surgery • VATS • Elderly

Early-stage non–small cell lung cancer (NSCLC) refers to stage I or stage II disease. Although patients with lung cancer who meet this criterion have the highest 5-year survival and lowest recurrence rates, their prognosis is still poor relative to other early-stage cancers. In patients with early-stage NSCLC, the ability to achieve complete surgical resection remains the most definitive treatment in current medical practice. Surgically resected stage I NSCLC has only a 70% 5-year survival and a 55% to 75% recurrence rate.[1–4] Five-year survival rates after surgical resection decrease to 40% to 50% for stage II disease.[5] The large database informing the most recent international lung cancer staging system demonstrated 5-year survival rates for stages IA, IB, IIA, and IIB of 73%, 58%, 46%, and 36%, respectively.[4] Unfortunately, lung cancer is detected in an advanced stage in approximately 70% of patients, making it one of the leading causes of death in America, with only a 16% overall 5-year survival rate.[6]

The past decade has witnessed a litany of advances in the treatment of early-stage lung cancer. In the past, patients who were inoperable due to poor lung function were relegated to few options with dismal survival results. Now, more options are available, including technologic advances in chest radiotherapy, a growing interest in the utility of sublobar resections, and an increase in the use of video-assisted thoracoscopic surgery (VATS).

Lung cancer screening has also undergone significant change during the past decade. The National Lung Screening Trial compared chest radiograph with low-dose helical chest CT in screening for lung cancer in 53,000 older patients with extensive (>30 pack-year) smoking history. The trial was stopped early due to a 20% reduction in lung cancer death among patients screened with CT scan compared with those screened with chest radiograph.[7] In the trial, the majority of patients was diagnosed at early stage; 93% of patients with stage I lung cancer detected by CT scan and 88% of patients with stage I lung cancer detected by chest radiograph underwent surgery with curative intent.[7]

One of the most important advances during the past decade was the development and implementation of the 7th edition of the international lung cancer stage classification system. The effect of tumor size on survival was studied in detail and incorporated in defining the new T descriptors. Additional size criteria for primary tumors (2, 5, and 7 cm) further subdivide previous cutoff values. T1 is now divided into T1a ($\leq$2 cm) and T1b (>2 cm but $\leq$3 cm). T2 is divided into T2a (>3 cm but $\leq$5 cm) and T2b (>5 cm but $\leq$7 cm). Tumors greater than 7 cm are now considered T3 because this group of patients have survival rates comparable to other definitions of T3.[4]

There is a growing recognition that smaller tumors ($\leq$2 cm) have a more favorable prognosis,

---

The authors have nothing to disclose.
[a] Division of Pulmonary and Critical Care Medicine, Medical University of South Carolina, 96 Jonathan Lucas Street, CSB 812, Charleston, SC 29425, USA
[b] Division of Surgery, Medical University of South Carolina, Ashley River Tower, 25 Courtenay Drive, MSC 295, Charleston, SC 29425, USA
* Corresponding author.
E-mail address: silvestr@musc.edu

Clin Chest Med 32 (2011) 827–838
doi:10.1016/j.ccm.2011.08.009
0272-5231/11/$ – see front matter © 2011 Elsevier Inc. All rights reserved.

prompting an increased consideration of sublobar as opposed to lobar resections for this group. Additionally, the past decade has witnessed the development and application of lung stereotactic radiation in nonsurgical candidates as well as the demonstration of benefit of adjuvant chemotherapy in patients with large stage IB and stage II NSCLC.[8]

LOBECTOMY VERSUS SUBLOBAR RESECTION

The first lung cancer surgeries involved complete pneumonectomies and frequently resulted in death.[9] As technology improved, surgery has evolved and become vastly safer and more effective. Patients now have additional surgical options, including lobectomy (the surgical removal of one complete lobe and its lymph nodes) and sublobar resection (anatomic segmentectomy or wedge resection). The surgical approach may be open thoracotomy or VATS. Despite the advances in surgery for early-stage lung cancer over the past decade, questions remain, such as whether lobectomy is uniformly superior to sublobar resection. The two procedures often differ with regard to the extent of parenchymal lymph node sampling and potentially the adequacy of surgical margins. The two procedures also have been associated with different mortality and/or recurrence rates.

Sublobar resections are typically used in patients who have an impaired pulmonary reserve and would not tolerate a full lobectomy. (See the articles by Von Groote-Bidlingmaier and colleagues and Mehta and colleagues elsewhere in this issue for further discussion of this evaluation.) These procedures can be done via open thoracotomy or VATS.[10] Wedge resections are most often recommended for smaller tumors (<2 cm) that are peripheral in location.[10] The tumor is resected without regard for anatomic bronchial segments and fissures. The benefits are preservation of lung volume and less perioperative morbidity and mortality. The major disadvantages of wedge resection are that N1 (intrapulmonary) lymph node sampling is not possible and that assessment of the surgical margin between staple line and tumor is difficult, leaving open the potential that it may be inadequate. Both of these issues may increase the possibility of higher rates of recurrence.[11] Segmentectomy refers to removal of an entire anatomic bronchial segment. It involves a detailed dissection of the bronchial segment and pulmonary arterial supply.[10,11] Performing a segmentectomy is more of a technical challenge for surgeons; its benefit is that it allows adequate lymph node sampling while preserving lung volume and function.[11]

In general, lobectomy is considered a superior approach when compared with sublobar resection. Debate continues on this topic, however. The discussion has been muddied by many and often conflicting studies comparing lobectomy with sublobar resections that did not separate the types of sublobar resections (segmentectomy or wedge resection) and that included high-risk patients who underwent sublobar resection because they could not tolerate a lobectomy.

To date, there has been a single prospective randomized study comparing lobectomy with sublobar resection for patients with NSCLC. In 1995, the Lung Cancer Study Group (LCSG) showed that in patients with peripheral early-stage (T1N0) NSCLC, lobectomy was superior to limited resection, which was defined as wedge resection or segmentectomy.[12] The study included 247 patients. In cases in which wedge or segmental resections were performed, there was a 3-fold increase in local recurrence, a 75% increase in combined local and distant recurrence ($P = .02$), and a 50% increase in death in comparison to lobectomies, although this did not reach statistical significance ($P = .09$). Based on this landmark study, the standard of care for individuals with peripheral early-stage NSCLC (T1N0) is lobectomy with lymph node sampling. Subsequent studies have supported the LCSG findings. In a large retrospective review of the Surveillance, Epidemiology, and End Results (SEER) database of 10,761 patients, there was a statistically significant difference in 5-year survival rates for patients who underwent lobectomy versus sublobar resection (61% vs 44%) in patients with stage IA NSCLC.[13] As with the LCSG study, wedge resection and segmentectomy were combined in this analysis.

Not all studies have concluded that lobectomy is superior to sublobar resction, with some retrospective studies reporting reporting similar survival rates in the two groups. In a series of 784 patients who underwent lung resection for stage I NSCLC, no difference in disease-free survival was noted between patients who had wedge resection or segmentectomy compared with lobectomy.[14] Although there was a difference in 5-year survival favoring lobectomy, the investigators speculated that patients with sublobar resections may have died earlier due to their underlying comorbid diseases, because patients underwent sublobar resection only if they were determined to be high-risk candidates for lobectomy due to decreased cardiopulmonary reserve.[14] Other studies of high-risk patients who underwent sublobar resection instead of lobectomy have had similar results, with 2-year and 5-year survival rates comparable between the two groups.[15,16] Given that these studies have been retrospective, and in light of the inconsistent findings in the literature comparing survival between surgical types, lobectomy with lymph node sampling remains the standard of care in patients who are medically fit for such an operation, with sublobar resections typically reserved for situations when lobectomy is not possible.

In some studies where sublobar resection was further separated into segmentectomy and wedge resection, there have been no statistically significant differences in 5-year survival rates between segmentectomy and lobectomy.[17,18] A recent large single-institution retrospective study comparing anatomic segmentectomy with lobectomy for stage I NSCLC showed no difference in operative morbidity or mortality between the two surgical approaches.[19] Furthermore, there was no difference in overall or disease-free survival between the two groups, although the mean follow-up time seemed limited in the segmentectomy group. A surgical margin of 1 cm seemed important for preventing a local recurrence. In a study evaluating tumor size and survival after various types of surgery, there was no statistical difference between lobectomy and segmentectomy for tumors between 2.1 cm to 3 cm in diameter, with 5-year survival rates of 87% and 85%, respectively.[20] For tumors greater than 3 cm, however, lobectomy had a 5-year survival rate of 81% compared with 63% with segmentectomy.[20] These findings suggest that segmentectomy may be a reasonable alternative to lobectomy for small early-stage tumors but that lobectomy remains the treatment of choice for larger cancers. In the absence of a randomized trial comparing lobectomy with segmentectomy for treatment of early-stage NSCLC, however, lobectomy remains the standard approach.

In contrast to the findings with anatomic segmentectomy, lobectomy has been shown to have a statistically significant 5-year survival advantage compared with wedge resection.[12,20,21] This may be in part because surgeons are better able to visualize and remove tumors and lymph nodes with lobectomy than with wedge resection.[11]

In comparing anatomic segmentectomy with wedge resection, the literature shows that there is a lower rate of cancer recurrence with the former. In an analysis of patients undergoing sublobar resections for early-stage lung cancer, the 5-year survival rate with segmentectomy for tumors less than 2 cm was 96% compared with 85% with wedge resection.[20] The difference in 5-year survival was even more evident with tumors between 2.1 cm to 3 cm in size (85% compared with 40%).[20]

Tumor size thus seems an important factor in the choice of surgical approach for the treatment of early-stage NSCLC. The survival advantage and decrease in recurrence rate associated with a more extensive resection are likely due to a combination of factors. First, the number of lymph nodes that can be sampled varies with the type of surgery. During a segmentectomy, the dissection of the bronchial tree exposes lymph nodes that are routinely resected. Conversely, these intraparenchymal lymph nodes are not visualized or sampled during wedge resection.[22] A second factor affecting survival with sublobar resection is the width of the surgical resection margin around the removed tumor. A surgical margin greater than 1 cm is more likely to be achieved with segmentectomy than with wedge resection.[23] To minimize the risk of recurrence, some surgeons advocate that in sublobar resection the surgical margin width should be greater than the tumor diameter.[24]

In comparing recurrence rates among patients undergoing various degrees of resection for early-stage lung cancer, physicians must continue to refer back to the LCSG study, which identified a 3-fold increase in cancer recurrence with wedge resection and greater than 2-fold increase in recurrence with anatomic segmentectomy compared with lobectomy. Other studies have reported recurrence rates of 2% to 9% with lobectomy compared with 19% to 22% with segmentectomy or wedge resection.[21,25,26]

It is also important to consider the contribution of adequate mediastinal lymph node evaluation in interpreting outcomes associated with surgical resection of early-stage lung cancer. In patients with stage I NSCLC who underwent sublobar resection (wedge resection or segmentectomy), recurrence rates as high as 50% have been reported in those patients who did not have mediastinal lymphadenectomy compared with 5% in those who did.[27] This highlights the importance of the mediastinal lymph node evaluation in patients undergoing curative surgery for early-stage lung cancer.[27]

In summary, lobectomy with lymphadenectomy is recommended as optimal curative intent therapy for patients with early-stage NSCLC who are appropriate surgical candidates for such a procedure. Sublobar resection, in particular anatomic segmentectomy, should be considered for patients who are suboptimal candidates for lobectomy due to limited pulmonary reserve or other medical comorbidities (**Table 1**). Controversies in this area deserve further study. It is unclear whether lobectomy with lymphadenectomy is superior to anatomic segmentectomy with

Table 1
Advantages and disadvantages of surgeries for early-stage lung cancer

Surgery	Advantages	Disadvantages
1. Lobectomy	• Lowest recurrence rate • Entire tumor and lymph nodes removed	• Greater loss of lung function • More extensive and lengthier procedure
2. Segmentectomy	• Preservation of lung function • Low recurrence rate • Better tolerated in patients with comorbid medical conditions • Greater number of lymph node dissected than wedge resection • Better surgical margin compared with wedge resection	• Technically challenging • Recurrence rate not clearly equal to lobectomy
3. Wedge resection	• Preservation of lung function • Better tolerated in patients with comorbid medical conditions • Shorter operative time	• Highest recurrence rate • Lung tissue removed with disregard to anatomy • Surgical margins may be less sufficient • Cannot remove intrapulmonary (N1) lymph nodes • Mediastinal lymph node dissection often limited or not performed

lymphadenectomy, particularly in patients with small (T1a) tumors, and this is a topic of current active study. A recent report using the SEER database evaluated survival after lobectomy or limited resection in patients with stage IA NSCLC with tumors less than or equal to 1 cm size and found no difference in survival between the two procedures.[28] This finding is of particular interest when considering that lung cancer screening with low-dose CT scanning will likely increase the number of these very small cancers that are identified.

VIDEO-ASSISTED THORACOSCOPIC SURGERY

The past decade has seen an increase in the use of VATS for early-stage lung cancer. In 2006, there were approximately 40,000 lobectomies performed, and VATS was used in only 2000 (5%) of those cases.[29] This percentage has increased yearly since the initial description of VATS in 1992. Initially VATS was used only for wedge resections; however, as the technology has advanced, more surgeons are increasingly facile with VATS for lobectomy and segmentectomy.

Despite its increasing popularity, there is reluctance among many in the surgical community to change their practice patterns, which may reflect the steep learning curve and technical challenges associated with the VATS approach. There is substantial evidence available demonstrating that VATS lobectomy for early-stage lung cancer is an equivalent oncological operation to lobectomy by open thoracotomy, with equal long-term

survival rates. In addition, many studies have suggested that VATS results in decreased morbidity, decreased length of hospitalization, and a more rapid return to baseline functional levels compared with open procedures. Definitive evidence that VATS is superior to open lobectomy is lacking, however, and changes in practice will likely reflect changing generations of surgeons with more familiarity and training in thoracoscopic surgery rather than the accumulation of such evidence.

There does not seem to be a difference between VATS and open procedures in 5-year survival rates for surgically resected early-stage NSCLC. In the current largest review of a single-center experience that included 1100 patients, McKenna and colleagues[29] found that their 5-year survival rate with VATS for early-stage NSCLC was comparable with most contemporary series of patient undergoing open lobectomy. Other single-institution reviews have also shown similar 5-year survival rates between VATS and open lobectomy.[30–33] In a multicenter review performed in Japan, the 5-year survival rate for patients with early-stage NSCLC was not statistically significant between the two groups: 97% with open lobectomy versus 96% with VATS.[34] Other studies have reported no statistically significant differences in locoregional recurrence with VATS compared with conventional lobectomy.[29,34,35]

The perioperative mortality rates with VATS and conventional open thoracotomy are similar.[35,36] Initially, skeptics of VATS questioned whether an adequate lymph node dissection could be performed, but it is clear that lymph node dissection performed via VATS can be performed as thoroughly as with an open approach.[37,38] Shortly after the initiation of VATS, a randomized study compared VATS lobectomy with open lobectomy and found no difference in duration of chest tube drainage, length of hospital stay, recovery time, or a decrease in post-thoracotomy pain.[39] Since that time, however, several studies have reported significantly shorter hospital length of stay, less postoperative pain and pain medication use, fewer hospital readmissions, shorter recuperation time, shorter chest tube drainage duration, and better preservation of preoperative performance status with VATS.[34,40–43] The procedure is associated with smaller chest wall incisions and consequently less inflammation, which may contribute to diminished postoperative discomfort and shorter length of stay.[34] VATS causes fewer inflammatory markers to be released compared with conventional open lobectomies.[37,44]

All of the above factors should be considered in choosing the type of surgery to perform for early-stage NSCLC. This may be of particular importance in patients who are anticipated to have treatment with postoperative chemotherapy, because recuperation after surgery often has an impact on the timing of adjuvant therapy. Petersen and colleagues[45] demonstrated that patients undergoing VATS resections had fewer delays in the delivery of adjuvant chemotherapy and additionally that these patients were more often able to tolerate the prescribed dose of chemotherapy without interruption.

VATS is more likely to be performed in large academic centers with higher surgical volume and dedicated thoracic surgeons.[36,46] The Society of Thoracic Surgeons is composed of predominantly board-certified thoracic surgeons (220 of the 225 members). In a review of the Society of Thoracic Surgeons database, 22% of all lobectomies in 2004 were performed via VATS, with that percentage increasing to 32% in 2006.[47] Of all thoracic surgeries in the United States, 36% are performed by general surgeons, who typically do not have extensive training or experience with VATS.[48] It has been demonstrated that thoracic surgical procedures performed by general surgeons are associated with higher mortality and morbidity, and longer length of stay than are observed with specialty trained thoracic surgeons.[49,50] The reasons for these differences are likely multifactorial. General surgeons have less exposure and perform fewer thoracic surgeries during their training. In addition, a lower postoperative mortality with lung cancer resection is observed in centers performing a higher volume of cases.[47,51] Both factors likely contribute

to the lower mortality and morbidity seen in high-volume centers with specialty trained thoracic surgeons.[36,47,51]

Tumor location and size factor into whether VATS can be feasibly performed. Large tumors (>6 cm in diameter) may necessitate an open approach because of the challenge of manipulating such a bulky tumor with VATS instruments and also because of the practical consideration that a larger incision is required to get a large tumor out of the chest. Although a central tumor location is not necessarily a barrier to a VATS approach, these tumors are often approached with an open thoracotomy because a tactile approach may be needed to ensure adequate surgical margins.

In summary, substantial evidence demonstrates that VATS lobectomy is an appropriate alternative to open lobectomy when performed by experienced hands in centers with adequate thoracic surgical volume. VATS seems to have equivalent oncologic outcomes when compared with open thoracotomy. The decision of which procedure should be chosen for curative intent surgery for early-stage NSCLC should be based on the experience of individual surgeons, the experience of the operating institution, and patient anatomic considerations.

TUMOR SIZE AND SURVIVAL AFTER RESECTION

There is an increased risk of lung cancer mortality with larger tumors, even in patients undergoing successful resection.[52] Since its inception, TNM staging has served to provide a common descriptive language as well as important prognostic information for patients with solid tumors, including NSCLC.[53,54] Over the past decade, there has been a great deal of interest in the effect of tumor size, even within the same stage, because there is an association between tumor size and survival.[4,55–57] Patients with resected small tumors (<2 cm) are well described as having a better 5-year survival than patients whose tumors measure 2.1 cm to 3 cm.[13] This effect of tumor size on survival was one of the driving forces for change in the lung cancer staging system. The current 7th edition of the TNM staging classification for lung cancer identified new cutpoints for the size of the primary tumor at 2 cm, 3 cm, 5 cm, and 7 cm. Goldstraw and colleagues[4] reclassified more than 13,000 cases of tumors originally staged by the previous 6th edition of the staging system and demonstrated that median 5-year survival was affected by placement in a different stage. For example, patients who had tumors of 6 cm and no lymph node involvement were classified as T2N0, stage IB in the old system, with a group 5-year survival of 54%. In the new system, however, these were reclassified as T2bN0, stage IIA, with a group projected 5-year survival of 46%. Tumors greater than 7 cm in diameter with ipsilateral hilar lymph node involvement were staged T2N1, stage IIB in the 6th edition, with a 5-year survival of 38%. In the 7th edition, these tumors would be classified as T3N1 (stage IIIA) with a 5-year survival of 24%. The new changes in the T descriptor in addition to other changes in the staging classification system represent a major advance in lung cancer management and should enhance the ability to more accurately group and characterize patients based on the anatomic description of their cancers.

AGE AND SURVIVAL AFTER RESECTION

Traditionally, lung cancer operations have been avoided in the older geriatric population due to concerns related to the likelihood of increased morbidity and mortality. Some studies have shown a higher mortality rate in elderly patients undergoing surgery for early-stage NSCLC, suggesting that age is an independent predictor of survival.[13,58] Other studies have demonstrated, however, that lung cancer surgery for elderly patients is a reasonably safe and viable option. As is true for all patients, lung cancer surgical outcomes in older individuals are dependent on their performance status and comorbid conditions.[59,60] It has been repeatedly demonstrated that elderly patients with good performance status and no comorbid conditions have postoperative outcomes similar to those of their younger counterparts. For example, there was no difference in 5-year survival in 133 Japanese elderly patients (age greater than 75) who underwent either lobectomy or sublobar surgery for stage I NSCLC and also no difference in the postoperative complication rate.[61,62] Similarly, a study in the Netherlands analyzed approximately 2000 patients over age 80 who were diagnosed with stage I or II NSCLC during a period of 15 years, of whom 6% (124 patients) underwent surgical intervention. The survival rate in the resected patients after 1 year was 83% and after 5 years was 47%, which is comparable with outcomes of surgery in other age demographics in the Netherlands.[63] Only a minority of the elderly patients in this study was treated surgically. The fact that they did so well emphasizes that appropriate patient selection is important in optimizing outcomes but also raises the question as to whether more of the elderly patients in that cohort might have benefited from a surgical approach.

Based on these and other studies, there should be no absolute age cutoff for surgery in patients with early-stage NSCLC. This recommendation is clear in the American College of Chest Physicians evidence-based guidelines for lung cancer.[64] Each case should be individualized, and patient comorbidities, functional status, and personal beliefs taken into account before deciding whether or not surgery is an appropriate recommendation.

SMALL CELL LUNG CANCER

Approximately 13% of all lung cancers diagnosed are SCLC histology.[65] During the past 10 years, the philosophy of treatment of limited-stage small cell lung cancer (SCLC) has changed (see the article by Neal and colleagues elsewhere in this issue). SCLC tends to progress rapidly and is typically diagnosed after it has metastasized to other sites.[66] Like NSCLC, SCLC is staged by the TNM paradigm, but the traditional classification of "limited" or "extensive" stage continues to have practical use. Limited-stage SCLC is defined as disease confined to one hemothorax, the mediastinum, and supraclavicular lymph nodes, with the entire extent of disease able to be included in one radiotherapy field. SCLC beyond limited stage is defined as extensive disease. Traditionally, treatment of limited-stage SCLC has been combination chemotherapy and radiation therapy.[67] Although current guidelines state that there is not enough evidence to categorically offer surgery to limited-stage SCLC patients, consideration is often given to resection with adjuvant chemotherapy for patients who have small tumors and are node negative. In these cases, patients should undergo a thorough evaluation to confirm that disease is truly confined to the primary site, typically with mediastinoscopy, brain imaging, abdominal imaging, and bone scan before surgery.[68]

Yu and colleagues[69] reviewed 1560 patients with SCLC from the SEER database, of whom 247 underwent lobectomy for stage I disease (primary tumor <3 cm diameter without other disease). Of those, 205 patients did not undergo radiation therapy, with 3-year and 5-year survival rates of 58% and 50%, respectively. There was no difference in survival when compared with patients who did undergo postoperative radiation therapy ($P = .90$).[69] The median survival of patients who underwent surgery for localized SCLC (defined as T1-T2 NX-N0) was an impressive 65 months, with a 5-year overall survival rate of 52%.[67] These results suggest that patient with early localized SCLC may benefit from curative intent surgery with adjuvant chemotherapy, with or without radiation therapy.[65]

CHEMOTHERAPY

Treatment regimens involving early-stage NSCLC concentrate on surgical removal of the tumor. In recent years there have been many trials published on the role of adjuvant chemotherapy (4–8 weeks after surgery) for early-stage NSCLC (see the article by Gettinger and Lynch elsewhere in this issue). Before the use of platinum-based chemotherapy there was no survival advantage to adjuvant chemotherapy, so it was not routinely used. More recent studies with the use of platinum-based adjuvant chemotherapy, in particular cisplatin, however, seem to demonstrate a reduction in mortality.[70]

There have been 4 large trials published in the past decade that have confirmed the usefulness of adjuvant chemotherapy in early-stage NSCLC. All of the trials incorporated cisplatin-based chemotherapy regimens. The survival benefit seen in these studies was observed predominantly in stage II lung cancer as opposed to stages IA or IB. The Lung Adjuvant Cisplatin Evaluation (LACE) trial was a meta-analysis of these trials, inclusive of 4500 patients. The LACE trial showed that patients with stage II NSCLC who received adjuvant chemotherapy had a 5% decrease in risk of death at 5 years compared with patients who received no chemotherapy. In contrast, patients with stage IA disease who received chemotherapy had worse outcomes than those who did not receive chemotherapy, and there was no survival advantage in patients with stage IB disease who received chemotherapy.[71]

The Adjuvant Navelbine International Trialist Association (ANITA) trial examined the impact of adjuvant chemotherapy in patients with stages IB, II, and III NSCLC.[72] Stages II and III patients who received adjuvant chemotherapy demonstrated improved survival (66 months compared with 44 months), with an 8.6% increase in overall survival at 5 years compared with those who received no chemotherapy.[72] This study showed that there was no benefit in using adjuvant chemotherapy in patients with stage IB disease.[72]

Two other trials, the JBR trial and International Adjuvant Lung Trial (IALT), showed similar results. Both studies demonstrated a survival advantage in patients with stage II disease who received adjuvant chemotherapy as opposed to no chemotherapy.[73,74] In the JBR trial, patients with stage II disease who received adjuvant chemotherapy had a 5-year survival rate of 59% compared with 44% in those who received no chemotherapy.[73]

Based on these results, the standard of care in patients with stage II disease is surgical resection followed by adjuvant chemotherapy.[75] The role of adjuvant chemotherapy in stage IB lung cancer remains controversial. None of the aforementioned trials found a survival advantage in patients with stage IB who received adjuvant chemotherapy.[71–74] Another landmark trial, however, cancer and leukemia group B (CALGB) 9633, which examined patients solely with stage IB disease, initially showed a survival advantage in patients who had resection and adjuvant chemotherapy,[8] and on the basis of this advantage the trial was stopped early. After the ANITA, JBR, and IALT trials failed to confirm this benefit, however, CALGB 9633 was reviewed with more longitudinal data, and no statistical significance in survival after 74 months (ie, beyond the original 5-year survival benchmark) was observed in patients who received chemotherapy compared with those that did not.[8] A subgroup analysis noted that in patients with tumors greater than 4 cm in size (stage IB), a 31% increase in disease-free survival in patients who received adjuvant chemotherapy compared with those who did not was identified.[8]

To summarize, the recommendation that adjuvant chemotherapy is recommended for patients with stage II NSCLC does represent a substantive change in practice over the past decade. In contrast, the treatment approach for patients with stage IB lung cancer has not changed. The American Society of Clinical Oncology does not recommend adjuvant chemotherapy in these patients.[75] Based on the results of the CALGB 9633 trial, however, there may be a role for adjuvant chemotherapy in select patients with stage IB NSCLC with large tumors (>4 cm). Furthermore, the new staging system adds a further level of complexity because patients with tumors greater than 5 cm in diameter with no lymph node involvement are now classified as stage IIA; whether or not they may benefit from adjuvant chemotherapy is a subject for future study.

ADVANCES IN CHEST RADIOTHERAPY

Approximately 25% of all patients with early-stage NSCLC are medically inoperable.[76] Because most patients diagnosed with lung cancer are current or former smokers, many have chronic obstructive pulmonary disease and other medical comorbidities. These patients may be deemed medically inoperable because of projected high rates of complications and death. Patients also may be considered inoperable due to severe heart disease and poor performance status. Patients further may simply decline surgery for personal reasons; these patients are typically treated as if they were medically inoperable. Follow-up of these patients through the SEER database demonstrates that they have a median survival of 14 months.[77] The 5-year survival rate of patients treated with supportive care alone is less than 10%.[78]

In the past, the only option for patients who declined surgery or who were medically inoperable was radiation therapy. These patients were given 1 to 3 Gyper fraction for 4 to 7 weeks for a total dose of 20 to 80 Gy.[79] The local recurrence rate (ie, tumor recurrence at the site that was irradiated) varied from 6.4% to 70%.[79] The 3-year recurrence rate was in the range of 60% to 67%,[79] whereas 5-year survival rates varied from 0% to 42%.[80,81] Given these statistics, it is evident that conventional radiation therapy for early-stage NSCLC has a high local relapse rate and a low 5-year survival.[78] The patients who benefit most from conventional radiation therapy are those with smaller tumors and those who receive higher doses of radiation to the tumor.[80]

Perhaps the greatest advancement in the past 10 years for early-stage NSCLC has been the use of stereotactic body radiation therapy (SBRT) in patients who are deemed medically inoperable or refuse surgery. SBRT is a method in which high doses of radiation (>15 Gy/fraction) are delivered to a tumor in 5 or fewer sessions over 1 to 2 weeks.[80] The radiation is transported via 6 to 12 radiation beams that all converge onto the tumor, which allows the targeting of a greater amount of radiation to the tumor while sparing the skin and normal surrounding lung tissue.[82]

The Radiation Therapy Oncology Group recently published 3-year results on 55 patients with early-stage NSCLC treated with SBRT.[83] They demonstrated that local control at 3 years was 90%, with a 3-year disease-free survival rate of 48%. The 3-year primary tumor control in this study was an impressive 97%, which is 2-fold greater than that of conventional radiation therapy.[83] There are some limitations to the use of SBRT. It is a newer treatment option that is not available in all centers and can only be done in tumors up to 5 cm, because the radiation dose becomes rate limiting. Furthermore, there is limited information on the relapse rate after 3 years. The largest trial to date has follow-up only out to 3 years.[78,83] Another limitation is that SBRT cannot be used in centrally located tumors due to an 11-fold risk of developing severe radiation toxicity and increased risk of life-threatening bleeding compared with its relative safety in peripheral tumors.[84]

Most studies that have been completed for SBRT for lung cancer have been performed in patients who are medically inoperable. Given the impressive short term SBRT results in patients with early-stage NSCLC, there is growing interest in studying its use in patients who are surgical candidates. There is an ongoing trial in the Netherlands randomizing patients to either surgery or SBRT for stage I NSCLC that examines local and regional control at 2 and 5 years. There is hope that this study will build on work already completed in Japan, in which a subgroup analysis showed that patients who were medically operable or refused surgery and who were treated with SBRT had a 5-year survival rate of 71%.[85,86]

Table 2
Advantages and disadvantages of radiotherapy for early-stage lung cancer

Radiotherapy	Advantages	Disadvantages
1. Conventional radiation therapy	• Widely available	• High relapse rate • Low 5-year survival • Requires 4–7 weeks for completion
2. Stereotactic body radiation therapy	• Completed within a few treatments • Good local control at 3 years • Can perform in patient with comorbid conditions • Can perform in patients who decline surgery • Can perform in tumors up to 5 cm in size	• Limited data available on relapse rates after 3–5 years • Limited availability • Cannot perform in centrally located tumors
3. Radiofrequency ablation	• Completed in one session • Good local control at 2 years • Can perform in patients with comorbid conditions • Can perform in patients who decline surgery	• Limited data available on relapse rates after 3–5 years • Limited availability • Best for tumors <3 cm in size • Cannot perform in centrally located tumors • High rate of pneumothorax

Table 3
Five-year survival and locoregional relapse rate after various therapies for early-stage non–small cell lung cancer

Treatment Modality	5-Year Survival	Locoregional Relapse Rate
Lobectomy	47%–90%[92]	2%–28%[14,26]
Segmentectomy	57%–85%[17,20]	8%–29%[14,92]
Wedge resection	27%–84%[17,20]	15%–55%[22,92]
Conventional radiotherapy	0%–42%[81]	60%–67%[79]
Stereotactic body radiation therapy	48%–71% at 3 years[83,85]	22% at 3 years[83]
Radiofrequency ablation	48%–70% at 2 years[87]	25%–64% at 2 years[87]

Radiotherapy advances from the past decade also include the use of radiofrequency ablation (RFA) for treatment of lung tumors (see **Table 2** for a comparison of radiation therapy modalities). Despite no controlled studies that compare lung ablation with surgery or radiation, RFA has become more accepted. Performing RFA is similar to performing a CT-guided lung biopsy. Patients are placed in a CT scanner and sedated, and an RFA probe is placed into the tumor. The probe contains stainless steel electrodes that protrude outwards into the tumor; heat is transmitted to the tumor for a set amount of time (dependent on the size of the tumor) to achieve coagulation necrosis. Once the electrodes have cooled, the probe is removed and the track from the tumor to the skin is ablated to prevent bleeding and tumor cell dissemination.[87] Results depend on the size of the tumor, with 64% 2-year local control in tumors less than 3 cm in size but only 25% in tumors greater than 3 cm.[88] Although data are limited to small series, the overall survival with RFA at all stages at 1 year is 70% and at 2 years is 48%, both of which are superior to conventional radiation therapy.[87] The disadvantage of RFA is an approximately 30% rate of pneumothorax,[89,90] related to the trocar and probe passing through normal lung tissue to reach the tumor. RFA is also limited by tumor size and location; tumors located within 1 cm of hilar structures are associated with increased risk of incomplete ablation and damage to bronchovascular structures, potentially leading to hemothorax.[91] These considerations contribute to limited use of RFA for the treatment of NSCLC.

SUMMARY

Emerging from the past decade, there has been a diversification of options for the treatment of early-stage lung cancer (**Table 3**). VATS is now more widely performed, with oncologic outcomes equivalent to those with open thoracotomy.

Although lobectomy remains the standard approach to surgical resection, lesser resections, such as segmentectomy and wedge resection, are considerations for some patients. Advances in surgical, radiation, and medical therapies continue to evolve. Future research questions will focus on comparing long-term outcomes with these modalities, including survival, as well as patient-centered endpoints, such as quality of life.

REFERENCES

1. Mountain CF. Revisions in the international system for staging lung cancer. Chest 1997;111(6):1710–7.
2. Pairolero PC, Williams DE, Bergstralh EJ, et al. Postsurgical stage I bronchogenic carcinoma: morbid implications of recurrent disease. Ann Thorac Surg 1984;38(4):331–8.
3. Feld R, Rubinstein LV, Weisenberger TH. Sites of recurrence in resected stage I non-small-cell lung cancer: a guide for future studies. J Clin Oncol 1984;2(12):1352–8.
4. Goldstraw P, Crowley J, Chansky K, et al. The IASLC Lung Cancer Staging Project: proposals for the revision of the TNM stage groupings in the forthcoming (seventh) edition of the TNM Classification of malignant tumours. J Thorac Oncol 2007;2(8):706–14.
5. Scott WJ, Howington J, Feigenberg S, et al. Treatment of non-small cell lung cancer stage I and stage II: ACCP evidence-based clinical practice guidelines (2nd edition). Chest 2007;132(Suppl 3):234S–42S.
6. Jemal A, Siegel R, Xu J, et al. Cancer statistics, 2010. CA Cancer J Clin 2010;60(5):277–300.
7. The National Lung Screening Trial Research Team. Reduced lung-cancer mortality with low-dose computed tomographic screening. N Engl J Med 2011;365(5):395–409. [Epub ahead of print].
8. Strauss GM, Herndon JE 2nd, Maddaus MA, et al. Adjuvant paclitaxel plus carboplatin compared with observation in stage IB non-small-cell lung cancer: CALGB 9633 with the Cancer and Leukemia Group B, Radiation Therapy Oncology Group, and North

Central Cancer Treatment Group Study Groups. J Clin Oncol 2008;26(31):5043–51.

9. Graham EA. The first total pneumonectomy. Tex Cancer Bull 1949;2(1):2–4.

10. Paul S, Port J. Limited resection for non-small cell lung cancer. Chest Physician 2010;5(6):13–4.

11. Narsule CK, Ebright MI, Fernando HC. Sublobar versus lobar resection: current status. Cancer J 2011;17(1):23–7.

12. Ginsberg RJ, Rubinstein LV. Randomized trial of lobectomy versus limited resection for T1 N0 non-small cell lung cancer. Lung Cancer Study Group. Ann Thorac Surg 1995;60(3):615–22 [discussion: 622–23].

13. Chang MY, Mentzer SJ, Colson YL, et al. Factors predicting poor survival after resection of stage IA non-small cell lung cancer. J Thorac Cardiovasc Surg 2007;134(4):850–6.

14. El-Sherif A, Gooding WE, Santos R, et al. Outcomes of sublobar resection versus lobectomy for stage I non-small cell lung cancer: a 13-year analysis. Ann Thorac Surg 2006;82(2):408–15 [discussion: 415–16].

15. Errett LE, Wilson J, Chiu RC, et al. Wedge resection as an alternative procedure for peripheral broncho-genic carcinoma in poor-risk patients. J Thorac Cardiovasc Surg 1985;90(5):656–61.

16. Pastorino U, Valente M, Bedini V, et al. Limited resection for Stage I lung cancer. Eur J Surg Oncol 1991;17(1):42–6.

17. Miller DL, Rowland CM, Deschamps C, et al. Surgical treatment of non-small cell lung cancer 1 cm or less in diameter. Ann Thorac Surg 2002; 73(5):1545–50 [discussion: 1550–51].

18. Kondo D, Yamada K, Kitayama Y, et al. Peripheral lung adenocarcinomas: 10 mm or less in diameter. Ann Thorac Surg 2003;76(2):350–5.

19. Schuchert MJ, Pettiford BL, Keeley S, et al. Anatomic segmentectomy in the treatment of stage I non-small cell lung cancer. Ann Thorac Surg 2007;84(3):926–32 [discussion: 932–933].

20. Okada M, Nishio W, Sakamoto T, et al. Effect of tumor size on prognosis in patients with non-small cell lung cancer: the role of segmentectomy as a type of lesser resection. J Thorac Cardiovasc Surg 2005;129(1):87–93.

21. Landreneau RJ, Sugarbaker DJ, Mack MJ, et al. Wedge resection versus lobectomy for stage I (T1 N0 M0) non-small-cell lung cancer. J Thorac Cardiovasc Surg 1997;113(4):691–8 [discussion 698–700].

22. Sienel W, Dango S, Kirschbaum A, et al. Sublobar resections in stage IA non-small cell lung cancer: segmentectomies result in significantly better cancer-related survival than wedge resections. Eur J Cardiothorac Surg 2008;33(4):728–34.

23. El-Sherif A, Fernando HC, Santos R, et al. Margin and local recurrence after sublobar resection of non-small cell lung cancer. Ann Surg Oncol 2007; 14(8):2400–5.

24. Sawabata N, Ohta M, Matsumura A, et al. Optimal distance of malignant negative margin in excision of nonsmall cell lung cancer: a multicenter prospective study. Ann Thorac Surg 2004;77(2):415–20.

25. Warren WH, Faber LP. Segmentectomy versus lobectomy in patients with stage I pulmonary carcinoma. Five-year survival and patterns of intrathoracic recurrence. J Thorac Cardiovasc Surg 1994; 107(4):1087–93 [discussion: 1093–94].

26. Campione A, Ligabue T, Luzzi L, et al. Comparison between segmentectomy and larger resection of stage IA non-small cell lung carcinoma. J Cardiovasc Surg (Torino) 2004;45(1):67–70.

27. Martini N, Bains MS, Burt ME, et al. Incidence of local recurrence and second primary tumors in resected stage I lung cancer. J Thorac Cardiovasc Surg 1995;109(1):120–9.

28. Kates M, Swanson S, Wisnivesky JP. Survival following lobectomy and limited resection for the treatment of stage I non-small cell lung cancer <=1 cm in size: a review of SEER data. Chest 2011;139(3):491–6.

29. McKenna RJ Jr, Houck W, Fuller CB. Video-assisted thoracic surgery lobectomy: experience with 1,100 cases. Ann Thorac Surg 2006;81(2):421–5 [discussion: 425–6].

30. Sugi K, Kaneda Y, Esato K. Video-assisted thoracoscopic lobectomy achieves a satisfactory long-term prognosis in patients with clinical stage IA lung cancer. World J Surg 2000;24(1):27–30 [discussion: 30–1].

31. Koizumi K, Haraguchi S, Hirata T, et al. Video-assisted lobectomy in elderly lung cancer patients. Jpn J Thorac Cardiovasc Surg 2002;50(1):15–22.

32. Sakuraba M, Miyamoto H, Oh S, et al. Video-assisted thoracoscopic lobectomy vs. conventional lobectomy via open thoracotomy in patients with clinical stage IA non-small cell lung carcinoma. Interact Cardiovasc Thorac Surg 2007;6(5):614–7.

33. Yamamoto K, Ohsumi A, Kojima F, et al. Long-term survival after video-assisted thoracic surgery lobectomy for primary lung cancer. Ann Thorac Surg 2010;89(2):353–9.

34. Shigemura N, Akashi A, Funaki S, et al. Long-term outcomes after a variety of video-assisted thoracoscopic lobectomy approaches for clinical stage IA lung cancer: a multi-institutional study. J Thorac Cardiovasc Surg 2006;132(3):507–12.

35. Yan TD, Black D, Bannon PG, et al. Systematic review and meta-analysis of randomized and nonrandomized trials on safety and efficacy of video-assisted thoracic surgery lobectomy for early-stage non-small-cell lung cancer. J Clin Oncol 2009;27(15):2553–62.

36. Farjah F, Wood DE, Mulligan MS, et al. Safety and efficacy of video-assisted versus conventional lung resection for lung cancer. J Thorac Cardiovasc Surg 2009;137(6):1415–21.

37. Inada K, Shirakusa T, Yoshinaga Y, et al. The role of video-assisted thoracic surgery for the treatment of

lung cancer: lung lobectomy by thoracoscopy versus the standard thoracotomy approach. Int Surg 2000;85(1):6–12.

38. Sagawa M, Sato M, Sakurada A, et al. A prospective trial of systematic nodal dissection for lung cancer by video-assisted thoracic surgery: can it be perfect? Ann Thorac Surg 2002;73(3):900.

39. Kirby TJ, Mack MJ, Landreneau RJ, et al. Lobectomy—video-assisted thoracic surgery versus muscle-sparing thoracotomy. A randomized trial. J Thorac Cardiovasc Surg 1995;109(5):997–1001 [discussion: 1001–2].

40. Handy JR Jr, Asaph JW, Douville EC, et al. Does video-assisted thoracoscopic lobectomy for lung cancer provide improved functional outcomes compared with open lobectomy? Eur J Cardiothorac Surg 2010;37(2):451–5.

41. Ohbuchi T, Morikawa T, Takeuchi E, et al. Lobectomy: video-assisted thoracic surgery versus posterolateral thoracotomy. Jpn J Thorac Cardiovasc Surg 1998;46(6):519–22.

42. Scott WJ, Allen MS, Darling G, et al. Video-assisted thoracic surgery versus open lobectomy for lung cancer: a secondary analysis of data from the American College of Surgeons Oncology Group Z0030 randomized clinical trial. J Thorac Cardiovasc Surg 2010;139(4):976–81 [discussion 981–3].

43. Swanson SJ, Herndon JE 2nd, D'Amico TA, et al. Video-assisted thoracic surgery lobectomy: report of CALGB 39802—a prospective, multi-institution feasibility study. J Clin Oncol 2007;25(31):4993–7.

44. Nagahiro I, Andou A, Aoe M, et al. Pulmonary function, postoperative pain, and serum cytokine level after lobectomy: a comparison of VATS and conventional procedure. Ann Thorac Surg 2001;72(2):362–5.

45. Petersen RP, Pham D, Burfeind WR, et al. Thoracoscopic lobectomy facilitates the delivery of chemotherapy after resection for lung cancer. Ann Thorac Surg 2007;83(4):1245–9 [discussion: 1250].

46. Yim AP, Landreneau RJ, Izzat MB, et al. Is video-assisted thoracoscopic lobectomy a unified approach? Ann Thorac Surg 1998;66(4):1155–8.

47. Boffa DJ, Allen MS, Grab JD, et al. Data from the society of thoracic surgeons general thoracic surgery database: the surgical management of primary lung tumors. J Thorac Cardiovasc Surg 2008;135(2):247–54.

48. Goodney PP, Lucas FL, Stukel TA, et al. Surgeon specialty and operative mortality with lung resection. Ann Surg 2005;241(1):179–84.

49. Silvestri GA, Handy J, Lackland D, et al. Specialists achieve better outcomes than generalists for lung cancer surgery. Chest 1998;114(3):675–80.

50. Schipper PH, Diggs BS, Ungerleider RM, et al. The influence of surgeon specialty on outcomes in general thoracic surgery: a national sample 1996 to 2005. Ann Thorac Surg 2009;88(5):1566–72 [discussion 1572–73].

51. Bach PB, Cramer LD, Schrag D, et al. The influence of hospital volume on survival after resection for lung cancer. N Engl J Med 2001;345(3):181–8.

52. Lyons G, Quadrelli S, Silva C, et al. Analysis of survival in 400 surgically resected non-small cell lung carcinomas: towards a redefinition of the T factor. J Thorac Oncol 2008;3(9):989–93.

53. Pelletier MP, Edwardes MD, Michel RP, et al. Prognostic markers in resectable non-small cell lung cancer: a multivariate analysis. Can J Surg 2001;44(3):180–8.

54. Strauss GM. Prognostic markers in resectable non-small cell lung cancer. Hematol Oncol Clin North Am 1997;11(3):409–34.

55. Sobin L, Wittekind C, editors. International union against cancer. Lung tumours. TNM classification of malignant tumors. New York: Wiley-Liss; 2002. p. 103.

56. Carbone E, Asamura H, Takei H, et al. T2 tumors larger than five centimeters in diameter can be upgraded to T3 in non-small cell lung cancer. J Thorac Cardiovasc Surg 2001;122(5):907–12.

57. Naruke T, Tsuchiya R, Kondo H, et al. Prognosis and survival after resection for bronchogenic carcinoma based on the 1997 TNM-staging classification: the Japanese experience. Ann Thorac Surg 2001;71(6):1759–64.

58. Mery CM, Pappas AN, Bueno R, et al. Similar long-term survival of elderly patients with non-small cell lung cancer treated with lobectomy or wedge resection within the surveillance, epidemiology, and end results database. Chest 2005;128(1):237–45.

59. Sawada S, Komori E, Nogami N, et al. Advanced age is not correlated with either short-term or long-term postoperative results in lung cancer patients in good clinical condition. Chest 2005;128(3):1557–63.

60. Zapatero J, Flandes J, Salvatierra S, et al. Thoracotomy in patients over 70 years old. Monaldi Arch Chest Dis 1994;49(4):298–301.

61. Okami J, Ito Y, Higashiyama M, et al. Sublobar resection provides an equivalent survival after lobectomy in elderly patients with early lung cancer. Ann Thorac Surg 2010;90(5):1651–6.

62. Ikeda N, Hayashi A, Iwasaki K, et al. Surgical strategy for non-small cell lung cancer in octogenarians. Respirology 2007;12(5):712–8.

63. Brokx HA, Visser O, Postmus PE, et al. Surgical treatment for octogenarians with lung cancer: results from a population-based series of 124 patients. J Thorac Oncol 2007;2(11):1013–7.

64. Alberts WM. Diagnosis and management of lung cancer executive summary: ACCP evidence-based clinical practice guidelines (2nd edition). Chest 2007;132:1S–19S.

65. Govindan R, Page N, Morgensztern D, et al. Changing epidemiology of small-cell lung cancer in the United States over the last 30 years: analysis

of the surveillance, epidemiologic, and end results database. J Clin Oncol 2006;24(28):4539–44.

66. Shepherd FA. Surgery for limited stage small cell lung cancer: time to fish or cut bait. J Thorac Oncol 2010;5(2):147–9.

67. Schreiber D, Rineer J, Weedon J, et al. Survival outcomes with the use of surgery in limited-stage small cell lung cancer: should its role be re-evaluated? Cancer 2010;116(5):1350–7.

68. Simon GR, Turrisi A, American College of Chest Physicians. Management of small cell lung cancer: ACCP evidence-based clinical practice guidelines (2nd edition). Chest 2007;132(Suppl 3):324S–39S.

69. Yu JB, Decker RH, Detterbeck FC, et al. Surveillance epidemiology and end results evaluation of the role of surgery for stage I small cell lung cancer. J Thorac Oncol 2010;5(2):215–9.

70. Chemotherapy in non-small cell lung cancer: a meta-analysis using updated data on individual patients from 52 randomised clinical trials. Non-small Cell Lung Cancer Collaborative Group. BMJ 1995;311(7010):899–909.

71. Pignon JP, Tribodet H, Scagliotti GV, et al. Lung adjuvant cisplatin evaluation: a pooled analysis by the LACE Collaborative Group. J Clin Oncol 2008; 26(21):3552–9.

72. Douillard JY, Rosell R, De Lena M, et al. Adjuvant vinorelbine plus cisplatin versus observation in patients with completely resected stage IB-IIIA non-small-cell lung cancer (Adjuvant Navelbine International Trialist Association [ANITA]): a randomised controlled trial. Lancet Oncol 2006;7(9):719–27.

73. Winton T, Livingston R, Johnson D, et al. Vinorelbine plus cisplatin vs. observation in resected non-small-cell lung cancer. N Engl J Med 2005;352(25):2589–97.

74. Arriagada R, Bergman B, Dunant A, et al. Cisplatin-based adjuvant chemotherapy in patients with completely resected non-small-cell lung cancer. N Engl J Med 2004;350(4):351–60.

75. Pisters KM, Evans WK, Azzoli CG, et al. Cancer Care Ontario and American Society of Clinical Oncology adjuvant chemotherapy and adjuvant radiation therapy for stages I-IIIA resectable non small-cell lung cancer guideline. J Clin Oncol 2007;25(34): 5506–18.

76. Bach PB, Cramer LD, Warren JL, et al. Racial differences in the treatment of early-stage lung cancer. N Engl J Med 1999;341(16):1198–205.

77. Wisnivesky JP, Bonomi M, Henschke C, et al. Radiation therapy for the treatment of unresected stage I-II non-small cell lung cancer. Chest 2005;128(3): 1461–7.

78. Fakiris AJ, McGarry RC, Yiannoutsos CT, et al. Stereotactic body radiation therapy for early-stage non-small-cell lung carcinoma: four-year results of a prospective phase II study. Int J Radiat Oncol Biol Phys 2009;75(3):677–82.

79. Qiao X, Tullgren O, Lax I, et al. The role of radiotherapy in treatment of stage I non-small cell lung cancer. Lung Cancer 2003;41(1):1–11.

80. Powell JW, Dexter E, Scalzetti EM, et al. Treatment advances for medically inoperable non-small-cell lung cancer: emphasis on prospective trials. Lancet Oncol 2009;10(9):885–94.

81. Rowell NP, Williams CJ. Radical radiotherapy for stage I/II non-small cell lung cancer in patients not sufficiently fit for or declining surgery (medically inoperable): a systematic review. Thorax 2001; 56(8):628–38.

82. Nguyen NP, Garland L, Welsh J, et al. Can stereotactic fractionated radiation therapy become the standard of care for early stage non-small cell lung carcinoma. Cancer Treat Rev 2008;34(8):719–27.

83. Timmerman R, Paulus R, Galvin J, et al. Stereotactic body radiation therapy for inoperable early stage lung cancer. JAMA 2010;303(11):1070–6.

84. Timmerman R, McGarry R, Yiannoutsos C, et al. Excessive toxicity when treating central tumors in a phase II study of stereotactic body radiation therapy for medically inoperable early-stage lung cancer. J Clin Oncol 2006;24(30):4833–9.

85. Onishi H, Shirato H, Nagata Y, et al. Hypofractionated stereotactic radiotherapy (HypoFXSRT) for stage I non-small cell lung cancer: updated results of 257 patients in a Japanese multi-institutional study. J Thorac Oncol 2007;2(7 Suppl 3):S94–100.

86. Onishi H, Shirato H, Nagata Y, et al. Stereotactic Body Radiotherapy (SBRT) for operable stage I non-small-cell lung cancer: can SBRT be comparable to surgery? Int J Radiat Oncol Biol Phys 2010. [Epub ahead of print].

87. Lencioni R, Crocetti L, Cioni R, et al. Response to radiofrequency ablation of pulmonary tumours: a prospective, intention-to-treat, multicentre clinical trial (the RAPTURE study). Lancet Oncol 2008;9(7):621–8.

88. Gewanter RM, Rosenzweig KE, Chang JY, et al. ACR Appropriateness Criteria: nonsurgical treatment for non-small-cell lung cancer: good performance status/definitive intent. Curr Probl Cancer 2010; 34(3):228–49.

89. Steinke K, Sewell PE, Dupuy D, et al. Pulmonary radiofrequency ablation—an international study survey. Anticancer Res 2004;24(1):339–43.

90. Lanuti M, Sharma A, Digumarthy SR, et al. Radiofrequency ablation for treatment of medically inoperable stage I non-small cell lung cancer. J Thorac Cardiovasc Surg 2009;137(1):160–6.

91. Gomez FM, Palussiere J, Santos E, et al. Radiofrequency thermocoagulation of lung tumours. Where we are, where we are headed. Clin Transl Oncol 2009;11(1):28–34.

92. Blasberg JD, Pass HI, Donington JS. Sublobar resection: a movement from the Lung Cancer Study Group. J Thorac Oncol 2010;5(10):1583–93.

A Decade of Advances in Treatment for Advanced Non–Small Cell Lung Cancer

Scott Gettinger, MD[a],*, Thomas Lynch, MD[b]

KEYWORDS

- Lung cancer • Personalized • Targeted
- Epidermal growth factor receptor • ERCC1
- Anaplastic lymphoma kinase

Lung cancer continues to be the leading cause of cancer-related mortality in the United States and worldwide. An estimated 220,520 patients were diagnosed with lung cancer in the United States in 2010, with 157,300 deaths attributed to the disease.[1] This cancer accounts for more cancer-related deaths than breast, prostate, and colorectal cancers combined. The high mortality rate is largely related to advanced stage of disease at discovery, with more than 50% of patients presenting with metastatic disease. This rate may decline in the next decade, because more early-stage lung cancers will be detected if computed tomography (CT) screening for high-risk individuals becomes widely accepted. Recently, the National Lung Screening Trial (NLST), which randomized individuals with at least a 30-pack-year smoking history to screening chest radiograph or CT, reported a 20% reduction in lung cancer mortality in those undergoing screening CT scans.[2] The topic of lung cancer screening is discussed in more detail in the article by Midthun elsewhere in this issue.

The leading cause of lung cancer continues to be cigarette smoking; however, roughly 10% to 15% of lung cancer patients in the United States have no history of smoking.[3] This amounts to approximately 30,000 never-smokers with lung cancer annually in the United States, more than the number of cases of multiple myeloma, chronic myelogenous leukemia, acute leukemia, sarcoma, or cancers of the brain, esophagus, stomach, liver, or cervix. National efforts continue to focus on smoking cessation; however, the percentage of current smokers in the United States has not changed since 2004, after a significant gradual decline from 1997.[4] It is currently estimated that approximately 20% of adults in America continue to smoke. Other potential causes of lung cancer, including radon gas and asbestos, have also been the focus of national agencies, with specific recommendations concerning radon mitigation and asbestos abatement issued by the Environmental Protection Agency.

For those with lung cancer, the last 10 years have seen small but real advances in both curative intent and palliative therapies. This review will focus on systemic therapies for advanced incurable non–small cell lung cancer (NSCLC), detailing changes in practice and emerging discoveries in advanced disease. Advances in the treatment of early stage NSCLC will be discussed elsewhere

No funding was provided for the preparation of this article. Dr Lynch has provided consulting services to Merck, Boehringer-Ingelheim, and Supergen as well as serving on the Board of Directors of Infinity Pharmaceuticals. He is a holder of a patent for EGFR testing from Partners Healthcare.

[a] Division of Medical Oncology, Yale University School of Medicine, 333 Cedar Street, FMP 127, New Haven, CT 06520, USA
[b] Division of Medical Oncology, Yale University School of Medicine, Yale Cancer Center, Smilow Cancer Hospital at Yale-New Haven, 333 Cedar Street, New Haven, CT 06520, USA
* Corresponding author.
E-mail address: scott.gettinger@yale.edu

Clin Chest Med 32 (2011) 839–851
doi:10.1016/j.ccm.2011.08.017
0272-5231/11/$ – see front matter © 2011 Published by Elsevier Inc.

in this issue in an article by Paoletti and colleagues. Therapies for small cell lung cancer will be additionally reviewed in the article by Neal and colleagues.

ADVANCES IN CHEMOTHERAPY
Choosing Therapy Based on Histology

NSCLC is subclassified by histology into adenocarcinoma, squamous cell carcinoma, and large cell carcinoma.[5] Adenocarcinoma has surpassed squamous cell histology in the United States as the most common type of NSCLC, possibly related to the introduction of low-tar filter cigarettes in the 1960s, whereas large cell carcinoma continues to be rare.[6] Up until the early 2000s, the distinction between squamous cell carcinoma and adenocarcinoma was not relevant, because treatment options for both were identical. As such, the classification of a tumor as non–small cell lung cancer not otherwise specified (NSCLC-NOS) previously sufficed, but has recently been met with consternation from medical oncologists, who are increasingly prescribing therapies based on the distinction between squamous and nonsquamous cell NSCLC histology.

Bevacizumab

In 2006, the United States Food and Drug Administration (FDA) approved the antiangiogenesis agent bevacizumab (Avastin), a monoclonal antibody to vascular endothelial growth factor (VEGF), for use in patients with advanced nonsquamous cell NSCLC. Approval came after a large phase 3 trial comparing standard first-line chemotherapy with carboplatinum and paclitaxel to identical therapy with the addition of bevacizumab demonstrated a significant improvement in median survival (MS) to 12.2 months.[7] The 1-year survival rate was 51%, with 20% of patients surviving 2 years. The trial was restricted to patients with nonsquamous cell histology because early clinical trial data suggested an increased incidence of fatal hemoptysis in patients with squamous cell NSCLC.[8] There is no clear explanation for this association, although one hypothesis has been that squamous cell carcinoma of the lung may be exquisitely sensitive to the effects of VEGF antagonism, with bleeding from tumor-associated blood vessels as the tumor shrinks. This association may also relate to the tendency for squamous cell carcinoma of the lung to cavitate. A retrospective analysis from the two randomized clinical trials evaluating the addition of bevacizumab to carboplatinum and paclitaxel suggested an increased incidence of significant hemoptysis with bevacizumab in those tumors

that cavitated, independent of histology, although the number of events was small.[9] Central location of lesions did not appear to be predictive of hemoptysis in these trials, but again, the small number of cases limits conclusions.

Pemetrexed

The other drug that is presently FDA approved based on NSCLC histology is pemetrexed (Alimta), an antifolate chemotherapy targeting multiple enzymes involved in folate metabolism, including thymidylate synthase (TS). Pemetrexed initially received approval in 2004 as second-line therapy for patients with advanced NSCLC, regardless of NSCLC histology. The approval was based on the results of a phase 3 trial comparing docetaxel, the standard second-line therapy at the time, with pemetrexed.[10] Efficacy was similar with both regimens; however, toxicity favored pemetrexed with less neutropenia and alopecia. In 2008 this indication was modified, restricting pemetrexed to use only in patients with nonsquamous cell histology. The FDA reached this decision after reviewing subset analyses by histology in this trial and additionally from a phase 3 first-line trial with pemetrexed.[11] The former was unplanned, and reported a small survival advantage with pemetrexed in patients with nonsquamous cell carcinoma (MS 9.3 months vs 8 months; $P = .048$), whereas patients with squamous cell histology fared better with docetaxel (MS 7.4 months vs 6.2 months; $P = .018$).[12] Given the small size of the trial with an unplanned subset analysis, conclusions from this alone would not justify a change of indication. However, a preplanned subset analysis from a larger phase 3 trial comparing first-line therapy with cisplatin and pemetrexed with cisplatin and gemcitabine in 1725 patients also suggested a survival benefit by histology.[11] Although neither regimen seemed superior overall, nonsquamous cell histology predicted for survival benefit with the pemetrexed-containing regimen (n = 1000; hazard ratio [HR] 0.81, 95% confidence interval [CI] 0.7–0.94; $P = .005$); whereas patients with squamous cell histology appeared to do better with the gemcitabine-containing regimen (n = 473; HR 1.23, 95% CI 1.0–1.51; $P = .05$). This trial led to the second FDA indication of pemetrexed with cisplatin in patients with chemo-naïve advanced nonsquamous cell NSCLC. An even more compelling argument for a histology effect came from a subsequent trial evaluating maintenance pemetrexed.[13] Patients who received 4 cycles of standard platinum-based doublet therapy for advanced NSCLC without evidence of progression were randomized in a 2:1 ratio to pemetrexed (n = 441) or placebo (n = 221). The trial found a 2.8-month improvement in MS with pemetrexed (10.6 to 13.4 months; $P = .012$). However, a pre-planned analysis by histology found no benefit with pemetrexed in patients with squamous cell carcinoma (n = 182), with an HR of 1.07 (95% CI 0.49–0.73; $P = .678$). In the remaining 481 patients with nonsquamous cell histology, MS was improved by 5 months with pemetrexed (10.3 months vs 15.5 months with HR 0.70, 95% CI 0.56–0.88; $P = .002$). These results led to the third FDA indication for pemetrexed as maintenance therapy in patients with advanced nonsquamous cell NSCLC.

Predictive Molecular Markers: ERCC1, RRM1, BRCA1/RAP80, and TS

Admittedly, histology is a somewhat crude way to personalize therapy in the era of molecular oncology. Furthermore, medical oncologists are often only provided a diagnosis of NSCLC without further characterization from pathology. Although immunohistochemical (IHC) stains, such as p63 and CK 5/6 (both squamous cell markers) and TTF-1 (thyroid transcription factor-1, suggestive of adenocarcinoma), are increasingly being used in attempts to distinguish squamous cell from non-squamous cell NSCLC, a diagnosis of nonsqua-mous cell NSCLC cannot always be achieved. In time, this distinction will likely become less impor-tant, with reliance on predictive biomarkers rather than histology to select optimal chemotherapy. To date several potential biomarkers have been iden-tified, with a handful being evaluated prospectively in clinical trials. These include excision repair cross-complementing 1 (ERCC1), ribonucleotide reductase subunit M1 (RRM1), breast cancer 1 (BRCA1), and TS.

Excision repair cross-complementing 1

The ERCC1 gene encodes the $5'$ endonuclease of the nuclear excision repair (NER) complex, the primary DNA repair mechanism that removes damaged nucleotide bases in mammalian cells. In addition to protecting normal cells from endogenous and environmental toxins, NER also mediates resistance of several malignancies to different chemotherapies, including cisplatinum and carboplatinum. Platinum compounds exert their cytotoxic effect by covalently binding to DNA, forming adducts that distort DNA. An intact NER pathway is essential to repair such damage and prevent apoptosis.

Levels of tumor ERCC1 appear to be predictive of sensitivity to platinum chemotherapies, as well as being prognostic in the clinic. Retrospective biomarker studies have demonstrated that high levels of ERCC1 as measured by IHC or reverse-transcription polymerase chain reaction (RT-PCR) are associated with better prognosis after surgery for early-stage lung cancer.[14,15] One explanation for this has been that enhanced ERCC1 activity may limit further molecular events in tumor cells, leading to a less aggressive phenotype. This observation is supported by a large retrospective analysis of the International Adjuvant Lung Trial (IALT), the first randomized study demonstrating a survival benefit with chemotherapy after complete resection of stage I to III NSCLC.[15] Patients in the trial were randomized to receive cisplatin-based doublet chemotherapy or obser-vation. There was a 4% absolute improvement in overall survival with chemotherapy. However, in the population of patients with ERCC1-positive tumors by IHC (n = 355), there was no benefit observed with chemotherapy. These patients overall had a better prognosis than those with ERCC1-negative tumors, with 5-year survival rates of 46% in the observation arm (n = 170) compared with 39% (n = 202), respectively (HR 0.66, 95% CI 0.49–0.90; $P = .009$). Whether they would have benefited from a nonplatinum chemotherapy doublet is uncertain; but the benefit of any chemo-therapy would be expected to be less, considering the better overall prognosis. Conversely, those with ERCC1-negative tumors (n = 426) survived longer if given chemotherapy, with a 5-year survival rate of 47% in the treated group versus 39% in the untreated group (HR 0.65, 95% CI 0.50–0.86, $P = .002$).

In the metastatic setting, the potential value of ERCC1 in selecting chemotherapy has been eval-uated retrospectively in several studies. A recent meta-analysis of 12 such studies reported that both response and survival in patients treated with platinum-based chemotherapy were superior in patients with low ERCC1 expression by IHC or RT-PCR.[16] A total of 865 patients were included in this meta-analysis, with a response rate of 47% in ERCC1 low/negative tumors compared with 28% in ERCC1 high/positive tumors (odds ratio 0.48, 95% CI 0.35–0.64; $P<.00001$). MS was 74 versus 45 weeks, respectively (median ratio 0.77, 95% CI 0.47–1.01; $P<.00001$). Although comparison is limited in such an analysis, IHC seemed better than RT-PCR in predicting the response rate. Based on encouraging results from individual retrospective studies, the Spanish Lung Cancer Group (SLCG) conducted a prospec-tive phase 3 trial randomizing patients with meta-static NSCLC to first-line standard chemotherapy with docetaxel and cisplatin or to a genotypic arm that selected therapy based on ERCC1 mRNA expression.[17] Those with low tumor levels received cisplatin and docetaxel, whereas patients with high tumor expression were administered docetaxel and gemcitabine. The response rate in the control arm was 39% compared with 51% in the genotypic arm (n = 346; P = .02). Additional ongoing prospective trials are listed in **Table 1** and are discussed later.

Ribonucleotide reductase M1

The RRM1 gene encodes the regulatory subunit of ribonucleotide reductase, an enzyme that is required for DNA synthesis and repair, catalyzing the biosynthesis of deoxyribonucleosides from the corresponding ribonucleotides. Like ERCC1, expression of RRM1 has been associated with prognosis in NSCLC, with longer survival reported in patients with high expression by IHC and RT-PCR.[18,19] RRM1 is also a molecular target of gemcitabine, an antimetabolite that has proven activity in several malignancies including NSCLC. Preclinical studies[19,20] and retrospective analyses[21–23] from clinical trials have in turn indicated RRM1 expression to be a strong predictor of therapeutic efficacy with gemcitabine-based chemotherapy.

The value of RRM1 as a marker for sensitivity to gemcitabine has been prospectively evaluated in a phase 2 feasibility study conducted at the Moffitt Cancer Center.[24] A total of 53 patients with chemo-naïve advanced NSCLC were treated with doublet chemotherapy based on mRNA expression of both RRM1 and ERCC1. In patients with tumors showing high RRM1 expression by RT-PCR, gemcitabine was not given. Patients were then further divided into those with high and low expression of ERCC1; patients with high expression did not receive cisplatin. Although the purpose of the study was to assess the feasibility

Table 1
Selected ongoing randomized non–small cell lung cancer clinical trials prospectively evaluating predictive biomarkers for chemotherapy

Sponsor (Location) Identifier	Stage	Phase	Primary End Point/ Planned Number	Biomarker	Method	Control Arm	Customized Therapy
First-line therapy for advanced NSCLC							
H Lee Moffitt Cancer Center (USA) NCT00499109 MADeIT	IIIB/IV	3	PFS 267	ERCC1 RRM1	AQUA (protein)	GC	GC DC GD VD
SLCG (Spain) NCT00617656 BREC	IIIB/IV	3	TTP 480	BRCA1 RAP80	RT-PCR (mRNA)	DP	DP GP D
Yonsei U. (Korea) NCT00736814	IIIB/IV	R2	RR 117	ERCC1 RRM1	RT-PCR	DC	DC GC GD VD
Postoperative (adjuvant) chemotherapy							
IFCT (France) NCT00775385 TASTE	II/IIIA	2/3	Feasibility 108	EGFR ERCC1	Sequence (DNA mut) IHC	PemP	Erlotinib PemP Observation
SLCG (Spain) NCT00478699 SCAT	II/IIIA	3	OS 432	BRCA1	RT-PCR	DP	DP GP D
ITACA (Italy/ Germany)	I–IIIA	3	OS 700	ERCC1 TS	RT-PCR	DP[a] GP VP	PemP GP Pem Taxane

Abbreviations: AQUA, automated quantitative analysis; BREC, BRAC1/RAP80 expression customization; C, carboplatin; D, docetaxel; G, gemcitabine; ITACA, International Tailored Chemotherapy Adjuvant; MADeIt, Molecular Analysis-Directed Individualized Therapy; NSCLC, non–small cell lung cancer; OS, overall survival; P, cisplatinum; Pem, pemetrexed; PFS, progression free survival; R, randomized; RR, response rate; RT-PCR, reverse-transcription polymerase chain reaction; SCAT, Spanish Customized Adjuvant Treatment; TASTE, Tailored Post Surgical Therapy in Early-Stage NSCLC; TTP, time to progression; V, vinorelbine.
[a] Investigator choice of listed chemotherapy options on control arm.

of molecularly directed therapy, with only a small number of patients treated, response and survival data were encouraging, with an overall response rate of 44%, MS of 13.3 months, and 1-year survival rate of 59%.

Ongoing trials evaluating ERCC1/RRM1 Based on the data discussed above, a handful of randomized trials have been launched to prospectively test the predictive value of both RRM1 and ERCC1 (see **Table 1**). Some of these trials are being conducted in the adjuvant setting, after surgery, where two additional questions are also being considered: Is there a population of patients with stage I NSCLC who would benefit from adjuvant chemotherapy and, conversely, are there patients with node-positive disease who may not benefit from traditional adjuvant chemotherapy? To date, the role of chemotherapy in patients with node-negative NSCLC has not been established, although there is a suggestion that larger tumors, particularly those at least 4 cm in size, may benefit from chemotherapy.[25] The Southwest Oncology Group is conducting a pilot study in this population, in which patients with completely resected stage I NSCLC (per AJCC 6th edition[26]) with T1 tumors 2 cm or larger will only receive adjuvant chemotherapy if their tumors are found to have low protein expression of ERCC1 or RRM1 (NCT00792701). This is a feasibility trial, and interpretation of results will be limited by both the prognostic and predictive value of these biomarkers. If there is a signal from this study, additional trials may randomize only patients with low expression of ERCC1 and tumors between 2 and 4 cm in size to adjuvant chemotherapy or observation, or those with high expression of ERCC1 and tumors larger than 4 cm without nodal involvement to chemotherapy or observation.

Breast cancer 1/Receptor-associated protein 80
BRCA1 is a tumor suppressor gene that encodes the breast cancer type 1 susceptibility protein. One of the major functions of BRCA1 is to help repair damaged DNA, in particular, correcting double-strand breaks by participating in homologous recombination, a process for which nucleotide sequences are used from a sister chromatid as a template for repair.[27] BRCA1 is also thought to be involved in transcription-coupled NER.[28] The importance of BRCA1 is perhaps best illustrated in women with germline BRCA1 mutations. Approximately 65% of these women will develop breast cancer by the age of 70 years, and an estimated 39% will develop ovarian cancer.[29,30]

BRCA-1 has also emerged as a potential predictive biomarker for chemotherapy, with decreased expression associated with cisplatin sensitivity, and increased expression predictive of benefit from antimicrotubulin agents, such as taxanes.[31–34] These observations led to a phase 2 trial using BRCA1 mRNA expression to guide therapy in patients with epidermal growth factor receptor (EGFR) wild-type advanced NSCLC. A total of 123 patients were stratified to gemcitabine/cisplatin (low BRCA1), docetaxel/cisplatin (intermediate BRCA1), or docetaxel alone (high BRCA1).[35] Response rates/MS were 25%/11 months (low BRCA1); 46%/9 months (intermediate BRCA1); and 42%/11 months (high BRCA1), respectively. An exploratory analysis of this study further evaluated another potential biomarker, receptor-associated protein 80 (RAP80), a nuclear protein required for the accumulation of BRCA1 to sites of DNA breaks.[36–38] Eleven patients were evaluable with low expression of both BRCA1 and RAP80; although the number of patients was small, the outcome of this group was impressive, with MS not reached and time to progression of 14 months. However, the prognostic impact of these biomarkers needs to be considered, with limited data suggesting that high levels of BRCA1 are associated with a poorer prognosis in early-stage lung cancer.[39] The response rate in the patients with low BRCA1/RAP80 was not provided. Based on encouraging findings from this trial, the SLCG is currently conducting a phase 3 trial comparing standard first-line chemotherapy for advanced NSCLC to customized therapy based on BRCA1 and RAP80 mRNA levels (BREC trial) (see **Table 1**).

Thymidylate synthase
TS is a key enzyme in folate metabolism, which is essential for the generation of thymidine monophosphate required for DNA synthesis and repair. TS is a major target of several chemotherapies, including pemetrexed, and is currently being evaluated as a predictive biomarker of benefit with pemetrexed in patients with nonsquamous cell NSCLC. This approach is supported by preclinical studies correlating high expression of TS with resistance to pemetrexed, and low levels with chemosensitivity to pemetrexed.[40–42] High expression of TS typically seen in squamous cell NSCLC[43] has been hypothesized to explain, at least partly, the lack of activity seen with pemetrexed in patients with this histologic subtype of NSCLC. The predictive power of TS expression will be tested prospectively in the EPIC trial (Elderly and Poor Performance Status Individualized Chemotherapy trial), in which patients

with chemo-naïve advanced NSCLC will be randomized to standard therapy or individualized therapy based on mRNA levels of TS, ERCC1, and RRM1.

MOLECULAR THERAPY

To date, three molecular targets have been validated in the treatment of advanced NSCLC: EGFR, anaplastic lymphoma kinase (ALK), and VEGF. The benefit of bevacizumab, a monoclonal antibody to VEGF, has been discussed previously, and this section will focus on EGFR and ALK.

Epidermal Growth Factor Receptor

The EGFR is a transmembrane protein composed of an extracellular ligand binding domain and an intracellular tyrosine kinase (**Fig. 1**). Activation of this receptor by ligand binding leads to receptor dimerization and autophosphorylation of the intracellular tyrosine kinase domain. This activated receptor complex in turn initiates a cascade of intracellular signaling resulting in cellular proliferation, inhibition of apoptosis, angiogenesis, and

metastasis.[44] Because the EGFR is aberrantly expressed in 40% to 90% of NSCLCs, it became an attractive target for drug development in the 1990s.[45]

Two oral, small-molecule EGFR tyrosine kinase inhibitors (TKI), gefitinib (Iressa) and erlotinib (Tarceva), have been developed in parallel over the last decade. Gefitinib received FDA approval first, based on two phase 2 trials reporting encouraging response rates, symptom control, and survival in previously treated patients with advanced NSCLC.[46,47] However, the results of a confirmatory phase 3 trial failed to show a survival advantage with gefitinib compared with best supportive care alone, and gefitinib lost its FDA indication in 2005, with use limited to those who were already benefiting from the drug.[48] Erlotinib fared better, with a positive phase 3 trial randomizing patients with advanced NSCLC to salvage erlotinib or best supportive care alone.[49] MS was improved by 2 months with better quality of life, and erlotinib was FDA approved for use as second-line or third-line treatment in 2004. Recently, the FDA indication for erlotinib was

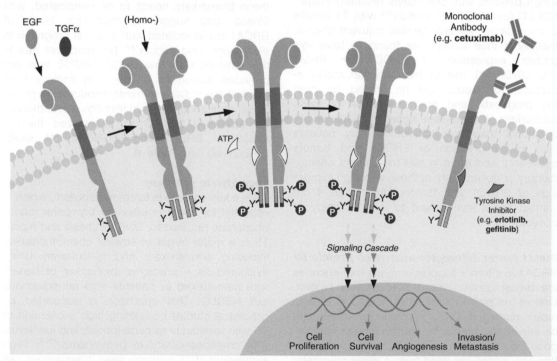

Fig. 1. Epidermal growth factor receptor (EGFR) activation and inhibition. The EGFR is a transmembrane protein that is activated by ligand binding (eg, EGF or TGFα), resulting in dimerization with another EGFR (homo) or related receptor (hetero) and autophosphorylation of the EGFR intracellular tyrosine kinase domain. This activated complex in turn initiates a cascade of intracellular signaling resulting in cellular proliferation, inhibition of apoptosis, angiogenesis, and metastases. The EGFR is inhibited by both monoclonal antibodies (eg, cetuximab) to the extracellular ligand-binding portion and small-molecule adenosine triphosphate (ATP) competitive inhibitors (eg, erlotinib and gefitinib) of the intracellular tyrosine kinase domain. EGF, epidermal growth factor; TGFα, transforming growth factor α; Y, tyrosine residue; P, phosphate.

expanded to include maintenance erlotinib, based on modest survival results from the SATURN trial (Sequential Tarceva in Unresectable NSCLC).[50] This trial randomized patients with advanced NSCLC, whose disease did not progress after standard first-line chemotherapy, to erlotinib or observation. Progression-free survival (PFS), the primary endpoint, was 12.3 weeks with erlotinib versus 11.1 weeks in the observation arm, with an HR of 0.71 (95% CI 0.62–0.82; $P<.0001$). A 1-month improvement in MS was reported with an HR of 0.81 (95% CI 0.7–0.95; $P = .0088$).

Cetuximab, a monoclonal antibody to EGFR, has also been evaluated in a phase 3 trial in patients with advanced NSCLC (the FLEX study).[51] A total of 1124 patients with chemo-naïve advanced NSCLC were randomized to standard chemotherapy or to the same therapy with cetuximab. Unlike previous trials finding no benefit when gefitinib or erlotinib was added to chemotherapy, the FLEX trial found a modest improvement in MS of 1.2 months with cetuximab (MS 11.3 months vs 10.1 months; HR 0.87, 95% CI 0.762–0.996; $P = .044$). The FDA is currently considering approval of this costly agent.

Predicting response to erlotinib/gefitinib

Well before erlotinib or gefitinib came to market, certain characteristics emerged as predictive of response, often dramatic and prolonged, to these agents. These included, adenocarcinoma histology, East Asian ancestry, female sex and, most importantly, no history of smoking. Considering the profound benefit seen in these patients, three separate research centers sequenced archived tumor tissue from responding patients and simultaneously discovered mutations in the tyrosine kinase domain of EGFR.[52–54] Both in-frame deletions in exon 19 and a specific missense mutation in exon 21 (L858R) were reported. Since this discovery, a growing database of patients with EGFR mutant NSCLC has been compiled, with recent phase 3 trials establishing an oral EGFR TKI as a first-line strategy over chemotherapy in patients with newly diagnosed EGFR-mutant advanced NSCLC.[55–58] Response rates in these trials range from 62% to 85%, with a PFS of 8.4 to 13.1 months. It is estimated that 10% to 15% of unselected patients in North America and Western Europe with NSCLC, and 50% of never-smokers with NSCLC, have EGFR-mutant tumors.[56,59–62]

Acquired resistance to EGFR TKI

Inevitably, most patients with EGFR-mutant advanced NSCLC develop resistance to gefitinib or erlotinib, generally within 1 year of starting treatment. Progression tends to be slow, and oncologists often choose to continue erlotinib for fear of rapid progression. This phenomenon was illustrated in a group of 10 patients with EGFR-mutant NSCLC with acquired resistance to erlotinib or gefitinib.[63] After baseline CT and positron emission tomography/CT scans, erlotinib or gefitinib was held for 3 weeks, at which time imaging was repeated. The same EGFR TKI was then restarted and imaging was repeated 3 weeks later. This small study found that stopping EGFR inhibition led to an increased rate of clinical and radiographic progression, which stabilized or improved on reinitiation of drug. Another approach to such patients has been to discontinue EGFR inhibition temporarily, with rechallenge after progression of disease on salvage chemotherapy. Re-responses in this situation are not uncommon, with one explanation being that without the selection pressure from the EGFR TKI, the resistant clone will fade.[64,65]

Much work has been done to elucidate mechanisms of acquired resistance to erlotinib and gefitinib (**Fig. 2**). It is estimated that at least 50% of such tumors harbor an additional EGFR mutation, the T790M mutation in exon 20, where a bulky methionine is substituted for threonine at position 790 on exon 20.[63,66–69] It was initially thought that the T790M mutation led to resistance simply by steric interference with drug binding in the adenosine triphosphate (ATP) pocket of EGFR; however, subsequent studies suggest that the introduction of this mutation leads to increased ATP affinity of the mutant EGFR receptor.[70,71] Because erlotinib and gefitinib are reversible ATP competitive inhibitors, restoring the ATP affinity of the mutant EGFR decreases its vulnerability to erlotinib or gefitinib. Another mechanism of acquired resistance to EGFR TKIs is amplification of the MET oncogene, which is identified in approximately 20% of cases, with some overlap with the T790M mutation.[72,73] Increased cell signaling through the MET kinase appears to circumvent EGFR inhibition, maintaining activation of downstream molecules. Identification of both MET amplification and the T790M EGFR mutation as mechanisms of acquired resistance to EGFR TKIs has allowed the development of clinical trials evaluating agents specifically targeting these events (**Table 2**). For example, a next-generation irreversible EGFR inhibitor that covalently binds to EGFR for resistance mediated by the T790M mutation, or combination therapy with an EGFR TKI and a MET inhibitor for tumors with MET amplification. Other potential mechanisms of acquired resistance are currently being investigated (eg, epithelial to mesenchymal transition, increased

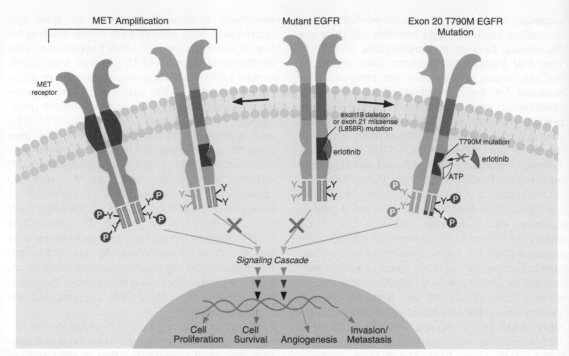

Fig. 2. Mechanisms of acquired resistance to geftinib/erlotinib. Two established mechanisms of acquired resistance to erlotinib and gefitinib include MET amplification and the T790M EGFR mutation. The former is found in approximately 20% of cases with such resistance, and is thought to circumvent EGFR inhibition by restoring activation of downstream molecules. T790M EGFR mutations are identified in 50% to 60% of cases, and are thought to increase ATP affinity of the mutant EGFR. Because erlotinib and gefitinib are reversible ATP competitive inhibitors, increasing the ATP affinity of the mutant EGFR decreases its vulnerability to these inhibitors. Y, tyrosine residue; P, phosphate.

insulin-like growth factor receptor 1 signaling, and transformation to small-cell histology) with clinical trials being developed to exploit such mechanisms.[69]

Anaplastic Lymphoma Kinase

The ALK was originally identified in 1994 as part of a chimeric protein found in large cell anaplastic lymphomas.[74,75] The fusion resulted

Table 2
Selected ongoing non–small cell lung cancer clinical trials in patients with acquired resistance to EGFR TKIs

Trial Sponsor/ Identifier	Phase	Agent/Design
Exelixis NCT00596648	1/2	XL-184: oral multikinase inhibitor including MET, VEGFR2 *plus/minus* Erlotinib
Boehringer NCT01090011	1	BIBW 2992 (Afatinib): oral irreversible inhibitor of EGFR/HER2 *plus* Cetuximab: monoclonal antibody to EGFR
Pfizer NCT01121575	1	PF00299804: oral irreversible inhibitor of EGFR/HER2 *plus/minus* Crizotinib: oral inhibitor of MET and ALK
Merrimack NCT00994123	1/2	MM-121: monoclonal antibody to HER3 *plus* Erlotinib
Northwest U (US) NCT01259089	1/2	AUY-922: intravenous heat shock protein 90 Inhibitor *plus* Erlotinib

from a translocation of the ALK gene on chromosome 2 to nucleophosmin (NPM) on chromosome 5, transforming cells driven by the constitutive tyrosine kinase activity of ALK. NPM-ALK rearrangements are thought to activate numerous cell-signaling pathways promoting tumorigenesis. The importance of ALK in lung cancer was only recently realized. In 2007, Japanese researchers first identified an ALK gene rearrangement in a patient with NSCLC.[76] RT-PCR demonstrated a translocation of the echinoderm microtubule-associated protein like 4 (EML4) gene on chromosome 2 with ALK. In a relatively short period, ALK has since been validated as a target in NSCLC.

Based on encouraging activity in two patients with ALK-rearranged NSCLC in a phase 1 dose escalation trial of crizotinib, a small-molecule MET and ALK inhibitor, an expansion cohort of 82 patients with ALK-rearranged lung cancer were treated with crizotinib.[77] A response rate of 57% was reported, with an additional 33% showing stability or regression not meeting strict criteria for response. PFS was not reached when the study results were published in 2010, with updated results at the European Society of Medical Oncology annual meeting reporting a median PFS of 9.2 months.[78] These encouraging results have led to an ongoing phase 3 trial of second-line crizotinib in comparison with standard chemotherapy, and a phase 2 trial of salvage crizotinib in patients not eligible for the phase 3 trial. In addition, a first-line randomized trial of standard chemotherapy versus crizotinib has recently been launched for patients with ALK-rearranged NSCLC.

Over the last 4 years, a growing database has provided some insight into the nature of ALK-rearranged lung cancer. It is estimated that 4% to 6% of patients with adenocarcinoma of the lung will be found to have an ALK-rearranged tumor, accounting for roughly 8000 to 10,000 patients annually in the United States. Patients tend to be never-smokers and, unlike EGFR-mutant lung cancer, this event seems to be more common in males. Among never-smokers with EGFR wild-type NSCLC, roughly a third will have a tumor driven by an ALK rearrangement.[79] Often, signet-ring cells are appreciated on pathologic review, and their presence should alert the clinician to the possibility of an ALK-rearranged tumor. Like EGFR-mutant lung cancer, acquired resistance to ALK inhibitors is beginning to be appreciated, with efforts now concentrating on elucidating the mechanisms of resistance. Two secondary mutations in the kinase domain of EML4-ALK in a patient with acquired resistance to crizotinib have already been reported, with one being in

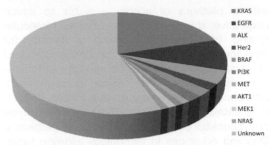

Fig. 3. Estimated frequency of driver mutations in non-small cell lung cancer.

the gatekeeper residue similar to the T790M mutation found in patients with acquired resistance to EGFR TKIs.[80] Several other potential mechanisms are currently being explored, and it is anticipated that clinical trials evaluating strategies to counteract acquired resistance will follow on the heels of such discovery.

Other NSCLC Driver Mutations

Both EGFR-mutant NSCLC and ALK-rearranged NSCLC are examples of tumors dependent primarily on one oncogenic event, similar to the BCR-ABL translocation in chronic myelogenous leukemia, KIT mutation in gastrointestinal stromal tumor and BRAF mutation in melanoma. Such reliance has led to the term oncogene addiction, with the potential for profound tumor regression if this oncogene can be successfully inhibited.[81] A handful of other driver mutations in NSCLC has been identified, and efforts are focusing on developing agents to target these events (**Fig. 3**).[82–84] The most common driver mutation in NSCLC is KRAS, and investigators continue to evaluate anti-KRAS strategies. This target has proved to be elusive, though, and several anti-KRAS agents have failed in the clinic to date. Other driver mutations include HER2, BRAF, PI3K, and MEK. Of course, most NSCLCs are not likely to depend on one molecular event, and a cocktail of targeted therapies will be required to halt the progression of these tumors at the molecular level.

SUMMARY

The last decade has seen small but significant advances in the treatment of advanced NSCLC cancer. A plateau in the effectiveness of chemotherapy has clearly been reached, and refinement in such therapy will require further identification and validation of predictive biomarkers. The promise of targeted therapy has been realized in small molecular cohorts of patients with NSCLC, and other such groups are emerging with a plethora of agents available to inhibit respective driver mutations. Routine molecular testing to assist in choosing a therapy for advanced NSCLC is now becoming standard practice. For patients without one dominant mutation characterizing their tumor, a customized approach will likely require identification of multiple pathways essential to the tumor phenotype and a cocktail of agents targeting these pathways. Ongoing advances in technology allowing rapid, sophisticated evaluation of both proteins and genes should help realize the ultimate goal of individualizing therapy for every patient diagnosed with lung cancer.

REFERENCES

1. Jemal A, Siegel R, Xu J, et al. Cancer Statistics, 2010. CA Cancer J Clin 2010;60(5):277–300.
2. Available at: http://www.cancer.gov/newscenter/pressreleases/2011/NLSTresultsRel. Accessed April 1, 2011.
3. Wakelee HA, Chang ET, Gomez SL, et al. Lung cancer incidence in never smokers. J Clin Oncol 2007;25(5):472–8.
4. Barnes PM, Heyman KM, Freeman G, et al. Early release of selected estimates based on data from the 2009 National Health Interview Survey. Hyattsville (MD): National Center for Health Statistics; 2010. Available at: http://www.cdc.gov/nchs/nhis.htm. Accessed August 27, 2011.
5. Beasley MB, Brambilla E, Travis WD. The 2004 World Health Organization classification of lung tumors. Semin Roentgenol 2005;40(2):90–7.
6. Altekruse SF, Kosary CL, Krapcho M. SEER Cancer Statistics Review, 1975-2007. National Cancer Institute; 2010. Available at: http://seer.cancer.gov/csr/1975_2007/. Accessed April 1, 2011.
7. Sandler A, Gray R, Perry MC, et al. Paclitaxel-carboplatin alone or with bevacizumab for non-small-cell lung cancer. N Engl J Med 2006;355(24):2542–50.
8. Johnson DH, Fehrenbacher L, Novotny WF, et al. Randomized phase II trial comparing bevacizumab plus carboplatin and paclitaxel with carboplatin and paclitaxel alone in previously untreated locally advanced or metastatic non-small-cell lung cancer. J Clin Oncol 2004;22(11):2184–91.
9. Sandler AB, Schiller JH, Gray R, et al. Retrospective evaluation of the clinical and radiographic risk factors associated with severe pulmonary hemorrhage in first-line advanced, unresectable non-small-cell lung cancer treated with Carboplatin and Paclitaxel plus bevacizumab. J Clin Oncol 2009; 27(9):1405–12.
10. Hanna N, Shepherd FA, Fossella FV, et al. Randomized phase III trial of pemetrexed versus docetaxel in patients with non-small-cell lung cancer

previously treated with chemotherapy. J Clin Oncol 2004;22(9):1589–97.
11. Scagliotti GV, Parikh P, von Pawel J, et al. Phase III study comparing cisplatin plus gemcitabine with cisplatin plus pemetrexed in chemotherapy-naive patients with advanced-stage non-small-cell lung cancer. J Clin Oncol 2008;26(21):3543–51.
12. Petersen P, Park K, Fossella FV, et al. Is pemetrexed more effective in adenocarcinoma and large cell lung cancer than in squamous cell carcinoma? A retrospective analysis of a phase III trial of pemetrexed versus docetaxel in previously treated patients with advanced non-small cell lung cancer (NSCLC). 12th World Conference on Lung Cancer. J Thorac Oncol 2007;P2:328.
13. Ciuleanu T, Brodowicz T, Zielinski C, et al. Maintenance pemetrexed plus best supportive care versus placebo plus best supportive care for non-small-cell lung cancer: a randomised, double-blind, phase 3 study. Lancet 2009;374(9699):1432–40.
14. Simon GR, Sharma S, Cantor A, et al. ERCC1 expression is a predictor of survival in resected patients with non-small cell lung cancer. Chest 2005;127(3):978–83.
15. Olaussen KA, Dunant A, Fouret P, et al. DNA repair by ERCC1 in non-small-cell lung cancer and cisplatin-based adjuvant chemotherapy. N Engl J Med 2006;355(10):983–91.
16. Chen S, Zhang J, Wang R, et al. The platinum-based treatments for advanced non-small cell lung cancer, is low/negative ERCC1 expression better than high/positive ERCC1 expression? A meta-analysis. Lung Cancer 2010;70(1):63–70.
17. Cobo M, Isla D, Massuti B, et al. Customizing cisplatin based on quantitative excision repair cross-complementing 1 mRNA expression: a phase III trial in non-small-cell lung cancer. J Clin Oncol 2007;25(19):2747–54.
18. Zheng Z, Chen T, Li X, et al. DNA Synthesis and Repair Genes RRM1 and ERCC1 in Lung Cancer. N Engl J Med 2007;356(8):800–8.
19. Bepler G, Kusmartseva I, Sharma S, et al. RRM1 modulated in vitro and in vivo efficacy of gemcitabine and platinum in non–small-cell lung cancer. J Clin Oncol 2006;24(29):4731–7.
20. Davidson JD, Ma L, Flagella M, et al. An increase in the expression of ribonucleotide reductase large subunit 1 is associated with gemcitabine resistance in non-small cell lung cancer cell lines. Cancer Res 2004;64(11):3761–6.
21. Rosell R, Scagliotti G, Danenberg KD, et al. Transcripts in pretreatment biopsies from a three-arm randomized trial in metastatic non-small-cell lung cancer. Oncogene 2003;22(23):3548–53.
22. Souglakos J, Boukovinas I, Taron M, et al. Ribonucleotide reductase subunits M1 and M2 mRNA expression levels and clinical outcome of lung

adenocarcinoma patients treated with docetaxel/gemcitabine. Br J Cancer 2008;98(10):1710–5.

23. Bepler G, Sommers KE, Cantor A, et al. Clinical efficacy and predictive molecular markers of neoadjuvant gemcitabine and pemetrexed in resectable non-small cell lung cancer. J Thorac Oncol 2008; 3(10):1112–8.

24. Simon G, Sharma A, Li X, et al. Feasibility and efficacy of molecular analysis-directed individualized therapy in advanced non-small-cell lung cancer. J Clin Oncol 2007;25(19):2741–6.

25. Strauss GM, Herndon JE 2nd, Maddaus MA, et al. Adjuvant paclitaxel plus carboplatin compared with observation in stage IB non-small-cell lung cancer: CALGB 9633 with the Cancer and Leukemia Group B, Radiation Therapy Oncology Group, and North Central Cancer Treatment Group Study Groups. J Clin Oncol 2008;26(31):5043–51.

26. Mountain CF. Revisions in the international system for staging lung cancer. Chest 1997;111(6):1710–7.

27. Powell SN, Kachnic LA. Roles of BRCA1 and BRCA2 in homologous recombination, DNA replication fidelity and the cellular response to ionizing radiation. Oncogene 2003;22(37):5784–91.

28. Le Page F, Randrianarison V, Marot D, et al. BRCA1 and BRCA2 are necessary for the transcription-coupled repair of the oxidative 8-oxoguanine lesion in human cells. Cancer Res 2000; 60(19):5548–52.

29. Antoniou A, Pharoah PD, Narod S, et al. Average risks of breast and ovarian cancer associated with BRCA1 or BRCA2 mutations detected in case Series unselected for family history: a combined analysis of 22 studies. Am J Hum Genet 2003; 72(5):1117–30.

30. Antoniou AC, Cunningham AP, Peto J, et al. The BOADICEA model of genetic susceptibility to breast and ovarian cancers: updates and extensions. Br J Cancer 2008;98(8):1457–66.

31. Taron M, Rosell R, Felip E, et al. BRCA1 mRNA expression levels as an indicator of chemoresistance in lung cancer. Hum Mol Genet 2004;13(20): 2443–9.

32. Quinn JE, Kennedy RD, Mullan PB, et al. BRCA1 functions as a differential modulator of chemotherapy-induced apoptosis. Cancer Res 2003;63(19):6221–8.

33. Quinn JE, James CR, Stewart GE, et al. BRCA1 mRNA expression levels predict for overall survival in ovarian cancer after chemotherapy. Clin Cancer Res 2007;13(24):7413–20.

34. Stordal B, Davey R. A systematic review of genes involved in the inverse resistance relationship between cisplatin and paclitaxel chemotherapy: role of BRCA1. Curr Cancer Drug Targets 2009; 9(3):354–65.

35. Rosell R, Perez-Roca L, Sanchez JJ, et al. Customized treatment in non-small-cell lung cancer based on EGFR mutations and BRCA1 mRNA expression. PLoS One 2009;4(5):e5133.

36. Wang B, Matsuoka S, Ballif BA, et al. Abraxas and RAP80 form a BRCA1 protein complex required for the DNA damage response. Science 2007; 316(5828):1194–8.

37. Sobhian B, Shao G, Lilli DR, et al. RAP80 targets BRCA1 to specific ubiquitin structures at DNA damage sites. Science 2007;316(5828): 1198–202.

38. Kim H, Chen J, Yu X. Ubiquitin-binding protein RAP80 mediates BRCA1-dependent DNA damage response. Science 2007;316(5828):1202–5.

39. Rosell R, Skrzypski M, Jassem E, et al. BRCA1: a novel prognostic factor in resected non-small-cell lung cancer. PLoS One 2007;2(11):e1129.

40. Sigmond J, Backus HH, Wouters D, et al. Induction of resistance to the multitargeted antifolate Pemetrexed (ALIMTA) in WiDr human colon cancer cells is associated with thymidylate synthase overexpression. Biochem Pharmacol 2003;66(3):431–8.

41. Giovannetti E, Mey V, Nannizzi S, et al. Cellular and pharmacogenetics foundation of synergistic interaction of pemetrexed and gemcitabine in human non-small-cell lung cancer cells. Mol Pharmacol 2005; 68(1):110–8.

42. Hanauske AR, Eismann U, Oberschmidt O, et al. In vitro chemosensitivity of freshly explanted tumor cells to pemetrexed is correlated with target gene expression. Invest New Drugs 2007;25(5):417–23.

43. Ceppi P, Volante M, Saviozzi S, et al. Squamous cell carcinoma of the lung compared with other histotypes shows higher messenger RNA and protein levels for thymidylate synthase. Cancer 2006; 107(7):1589–96.

44. Olayioye MA, Neve RM, Lane HA, et al. The ErbB signaling network: receptor heterodimerization in development and cancer. EMBO J 2000;19(13): 3159–67.

45. Isobe T, Herbst RS, Onn A. Current management of advanced non-small cell lung cancer: targeted therapy. Semin Oncol 2005;32(3):315–28.

46. Kris MG, Natale RB, Herbst RS, et al. Efficacy of gefitinib, an inhibitor of the epidermal growth factor receptor tyrosine kinase, in symptomatic patients with non-small cell lung cancer: a randomized trial. JAMA 2003;290(16):2149–58.

47. Fukuoka M, Yano S, Giaccone G, et al. Multi-institutional randomized phase II trial of gefitinib for previously treated patients with advanced non-small-cell lung cancer (The IDEAL 1 Trial) [corrected]. J Clin Oncol 2003;21(12):2237–46.

48. Thatcher N, Chang A, Parikh P, et al. Gefitinib plus best supportive care in previously treated patients with refractory advanced non-small-cell lung cancer: results from a randomised, placebo-controlled, multicentre study (Iressa Survival

Evaluation in Lung Cancer). Lancet 2005;366(9496): 1527–37.

49. Shepherd FA, Rodrigues Pereira J, Ciuleanu T, et al. Erlotinib in previously treated non-small-cell lung cancer. N Engl J Med 2005;353(2):123–32.

50. Cappuzzo F, Ciuleanu T, Stelmakh L, et al. Erlotinib as maintenance treatment in advanced non-small-cell lung cancer: a multicentre, randomised, placebo-controlled phase 3 study. Lancet Oncol 2010;11(6):521–9.

51. Pirker R, Pereira JR, Szczesna A, et al. Cetuximab plus chemotherapy in patients with advanced non-small-cell lung cancer (FLEX): an open-label rando-mised phase III trial. Lancet 2009;373(9674): 1525–31.

52. Lynch TJ, Bell DW, Sordella R, et al. Activating mutations in the epidermal growth factor receptor underlying responsiveness of non-small-cell lung cancer to gefitinib. N Engl J Med 2004;350(21): 2129–39.

53. Paez JG, Janne PA, Lee JC, et al. EGFR mutations in lung cancer: correlation with clinical response to ge-fitinib therapy. Science 2004;304(5676):1497–500.

54. Pao W, Miller V, Zakowski M, et al. EGF receptor gene mutations are common in lung cancers from "never smokers" and are associated with sensitivity of tumors to gefitinib and erlotinib. Proc Natl Acad Sci U S A 2004;101(36):13306–11.

55. Mok TS, Wu YL, Thongprasert S, et al. Gefitinib or carboplatin-paclitaxel in pulmonary adenocarci-noma. N Engl J Med 2009;361(10):947–57.

56. Maemondo M, Inoue A, Kobayashi K, et al. Gefitinib or chemotherapy for non-small-cell lung cancer with mutated EGFR. N Engl J Med 2010;362(25):2380–8.

57. Mitsudomi T, Morita S, Yatabe Y, et al. Gefitinib versus cisplatin plus docetaxel in patients with non-small-cell lung cancer harbouring mutations of the epidermal growth factor receptor (WJTOG3405): an open label, randomised phase 3 trial. Lancet On-col 2010;11(2):121–8.

58. Zhou C, Wu YL, Chen G, et al. Efficacy results from the randomised phase III OPTIMAL (CTONG 0802) study comparing first-line erlotinib versus carbopla-tin plus gemcitabine, in chinese advanced non-small-cell lung cancer patients with EGFR activating mutations ESMO 2010 [abstract LBA13]. Program and abstracts of the 35th European Society of Medical Oncology Congress 2010. Milan (Italy): European Society of Medical Oncology 2010 Abstract LBA 13.

59. Pao W, Miller VA. Epidermal growth factor receptor mutations, small-molecule kinase inhibitors, and non-small-cell lung cancer: current knowledge and future directions. J Clin Oncol 2005;23(11):2556–68.

60. Pham D, Kris MG, Riely GJ, et al. Use of cigarette-smoking history to estimate the likelihood of muta-tions in epidermal growth factor receptor gene

exons 19 and 21 in lung adenocarcinomas. J Clin Oncol 2006;24(11):1700–4.

61. Shigematsu H, Lin L, Takahashi T, et al. Clinical and biological features associated with epidermal growth factor receptor gene mutations in lung cancers. J Natl Cancer Inst 2005;97(5):339–46.

62. Rosell R, Moran T, Queralt C, et al. Screening for epidermal growth factor receptor mutations in lung cancer. N Engl J Med 2009;361(10):958–67.

63. Riely GJ, Kris MG, Zhao B, et al. Prospective assessment of discontinuation and reinitiation of er-lotinib or gefitinib in patients with acquired resis-tance to erlotinib or gefitinib followed by the addition of everolimus. Clin Cancer Res 2007; 13(17):5150–5.

64. Kurata T, Tamura K, Kaneda H, et al. Effect of re-treatment with gefitinib ('Iressa', ZD1839) after acquisition of resistance. Ann Oncol 2004;15(1): 173–4.

65. Yano S, Nakataki E, Ohtsuka S, et al. Retreatment of lung adenocarcinoma patients with gefitinib who had experienced favorable results from their initial treatment with this selective epidermal growth factor receptor inhibitor: a report of three cases. Oncol Res 2005;15(2):107–11.

66. Kobayashi S, Boggon TJ, Dayaram T, et al. EGFR mutation and resistance of non-small-cell lung cancer to gefitinib. N Engl J Med 2005;352(8): 786–92.

67. Pao W, Miller VA, Politi KA, et al. Acquired resistance of lung adenocarcinomas to gefitinib or erlotinib is associated with a second mutation in the EGFR kinase domain. PLoS Med 2005;2(3):e73.

68. Arcila ME, Oxnard GR, Nafa K, et al. Rebiopsy of lung cancer patients with acquired resistance to EGFR inhibitors and enhanced detection of the T790M mutation using a locked nucleic acid-based assay. Clin Cancer Res 2011;17(5): 1169–80.

69. Sequist LV, Waltman BA, Dias-Santagata D, et al. Genotypic and histological evolution of lung cancers acquiring resistance to EGFR inhibitors. Sci Transl Med 2011;3(75):75ra26.

70. Yun CH, Mengwasser KE, Toms AV, et al. The T790M mutation in EGFR kinase causes drug resistance by increasing the affinity for ATP. Proc Natl Acad Sci U S A 2008;105(6):2070–5.

71. Sos ML, Rode HB, Heynck S, et al. Chemogenomic profiling provides insights into the limited activity of irreversible EGFR Inhibitors in tumor cells express-ing the T790M EGFR resistance mutation. Cancer Res 2010;70(3):868–74.

72. Bean J, Brennan C, Shih JY, et al. MET amplification occurs with or without T790M mutations in EGFR mutant lung tumors with acquired resistance to gefi-tinib or erlotinib. Proc Natl Acad Sci U S A 2007; 104(52):20932–7.

73. Engelman JA, Zejnullahu K, Mitsudomi T, et al. MET amplification leads to gefitinib resistance in lung cancer by activating ERBB3 signaling. Science 2007;316(5827):1039–43.

74. Morris SW, Kirstein MN, Valentine MB, et al. Fusion of a kinase gene, ALK, to a nucleolar protein gene, NPM, in non-Hodgkin's lymphoma. Science 1994; 263(5151):1281–4.

75. Shiota M, Fujimoto J, Semba T, et al. Hyperphosphorylation of a novel 80 kDa protein-tyrosine kinase similar to Ltk in a human Ki-1 lymphoma cell line, AMS3. Oncogene 1994;9(6):1567–74.

76. Soda M, Choi YL, Enomoto M, et al. Identification of the transforming EML4-ALK fusion gene in non-small-cell lung cancer. Nature 2007;448(7153): 561–6.

77. Kwak EL, Bang YJ, Camidge DR, et al. Anaplastic lymphoma kinase inhibition in non-small-cell lung cancer. N Engl J Med 2010;363(18):1693–703.

78. Camidge DR, Bang YJ, Iafrate AJ, et al. Clinical activity of crizotinib (PF-02341066), in ALK-positive patients with advanced non-small cell lung cancer [abstract 366PD]. Program and abstracts of the 35th European Society of Medical Oncology Congress 2010. Milan (Italy): European Society of Medical Oncology; 2010.

79. Shaw AT, Yeap BY, Mino-Kenudson M, et al. Clinical features and outcome of patients with non-small-cell lung cancer who harbor EML4-ALK. J Clin Oncol 2009;27(26):4247–53.

80. Choi YL, Soda M, Yamashita Y, et al. EML4-ALK mutations in lung cancer that confer resistance to ALK inhibitors. N Engl J Med 2010;363(18):1734–9.

81. Weinstein IB. Cancer. Addiction to oncogenes—the Achilles heal of cancer. Science 2002;297(5578): 63–4.

82. Pao W, Iafrate AJ, Su Z. Genetically informed lung cancer medicine. J Pathol 2011;223(2):230–40.

83. Pao W, Girard N. New driver mutations in non-small-cell lung cancer. Lancet Oncol 2011;12(2): 175–80.

84. Molecular Profiling of Lung Cancer. Available at: http://www.vicc.org/mycancergenome/nsclc/. Accessed April 1, 2011.

Current Management of Small Cell Lung Cancer

Joel W. Neal, MD, PhD[a],*, Matthew A. Gubens, MD[b],
Heather A. Wakelee, MD[a]

KEYWORDS

- Small cell lung cancer • Limited stage • Advanced stage
- Chemotherapy

In 2010, approximately 222,000 cases of lung and bronchus cancers were anticipated to be diagnosed in the United States,[1] and worldwide, lung cancer is the eighth most common cause of death, killing an estimated 1.3 million people in 2004.[2] Small cell lung cancer (SCLC) is a high-grade, neuroendocrine carcinoma of the lung, named for its histologically distinct features, including small cells with sparse cytoplasm, fine chromatin, nuclear molding, and the presence of markers of neuroendocrine differentiation such as synaptophysin and chromogranin A. In the United States, SCLC accounts for a shrinking percentage of lung cancers, from 17% in 1986 to 13% in 2002, with non–small cell lung cancer (NSCLC) making up most of the remaining fraction.[3] This decreasing incidence may be a result of recent advances in public health measures, such as antismoking campaigns and bans on smoking in the workplace and other public places.[4] Because improvements in survival among patients with SCLC have been only modest over the last 30 years, the best way to eliminate morbidity from this disease may be through prevention.[3]

CLINICAL PRESENTATION AND STAGING

Presenting symptoms of SCLC are usually related to the tumor burden or effects of metastatic disease burden. Most disease presents in the central airways and mediastinum, leading to cough, shortness of breath, chest pain, hemoptysis, and compression of the superior vena cava. Common manifestations of metastatic disease include fatigue, anorexia, weight loss, headaches, and neurologic symptoms, with less than 10% of patients being asymptomatic at the time of presentation.[5] SCLC also has a propensity to cause paraneoplastic syndromes in up to 40% of patients as a result of release of peptide hormones. These syndromes include hyponatremia from inappropriate antidiuretic hormone secretion and Cushing syndrome from tumor-derived adrenocorticotropic hormone production. Less frequently, antigenic similarity to nervous system proteins triggers inappropriate autoimmune reactions, leading to neuromuscular disorders such as proximal motor weakness from Lambert-Eaton myasthenic syndrome, encephalomyelitis from anti-Hu antibodies, or cerebellar degeneration from anti-Purkinje cell antibodies.[6] Although the hormone-mediated paraneoplastic syndromes often respond to effective anticancer therapy, the antibody-mediated neurologic disorders often persist even despite disease response.

Although the *American Joint Commission on Cancer, Seventh Edition* staging criteria include both NSCLC and SCLC,[7] in clinical practice few SCLCs are diagnosed as small, peripheral solitary nodules with lymph nodes isolated to the lung

Funding Support: Dr Neal receives clinical trial support from Genentech; Dr Gubens has no competing interests to disclose; Dr Wakelee receives clinical trial support from Genentech, Celgene, Novartis, and Pfizer.

[a] Stanford Cancer Institute, Department of Medicine, Stanford University, 875 Blake Wilbur Drive, Stanford, CA 94305-5826, USA
[b] Thoracic Oncology, University of California, San Francisco, 1600 Divisadero Street, A738, San Francisco, CA 94115-1770, USA
* Corresponding author.
E-mail address: jwneal@stanford.edu

Clin Chest Med 32 (2011) 853–863
doi:10.1016/j.ccm.2011.07.002
0272-5231/11/$ – see front matter © 2011 Elsevier Inc. All rights reserved.

(stage I–IIB). In contrast, the 2-stage Veterans Administration Lung Study Group staging system is a useful and simple staging system. Limited stage (LS) is disease contained within 1 hemithorax, including the primary tumor, mediastinal nodes, and ipsilateral supraclavicular disease. Extensive stage (ES) is disease that cannot be contained in a single radiotherapy portal, including overtly metastatic disease. Historically the staging workup included computed tomography (CT) scan of the torso, bone scan, brain magnetic resonance imaging or CT with contrast, and occasionally a bone marrow biopsy. [18F]fluorodeoxyglucose positron emission tomography/CT scans are sufficiently sensitive to replace the bone scan and biopsy, but cannot substitute for dedicated brain imaging. With modern staging tools, the proportion of patients diagnosed with ES-SCLC has increased from 50% to 75% over the last 30 years, but the prognosis of patients has changed minimally. The median overall survival (OS) in LS disease is approximately 20 months, with expected 5-year survival less than 15%. In ES disease the expected median survival is only 8 to 12 months, and less than 2% of patients survive past 5 years.[4] Therefore, it is hoped that ongoing clinical research will yield important advances in the treatment of SCLC.

STANDARD TREATMENT OF SCLC

The treatment of LS-SCLC involves multimodality therapy with concurrent thoracic radiotherapy and chemotherapy with cisplatin and etoposide,[8] based on a meta-analysis that showed a 14% reduction in the mortality of LS patients treated with radiotherapy in addition to chemotherapy.[9] Some treatment paradigms that have incrementally improved on this backbone of concurrent chemoradiation include the commencement of radiotherapy early in the course of treatment, consideration of twice-daily thoracic radiation over a shorter total course, and the use of prophylactic cranial irradiation (PCI) in selected patients. Addressing the optimal timing of initiation of radiation, a meta-analysis published in 2007 reported a significant OS benefit when radiotherapy started within 9 weeks of chemotherapy or before the third cycle of chemotherapy, particularly in patients who received hypofractionated (twice-daily) courses of radiation.[10] One commonly used schedule is twice-daily thoracic radiation given in 1.5-Gy fractions to 45 Gy over 3 weeks, based on a study among 419 patients that showed an improvement in median survival from 19 months to 23 months among patients receiving the accelerated course.[11] However, 1 criticism is that 45 Gy may be an inadequate dose of radiation,

compared with the more typical 60 to 70 Gy. To help address this question, another trial used a treatment break midway through in the hypofractionated arm to try to make the biologic effective doses more similar, and did not report a survival difference between the groups.[12] Therefore, the adoption of twice-daily radiotherapy in LS-SCLC has been limited. To provide more conclusive evidence regarding the best radiotherapy approach, an ongoing 3-arm intergroup trial randomizes patients to twice-daily standard radiation to 45 Gy, daily radiation to 70 Gy, or a hybrid of the 2 techniques (NCT00632853).

After completion of chemoradiotherapy, PCI should be considered in patients with systemic disease control and no evidence of metastases on repeat cranial imaging. A meta-analysis included 987 patients and reported a 5% absolute increase in the rate of 3-year survival in patients who received PCI as well as a decrease in the risk of brain metastases.[13] Doses of radiation used for PCI are generally lower than full treatment doses in patients with known brain metastases.

Although the single prospective randomized clinical trial that evaluated the role of surgery in SCLC reported no benefit for resection in patients who achieved a response to chemotherapy,[14] a recent retrospective review showed impressive 1-year and 5-year survival times of 75% and 50% among 59 patients who had undergone complete surgical resection.[15] Surgery seems to be most appropriately restricted to patients presenting with extremely limited disease (ie, clinical stage I by the American Joint Commission on Cancer criteria). Adjuvant chemotherapy and PCI should be considered in all patients who undergo surgical resection.

The standard treatment of ES-SCLC consists of chemotherapy alone, generally cisplatin or carboplatin plus etoposide for up to 6 cycles, followed by watchful waiting.[16] Even patients with an Eastern Cooperative Oncology Group (ECOG) performance status of 3 or 4 as a result of disease should be considered for treatment with chemotherapy, because response rates to chemotherapy exceed 75% and clinical improvement can be observed within a few days. After initial chemotherapy, PCI is recommended, as in LS disease, as a result of an improvement in 1-year OS of 15%.[17] However, mounting evidence suggests that PCI increases the chances of hair loss, fatigue, and cognitive impairment, and therefore may hinder quality of life in patients.[18] Despite rapid and impressive responses to initial chemotherapy, virtually all patients eventually relapse. The choice of subsequent treatment depends on the duration and magnitude of response to platinum-based chemotherapy. Patients with an initial response to treatment lasting more than 3 months from the completion of chemotherapy are considered chemotherapy sensitive. These patients have about a 25% chance of response to second-line treatment, in contrast with patients without an initial response or earlier relapse, who are considered refractory to chemotherapy and have a less than 10% chance of response. In patients with disease control for 12 months or more from the time of initial treatment, a second course of a platinum/etoposide regimen often can achieve disease control, although for a more limited period. Otherwise, salvage chemotherapy generally consists of non-platinum single-agent chemotherapy drugs; agents with efficacy in SCLC include camptothecins, taxanes, and gemcitabine. In the United States, topotecan is approved for the treatment of patients based on a phase III trial that showed a 25% response rate and more symptomatic improvement compared with a more toxic regimen of cyclophosphamide, doxorubicin, and vincristine.[19] An oral version of topotecan has also been approved with similar efficacy.[20,21] Other single agents can be used sequentially, with diminishing response rates and duration of response depending on the line of therapy, with few patients achieving disease control after the third line of treatment.[15,16] Therefore, most clinical trials of novel therapies are initially designed for patients with ES disease, with the goal that active drugs could be subsequently tested in the LS setting. The remainder of this article focuses on phase II and III clinical trials involving novel chemotherapeutics and targeted therapies in ES-SCLC.

RECENT CLINICAL TRIALS INVOLVING CHEMOTHERAPY
Irinotecan

Several older trials investigated alternatives to platinum plus etoposide, but failed to show superiority. For example, even although gemcitabine has single-agent activity in relapsed, refractory, and resistant SCLC,[22,23] carboplatin plus gemcitabine showed no additional efficacy over cisplatin/etoposide.[24] Similarly, phase III trials involving the addition of a third drug, including ifosfamide, epirubicin, or paclitaxel, to cisplatin and etoposide have all reported increased toxicity but no survival benefit.[25–27] However, a camptothecin, irinotecan, did show early promise as a replacement for etoposide in first-line treatment of ES-SCLC (Table 1).

A phase II study initially suggested activity of the topoisomerase I inhibitor topotecan, with response rates of 38% in sensitive patients and 6% in refractory patients,[28] and topotecan is approved for use in the United States in recurrent SCLC. Based on

this finding, the related agent irinotecan was paired with platinum agents in the frontline setting. In Japan, a phase III study in 2002 compared cisplatin/etoposide treatment with cisplatin and irinotecan. This study was terminated early because of an improvement in median OS in patients receiving irinotecan (60 mg/m^2 irinotecan given on days 1, 8, and 15 of a 3-week cycle) (12.8 months) compared with patients receiving etoposide (9.4 months).[29] Although this regimen was adopted as standard of care in Japan, concern remained that these results may not be applicable to Western countries. Therefore, 3 subsequent phase III studies were conducted using similar regimens. In the first, a modified dosing schedule of irinotecan (65 mg/m^2) was used, giving drug on days 1 and 8 of a 3-week cycle. Among 331 patients randomized in a 1:2 fashion to etoposide or irinotecan, no survival difference was observed, with 9.3 months on irinotecan and 10.2 months on etoposide. Another phase III trial was conducted with the same irinotecan dosing as in the Japanese study.[30] Among 651 patients, this trial also showed no difference in survival (9.9 months for irinotecan and 9.1 months for etoposide, $P = .71$), with more diarrhea on the irinotecan arm and more hematological toxicity on the etoposide arm. In a third trial, the more commonly used platinum chemotherapeutic carboplatin (area under the curve of 5 mg-min/mL) was combined with irinotecan (50 mg/m^2) on days 1, 8, and 15, and these were compared with carboplatin and etoposide. Of 216 evaluable patients, median survival was 10 months among patients receiving irinotecan and 9 months among patients receiving etoposide.[31] Platinum plus irinotecan is an acceptable alternative to platinum plus etoposide in the first-line treatment of ES-SCLC, but superiority and impressive median survival time of more than 12 months were not replicated in 3 subsequent Western trials.

Amrubicin

Amrubicin is a novel anthracycline derivative with antitumor activity based on inhibition of DNA topoisomerase II.[32] In contrast to the related compound doxorubicin, amrubicin has not been associated with cumulative cardiotoxicity in animal models or in subsequent human studies, but does have neutropenia as a dose-limiting toxicity.[33,34] Amrubicin has been approved in Japan for use in SCLC and NSCLC since 2006 based on promising phase II studies.[35] As a single agent in the first-line setting, amrubicin had a 75% response rate among 35 previously untreated patients,[36] and had an 89% response rate in combination with carboplatin in an elderly population.[37] A more recent study in

Table 1
Recent randomized clinical trials of chemotherapy in SCLC

Trial and Population	Agents	Patients (n)	Response Rate (%)	PFS (mo)	OS (mo)
JCOG 9511[29]	Cisplatin/**irinotecan**	75	84[a]	6.9[a]	12.8[a]
First-line	Cisplatin/etoposide	77	68	4.8	9.4
Hanna et al[86]	Cisplatin/**irinotecan**	221	48	4.1	9.3
First-line	Cisplatin/etoposide	110	44	4.6	10.2
SWOG S0124[30]	Cisplatin/**irinotecan**	324	60	5.8	9.9
First-line	Cisplatin/etoposide	327	57	5.2	9.1
Schmittel et al[31]	Carboplatin/**irinotecan**	106	54	6.0	10.0
First-line	Carboplatin/etoposide	110	52	6.0	9.0
North Japan 0402[41]	**Amrubicin**	29	38[a]	3.5	8.1
Relapsed/refractory	Topotecan	30	13	2.2	8.4
Jotte et al[45]	**Amrubicin**	50	44[a]	4.5	9.2
Relapsed/refractory, chemosensitive	Topotecan	26	15	3.3	7.6
SPEAR[51]	**Picoplatin**	268	4	2.1[a]	4.8
Refractory or resistant second-line	Best supportive care	133	0	1.5	4.6
GALES (Global Analysis of Pemetrexed in SCLC)[56]	Carboplatin/**pemetrexed**	453	31	3.8	8.1
First-line	Carboplatin/etoposide	455	52[a]	5.4[a]	10.6[a]
ACT-1[46]	**Amrubicin**	424	31[a]	4.1	7.5
Sensitive or refractory second-line	Topotecan	213	17	4.0	7.8

Boldface type, investigational agent.
[a] Statistically superior value in comparison with opposite arm, $P<.05$.

Table 2
Recent randomized clinical trials of antiangiogenic therapies in SCLC

Trial and Population	Agents	Patients (n)	Response Rate (%)	PFS (mo)	OS (mo)
Pujol et al[62]	Thalidomide	49	N/A	6.6	11.7
First-line with chemo, delayed start	Placebo	43	N/A	6.4	8.7
Lee et al[63]	Carboplatin/etoposide/thalidomide	177	80	7.6[a]	12.1
First-line LS	Carboplatin/etoposide/placebo	191	76	7.6[a]	13.1
Lee et al[63]	Carboplatin/etoposide/thalidomide	188	68	7.6[a]	8.0[b]
First-line ES	Carboplatin/etoposide/placebo	168	80	7.6[a]	9.1
SALUTE[70]	Platinum/etoposide/bevacizumab	50	48	5.5[b]	9.4
First-line	Platinum/etoposide/placebo	52	58	4.4	10.9

Abbreviation: N/A, not applicable (performed in patients selected for initial response).
[a] For combined LS and ES-SCLC groups; PFS not reported by stage.
[b] Statistically superior value with $P<.05$.

elderly patients was terminated early because of a 10% higher treatment-related death rate in the amrubicin arm, compared with carboplatin/etoposide, although there were no statistically significant differences between the 2 arms with respect to response, progression, survival, or quality of life.[38] The West Japan Thoracic Oncology Group investigated adding 3 cycles of amrubicin sequentially after 3 cycles of cisplatin and irinotecan in a single-arm phase II study, finding an overall response rate of 79% with 1 complete response among 45 patients. Median PFS was 6.5 months and OS was 15.4 months. Only 64% of patients were able to complete the entire planned course of treatment, with myelosuppression as the dominant toxicity.[39]

However, most development of amrubicin has been as a second-line agent. A phase II study of second-line use of amrubicin by the Thoracic Oncology Research Group in Japan (study 0301) showed a response rate of 52% among 44 platinum-sensitive patients and a 50% response rate among 16 platinum-refractory patients.[40] The North Japan Lung Cancer Study Group 0402 Trial randomized 60 patients (36 sensitive and 23 refractory) to amrubicin or topotecan as second-line treatment, with response rates of 38% in the amrubicin arm versus 13% for topotecan.[41] Recent single-arm phase II trials in Japan also piloted amrubicin in combination with other chemotherapy in the relapsed setting, and showed a 58% response rate using amrubicin plus carboplatin,[42] and a 43% response rate using amrubicin plus topotecan.[43] In a Western population, 75 patients with platinum-refractory SCLC were treated in a single-arm phase II study with amrubicin, with a lower response rate of 21% and a median OS of 6.0 months.[44] However, in a subsequent randomized phase II study in the United States comparing amrubicin with topotecan in 76 chemosensitive relapsed patients, results were closer to the Japanese data, with significantly higher response rate for amrubicin (44% vs 15%, $P = .21$), and trend toward better progression-free survival (PFS) (4.5 vs 3.3 months) and OS (9.2 vs 7.6 months).[45] Results of the international phase III ACT-1 trial were recently reported, in which 637 patients with sensitive or refractory SCLC were randomized in a 2:1 fashion to amrubicin versus topotecan.[46] Unfortunately, for amrubicin as compared with topotecan, there was an increase in response rate (31% vs 17%) but no difference in PFS (4.1 vs 4.0 months) or overall survival (7.5 vs 7.8 months). There was a trend toward an overall survival benefit among the 295 patients with refractory disease (6.2 vs 5.7 mo, HR 0.77, p = 0.047), but this small 15 day improvement may not be a clinically relevant difference. The future of this agent, which had received FDA "fast track" status in 2008, is uncertain at present.

Picoplatin

Picoplatin is an analogue of cisplatin that includes a large picoline ring intended to reduce susceptibility to certain mechanisms of platinum resistance.[47] Myelosuppression is the dose-limiting toxicity, with thrombocytopenia more common than neutropenia. Ototoxicity and nephrotoxicity are infrequent.[48] In a single-arm phase II trial of 37 patients, a response rate of 15% was observed among platinum-resistant patients and 8% among platinum-sensitive patients, with survival of 6.3 and 8.2 months, respectively.[49] In another trial of relapsed and refractory patients, treatment with picoplatin produced just a 4% response rate, although the disease control rate was 43% and median survival was 6.3 months.[50] Results were recently reported from the phase III SPEAR (Study of Picoplatin Efficacy After Relapse) trial, which randomized 401 relapsed or refractory patients to picoplatin or best supportive care.[51] The median survival time was similar between the groups: 4.8 months for picoplatin versus 4.6 months for BSC. However, a subgroup analysis revealed a modest survival advantage among platinum-refractory patients, with a significantly different median survival time of 4.9 months versus 4.3 months. Given the small magnitude of this difference and the failure to show improvement in OS, further development of picoplatin in SCLC is unlikely.

Pemetrexed

Pemetrexed is a multitargeted antimetabolite chemotherapy that inhibits essential enzymes for tumor nucleotide metabolism such as thymidylate synthase.[52] Pemetrexed has been shown to be effective and well tolerated in the treatment of NSCLC of adenocarcinoma histology.[53,54] In SCLC, a phase II study reported that the combination of pemetrexed with either cisplatin or carboplatin appeared tolerable, with a median OS of 10.4 months.[55] Based on this finding, a randomized phase III trial was conducted to compare carboplatin/etoposide with carboplatin/pemetrexed. An interim safety analysis halted enrollment halfway through because of inferior survival in the pemetrexed arm. Among 453 patients treated with carboplatin and pemetrexed, the response rate was 31% and OS was 8.1 months, compared with response rate of 52% and OS of 10.6 months in the carboplatin/etoposide arm.[56]

Even in relapsed or refractory patients, pemetrexed has minimal activity, with a response rate of less than 1%.[57] This situation may be because of the relatively higher expression of 1 target of pemetrexed, thymidylate synthase, compared with either the adenocarcinoma or squamous histologic subtypes of NSCLC.[58] Given the potential inferiority, the use of pemetrexed in SCLC is not recommended outside the scope of a clinical trial.

TARGETED THERAPIES
Thalidomide

Thalidomide is a small molecule with antitumor activity that may result from antiangiogenic effects, thereby depriving solid tumors of a blood supply.[59] In ES-SCLC, thalidomide has been tested in the frontline setting in several clinical trials. In a small phase II trial, thalidomide with carboplatin and etoposide yielded a response rate of 68%, with PFS of 8.1 months and median OS of 10.1 months and appeared to be safe.[60] A second phase II trial of a different design used maintenance thalidomide immediately after first-line chemotherapy. Although response rates were not meaningful in this study, the median OS was 12.8 months (Table 2).[61]

Based on these promising results and demonstration of tolerability, there were 2 randomized trials. One trial used a French backbone of cisplatin, etoposide, cyclophosphamide, and epirubicin for 2 cycles, followed by continuation of chemotherapy with the addition of thalidomide, 400 mg daily, or placebo.[62] In this relatively small trial of 92 patients, those who received thalidomide had a numerically better, but not statistically significant, median OS of 11.7 months compared with 8.7 months among patients treated with placebo ($P = .16$). To confirm this trend in a larger setting, another trial randomized 724 patients with both ES-SCLC and LS-SCLC to thalidomide (200 mg daily) or placebo.[63] This study showed no survival difference between the treatment groups with LS disease, but among patients with ES-SCLC, the median OS was significantly worse in patients treated with thalidomide (8.0 months) compared with patients treated with placebo (9.1 months). The patients treated with thalidomide had almost a 20% incidence of thrombotic events, including deep venous thrombosis and pulmonary embolism, compared with 10% in the placebo group, suggesting this difference in survival may have been related to side effects. Thalidomide was also associated with a higher incidence of grade 3 or 4 neuropathy in this trial, leading to the conclusion that thalidomide should be avoided in the treatment of SCLC.

Antiangiogenesis Agents: Bevacizumab

Treatment with bevacizumab, a monoclonal antibody that targets vascular endothelial growth factor (VEGF), results in deprivation of a growth factor that is necessary to support the growth of macroscopic tumors.[64] In NSCLC, the addition of bevacizumab to carboplatin and paclitaxel improves OS.[65] In SCLC, the ECOG 3501 single-arm phase II trial tested the addition of bevacizumab to cisplatin/etoposide in 63 patients, with a response rate of 63%, PFS of 4.7 months, and median OS of 10.9 months. One patient experienced a grade 3 pulmonary hemorrhage.[66] Two single-arm phase II trials also were conducted combining bevacizumab with platinum and irinotecan. One used carboplatin in the combination with a response rate of 84%, a median PFS of 9.1 months, and a median OS of 12.1 months,[67] whereas a larger study using cisplatin showed a response rate of 75%, a median PFS of 7.1 months, and median OS of 11.7 months.[68] Bevacizumab was also incorporated into the treatment of LS-SCLC in combination with radiation and carboplatin/irinotecan-based chemotherapy. Among 29 treated patients, 2 developed tracheoesophageal fistulae, 1 fatal, and a third patient died of aerodigestive hemorrhage, prompting early closure of the study and a recommendation to avoid bevacizumab in the setting of concurrent radiotherapy.[69] However, randomized clinical trials have been conducted only with the platinum/etoposide backbone. In the SALUTE (Study of Bevacizumab in Previously Untreated Extensive-Stage Small-Cell Lung Cancer) phase II trial, 102 patients were randomized to 4 cycles of treatment with carboplatin or cisplatin and etoposide, with and without bevacizumab. In a preliminary report of this trial, patients who received bevacizumab had a significantly better PFS (5.5 months vs 4.4 months without bevacizumab).[70] However, patients who received chemotherapy plus bevacizumab had no difference in OS (9.4 months) compared with patients who received chemotherapy plus placebo (10.9 months). Based on this finding, there are no reported plans for a phase III trial randomized trial of bevacizumab in SCLC.

Antiangiogenic Tyrosine Kinase Inhibitors

Sorafenib, a small molecule tyrosine kinase inhibitor, has antiangiogenic and antiproliferative properties based on its ability to inhibit B-raf and the VEGF receptors VEGFR1, 2, and 3. Sorafenib has been tested in several different solid tumors and has proven efficacy in renal cell carcinoma and hepatocellular carcinoma.[71,72] Toxicities typically include fatigue, rash, hand-foot syndrome, and gastrointestinal disorders. This drug seems to have modest activity in SCLC, as shown by a phase II trial.[73] Among 38 patients with platinum-sensitive disease, 4 partial responses were seen (11% response rate), with PFS of 2.2 months and OS of 5.3 months. Among 45 patients with platinum-refractory disease, the response rate was 2%, with PFS of 2.0 months and OS of 6.7 months. Although this study did not show sufficient signal to further pursue development of single-agent sorafenib in SCLC, a phase I/II trial is ongoing in combination with chemotherapy (NCT00726986).

Sunitinib is another tyrosine kinase inhibitor that inhibits the VEGFR, platelet-derived growth factor (PDGF) receptor, and the KIT receptors. Two front-line clinical trials are currently in the enrollment phase, including a randomized phase II cooperative group study in combination with platinum/etoposide (NCT00453154), and a trial in patients with stable disease as a maintenance agent after initial chemotherapy (NCT00616109). A phase II study is also being conducted with the related VEGFR, PDGF, and c-kit inhibitor, pazopanib, in patients with relapsed or refractory disease (NCT01253369). These phase II studies will ideally help to define the role of VEGF inhibitors in the treatment of SCLC.

Other Agents

As the molecular pathways leading to tumorigenesis in SCLC have been elucidated, efforts have been made to incorporate targeted agents into clinical trials. Some specific pathways of interest include apoptosis, the mTOR (mammalian target of rapamycin) signaling pathway, and the hedgehog (Hh) signaling pathway as possible targets.

Avoidance of normal programmed cell death (apoptosis) is 1 mechanism of resistance to chemotherapy, and the Bcl-2 protein seems to mediate resistance to chemotherapy-induced apoptosis in many SCLCs.[74] Navitoclax (ABT-263) is a small molecule that acts as a BH3 mimetic, thereby lowering the cellular threshold for apoptosis by inhibiting Bcl-2. In a phase I safety study, including 29 patients with relapsed or refractory SCLC and pulmonary carcinoid, 8 patients had stable disease and 1 patient with SCLC had a response that lasted 2 years.[75] Up to 40% of patients experienced diarrhea, nausea, vomiting, and fatigue. With some evidence of activity in this study, ongoing development includes a trial to investigate the safety of the combination of navitoclax together with cisplatin and etoposide (NCT00878449).

An alternative, but unproductive strategy that was attempted to target Bcl-2 was the antisense oligonucleotide, oblimersen, which appeared safe in combination with chemotherapy in phase I studies.[76] However, in a small randomized phase II

study of 56 patients, survival was worse in patients receiving oblimersen compared with placebo with carboplatin and etoposide, suggesting that further development will not take place.[77]

The mTOR and PI3K/AKT kinase signaling pathways are also active in many malignancies and regulate processes from cellular proliferation to control of apoptosis. Everolimus is a rapamycin derivative that inhibits mTOR that is approved by the US Food and Drug Administration for treatment of advanced kidney cancer. In SCLC, an early report of a phase II trial showed some activity in patients with relapsed and refractory disease. Among 35 evaluable patients, there was 1 patient who responded and 8 patients with stable disease, with median PFS of 1.4 months and median OS of 5.5 months.[78] There is an ongoing frontline clinical trial with everolimus in combination with carboplatin and etoposide (NCT00466466); based on the final results from these studies further development will be determined.

The Hh signaling pathway is critical for normal growth and development, and many lung cancer cell lines are dependent on this pathway for survival.[79] Hh signaling may be critical for the survival and self-renewal of a small number of cancer stem cells, which are often resistant to chemotherapy and may be responsible for tumor resistance in SCLC.[80] Derivatives of a naturally occurring inhibitor of this pathway, cyclopamine, have elicited remarkable responses in patients with metastatic basal cell cancer and medulloblastoma.[81,82] In SCLC, an ongoing cooperative group clinical trial, ECOG 1508, is a first-line study with cisplatin and etoposide, in combination with either the Hh inhibitor GDC0449 or the insulinlike growth factor 1 receptor (IGF-1R) antibody cixutumumab (NCT00887159). The addition of the IGF-1R antibody based on preclinical evidence inhibition of this pathway may potentiate chemotherapy, epidermal growth factor receptor inhibitors, and even radiation effects in lung cancer cell lines.[83–85] This trial may show whether inhibitors of either of these pathways have activity in SCLC.

SUMMARY

Despite numerous clinical trials and excellent responses to first-line chemotherapy, there have been few substantial clinical advances in the treatment of ES SCLC over the last 30 years. Irinotecan is an active agent both in combination with platinum agents and in the second-line setting, but pemetrexed and picoplatin seem to be relatively ineffective. The novel anthracycline amrubicin showed early promise in small clinical trials, but unfortunately was not superior to topotecan.

Inhibitors of angiogenesis, although conceptually promising, have not yielded additional clinical benefit. It is hoped that future advances in the biology of the disease will lead to the development of effective targeted therapies.

REFERENCES

1. American Cancer Society. Cancer facts & figures 2010. Atlanta (GA): American Cancer Society; 2010.
2. Mathers C, Fat DM. The global burden of disease: 2004 update. Geneva (Switzerland): WHO Press; 2004.
3. Govindan R, Page N, Morgensztern D, et al. Changing epidemiology of small-cell lung cancer in the United States over the last 30 years: analysis of the surveillance, epidemiologic, and end results database. J Clin Oncol 2006;24(28):4539–44.
4. Lally BE, Urbanic JJ, Blackstock AW, et al. Small cell lung cancer: have we made any progress over the last 25 years? Oncologist 2007;12(9):1096–104.
5. Dowell JE. Small cell lung cancer: are we making progress? Am J Med Sci 2010;339(1):68–76.
6. Dropcho EJ. Update on paraneoplastic syndromes. Curr Opin Neurol 2005;18(3):331–6.
7. Goldstraw P, Crowley J, Chansky K, et al. The IASLC Lung Cancer Staging Project: proposals for the revision of the TNM stage groupings in the forthcoming (seventh) edition of the TNM Classification of malignant tumours. J Thorac Oncol 2007;2(8): 706–14.
8. Stinchcombe TE, Gore EM. Limited-stage small cell lung cancer: current chemoradiotherapy treatment paradigms. Oncologist 2010;15(2):187–95.
9. Pignon JP, Arriagada R, Ihde DC, et al. A meta-analysis of thoracic radiotherapy for small-cell lung cancer. N Engl J Med 1992;327(23):1618–24.
10. Fried DB, Morris DE, Poole C, et al. Systematic review evaluating the timing of thoracic radiation therapy in combined modality therapy for limited-stage small-cell lung cancer. J Clin Oncol 2004; 22(23):4837–45.
11. Turrisi AT 3rd, Kim K, Blum R, et al. Twice-daily compared with once-daily thoracic radiotherapy in limited small-cell lung cancer treated concurrently with cisplatin and etoposide. N Engl J Med 1999; 340(4):265–71.
12. Schild SE, Bonner JA, Shanahan TG, et al. Long-term results of a phase III trial comparing once-daily radiotherapy with twice-daily radiotherapy in limited-stage small-cell lung cancer. Int J Radiat Oncol Biol Phys 2004;59(4):943–51.
13. Auperin A, Arriagada R, Pignon JP, et al. Prophylactic cranial irradiation for patients with small-cell lung cancer in complete remission. Prophylactic Cranial Irradiation Overview Collaborative Group. N Engl J Med 1999;341(7):476–84.
14. Lad T, Piantadosi S, Thomas P, et al. A prospective randomized trial to determine the benefit of surgical resection of residual disease following response of small cell lung cancer to combination chemotherapy. Chest 1994;106(Suppl 6):320S–3S.
15. Lim E, Belcher E, Yap YK, et al. The role of surgery in the treatment of limited disease small cell lung cancer: time to reevaluate. J Thorac Oncol 2008;3(11):1267–71.
16. Evans WK, Shepherd FA, Feld R, et al. VP-16 and cisplatin as first-line therapy for small-cell lung cancer. J Clin Oncol 1985;3(11):1471–7.
17. Slotman B, Faivre-Finn C, Kramer G, et al. Prophylactic cranial irradiation in extensive small-cell lung cancer. N Engl J Med 2007;357(7):664–72.
18. Slotman BJ, Mauer ME, Bottomley A, et al. Prophylactic cranial irradiation in extensive disease small-cell lung cancer: short-term health-related quality of life and patient reported symptoms–results of an international Phase III randomized controlled trial by the EORTC Radiation Oncology and Lung Cancer Groups. J Clin Oncol 2008;27(1):78–84.
19. von Pawel J, Schiller JH, Shepherd FA, et al. Topotecan versus cyclophosphamide, doxorubicin, and vincristine for the treatment of recurrent small-cell lung cancer. J Clin Oncol 1999;17(2):658–67.
20. Eckardt JR, von Pawel J, Pujol JL, et al. Phase III study of oral compared with intravenous topotecan as second-line therapy in small-cell lung cancer. J Clin Oncol 2007;25(15):2086–92.
21. O'Brien ME, Ciuleanu TE, Tsekov H, et al. Phase III trial comparing supportive care alone with supportive care with oral topotecan in patients with relapsed small-cell lung cancer. J Clin Oncol 2006; 24(34):5441–7.
22. Masters GA, Declerck L, Blanke C, et al. Phase II trial of gemcitabine in refractory or relapsed small-cell lung cancer: Eastern Cooperative Oncology Group Trial 1597. J Clin Oncol 2003;21(8):1550–5.
23. van der Lee I, Smit EF, van Putten JW, et al. Single-agent gemcitabine in patients with resistant small-cell lung cancer. Ann Oncol 2001;12(4):557–61.
24. Lee SM, James LE, Qian W, et al. Comparison of gemcitabine and carboplatin versus cisplatin and etoposide for patients with poor-prognosis small cell lung cancer. Thorax 2009;64(1):75–80.
25. Loehrer PJ Sr, Ansari R, Gonin R, et al. Cisplatin plus etoposide with and without ifosfamide in extensive small-cell lung cancer: a Hoosier Oncology Group study. J Clin Oncol 1995;13(10):2594–9.
26. Pujol JL, Daures JP, Riviere A, et al. Etoposide plus cisplatin with or without the combination of 4'-epidoxorubicin plus cyclophosphamide in treatment of extensive small-cell lung cancer: a French Federation of Cancer Institutes multicenter phase III randomized study. J Natl Cancer Inst 2001;93(4):300–8.
27. Niell HB, Herndon JE 2nd, Miller AA, et al. Randomized phase III intergroup trial of etoposide and

cisplatin with or without paclitaxel and granulocyte colony-stimulating factor in patients with extensive-stage small-cell lung cancer: Cancer and Leukemia Group B Trial 9732. J Clin Oncol 2005;23(16):3752–9.

28. Ardizzoni A, Hansen H, Dombernowsky P, et al. Topotecan, a new active drug in the second-line treatment of small-cell lung cancer: a phase II study in patients with refractory and sensitive disease. The European Organization for Research and Treatment of Cancer Early Clinical Studies Group and New Drug Development Office, and the Lung Cancer Cooperative Group. J Clin Oncol 1997; 15(5):2090–6.

29. Noda K, Nishiwaki Y, Kawahara M, et al. Irinotecan plus cisplatin compared with etoposide plus cisplatin for extensive small-cell lung cancer. N Engl J Med 2002;346(2):85–91.

30. Lara PN, Natale R, Crowley J, et al. Phase III trial of irinotecan/cisplatin compared with etoposide/cisplatin in extensive-stage small-cell lung cancer: clinical and pharmacogenomic results from SWOG S0124. J Clin Oncol 2009;27(15):2530–5.

31. Schmittel A, Sebastian M, Fischer von Weikersthal L, et al. A German multicenter, randomized phase III trial comparing irinotecan-carboplatin with etoposide-carboplatin as first-line therapy for extensive-disease small-cell lung cancer. Ann Oncol 2011; 22(8):1798–804.

32. Hanada M, Mizuno S, Fukushima A, et al. A new antitumor agent amrubicin induces cell growth inhibition by stabilizing topoisomerase II-DNA complex. Jpn J Cancer Res 1998;89(11):1229–38.

33. Noda T, Watanabe T, Kohda A, et al. Chronic effects of a novel synthetic anthracycline derivative (SM-5887) on normal heart and doxorubicin-induced cardiomyopathy in beagle dogs. Invest New Drugs 1998;16(2):121–8.

34. Inoue K, Ogawa M, Horikoshi N, et al. Phase I and pharmacokinetic study of SM-5887, a new anthracycline derivative. Invest New Drugs 1989;7(2–3): 213–8.

35. Ettinger DS. Amrubicin for the treatment of small cell lung cancer: does effectiveness cross the Pacific? J Thorac Oncol 2007;2(2):160–5.

36. Yana T, Negoro S, Takada M, et al. Phase II study of amrubicin in previously untreated patients with extensive-disease small cell lung cancer: West Japan Thoracic Oncology Group (WJTOG) study. Invest New Drugs 2007;25(3):253–8.

37. Inoue A, Ishimoto O, Fukumoto S, et al. A phase II study of amrubicin combined with carboplatin for elderly patients with small-cell lung cancer: North Japan Lung Cancer Study Group Trial 0405. Ann Oncol 2010;21(4):800–3.

38. Hida N, Okamoto H, Horai T, et al. Results of a randomized phase III study of single-agent amrubicin versus carboplatin and etoposide in elderly

patients with extensive-disease small cell lung cancer. Ann Oncol 2010;21(Suppl 8):[abstract: 442].

39. Kobayashi M, Matsui K, Iwamoto Y, et al. Phase II study of sequential triplet chemotherapy, irinotecan and cisplatin followed by amrubicin, in patients with extensive-stage small cell lung cancer: West Japan Thoracic Oncology Group Study 0301. J Thorac Oncol 2010;5(7):1075–80.

40. Onoda S, Masuda N, Seto T, et al. Phase II trial of amrubicin for treatment of refractory or relapsed small-cell lung cancer: Thoracic Oncology Research Group Study 0301. J Clin Oncol 2006;24(34):5448–53.

41. Inoue A, Sugawara S, Yamazaki K, et al. Randomized phase II trial comparing amrubicin with topotecan in patients with previously treated small-cell lung cancer: North Japan Lung Cancer Study Group Trial 0402. J Clin Oncol 2008;26(33):5401–6.

42. Hirose T, Nakashima M, Shirai T, et al. Phase II trial of amrubicin and carboplatin in patients with sensitive or refractory relapsed small-cell lung cancer. Lung Cancer 2011;73(3):345–50.

43. Nogami N, Hotta K, Kuyama S, et al. A phase II study of amrubicin and topotecan combination therapy in patients with relapsed or extensive-disease small-cell lung cancer: Okayama Lung Cancer Study Group Trial 0401. Lung Cancer 2011 [in press].

44. Ettinger DS, Jotte R, Lorigan P, et al. Phase II study of amrubicin as second-line therapy in patients with platinum-refractory small-cell lung cancer. J Clin Oncol 2010;28(15):2598–603.

45. Jotte R, Conkling P, Reynolds C, et al. Randomized phase II trial of single-agent amrubicin or topotecan as second-line treatment in patients with small-cell lung cancer sensitive to first-line platinum-based chemotherapy. J Clin Oncol 2011;29(3):287–93.

46. Jotte R, Pawel JV, Spigel DR, et al. Randomized phase III trial of amrubicin versus topotecan (Topo) as second-line treatment for small cell lung cancer (SCLC). J Clin Oncol 2011;29(Suppl):[abstract: 7000].

47. Kelland L. The resurgence of platinum-based cancer chemotherapy. Nat Rev Cancer 2007;7(8): 573–84.

48. Beale P, Judson I, O'Donnell A, et al. A Phase I clinical and pharmacological study of cis-diamminedichloro(2-methylpyridine) platinum II (AMD473). Br J Cancer 2003;88(7):1128–34.

49. Treat J, Schiller J, Quoix E, et al. ZD0473 treatment in lung cancer: an overview of the clinical trial results. Eur J Cancer 2002;38(Suppl 8):S13–8.

50. Eckardt JR, Bentsion DL, Lipatov ON, et al. Phase II study of picoplatin as second-line therapy for patients with small-cell lung cancer. J Clin Oncol 2009;27(12):2046–51.

51. Ciuleanu T, Samarzjia M, Demidchik Y, et al. Randomized phase III study (SPEAR) of picoplatin plus best

supportive care (BSC) or BSC alone in patients (pts) with SCLC refractory or progressive within 6 months after first-line platinum-based chemotherapy. J Clin Oncol 2010;28(15s):[abstract: 7002].

52. Adjei AA. Pemetrexed (ALIMTA), a novel multitargeted antineoplastic agent. Clin Cancer Res 2004; 10(12 Pt 2):4276s–80s.

53. Scagliotti GV, Parikh P, von Pawel J, et al. Phase III study comparing cisplatin plus gemcitabine with cisplatin plus pemetrexed in chemotherapy-naive patients with advanced-stage non-small-cell lung cancer. J Clin Oncol 2008;26(21):3543–51.

54. Hanna N, Shepherd FA, Fossella FV, et al. Randomized phase III trial of pemetrexed versus docetaxel in patients with non-small-cell lung cancer previously treated with chemotherapy. J Clin Oncol 2004;22(9):1589–97.

55. Socinski MA, Weissman C, Hart LL, et al. Randomized phase II trial of pemetrexed combined with either cisplatin or carboplatin in untreated extensive-stage small-cell lung cancer. J Clin Oncol 2006;24(30):4840–7.

56. Socinski MA, Smit EF, Lorigan P, et al. Phase III study of pemetrexed plus carboplatin compared with etoposide plus carboplatin in chemotherapy-naive patients with extensive-stage small-cell lung cancer. J Clin Oncol 2009;27(28):4787–92.

57. Socinski MA, Raju RN, Neubauer M, et al. Pemetrexed in relapsed small-cell lung cancer and the impact of shortened vitamin supplementation lead-in time: results of a phase II trial. J Thorac Oncol 2008;3(11):1308–16.

58. Monica V, Scagliotti GV, Ceppi P, et al. Differential thymidylate synthase expression in different variants of large-cell carcinoma of the lung. Clin Cancer Res 2009;15(24):7547–52.

59. D'Amato RJ, Loughnan MS, Flynn E, et al. Thalidomide is an inhibitor of angiogenesis. Proc Natl Acad Sci U S A 1994;91(9):4082–5.

60. Lee SM, James L, Buchler T, et al. Phase II trial of thalidomide with chemotherapy and as maintenance therapy for patients with poor prognosis small-cell lung cancer. Lung Cancer 2008;59(3):364–8.

61. Dowlati A, Subbiah S, Cooney M, et al. Phase II trial of thalidomide as maintenance therapy for extensive stage small cell lung cancer after response to chemotherapy. Lung Cancer 2007; 56(3):377–81.

62. Pujol JL, Breton JL, Gervais R, et al. Phase III double-blind, placebo-controlled study of thalidomide in extensive-disease small-cell lung cancer after response to chemotherapy: an intergroup study FNCLCC cleo04 IFCT 00-01. J Clin Oncol 2007;25(25):3945–51.

63. Lee SM, Woll PJ, Rudd R, et al. Anti-angiogenic therapy using thalidomide combined with chemotherapy in small cell lung cancer: a randomized, double-blind, placebo-controlled trial. J Natl Cancer Inst 2009;101(15):1049–57.

64. Folkman J. Angiogenesis. Annu Rev Med 2006;57: 1–18.

65. Sandler A, Gray R, Perry MC, et al. Paclitaxel-carboplatin alone or with bevacizumab for non-small-cell lung cancer. N Engl J Med 2006;355(24):2542–50.

66. Horn L, Dahlberg SE, Sandler AB, et al. Phase II study of cisplatin plus etoposide and bevacizumab for previously untreated, extensive-stage small-cell lung cancer: Eastern Cooperative Oncology Group Study E3501. J Clin Oncol 2009;27(35):6006–11.

67. Spigel DR, Greco FA, Zubkus JD, et al. Phase II trial of irinotecan, carboplatin, and bevacizumab in the treatment of patients with extensive-stage small-cell lung cancer. J Thorac Oncol 2009; 4(12):1555–60.

68. Ready N, Dudek AZ, Wang XF, et al. CALGB 30306: a phase II study of cisplatin (C), irinotecan (I) and bevacizumab (B) for untreated extensive stage small cell lung cancer (ES-SCLC). J Clin Oncol 2010;25(18s):[abstract: 7563].

69. Spigel DR, Hainsworth JD, Yardley DA, et al. Tracheoesophageal fistula formation in patients with lung cancer treated with chemoradiation and bevacizumab. J Clin Oncol 2010;28(1):43–8.

70. Spigel D, Townley P, Waterhouse D, et al. SALUTE: a placebo-controlled, double-blind, multicenter, randomized, phase II study of bevacizumab in previously untreated extensive-stage small cell lung cancer (SCLC). J Thorac Oncol 2009;4(9 Suppl 1): S398:[abstract: D396.394].

71. Escudier B, Eisen T, Stadler WM, et al. Sorafenib in advanced clear-cell renal-cell carcinoma. N Engl J Med 2007;356(2):125–34.

72. Llovet JM, Ricci S, Mazzaferro V, et al. Sorafenib in advanced hepatocellular carcinoma. N Engl J Med 2008;359(4):378–90.

73. Gitlitz BJ, Moon J, Glisson BS, et al. Sorafenib in platinum-treated patients with extensive stage small cell lung cancer: a Southwest Oncology Group (SWOG 0435) phase II trial. J Thorac Oncol 2010; 5(11):1835–40.

74. Mortenson MM, Schlieman MG, Virudachalam S, et al. Reduction in BCL-2 levels by 26S proteasome inhibition with bortezomib is associated with induction of apoptosis in small cell lung cancer. Lung Cancer 2005;49(2):163–70.

75. Gandhi L, Camidge DR, Ribeiro de Oliveira M, et al. Phase I study of Navitoclax (ABT-263), a novel Bcl-2 family inhibitor, in patients with small-cell lung cancer and other solid tumors. J Clin Oncol 2011; 29(7):909–16.

76. Rudin CM, Kozloff M, Hoffman PC, et al. Phase I study of G3139, a bcl-2 antisense oligonucleotide, combined with carboplatin and etoposide in patients with small-cell lung cancer. J Clin Oncol 2004;22(6):1110–7.

77. Rudin CM, Salgia R, Wang X, et al. Randomized phase II study of carboplatin and etoposide with or without the bcl-2 antisense oligonucleotide oblimersen for extensive-stage small-cell lung cancer: CALGB 30103. J Clin Oncol 2008;26(6):870–6.

78. Kotsakis AP, Tarhini A, Petro D, et al. Phase II study of RAD001 (everolimus) in previously treated small cell lung cancer (SCLC). J Clin Oncol 2009; 27(15s):[abstract: 8107]. PMID: 21045083.

79. Watkins DN, Berman DM, Burkholder SG, et al. Hedgehog signalling within airway epithelial progenitors and in small-cell lung cancer. Nature 2003; 422(6929):313–7.

80. Zhao C, Chen A, Jamieson CH, et al. Hedgehog signalling is essential for maintenance of cancer stem cells in myeloid leukaemia. Nature 2009;458(7239): 776–9.

81. Rudin CM, Hann CL, Laterra J, et al. Treatment of medulloblastoma with hedgehog pathway inhibitor GDC-0449. N Engl J Med 2009;361(12):1173–8.

82. Von Hoff DD, LoRusso PM, Rudin CM, et al. Inhibition of the hedgehog pathway in advanced basal-cell carcinoma. N Engl J Med 2009;361(12):1164–72.

83. Lee YJ, Imsumran A, Park MY, et al. Adenovirus expressing shRNA to IGF-1R enhances the chemosensitivity of lung cancer cell lines by blocking IGF-1 pathway. Lung Cancer 2007;55(3):279–86.

84. Guix M, Faber AC, Wang SE, et al. Acquired resistance to EGFR tyrosine kinase inhibitors in cancer cells is mediated by loss of IGF-binding proteins. J Clin Invest 2008;118(7):2609–19.

85. Iwasa T, Okamoto I, Suzuki M, et al. Inhibition of insulin-like growth factor 1 receptor by CP-751,871 radiosensitizes non-small cell lung cancer cells. Clin Cancer Res 2009;15(16):5117–25.

86. Hanna N, Bunn PA Jr, Langer C, et al. Randomized phase III trial comparing irinotecan/cisplatin with etoposide/cisplatin in patients with previously untreated extensive-stage disease small-cell lung cancer. J Clin Oncol 2006;24(13):2038–43.

Gene Therapy for Lung Neoplasms

Anil Vachani, MD[a], Edmund Moon, MD[a],
Elliot Wakeam, MD[b], Andrew R. Haas, MD, PhD[a],
Daniel H. Sterman, MD[a], Steven M. Albelda, MD[a,*]

KEYWORDS

- Gene therapy • Immunotherapy
- Lung cancer • Mesothelioma

Approximately 20 years ago, advances in molecular genetics and gene transfer technology made the development of gene therapy (the modification of the genetic makeup of cells for therapeutic purposes) a clinical possibility. The disorders originally proposed as targets for gene therapy were the inherited, recessive disorders in which transfer of a normal copy of a single defective gene could potentially prevent or alter the course of a disease. Clear, but slow progress has been made in the areas of genetic diseases such as blindness[1] and inherited immune deficiencies.[2] It soon became apparent that the range of target diseases could be extended to acquired diseases, such as cancer, and many early-phase clinical trials have now been conducted in various malignancies. The good news is that most trials have shown good safety. The bad news is that there has been relatively limited efficacy.

Despite advances in chemotherapy, radiation therapy, and surgery for lung cancer, the 5-year survival rate remains poor at 15% and has improved only minimally over the last 2 decades. This situation coupled with the advances that have been made in the understanding of molecular events leading to cancer development has led to great interest in gene therapy approaches for thoracic malignancies. Lung cancer is usually metastatic at the time of diagnosis and thus requires systemic, rather than local, therapy.

Systemic therapy using gene therapy has remained largely impossible.

Malignant pleural mesothelioma (MPM) accounts for 80% of mesothelioma cases and usually presents in the fifth to seventh decade of life with dyspnea, pleural effusion, and nonpleuritic chest pain in the context of an asbestos exposure history. With a disease course affected only minimally by current treatments, MPM has a poor prognosis (median survival of 6–18 months) except in the rare cases in which it can be completely resected. MPM is a potentially good disease target for gene therapy because the thin layer of mesothelial and malignant cells offers a large surface area for efficient, rapid, and diffuse gene transfer.

The purpose of this article is to review the clinical experience in gene therapy for thoracic malignancies and to reflect on the future directions of this approach.

VECTORS USED IN GENE THERAPY

Gene delivery efficiency is an important requirement for successful gene therapy. To this end, various viral and nonviral vectors have been engineered, including replicating and nonreplicating viruses, bacteria, and liposomes.[3] Each varies in regards to the targeted cell type, DNA carrying capacity, in vivo gene transfer efficiency, and inflammatory response induced. Although no 1

This work was supported by Grant P01 CA66726 from the National Cancer Institute. A.V. is supported by NCI K07 CA111952.
The authors have nothing to disclose.
[a] Division of Pulmonary, Allergy & Critical Care Medicine, University of Pennsylvania, 3400 Spruce Street, Philadelphia, PA 19104, USA
[b] Department of Surgery, University of Toronto, 100 College Street, Toronto, ON M5G 1L5, Canada
* Corresponding author. University of Pennsylvania, 1016B Abramson Research Center, 3615 Civic Center Boulevard, Philadelphia, PA 19104-6160.
E-mail address: albelda@mail.med.upenn.edu

Clin Chest Med 32 (2011) 865–885
doi:10.1016/j.ccm.2011.08.006
0272-5231/11/$ – see front matter © 2011 Elsevier Inc. All rights reserved.

chestmed.theclinics.com

vector is suitable for all diseases, one can tailor the vector to the specific disease of interest.

Adenovirus

The most widely used vector is the recombinant, replication-incompetent adenovirus. Several characteristics of the adenoviral vector make it attractive for gene therapy for cancer (but not genetic diseases). It is able to transfect various target cell types, even when nondividing, with high efficiency rates, and is able to accomplish high-level but transient gene transfection.[4,5] Adenoviral-based delivery is accompanied by significant local and systemic inflammation: an early innate component involving a cytokine surge and a later acquired immune response involving neutralizing antibodies and cytotoxic lymphocytes. The safety record of adenoviral vectors in humans has been excellent.

Retrovirus

The principal advantages of this vector derive from its ability to accomplish efficient gene transfer in vitro in a broad range of targeted cells, with the capacity to achieve integration into the host genome and long-term expression. However, retroviral vectors can achieve gene transfer only to dividing cells and are labile in vivo because complement and other components inactivate the virion.

Lentiviruses

To circumvent the inability of retroviruses to infect nondividing cells, vector systems based on the lentivirus genus of retroviruses, which includes human immunodeficiency virus, have been developed.[6,7] Because these viruses are more complex than other retroviruses, and because of obvious safety concerns, development has been slow and cautious. We are not aware of the use of lentivirus yet for thoracic malignancies.

Adeno-Associated Virus

Another viral vector that has generated interest is the adeno-associated virus (AAV),[8,9] a defective parvovirus with a single-strand DNA genome and a naked protein coat. AAV has not been associated with any known human disease state, suggesting a significant safety margin for this vector.

Vaccinia/Fowlpox Vectors

Vaccinia is a double-stranded DNA virus the entire life cycle of which takes place within the cytoplasm of infected cells. Because of its role in the eradication of smallpox, it has been used extensively in humans and is safe. Vaccinia is being explored as a vector for delivery of cancer therapeutic genes, as a carrier for tumor antigens or immunostimulatory molecules to develop cancer vaccines, and as a replication-selective, tumor-specific oncolytic virus.[10,11] The related fowlpox vectors have been used primarily as cancer vaccines.

Nonviral Vectors

As an alternative to the viral vectors, a variety of nonviral vectors have also been developed for in vivo and in vitro gene delivery. Several general strategies have been developed to achieve this end, including liposomes, polymers, and molecular conjugates.[12,13] For the most part, these strategies seem to be less efficient than the various viral vectors described earlier and they do not result in prolonged transgene expression.

Antisense Therapy

Antisense therapy relies on inhibition of gene expression, accomplished with a targeted oligonucleotide delivered either intravenously or intratumorally, leading to diminished transcription of the complementary mRNA. The oligonucleotide is usually modified to enhance stability. More recently, siRNA has been used in preclinical models, but has not yet moved to clinical trials.

CLINICAL TRIALS IN LUNG CANCER

The number of potential cancer gene therapy strategies is limited only by the imagination of investigators and many have been proposed and tested in preclinical models. However, many fewer have been tested in clinical trials. These strategies are discussed below and summarized in **Tables 1–3**.

Replacement of Tumor Suppressor Genes

Tumor suppressor genes may undergo homozygous loss of function by a variety of mechanisms including mutation, deletion, and methylation, or a combination of these. The rationale for this approach is to use a gene therapy vector to encode a tumor suppressor gene that is mutated or absent in most lung cancers. Theoretically, replacement of a nonfunctional copy of a tumor suppressor gene could lead to suppression of tumor growth or tumor cell death in vivo.

Tumor-based p53 therapy
Cellular and animals studies have shown that replacement of the normal p53 tumor suppressor gene in tumor cells induced rapid cell death. The strategy of restoring wild-type p53 expression in

lung tumor cells has been evaluated in several early-phase clinical trials (see **Table 1**). In the earliest phase I study, a retrovirus vector carrying wild-type p53 was administered to 9 patients with lung cancer by direct intratumoral injection.[14] In 6 cases, there was evidence of increased apoptosis, and tumor regression at the site of injection was observed in 3 of the patients, but all 3 had progression of their disease at mediastinal or distant sites. This was the first study to show the feasibility of tumor suppressor gene replacement mediating local tumor regression.

Phase I studies of p53 replacement with adenoviral vectors (Ad) have also suggested clinical benefit with a few partial responses and several patients with stabilization of disease.[15–17] A large phase I study of Ad.p53 gene transfer delivered intratumorally combined with chemotherapy showed safety and evidence of increased apoptosis in transduced tumors when examined histologically.[18] A single-arm phase II study of intratumoral Ad.p53 in combination with radiation showed evidence of tumor regression in 63% (12 of 19) and was well tolerated.[19] However, in a phase II study in patients with at least 2 measurable lesions, there was no difference in response rates for lesions treated with Ad.p53/chemotherapy compared with chemotherapy alone, implying Ad.p53 provided little local benefit over chemotherapy.[20]

Keedy and colleagues[21] used repeated delivery of Ad.p53 by bronchoalveolar lavage (BAL) for patients with bronchioloalveolar carcinoma. BAL delivery resulted in transient expression of p53 in 19% (3 of 16), 2 of whom achieved stable disease. These results suggested that BAL could potentially be used for adenoviral delivery; however, there was considerable toxicity to this approach.

Guan and colleagues[22] performed a nonrandomized study with delivery of Ad.p53 alone or in combination with bronchial artery instillation (BAI) of chemotherapy (combination of fluorouracil, navelbine, or cisplatin). Ad.p53 delivery was performed via direct percutaneous delivery or via BAI. Results were encouraging for the indicator lesion with a 47% objective response rate in the combination group, and an improvement in time to progression when compared with BAI alone.

Although Ad.p53 has been approved for use in China, primarily based on studies of potential usefulness in head and neck cancers,[23] there are no current trials ongoing in the United States using this approach in lung cancer. In our opinion, the lack of a strong bystander effect coupled with the relatively low transfection efficiency of adenoviral vectors limits potential application in lung

cancer to treating local (ie, endobronchial) lesions unless more efficient vectors are developed.

FUS1 replacement

FUS1 is a novel tumor suppressor gene identified in the human chromosome 3p21.3 region where allele losses and genetic alterations occur early and frequently for many human cancers.[24] Expression of FUS1 protein is absent or reduced in most lung cancers and premalignant lung lesions. Restoration of wild-type FUS1 function in 3p21.3-deficient non–small cell lung carcinoma (NSCLC) cells significantly inhibits tumor cell growth by induction of apoptosis and alteration of cell cycle kinetics.[24] A phase I clinical trial is under way at MD Anderson Cancer Center (http://ClinicalTrials.gov, Identifier NCT0059605) to evaluate delivery of the FUS1 gene using repeated intravenous injection of liposomal particles. It will be interesting to determine the toxicity of this approach (injected DNA can activate toll-like receptors and induce inflammatory responses) and the efficiency of gene transfer to the lung.

Immunogene Therapy Approaches

Immunotherapy is based on the premise that there are intrinsic differences in the protein composition of tumor cells that allow the immune system to recognize tumor cells as foreign and kill them. However, established tumors have evolved many ways to evade or overwhelm the immune system, and thus some sort of exogenous stimulus is needed to enable the immune system to effectively eliminate tumor cells.[25]

Although immunotherapy is in its early stages of clinical development, there is now increasing evidence that a variety of cancer immunotherapy approaches can be highly effective under certain circumstances. Examples of successful approaches include: (1) vaccines (based on phase II and phase III data, the US Food and Drug Administration has recently approved Provenge, a prostate cancer vaccine),[26] (2) delivery of activating cytokines or chemokines into tumors, (3) adoptive T-cell transfer (dramatic antitumor responses using adoptive T-cell transfer have been shown in patients with melanoma[27] and Epstein-Barr virus lymphomas[28–30]), and (4) blockade of tumor immunosuppression (phase III data showing improved survival in patients with melanoma treated with a blocking antibody [ipilimumab] against the cytotoxic-T-lymphocyte-associated antigen 4 [CTLA-4], an immune checkpoint molecule that downregulates pathways of T-cell activation).[31]

Gene therapy approaches are becoming increasingly important in implementing immunotherapy.

Table 1
p53 gene therapy trials

Study	Phase	Histology	Total No. (No. Evaluable)	Vector	Delivery	Best Clinical Response (%)[a]	Additional Outcome Measures
Roth et al,[14] 1996	I	NSCLC	9 (7)	Retroviral p53	IT (single injection)	3 (33) with PR	All patients progressed at distant lesions 8 patients with evidence of gene transfer
Schuler et al,[15] 1998	I	NSCLC	15 (15)	Ad.p53	IT (single injection)	0 with PR 7 (47) with SD	6 patients with evidence of gene transfer
Swisher et al,[16] 1999	I	NSCLC	28 (25)	Ad.p53	IT (repeated injection)	2 (7) with PR 16 (57) with SD	18 patients with evidence of gene transfer
Nemunaitis et al,[18] 2000	I	NSCLC	24 (23)	Ad.p53	IT + cisplatin (up to 6 cycles)	2 (8) with PR 17 (71) with SD	6 patients with evidence of gene transfer
Schuler et al,[20] 2001	II	NSCLC	25 (25)[b]	Ad.p53	IT + chemotherapy (up to 3 cycles)	IT injected lesion: 13 (52) with PR Comparator lesion: 12 (48) with PR	No statistical difference between 2 groups 17 patients with evidence of gene transfer
Swisher et al,[19] 2003	II	NSCLC	19 (17)	Ad.p53	IT (3 injections) + radiation	1 (5) with CR 11 (58) with PR 3 (16) with SD	Biopsies of treated lesion 3 months after injection showed no viable tumor in 12 (63%) of 19 patients

Fujiwara et al,[17] 2006	NSCLC	15 (13)	Ad.p53	IT only, every 28 days (9 patients) IT + cisplatin, every cycle (6 patients)	1 (7) with PR 10 (66) with SD	The 1 PR was in Ad.p53 only group
Keedy et al,[21] 2008	BAC	29 (23)	Ad.p53	BAL, multiple instillations	16 (70) with SD	3 patients with evidence of gene transfer 8 patients with subjective improvement in pulmonary symptoms
Guan et al[22,c] 2009	NSCLC	58 (58)	Ad.p53	Vector only: IT injection or BAI Combo: vector + chemotherapy	Vector only: 15 (38) with PR, 8 (42) with SD Combo: 2 (11) with CR; 7 (37) with PR, 18 (46) with SD	No statistical difference in objective response between groups

Abbreviations: Ad, adenovirus; BAL, bronchoalveolar lavage; CR, complete response; IT, intratumoral; NSCLC, non–small cell lung cancer; PR, partial response; SD, stable disease.

a Best clinical response is noted for injected lesion only, unless otherwise noted.

b This study included patients who had 2 similar lesions, allowing for a comparison of the injected lesion with a comparator lesion.

c This study involved vector delivery by either by intratumoral injection or bronchial artery instillation (BAI); chemotherapy delivered via BAI.

Table 2
Immunogene therapy trials

Study	Phase	Histology	Total No. (No.Evaluable)	Vaccine	Delivery	Best Clinical Response (%)	Additional Outcome Measures
TGF-β							
Nemunaitis et al,[32] 2006	II[a]	NSCLC	75 (40)	Antisense gene-modified allogeneic tumor cell vaccine (belagenpumatucel-L)	Intradermal	Dose level 1: 1 of 11 (6) with PR Dose level 2: 3 of 11 (27) with PR Dose level 3: 2 of 13 (15) with PR	Dose-related overall survival differences were found between cohorts
Nemunaitis et al,[33] 2009	II	NSCLC	21 (20)	Belagenpumatucel-L	Intradermal	70% with SD	
GM-CSF							
Salgia et al,[34] 2003	I	NSCLC	37 (34)	Adenoviral modified autologous tumor cells engineered to secrete GM-CSF (GVAX)	Intradermal	1 (3) with MR 5 (15) with SD	Presence of CD4+/CD8+/CD20+ cell infiltration associated with tumor regression or disease stabilization
Nemunaitis et al,[35] 2004	I/II	NSCLC	83 (43)[b]	Adenoviral modified autologous tumor cells engineered to secrete GM-CSF (GVAX)	Intradermal	3 (9) with CR, 1 (3) with PR, 2 (6) with MR 7 (21) with SD	Vaccine associated GM-CSF secretion was associated with improvement in overall survival
Nemunaitis et al,[36] 2006	I/II	NSCLC	86 (49)	Autologous tumor cells with bystander cell line genetically modified to secrete GM-CSF (bystander GVAX)	Intradermal	No CR/PR, 4 (8) with MR 7 (14) with SD	Progression-free survival and median survival was better for subjects with injection site reactions
B7.1/HLA-A							
Raez et al,[37] 2004	I	NSCLC	19 (19)	AD100 adenocarcinoma cell line modified to express HLA-A1/A2 and B7	Subcutaneous	1 (7) with PR, 5 (26) with SD	Overall survival times ranging from 23 to 40+ months. 16 of 17 patients had a measurable CD8 response

α(1,3)galactosyltransferase

Study	Phase	Cancer	N (evaluable)	Vector/agent	Route	Response	Comments
Morris et al,[38] 2005	I	NSCLC	7 (7)	3 irradiated lung cancer cell lines modified by retroviral transfer of murine α(1,3) galactosyltransferase	Intradermal	No CR/PR, 4 (57) with SD	Data presented in abstract form only
p53							
Antonia et al,[39] 2006	II	SCLC	29 (29)	DC-Ad.p53	Intradermal	1 (3) with PR, 7 (24) with SD	Association between p53 specific T-cell response and response to second-line chemotherapy (after study)
MUC-1							
Ramlau et al,[41] 2008	II[a]	NSCLC	65 (53)	TG4010: vaccinia virus containing coding sequences for MUC-1 and IL-2 Arm 1: TG4010 + IV chemotherapy Arm 2: TG4010 alone (phase I), then TG4010 + IV chemotherapy (phase II)	Subcutaneous	Arm 1: 13 (35) with PR, 12 (32) with SD Arm 2: Phase I: 0 with PR, 2 (9.5) with SD Phase II: 1 (7%) with CR, 1 (7%) with PR	MUC-1 specific immune response was associated with longer time to disease progression and improved overall survival
L523S							
Nemunaitis et al,[42] 2006	I	NSCLC	13 (12)	pVAX/L523S (expressive plasmid) followed by Ad.L523S	Intramuscular	12 early-stage subjects (stage IB–IIB): median follow-up of 290 days: 2 recurrences; 1 second primary	Limited evidence of L523S-directed immune activation

Abbreviations: CR, complete response; IV, intravenous; NSCLC, non–small cell lung cancer; PR, partial response; SCLC, small cell lung cancer; SD, stable disease.

[a] Randomized phase II study.

[b] Response data in table is for 33 patients of the 43 evaluable.

Table 3
Antisense therapy trials

Study	Phase	Histology	Total No. (No. Evaluable)	Agent	Delivery	Best Clinical Response (%)	Additional Outcome Measures
Protein Kinase C (PKC)-α							
Villalona-Calero et al,[46] 2004	I/II	NSCLC	Phase II portion: 55 (49)	Antisense oligonucleotide to PKC-α (aprinocarsen)	IV aprinocarsen + IV gemcitabine/ cisplatin	Phase II: 1 (2) with CR, 15 with (31) with PR, 25 (49) with SD	Median overall survival of 8.9 mo
Vansteenkiste et al,[47] 2005	II[a]	NSCLC	Experimental arm: 9 (6) Control arm: 9 (9)	Aprinocarsen	IV aprinocarsen + IV gemcitabine/ cisplatin vs gemcitabine/ cisplatin alone	Experimental arm: 1 (17) with PR, 2 (34) with SD Control arm: 4 (44) with PR, 2 (22) with SD	Study terminated early because of publication of phase III study by Paz-Ares et al (2006)[49]
Ritch et al,[48] 2006	II	NSCLC	36 (29)	Aprinocarsen	IV aprinocarsen + IV gemcitabine/ cisplatin	9 (31) with PR, 11 (38) with SD	Median overall survival of 8.3 mo Severe thrombocytopenia in most patients
Paz-Ares et al,[49] 2006	III	NSCLC	Experimental arm: 342 (280) Control arm: 328 (289)	Aprinocarsen	IV aprinocarsen + IV gemcitabine/ cisplatin vs IV gemcitabine/ cisplatin alone	Experimental: 3 (1) with CR, 78 (28) with PR, 101 (36) with SD Control: 2 (1) with CR, 99 (34) with PR, 104 (36) with SD	Overall HR 1.05 (0.88–1.25)

c-Raf Kinase

Study	Phase	Tumor	No. (evaluable)	Agent	Treatment	Response	Comments
Coudert et al,[53] 2001	II	NSCLC, SCLC	NSCLC: 18 (15) SCLC: 8 (5)	Antisense oligonucleotide to c-Raf kinase (ISIS 5132)	Continuous 21-d IV infusion of ISIS 5132	0 CR/PR	c-Raf status not assessed

Bcl-2

Study	Phase	Tumor	No. (evaluable)	Agent	Treatment	Response	Comments
Rudin et al,[54] 2002	I	SCLC	12 (11)	Antisense oligonucleotide to Bcl-2 (G3139)	IV G3139 + IV paclitaxel	0 CR/PR, 2 (18) with SD	Suppression of Bcl-2 protein in PBMC noted in 1 pt with prolonged SD
Rudin et al,[55] 2004	I	SCLC	16 (14)	G3139	IV G139 + IV carboplatin/ etoposide	12 (86) with PR, 2 (14) with SD	No evidence of Bcl-2 suppression in PBMC
Rudin et al,[56] 2008	II[a]	SCLC	56 (48)	G3139	Arm A: IV cisplatin/ etoposide + IV G3139 Arm B: IV cisplatin/ etoposide alone	Arm A: 1 (2) with CR, 24 (59) with PR, 10 (24) with SD Arm B: 2 (13) with CR, 7 (47) with PR, 2 (13) with SD	Overall HR 2.1 (1.1–4.1)

Abbreviations: CR, complete response; HR, hazard ratio; IV, intravenous; NSCLC, non–small cell lung cancer; PBMC, peripheral blood mononuclear cells; PR, partial response; SCLC, small cell lung cancer; SD, stable disease.
[a] Randomized phase II study.

Specifically, gene therapy has been used to introduce tumor antigens directly, to introduce tumor antigens into dendritic cells (DC), to modify tumor cells used as vaccines, to introduce cytokines or chemokines into tumor cells in situ, and to introduce tumor-specificity to adoptively transferred T-cells. Several of these approaches have been tested in thoracic malignancies (see **Table 2**).

Gene-Modified Tumor Cell-Based Vaccination

Killed (usually irradiated) tumor cells that are then injected into patients as vaccines against recurrent cancer have been used for many years with only occasional success. Gene therapy has allowed investigators to modify these tumor cells (either autologous or allogeneic) to enhance immunogenicity.

Transforming growth factor β2 antisense vector modified cells

Increased levels of transforming growth factor β2 (TGF-β2) are associated with greater immunosuppression and with poorer prognosis in patients with NSCLC. In preclinical studies, delivery of an antisense gene targeting TGF-β2 to ex vivo tumor cells led to inhibition of cellular TGF-β2 expression and increased immunogenicity when these gene-modified tumor cells were used as a vaccine. This strategy of vaccination with irradiated tumor cells modified with a TGF-β2 antisense vector (belagenpumatucel-L) was evaluated in a phase II trial.[32] Each patient received 1 of 3 doses per month until disease progression. A dose-related survival advantage was observed with minimal toxicities. Differences in immunologic end points were also noted with increased cytokine (ie, interferon γ [IFN-γ], interleukin 6 [IL-6], IL-4) production and the development of HLA-antibody responses to the vaccine.

In a subsequent trial, 21 patients received belagenpumatucel-L at a single dose of 2.5×10^7 cells per month.[33] Stable disease was noted in 70%, but no complete or partial responses were observed. This compound is being evaluated in a phase III trial of patients with NSCLC.

Tumor cells genetically modified to secrete granulocyte-monocyte colony stimulating factor (GVAX)

Granulocyte-monocyte colony stimulating factor (GM-CSF) is a cytokine involved in the maturation and proliferation of myeloid progenitor cells and has been shown to stimulate proliferation, maturation, and migration of DC, which play a major role in induction of T-cell immune responses against cancer. Preclinical studies have shown that transfection of tumor cells with the GM-CSF gene markedly augmented the ability of these cells to induce antitumor immune responses.

Initial clinical trials in lung cancer used a patient-specific vaccine platform with intradermal vaccination of irradiated autologous tumor cells that were virally engineered to secrete GM-CSF.[34,35] In the first trial of metastatic NSCLC, GM-CSF was transduced into autologous tumor cells with the use of adenoviral vector before irradiation and patient vaccination.[34] A few clinical responses were observed and several lines of evidence suggested a strong immune response. In most patients, immunization elicited the development of a delayed hypersensitivity reaction to irradiated, autologous, nontransfected tumor cells. In a study that included both early-stage and late-stage patients, a similar strategy resulted in similarly promising results; several clinical responses were observed with similar evidence of immunologic outcomes.[35]

In an attempt to produce a vaccine with a more consistent rate of GM-CSF production, the next trial used a vaccine composed of unmodified, but irradiated autologous tumor cells mixed with a GM-CSF–secreting bystander cell line.[36] This approach eliminated the need for viral transduction and potentially allowed for more precise and higher rates of GM-CSF secretion. Although vaccine GM-CSF secretion with this approach was considerably higher than with the autologous vaccine, the frequency of vaccine site reactions, tumor responses, and survival were all less favorable with the bystander vaccine.

Based on lack of compelling evidence for efficacy in lung cancer and in other tumor types (such as prostate cancer) being studied, the GVAX (tumor cells genetically modified to secrete GM-CSF) approach has been abandoned in lung cancer, although studies in pancreatic cancer are ongoing.

B7.1/HLA vaccination

B7.1 (CD80) is responsible for costimulation of T cells during priming by an antigen-presenting cell (APC). Tumor cells transfected with B7.1 and foreign HLA molecules have been shown to stimulate an immune response leading to T-cell activation. The strategy of treatment with an allogeneic lung cancer cell line vaccine transfected with B7.1 and HLA-A1 or HLA-A2 was evaluated in a phase I trial of 19 patients with advanced NSCLC.[37] Overall, 1 patient had a partial response, and 5 had stable disease; however, the median overall survival in this group with a poor prognosis was an impressive 18 months. In the 6 responders, the CD8 T-cell titers to tumor cell stimulations remained increased up to 150 weeks after cessation of therapy. Based on the encouraging results of these trials in heavily pretreated patients, a trial is ongoing in patients with stage IIIB/IV disease who fail first-line chemotherapy (http://ClinicalTrials.gov, Identifier: NCT00534209).

α(1,3)Galactosyltransferase

The gene encoding α(1,3)-galactosyltransferase (αGT), which catalyzes the synthesis of αGal epitopes on glycoproteins and glycolipids, is inactive in humans but is functional in other mammalian cells. The human immune system produces anti-αGal antibodies, which is the major mechanism responsible for hyperacute rejection of xenotransplants. A phase I trial evaluated the use of allogeneic NSCLC tumor cells that were retrovirally modified to express αGT.[38] A total of 17 patients with advanced disease received up to 7 intradermal treatments, which were well tolerated and resulted in a 10-fold to 14-fold increase in serum anti-αGal titers. A total of 6 patients had prolonged stable disease. A phase II trial is under way at the National Cancer Institute (http://ClinicalTrials.gov, Identifier NCT-00075790).

Gene-Modified DC-Based Vaccination

DC are the most potent APCs in the immune system and have been used as vaccine vehicles. DC can be generated ex vivo from blood monocytes. One immunotherapy approach has been to load immature, phagocytic DC with antigen using purified protein, cell extracts, mRNA, or gene therapy vectors, mature the cells, and then inject these DC subcutaneously. A second approach has been to modify DC ex vivo with chemokines or cytokines and inject them directly into tumors where they can take up antigen, migrate to lymph nodes, and induce immune responses.

Ad.p53

Given that wild-type p53 protein has a brief half-life and is therefore present in low levels in normal cells, whereas mutant p53 has a significantly prolonged half-life and is present in greater quantities in tumor cells, p53 protein has been proposed as a good tumor antigen for a vaccine. Encouraging results with p53-based gene therapy have been attained with the combination of p53-transduced DC with standard chemotherapy.[39] In a phase I study, 29 patients with small cell lung cancer (SCLC) were vaccinated with DC transduced with Ad.p53, resulting in 1 partial response and 7 patients with stable disease. However, of the 21 patients receiving subsequent second-line chemotherapy, a 62% response rate was observed, considerably higher than the historical

response rate seen with second-line therapy in SCLC. A slight survival advantage (12.1 months vs 9.6 months) was observed for patients showing an immune response to vaccination. These results are promising, especially given the low survival rates and poor prognosis associated with advanced SCLC. A phase II trial is ongoing at H. Lee Moffitt Cancer Center (http://ClinicalTrials.gov, Identifier NCT00617409).

CCL21

CCL21 is a CC chemokine that is expressed at high levels in high endothelial venules and T-cell zones of spleen and lymph node, where it exerts potent attraction of naive T cells and mature DC, promoting T-cell activation.[40] Preclinical studies showed that DC transduced with CCL21 and injected into tumors had potent activity against lung cancers. A phase I clinical trial is ongoing at the University of California at Los Angeles in which DC derived from a leukopheresis sample are being transduced with an adenoviral vector encoding human CCL21 and then injected intratumorally under computed tomography (CT) guidance or bronchoscopy (http://ClinicalTrials.gov, Identifier NCT00601094). Results have not been published yet.

Vaccination Using Viral Vectors to Encode Tumor Antigens

Several trials have taken advantage of the strong innate and acquired immune responses to viruses by using viral vectors to encode tumor antigens to attempt to generate antitumor immune responses.

MUC-1 vaccination

MUC-1 is a tumor-associated mucin-type surface antigen normally found on epithelial cells in many tissues. Targeting of MUC-1 in lung cancer has been attempted in various ways including both gene and nongene therapy approaches. A vaccinia virus (VV) construct containing the coding sequences for MUC-1 and IL-2 (TG4010) was evaluated in a 2-arm phase II trial of 65 patients with stage IIIB/IV NSCLC.[41] All patients were required to have MUC-1 antigen expression on the primary tumor or a metastasis. Arm 1 consisted of upfront combination therapy with TG4010 and cisplatin/vinorelbine, whereas arm 2 used TG4010 monotherapy followed by combination therapy at progression. In arm 1 (44 patients), partial response was observed in 29.5%, with a 1-year survival rate of 53%. Arm 2 had 2 patients (of 21 total) with stable disease for more than 6 months with TG4010 monotherapy, but given the lack of efficacy this arm was closed early. MUC1-specific responses were measured with the enzyme-linked immunosorbent spot (ELISpot) assay (a method for measuring secretion of antigen-specific antibodies) and were observed in 57% of patients (12 of the 21) with either partial response or stable disease. In addition, 4 out of 5 patients who developed an ELISpot response during the study achieved disease control. Detectable MUC-1 specific responses were associated with significantly longer time to progression and overall survival. Based on the encouraging results of combination therapy, additional studies of TG4010 and chemotherapy are being performed in the first-line setting (http://ClinicalTrials.gov, identifier NCT00415818).

L523S vaccination

L523S is an immunogenic lung cancer antigen expressed in approximately 80% of lung cancer cells. In a phase I study, 13 patients with early-stage NSCLC (stage 1B, IIA, and IIB) were treated with 2 doses of intramuscular recombinant DNA (pVAX/L523S) followed by 2 doses of Ad.L523S given 4 weeks apart.[42] This vaccination schedule was used in an attempt to develop an immune response against the recombinant protein and thereby achieve a more substantial immune response to L523S. Although the regimen was well tolerated, only 1 patient showed a L523S-specific antibody response.

Adenovirus encoding B-galactosidase (Ad. β-gal)

Another strategy attempted early on in lung cancer was to use a replication deficient adenovirus containing the lacZ marker gene, which encodes the enzyme β-galactosidase (Ad. β-gal).[43] This initial dose-escalation trial was designed to investigate feasibility and tolerance of adenoviral vectors. Although B-galactosidase is not a true tumor antigen there was the possibility of antitumor responses as a result of antigen spreading from immune responses induced by the adenovirus or the transgene. A total of 12 patients with advanced lung cancer were treated with a single dose of Ad. β-gal and concomitant chemotherapy. One complete response was observed that lasted greater than 16 months after the last dose of gene therapy. Some patients at the highest dose level had CD4 and cytotoxic T-lymphocyte responses against both β-galactosidase and adenoviral particles.[44]

A separate group conducted 2 phase I studies of Ad. β-gal or Ad.IL-2 delivery in a total of 21 patients with NSCLC.[45] β-Galactosidase activity was measurable in most posttreatment biopsy samples; however, only low levels of IL-2 mRNA were detected. No clinical responses were noted.

Antisense Therapy

The rationale behind antisense therapy is that this technology offers the possibility of downregulating a wide variety of molecules that have been shown to promote lung cancer tumor growth. Antisense trials with 3 different targets have been published (see **Table 3**). The first used was aprinocarsen, a 20-mer oligonucleotide that binds to the mRNA for protein kinase C-α and inhibits its expression. Aprinocarsen was shown to be generally safe in patients with lung cancer, and had modest activity in combination with chemotherapy.[46–48] However, a phase III trial of chemotherapy with or without aprinocarsen as first-line therapy did not show enhanced survival and did show some toxicity.[49] Phase I studies in various patients who have advanced cancer with Raf antisense molecules showed a few patients with prolonged stable disease and 1 patient with a significant response.[50–52] Two phase II studies in lung cancer (total of 26 patients) failed to show any significant antitumor activity.[53] A third set of studies targeted Bcl-2, an apoptotic inhibitor that is overexpressed by many tumors including 80% to 90% of SCLCs and is associated with increased resistance to chemotherapy. Although 2 phase I trials had promising results,[54,55] a phase II study of standard chemotherapy with or without a bcl-2 antisense oligonucleotide (oblimersen) showed poorer overall survival in the experimental arm and greater hematologic toxicity.[56]

In general, these antisense approaches have not been successful. This finding is likely because the oligonucleotides even after modification are relatively unstable and thus difficult to deliver in adequate amounts and because in general they lack bystander effects. siRNA, which is more efficient, has promise, but still suffers from the same issues of adequate delivery to tumors and lack of bystander effects.

Clinical Trials Including Incidentally Treated Patients with Lung Cancer

Numerous other strategies have been used in cancer gene therapy and in some of these trials, patients with lung cancer have been included in either phase I or II studies. In this section, we examine some of these approaches and the results as they specifically pertain to lung cancer and the results of these strategies more generally.

Onyx-015

One additional approach to the use of p53 replacement has been the use of Onyx-015, an oncolytic adenovirus designed to replicate specifically in p53-mutant cells. When used alone, onyx-015 had limited efficacy, although some responses were noted in patients with head and neck cancer.[57,58] Onyx-015 has also been used in combination with Enbrel, a tumor necrosis factor (TNF)-α antagonist used to inhibit viral clearance. This study noted suppression of TNF-α secretion with some evidence of reduced viral clearance, but clinical efficacy was limited. Further trials are needed to evaluate higher Enbrel doses with potentially greater suppression of TNF-α.[59]

Carcinoembryonic antigen

Vaccine strategies have been devised by several groups that target carcinoembryonic antigen (CEA), a tumor marker known to be upregulated in many malignancies, particularly adenocarcinomas. The first such strategy used canarypox virus engineered to express both the costimulatory molecule B7 (to enhance response) and CEA.[60] In this phase I trial, 18 patients with metastatic tumors were treated including 3 with primary lung cancer. The vaccine was shown to be safe, but minimal clinical responses were noted in the patients with lung cancer.

A second phase I trial of a virally encoded CEA vaccine included 58 patients with advanced cancer, including 9 with primary lung cancer.[61] Eight cohorts received different combinations of 2 vectors (recombinant fowlpox and recombinant VV) and GM-CSF. The vaccines also encoded 3 costimulatory molecules to enhance immune response (B7, ICAM-1, and LFA-3, designated TRICOM). One patient with SCLC achieved a pathologic complete response, and significant immune responses were also observed. One-year survival was higher in patients with CEA-specific T-cell responses (83% vs 41%).

The CEA molecule has also been used in conjunction with gene-modified DC vaccination.[62] DC were transfected with a recombinant fowlpox vector encoding CEA and TRICOM. Although clinical responses were limited, immune responses were documented in most patients receiving DC-based anti-CEA therapy. Several ongoing phase II and III trials using the fowlpox-CEA/TRICOM vaccine are being conducted in patients with advanced NSCLC.

TNFerade

TNF-α is a proinflammatory cytokine that has been shown to possess direct cytotoxic effects on tumor endothelium and can increase procoagulant effect on tumor vasculature. In a phase I trial, 36 patients (including 5 with lung cancer) with accessible tumors were injected with adenoviral encoded TNF under the control of a radiation inducible promoter (TNFerade), followed by local radiation therapy.[63] A significant proportion of patients had objective tumor responses (43%), and in patients with synchronous lesions, TNFerade plus radiation was more efficacious than radiation alone. This approach effectively created high local levels of TNF-α for maximal antitumor effect without significant systemic toxicity. Other anti-TNF therapy trials that have included NSCLC have not noted significant clinical responses.[64]

Melanoma differentiation-associated gene (mda-7)

mda-7, also known as IL-24, is a tumor suppressor gene that can induce apoptosis in several cancer types. Cunningham and colleagues[50] performed a phase I trial in which 22 patients with advanced cancer were treated with intratumoral adenoviral-mda-7 (Ad.mda-7). Although response was evaluable in only 1 cohort of patients, all injected lesions showed intratumoral mda-7 DNA, RNA, and protein and apoptosis, as analyzed by TUNEL (terminal deoxynucleotidyl transferase dUTP nick end labeling) assay, correlated with MDA-7 protein expression. The 1 patient with lung cancer achieved stable disease and survived 180 days after treatment.

Clinical Trials in Mesothelioma and Malignant Pleural Disease

Gene therapy studies in MPM and malignant pleural disease has been facilitated because the pleural space is easily accessible and amenable to biopsy, allowing delivery of study vector/gene and fluid sampling to confirm successful gene transfer. Access and assessment of the pleural space have also been enhanced by the availability of indwelling tunneled pleural catheter systems. Accordingly, several groups have used a variety of gene therapy approaches in an attempt to improve treatment of these diseases (**Table 4**).

Suicide gene therapy

Suicide gene therapy involves transduction of tumor cells with a gene encoding for a specific enzyme that induces sensitivity to an otherwise benign agent. In essence, a prodrug is transformed into a toxic metabolite by the enzyme introduced into the cells with subsequent accumulation leading to tumor cell death or suicide.[65] An advantage of suicide gene therapy is the induction of a bystander effect: the killing of neighboring cells not transduced with the vector. A commonly studied suicide gene is the herpes simplex virus 1 thymidine kinase (HSVtk) gene, which makes transduced cells sensitive to the nucleoside analogue gancyclovir (GCV). GCV is metabolized poorly by mammalian cells and thus it is usually

Table 4
Mesothelioma gene therapy trials

Study	Phase	Histology	Total No. (No. Evaluable)	Agent	Delivery	Best Clinical Response (%)	Additional Outcome Measures
Suicide Gene Therapy							
Sterman et al,[67] 1998	I	MPM	21 (21)	Ad.HSV*tk* + IV GCV	Intrapleural: single dose	6 (29) with SD	Successful gene transfer in 11 patients
Sterman et al,[68] 2000	I	MPM	5 (5)	Ad.HSV*tk* + IV GCV + IV solumedrol	Intrapleural (Ad.HSV*tk*): single dose	N/A	Corticosteroids had no effect on cellular and humoral responses to Ad vector
Harrison et al,[70] 2000	I	MPM	16 (16)	PA1-STK (HSV*tk* gene modified ovarian cancer cell line) + IV GCV	Intrapleural: up to 3 doses	N/A	PA1-STK cells adhered preferentially to mesothelioma cells
Cytokine Gene Therapy							
Mukherjee et al,[71] 2000	I	MPM	6 (6)	VV expressing IL-2	Intratumoral: 3-12 doses	No significant tumor regression observed	VV-IL-2 mRNA detected for up to 3 weeks after each injection
Pitako et al,[72] 2003	I	MPM	14 (14)	Vero-IL-2 cells	Intratumoral: multiple doses	1 (7) with PR, 1 (7) with SD	7 patients with increased levels of serum IL-2 receptor
Sterman et al,[77] 2007	I	MPM MPE	MPM: 7 (7) MPE: 3 (3)	Ad.IFN-β	Intrapleural: single dose	1 (10) with CR, 2 (20) with PR, 4 (40) with SD	Successful gene transfer, induction of humoral/innate immune response
Sterman et al,[78] 2010	I	MPM MPE	MPM: 10 (10) MPE: 7 (7)	Ad.IFN-β	Intrapleural: 2 doses	3 (18) with PR/MR 11 (61) with SD	Successful gene transfer with first dose but not second, induction of humoral immune response
Sterman et al[80] 2011	I	MPM	9 (9)	Ad.IFN-α	Intrapleural: 2 doses	2 (22) PR, 4 (44) with SD	Ad.IFN-α induced higher levels of gene transfer than Ad.INF-β Induction of humoral/innate immune response

Abbreviations: Ad, adenovirus; CR, complete response; GCV, ganciclovir; IV, intravenous; MPE, malignant pleural effusion; MR, mixed response; N/A, not applicable; PR, partial response; SD, stable disease.

nontoxic. However, after conversion to GCV-monophosphate by HSV*tk*, it is metabolized rapidly by endogenous kinases to GCV-triphosphate, which acts as a potent inhibitor of DNA polymerase and competes with normal mammalian nucleosides for DNA replication.[65,66]

Sterman and colleagues[67–69] initiated a series of phase I clinical trials of adenovirus (Ad.HSV*tk*/GCV) gene therapy in patients with advanced MPM to assess toxicity, gene transfer efficiency, and immune response induction. After a single intrapleural administration of Ad.HSV*tk* vector, GCV was given intravenously twice daily for 2 weeks.

Trials using both a first-generation Ad vector and a more advanced-generation (E1/E4-deleted) adenoviral vector that allowed increased vector doses as a result of decreased contamination with high levels of replication-competent adenovirus were performed. Dose-related intratumoral HSV*tk* gene transfer was shown in 23 of 30 patients, with those treated at a dose equal to or greater than 3.2×10^{11} particle-forming units (pfu) having evidence of HSV*tk* protein expression at tumor surfaces and up to 30 to 50 cell layers deep. Overall, the therapy was well tolerated with minimal side effects, and dose-limiting toxicity was not reached. Antitumor antibodies and antiadenoviral immune responses, including high titers of antiadenoviral neutralizing antibody and proliferative T-cell responses, were generated in both serum and pleural fluid. Several clinical responses (ie, survival of more than 3 years) were seen at the higher dose levels, with 2 patients showing long periods of survival (1 7 years and 1 still alive after 10 years).[69] One of the 2 surviving patients had demonstrable reduction of tumor metabolic activity as assessed by serial [^{18}F]fluorodeoxyglucose (FDG) positron emission tomography (PET) scans over several months. This long response period was likely a result of induction of a secondary immune bystander effect of the Ad.HSV*tk*/GCV instillation.

Harrison and colleagues[70] conducted a phase I trial using irradiated ovarian carcinoma cells retrovirally transfected with HSV*tk* (PA1-STK cells) that were instilled intrapleurally followed by GCV for 7 days. Minimal side effects were seen and technetium 99m radiolabeled PA1-STK cells showed preferential adhesion to the tumor lining the chest wall. There were also some posttreatment increases in the percentage of CD8$^+$ T lymphocytes in the pleural fluid. However, no significant clinical responses were seen.

Cytokine gene therapy

The rationale for cytokine gene therapy is that high-level expression of immunostimulatory cytokines (such as IL-2, IL-12, TNF, GM-CSF, or IFN-α IFN-β, or IFN-γ) from tumor cells activates the immune system in situ, resulting in a more effective antitumor immune response without having to target specific antigens. The advantages of gene therapy over systemic administration of these agents includes lower toxicity, higher local concentrations, longer persistence of the cytokine, and advantages relating to cytokine secretion by the tumor cell itself.

Robinson and colleagues[71] conducted the first clinical trial of intratumoral cytokine gene delivery in patients with MPM using a recombinant partially replication-restricted VV that expressed the human IL-2 gene. Serial VV-IL-2 vector injections over a period of 12 weeks into chest wall lesions of 6 patients with advanced MPM resulted in minimal toxicity with no evidence of vector spread to patient contacts. Although no significant regression of tumor was seen, modest intratumoral T-cell infiltration was detected on posttreatment biopsy specimens. As measured by reverse transcriptase polymerase chain reaction, VV-IL-2 mRNA was detected in biopsy specimens for up to 6 days after injection (although declined to low levels by day 8) despite the generation of significant levels of anti-VV neutralizing antibodies.[71]

Vero cells, which are immortalized monkey fibroblasts capable of expressing human proteins, have also been studied as a cytokine delivery vector in humans. Fourteen patients with MPM received 4 courses of injections of Vero cells expressing IL-2. The treatment was well tolerated, with no significant adverse effects. Levels of circulating IL-2 were detected in half of the patients, with 1 patient showing transient tumor regression and 1 with disease stabilization for 4 months. To our knowledge, this approach is not being pursued further.[72]

Tan and colleagues[73] conducted a phase I clinical trial of 10 patients with malignant pleural effusions and persistent disease despite conventional therapy. Tumor-infiltrating lymphocytes acquired from the patients' effusions underwent retroviral-mediated IL-2 gene transfer before being infused back into the patients' chest cavities. The treatment was well tolerated, with transient mild fever being the most common adverse effect. Six of the 10 patients were effusion free for at least 4 weeks after treatment. One patient had both resolution of effusion as well as regression of the primary tumor.

Based on strong preclinical data,[74,75] a phase I Ad.IFN-β (Ad.IFN-β) dose-escalation trial in MPM (7 patients) and metastatic pleural malignancies (3 patients) was undertaken.[76,77] Gene transfer was detected in 7 of the 10 patients by measurement of pleural fluid IFN-β mRNA or protein. Antitumor immune responses, including humoral responses to known tumor antigens (eg, SV40 virus tag, mesothelin) and unknown tumor antigens were elicited in 7 of 10 patients. Four patients showed meaningful clinical responses defined as disease stability or partial regression on FDG-PET and CT imaging 2 months after vector administration.

In light of the encouraging results, a second study was performed with the aim of augmenting these immunologic and clinical responses.[78] Based on preclinical studies showing enhanced effects after 2 doses,[79] a second phase I trial involving 2 administrations of Ad.IFN-β (levels ranging from 3×10^{11} to 3×10^{12} viral particles) via an indwelling pleural catheter separated by 1 to 2 weeks was conducted in 17 patients (10 with MPM and 7 with malignant pleural effusions). Again, overall treatment was well tolerated, and antitumor humoral immune responses similar to that seen in the initial trials were induced. Several patients had meaningful clinical responses (mixed or partial responses) as determined by prevector and postvector delivery PET/CT scans. However, high antiadenoviral neutralizing antibodies titers were detected, even with a dose interval as short as 7 days, inhibiting effective gene transfer of the second dose.

A third phase I trial of Ad.IFN (α instead of β, solely as a result of changes in corporate sponsorship) has just been completed.[80] To avoid the effects of rapidly developing neutralizing antibodies to adenovirus, the protocol was modified to deliver the 2 Ad.IFN-α vector doses 3 days apart. Preliminary results show prolonged and high IFN-α protein expression in pleural fluid and serum. No clinical responses were seen in the 4 subjects with advanced disease. However,

evidence of disease stability or tumor regression was seen in the remaining 5 patients, including 1 dramatic example of partial tumor regression at sites not in contiguity with vector infusion (Fig. 1).

Based on preclinical studies showing synergy between Ad.IFN and systemic chemotherapy, our group at Penn has initiated a trial in which Ad.IFN-α is being administered in combination with first-line or second-line chemotherapy for patients with MPM. In addition, in light of animal studies showing a benefit of debulking surgery in combination with immunotherapy,[81] a neoadjuvant surgery trial involving vector administration to patients with MPM followed by maximal cytoreduction and adjuvant chemoradiotherapy is also being planned.

Tumor-based p53 therapy

There are 2 reports from China of using Ad.p53 to treat malignant effusions. Both studies noted more control of the effusion in patients who received the Ad.p53-based gene therapy, but did not report any data on tumor response rates or survival.[82,83] Thus, it is possible that this approach may have been useful only in achieving pleurodesis without any significant effect on the primary tumor.

SUMMARY AND FUTURE DIRECTIONS

In the past 2 decades, much experimentation using gene therapy has been carried out preclinically, and some clinical trials for thoracic malignancies have been performed. In general, these trials have shown safety, but only intermittent efficacy. In vivo gene transfer has been clearly achievable, but with the vectors currently available, it has been difficult to transduce more than a small percentage of tumor cells, and this is usually accomplished only by local injection. This

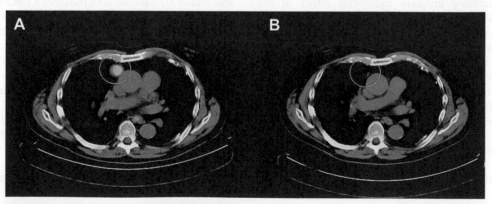

Fig. 1. Regression of mediastinal tumor after intrapleural Ad.IFN-α. (*A*) Pretreatment PET/CT image showing a pleural tumor nodule near the anterior mediastinum (*circled*). (*B*) Regression of nodule 6 months after treatment with Ad.IFN-α.

limitation has thus doomed the approaches that do not have strong bystander effects (ie, oncogene inactivation or replacement of tumor suppressor genes).

One potential approach that could avoid these problems is secretion of antitumor substances such as antiangiogenic agents. The development of vectors that can induce long-term in vivo expression, such as AAVs or lentiviruses, may make this feasible.

However, the primary direction of the field has been a shift toward immunogene therapy (**Fig. 2**). This strategy requires only enough gene transduction to stimulate an endogenous immune response and create a strong bystander effect. Promising approaches involve using gene therapy to stimulate antitumor responses by a vaccine or by delivering immunostimulatory cytokines. Although these strategies seem to be successful in initiating antitumor immune responses, investigators are beginning to recognize that they are limited by large tumor volumes and significant immunoinhibitory networks created by the tumors involving cytokines such as TGF-β, IL-10, prostaglandin E_2, and vascular endothelial cell growth factor and inhibitor cells such as T-regulatory cells and myeloid derived suppressor cells.[84] Future trials are likely to require combination approaches that stimulate the immune system, reduce tumor burden (surgery or chemotherapy), and inhibit the inhibitors (with agents such as cyclooxygenase 2 inhibitors or anti-CTLA-4 antibodies).

Another major direction of the field is to use adoptive transfer of gene-modified autologous lymphocytes that have been altered ex vivo by using retroviruses or lentiviruses to augment their ability to attack lung cancer or mesothelioma cells. This process can be achieved by transfection of T-cell receptors with altered specificity or by the introduction of totally artificial chimeric T-cell antigen receptors (CARs) that use single-chain antibody fragments to define antigen specificity and intracellular fragments of both the T-cell receptor and accessory molecules (such as CD28 or 4-1BB) to enhance activation.[85] A group at Baylor University has begun a clinical trial (see http://ClinicalTrials.gov, identifier NCT00889954) that is targeting HER-2-positive lung cancers with T cells directed to this antigen that have been modified with a chimeric receptor. These cells are also being modified to be resistant to TGF-β. Our group and a group at Memorial Sloan Kettering Cancer Center are designing CARs to target T cells to the tumor antigen mesothelin for use in the treatment of MPM. The approach has worked well in preclinical models,[86] and a clinical trial has been initiated at the University of Pennsylvania.

Gene therapy for lung cancer and MPM has not yet reached clinical practice. An appropriate analogy may be the development of monoclonal antibodies for which it took more than 20 years from discovery to clinical applications. Despite what some perceive as a slow start, we believe that progress is clearly being made and this

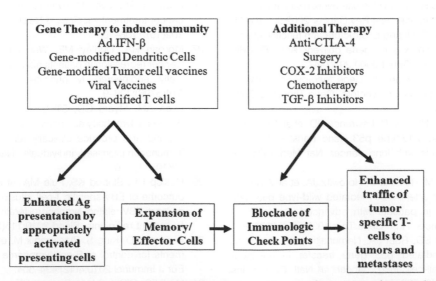

Fig. 2. Immunogene therapy paradigm. This approach relies on only enough gene transfer to induce immunity and generate a strong bystander effect. The antitumor immune responses are augmented by complementary approaches to target large tumor volumes or the immunosuppressive networks present in most tumors.

therapeutic tool will find its place in the anticancer armamentarium in the next decade.

REFERENCES

1. Maguire AM, Simonelli F, Pierce EA, et al. Safety and efficacy of gene transfer for Leber's congenital amaurosis. N Engl J Med 2008;358(21):2240–8.
2. Fischer A, Cavazzana-Calvo M. Gene therapy of inherited diseases. Lancet 2008;371(9629):2044–7.
3. Young LS, Searle PF, Onion D, et al. Viral gene therapy strategies: from basic science to clinical application. J Pathol 2006;208(2):299–318.
4. Bachtarzi H, Stevenson M, Fisher K. Cancer gene therapy with targeted adenoviruses. Expert Opin Drug Deliv 2008;5(11):1231–40.
5. Douglas JT. Adenoviral vectors for gene therapy. Mol Biotechnol 2007;36(1):71–80.
6. Breckpot K, Emeagi PU, Thielemans K. Lentiviral vectors for anti-tumor immunotherapy. Curr Gene Ther 2008;8(6):438–48.
7. Schambach A, Baum C. Clinical application of lentiviral vectors–concepts and practice. Curr Gene Ther 2008;8(6):474–82.
8. Daya S, Berns KI. Gene therapy using adeno-associated virus vectors. Clin Microbiol Rev 2008; 21(4):583–93.
9. Schultz BR, Chamberlain JS. Recombinant adeno-associated virus transduction and integration. Mol Ther 2008;16(7):1189–99.
10. Garber DA, O'Mara LA, Zhao J, et al. Expanding the repertoire of Modified Vaccinia Ankara-based vaccine vectors via genetic complementation strategies. PLoS One 2009;4(5):e5445.
11. Kirn DH, Thorne SH. Targeted and armed oncolytic poxviruses: a novel multi-mechanistic therapeutic class for cancer. Nat Rev Cancer 2009;9(1):64–71.
12. Chesnoy S, Huang L. Structure and function of lipid-DNA complexes for gene delivery. Annu Rev Biophys Biomol Struct 2000;29:27–47.
13. Niidome T, Huang L. Gene therapy progress and prospects: nonviral vectors. Gene Ther 2002;9(24): 1647–52.
14. Roth JA, Nguyen D, Lawrence DD, et al. Retrovirus-mediated wild-type p53 gene transfer to tumors of patients with lung cancer. Nat Med 1996;2(9): 985–91.
15. Schuler M, Rochlitz C, Horowitz JA, et al. A phase I study of adenovirus-mediated wild-type p53 gene transfer in patients with advanced non-small cell lung cancer. Hum Gene Ther 1998;9(14):2075–82.
16. Swisher SG, Roth JA, Nemunaitis J, et al. Adenovirus-mediated p53 gene transfer in advanced non-small-cell lung cancer. J Natl Cancer Inst 1999;91(9):763–71.
17. Fujiwara T, Tanaka N, Kanazawa S, et al. Multicenter phase I study of repeated intratumoral delivery of

adenoviral p53 in patients with advanced non-small-cell lung cancer. J Clin Oncol 2006;24(11): 1689–99.
18. Nemunaitis J, Swisher SG, Timmons T, et al. Adenovirus-mediated p53 gene transfer in sequence with cisplatin to tumors of patients with non-small-cell lung cancer. J Clin Oncol 2000;18(3):609–22.
19. Swisher SG, Roth JA, Komaki R, et al. Induction of p53-regulated genes and tumor regression in lung cancer patients after intratumoral delivery of adenoviral p53 (INGN 201) and radiation therapy. Clin Cancer Res 2003;9(1):93–101.
20. Schuler M, Herrmann R, De Greve JL, et al. Adenovirus-mediated wild-type p53 gene transfer in patients receiving chemotherapy for advanced non-small-cell lung cancer: results of a multicenter phase II study. J Clin Oncol 2001;19(6):1750–8.
21. Keedy V, Wang W, Schiller J, et al. Phase I study of adenovirus p53 administered by bronchoalveolar lavage in patients with bronchioloalveolar cell lung carcinoma: ECOG 6597. J Clin Oncol 2008;26(25): 4166–71.
22. Guan YS, Liu Y, Zou Q, et al. Adenovirus-mediated wild-type p53 gene transfer in combination with bronchial arterial infusion for treatment of advanced non-small-cell lung cancer, one year follow-up. J Zhejiang Univ Sci B 2009;10(5):331–40.
23. Peng Z. Current status of gendicine in China: recombinant human ad-p53 agent for treatment of cancers. Hum Gene Ther 2005;16(9):1016–27.
24. Ji L, Roth JA. Tumor suppressor FUS1 signaling pathway. J Thorac Oncol 2008;3(4):327–30.
25. Dunn GP, Bruce AT, Ikeda H, et al. Cancer immunoediting: from immunosurveillance to tumor escape. Nat Immunol 2002;3(11):991–8.
26. Brower V. Approval of Provenge seen as first step for cancer treatment vaccines. J Natl Cancer Inst 2010; 102(15):1108–10.
27. Morgan RA, Dudley ME, Wunderlich JR, et al. Cancer regression in patients after transfer of genetically engineered lymphocytes. Science 2006; 314(5796):126–9.
28. Leen AM, Myers GD, Sili U, et al. Monoculture-derived T lymphocytes specific for multiple viruses expand and produce clinically relevant effects in immunocompromised individuals. Nat Med 2006; 12(10):1160–6.
29. Heslop HE, Slobod KS, Pule MA, et al. Long-term outcome of EBV-specific T-cell infusions to prevent or treat EBV-related lymphoproliferative disease in transplant recipients. Blood 2010;115(5):925–35.
30. Brenner CD, King S, Przewoznik M, et al. Requirements for control of B-cell lymphoma by NK cells. Eur J Immunol 2010;40(2):494–504.
31. Hodi FS, O'Day SJ, McDermott DF, et al. Improved survival with ipilimumab in patients with metastatic melanoma. N Engl J Med 2010;363(8):711–23.

32. Nemunaitis J, Dillman RO, Schwarzenberger PO, et al. Phase II study of belagenpumatucel-L, a transforming growth factor beta-2 antisense gene-modified allogeneic tumor cell vaccine in non-small-cell lung cancer. J Clin Oncol 2006;24(29): 4721–30.

33. Nemunaitis J, Nemunaitis M, Senzer N, et al. Phase II trial of belagenpumatucel-L, a TGF-beta2 antisense gene modified allogeneic tumor vaccine in advanced non small cell lung cancer (NSCLC) patients. Cancer Gene Ther 2009;16(8):620–4.

34. Salgia R, Lynch T, Skarin A, et al. Vaccination with irradiated autologous tumor cells engineered to secrete granulocyte-macrophage colony-stimulating factor augments antitumor immunity in some patients with metastatic non-small-cell lung carcinoma. J Clin Oncol 2003;21(4):624–30.

35. Nemunaitis J, Sterman D, Jablons D, et al. Granulocyte-macrophage colony-stimulating factor gene-modified autologous tumor vaccines in non-small-cell lung cancer. J Natl Cancer Inst 2004;96(4):326–31.

36. Nemunaitis J, Jahan T, Ross H, et al. Phase 1/2 trial of autologous tumor mixed with an allogeneic GVAX vaccine in advanced-stage non-small-cell lung cancer. Cancer Gene Ther 2006;13(6):555–62.

37. Raez LE, Cassileth PA, Schlesselman JJ, et al. Allogeneic vaccination with a B7.1 HLA-A gene-modified adenocarcinoma cell line in patients with advanced non-small-cell lung cancer. J Clin Oncol 2004;22(14):2800–7.

38. Morris JC, Vahanian N, Janik JE, et al. Phase I study of an antitumor vaccination using alpha(1,3)galactosyltransferase expressing allogeneic tumor cells in patients with refractory or recurrent non-small cell lung cancer (NSCLC). J Clin Oncol 2005;23(16S): 2586.

39. Antonia SJ, Mirza N, Fricke I, et al. Combination of p53 cancer vaccine with chemotherapy in patients with extensive stage small cell lung cancer. Clin Cancer Res 2006;12(3 Pt 1):878–87.

40. Baratelli F, Takedatsu H, Hazra S, et al. Pre-clinical characterization of GMP grade CCL21-gene modified dendritic cells for application in a phase I trial in non-small cell lung cancer. J Transl Med 2008;6:38.

41. Ramlau R, Quoix E, Rolski J, et al. A phase II study of Tg4010 (mva-Muc1-Il2) in association with chemotherapy in patients with stage III/IV non-small cell lung cancer. J Thorac Oncol 2008;3(7):735–44.

42. Nemunaitis J, Meyers T, Senzer N, et al. Phase I trial of sequential administration of recombinant DNA and adenovirus expressing L523S protein in early stage non-small-cell lung cancer. Mol Ther 2006; 13(6):1185–91.

43. Tursz T, Cesne AL, Baldeyrou P, et al. Phase I study of a recombinant adenovirus-mediated gene transfer in lung cancer patients. J Natl Cancer Inst 1996;88(24):1857–63.

44. Molinier-Frenkel V, Le Boulaire C, Le Gal FA, et al. Longitudinal follow-up of cellular and humoral immunity induced by recombinant adenovirus-mediated gene therapy in cancer patients. Hum Gene Ther 2000;11(13):1911–20.

45. Griscelli F, Opolon P, Saulnier P, et al. Recombinant adenovirus shedding after intratumoral gene transfer in lung cancer patients. Gene Ther 2003;10(5): 386–95.

46. Villalona-Calero MA, Ritch P, Figueroa JA, et al. A phase I/II study of LY900003, an antisense inhibitor of protein kinase C-alpha, in combination with cisplatin and gemcitabine in patients with advanced non-small cell lung cancer. Clin Cancer Res 2004; 10(18 Pt 1):6086–93.

47. Vansteenkiste J, Canon JL, Riska H, et al. Randomized phase II evaluation of aprinocarsen in combination with gemcitabine and cisplatin for patients with advanced/metastatic non-small cell lung cancer. Invest New Drugs 2005;23(3):263–9.

48. Ritch P, Rudin CM, Bitran JD, et al. Phase II study of PKC-alpha antisense oligonucleotide aprinocarsen in combination with gemcitabine and carboplatin in patients with advanced non-small cell lung cancer. Lung Cancer 2006;52(2):173–80.

49. Paz-Ares L, Douillard JY, Koralewski P, et al. Phase III study of gemcitabine and cisplatin with or without aprinocarsen, a protein kinase C-alpha antisense oligonucleotide, in patients with advanced-stage non-small-cell lung cancer. J Clin Oncol 2006; 24(9):1428–34.

50. Cunningham CC, Holmlund JT, Schiller JH, et al. A phase I trial of c-Raf kinase antisense oligonucleotide ISIS 5132 administered as a continuous intravenous infusion in patients with advanced cancer. Clin Cancer Res 2000;6(5):1626–31.

51. Rudin CM, Holmlund J, Fleming GF, et al. Phase I trial of ISIS 5132, an antisense oligonucleotide inhibitor of c-Raf-1, administered by 24-hour weekly infusion to patients with advanced cancer. Clin Cancer Res 2001;7(5):1214–20.

52. Stevenson JP, Yao KS, Gallagher M, et al. Phase I clinical/pharmacokinetic and pharmacodynamic trial of the c-Raf-1 antisense oligonucleotide ISIS 5132 (CGP 69846A). J Clin Oncol 1999;17(7): 2227–36.

53. Coudert B, Anthoney A, Fiedler W, et al. Phase II trial with ISIS 5132 in patients with small-cell (SCLC) and non-small cell (NSCLC) lung cancer. A European Organization for Research and Treatment of Cancer (EORTC) early clinical studies group report. Eur J Cancer 2001;37 (17):2194–8.

54. Rudin CM, Otterson GA, Mauer AM, et al. A pilot trial of G3139, a bcl-2 antisense oligonucleotide, and paclitaxel in patients with chemorefractory small-cell lung cancer. Ann Oncol 2002;13(4):539–45.

55. Rudin CM, Kozloff M, Hoffman PC, et al. Phase I study of G3139, a bcl-2 antisense oligonucleotide, combined with carboplatin and etoposide in patients with small-cell lung cancer. J Clin Oncol 2004;22(6):1110–7.

56. Rudin CM, Salgia R, Wang X, et al. Randomized phase II study of carboplatin and etoposide with or without the bcl-2 antisense oligonucleotide oblimersen for extensive-stage small-cell lung cancer: CALGB 30103. J Clin Oncol 2008;26(6):870–6.

57. Nemunaitis J, Cunningham C, Buchanan A, et al. Intravenous infusion of a replication-selective adenovirus (ONYX-015) in cancer patients: safety, feasibility and biological activity. Gene Ther 2001; 8(10):746–59.

58. Nemunaitis J, Khuri F, Ganly I, et al. Phase II trial of intratumoral administration of ONYX-015, a replication-selective adenovirus, in patients with refractory head and neck cancer. J Clin Oncol 2001;19(2):289–98.

59. Nemunaitis J, Senzer N, Sarmiento S, et al. A phase I trial of intravenous infusion of ONYX-015 and enbrel in solid tumor patients. Cancer Gene Ther 2007;14(11):885–93.

60. Horig H, Lee DS, Conkright W, et al. Phase I clinical trial of a recombinant canarypoxvirus (ALVAC) vaccine expressing human carcinoembryonic antigen and the B7.1 co-stimulatory molecule. Cancer Immunol Immunother 2000;49(9):504–14.

61. Marshall JL, Gulley JL, Arlen PM, et al. Phase I study of sequential vaccinations with fowlpox-CEA (6D)-TRICOM alone and sequentially with vaccinia-CEA(6D)-TRICOM, with and without granulocyte-macrophage colony-stimulating factor, in patients with carcinoembryonic antigen-expressing carcinomas. J Clin Oncol 2005;23(4):720–31.

62. Morse MA, Clay TM, Hobeika AC, et al. Phase I study of immunization with dendritic cells modified with fowlpox encoding carcinoembryonic antigen and costimulatory molecules. Clin Cancer Res 2005;11(8):3017–24.

63. Senzer N, Mani S, Rosemurgy A, et al. TNFerade biologic, an adenovector with a radiation-inducible promoter, carrying the human tumor necrosis factor alpha gene: a phase I study in patients with solid tumors. J Clin Oncol 2004;22(4):592–601.

64. McLoughlin JM, McCarty TM, Cunningham C, et al. TNFerade, an adenovector carrying the transgene for human tumor necrosis factor alpha, for patients with advanced solid tumors: surgical experience and long-term follow-up. Ann Surg Oncol 2005; 12(10):825–30.

65. Tiberghien P. Use of suicide genes in gene therapy. J Leukoc Biol 1994;56(2):203–9.

66. Matthews T, Boehme R. Antiviral activity and mechanism of action of ganciclovir. Rev Infect Dis 1988; 10(Suppl 3):S490–4.

67. Sterman DH, Treat J, Litzky LA, et al. Adenovirus-mediated herpes simplex virus thymidine kinase/ganciclovir gene therapy in patients with localized malignancy: results of a phase I clinical trial in malignant mesothelioma. Hum Gene Ther 1998;9(7):1083–92.

68. Sterman DH, Molnar-Kimber K, Iyengar T, et al. A pilot study of systemic corticosteroid administration in conjunction with intrapleural adenoviral vector administration in patients with malignant pleural mesothelioma. Cancer Gene Ther 2000;7(12):1511–8.

69. Sterman DH, Recio A, Vachani A, et al. Long-term follow-up of patients with malignant pleural mesothelioma receiving high-dose adenovirus herpes simplex thymidine kinase/ganciclovir suicide gene therapy. Clin Cancer Res 2005;11(20):7444–53.

70. Harrison LH Jr, Schwarzenberger PO, Byrne PS, et al. Gene-modified PA1-STK cells home to tumor sites in patients with malignant pleural mesothelioma. Ann Thorac Surg 2000;70(2):407–11.

71. Mukherjee S, Haenel T, Himbeck R, et al. Replication-restricted vaccinia as a cytokine gene therapy vector in cancer: persistent transgene expression despite antibody generation. Cancer Gene Ther 2000;7(5):663–70.

72. Pitako J, Squiban P, Acres B. A randomized phase II single center study of gene transfer-based non-specific immunotherapy of malignant mesothelioma (MM) by intratumoral injections of an interleukin-2 producing vero cells. Proc Am Soc Clin Oncol 2003;22 [abstract: 920].

73. Tan Y, Xu M, Wang W, et al. IL-2 gene therapy of advanced lung cancer patients. Anticancer Res 1996;16(4A):1993–8.

74. Odaka M, Sterman DH, Wiewrodt R, et al. Eradication of intraperitoneal and distant tumor by adenovirus-mediated interferon-beta gene therapy is attributable to induction of systemic immunity. Cancer Res 2001;61(16):6201–12.

75. Odaka M, Wiewrodt R, DeLong P, et al. Analysis of the immunologic response generated by ad.IFN-beta during successful intraperitoneal tumor gene therapy. Mol Ther 2002;6(2):210–8.

76. Sterman DH, Gillespie CT, Carroll RG, et al. Interferon beta adenoviral gene therapy in a patient with ovarian cancer. Nat Clin Pract Oncol 2006; 3(11):633–9.

77. Sterman DH, Recio A, Carroll RG, et al. A phase I clinical trial of single-dose intrapleural IFN-beta gene transfer for malignant pleural mesothelioma and metastatic pleural effusions: high rate of anti-tumor immune responses. Clin Cancer Res 2007; 13(15 Pt 1):4456–66.

78. Sterman DH, Recio A, Haas AR, et al. A phase I trial of repeated intrapleural adenoviral-mediated interferon-beta gene transfer for mesothelioma and

metastatic pleural effusions. Mol Ther 2010;18(4): 852–60.

79. Lambright ES, Force SD, Lanuti ME, et al. Efficacy of repeated adenoviral suicide gene therapy in a localized murine tumor model. Ann Thorac Surg 2000;70(6):1865–70 [discussion: 1870–1].

80. Sterman DH, Haas AR, Moon E, et al. A phase I trial of intrapleural adenoviral-mediated interferon-alpha2b gene transfer for malignant pleural mesothelioma. Am J Respir Crit Care Med 2011. DOI:10.1164/rccm.201103-0554CR.

81. Kruklitis RJ, Singhal S, Delong P, et al. Immuno-gene therapy with interferon-beta before surgical debulking delays recurrence and improves survival in a murine model of malignant mesothelioma. J Thorac Cardiovasc Surg 2004;127(1):123–30.

82. Dong M, Li X, Hong LJ, et al. Advanced malignant pleural or peritoneal effusion in patients treated with recombinant adenovirus p53 injection plus cisplatin. J Int Med Res 2008;36(6):1273–8.

83. Zhao WZ, Wang JK, Li W, et al. Clinical research on recombinant human ad-p53 injection combined with cisplatin in treatment of malignant pleural effusion induced by lung cancer. Ai Zheng 2009;28(12): 1324–7 [in Chinese].

84. Kim R, Emi M, Tanabe K, et al. Tumor-driven evolution of immunosuppressive networks during malignant progression. Cancer Res 2006;66(11): 5527–36.

85. June CH. Adoptive T cell therapy for cancer in the clinic. J Clin Invest 2007;117(6):1466–76.

86. Carpenito C, Milone MC, Hassan R, et al. Control of large, established tumor xenografts with genetically retargeted human T cells containing CD28 and CD137 domains. Proc Natl Acad Sci U S A 2009; 106(9):3360–5.

Index

Note: Page numbers of article titles are in **boldface** type.

Clin Chest Med 32 (2011) 887–895
doi:10.1016/S0272-5231(11)00102-X
0272-5231/11/$ – see front matter © 2011 Elsevier Inc. All rights reserved.

United States Postal Service

Statement of Ownership, Management, and Circulation
(All Periodicals Publications Except Requestor Publications)

1. Publication Title	2. Publication Number	3. Filing Date
Clinics in Chest Medicine	0 0 0 - 7 0 6	9/16/11

4. Issue Frequency	5. Number of Issues Published Annually	6. Annual Subscription Price
Mar, Jun, Sep, Dec	4	$293.00

7. Complete Mailing Address of Known Office of Publication (Not printer) (Street, city, county, state, and ZIP+4®)

Elsevier Inc.
360 Park Avenue South
New York, NY 10010-1710

Contact Person
Amy S. Beacham

Telephone (Include area code)
215-239-3687

8. Complete Mailing Address of Headquarters or General Business Office of Publisher (Not printer)

Elsevier Inc., 360 Park Avenue South, New York, NY 10010-1710

9. Full Names and Complete Mailing Addresses of Publisher, Editor, and Managing Editor (Do not leave blank)

Publisher (Name and complete mailing address)

Kim Murphy, Elsevier, Inc., 1600 John F. Kennedy Blvd. Suite 1800, Philadelphia, PA 19103-2899

Editor (Name and complete mailing address)

Sarah Barth, Elsevier, Inc., 1600 John F. Kennedy Blvd. Suite 1800, Philadelphia, PA 19103-2899

Managing Editor (Name and complete mailing address)

Sarah Barth, Elsevier, Inc., 1600 John F. Kennedy Blvd. Suite 1800, Philadelphia, PA 19103-2899

10. Owner (Do not leave blank. If the publication is owned by a corporation, give the name and address of the corporation immediately followed by the names and addresses of all stockholders owning or holding 1 percent or more of the total amount of stock. If not owned by a corporation, give the names and addresses of the individual owners. If owned by a partnership or other unincorporated firm, give its name and address as well as those of each individual owner. If the publication is published by a nonprofit organization, give its name and address.)

Full Name	Complete Mailing Address
Wholly owned subsidiary of	4520 East-West Highway
Reed/Elsevier, US holdings	Bethesda, MD 20814

11. Known Bondholders, Mortgagees, and Other Security Holders Owning or Holding 1 Percent or More of Total Amount of Bonds, Mortgages, or Other Securities. If none, check box ☐ None

Full Name	Complete Mailing Address
N/A	

12. Tax Status (For completion by nonprofit organizations authorized to mail at nonprofit rates) (Check one)
The purpose, function, and nonprofit status of this organization and the exempt status for federal income tax purposes:
☐ Has Not Changed During Preceding 12 Months
☐ Has Changed During Preceding 12 Months (Publisher must submit explanation of change with this statement)

PS Form 3526, September 2007 (Page 1 of 3 (Instructions Page 3)) PSN 7530-01-000-9931 PRIVACY NOTICE: See our Privacy policy in www.usps.com

13. Publication Title	14. Issue Date for Circulation Data Below
Clinics in Chest Medicine	September 2011

15. Extent and Nature of Circulation		Average No. Copies Each Issue During Preceding 12 Months	No. Copies of Single Issue Published Nearest to Filing Date
a. Total Number of Copies (Net press run)		2044	1540
b. Paid Circulation (By Mail and Outside the Mail)	(1) Mailed Outside-County Paid Subscriptions Stated on PS Form 3541. (Include paid distribution above nominal rate, advertiser's proof copies, and exchange copies)	1045	962
	(2) Mailed In-County Paid Subscriptions Stated on PS Form 3541 (Include paid distribution above nominal rate, advertiser's proof copies, and exchange copies)		
	(3) Paid Distribution Outside the Mails Including Sales Through Dealers and Carriers, Street Vendors, Counter Sales, and Other Paid Distribution Outside USPS®	451	408
	(4) Paid Distribution by Other Classes Mailed Through the USPS (e.g. First-Class Mail®)		
c. Total Paid Distribution (Sum of 15b (1), (2), (3), and (4))		1496	1370
d. Free or Nominal Rate Distribution (By Mail and Outside the Mail)	(1) Free or Nominal Rate Outside-County Copies Included on PS Form 3541	62	46
	(2) Free or Nominal Rate In-County Copies Included on PS Form 3541		
	(3) Free or Nominal Rate Copies Mailed at Other Classes Through the USPS (e.g. First-Class Mail)		
	(4) Free or Nominal Rate Distribution Outside the Mail (Carriers or other means)		
e. Total Free or Nominal Rate Distribution (Sum of 15d (1), (2), (3) and (4))		62	46
f. Total Distribution (Sum of 15c and 15e)		1558	1416
g. Copies not Distributed (See instructions to publishers #4 (page #3))		486	124
h. Total (Sum of 15f and g)		2044	1540
i. Percent Paid (15c divided by 15f times 100)		96.02%	96.75%

16. Publication of Statement of Ownership

☐ If the publication is a general publication, publication of this statement is required. Will be printed in the **December 2011** issue of this publication. ☐ Publication not required

17. Signature and Title of Editor, Publisher, Business Manager, or Owner

Amy S. Beacham — Senior Inventory Distribution Coordinator

Date: September 16, 2011

I certify that all information furnished on this form is true and complete. I understand that anyone who furnishes false or misleading information on this form or who omits material or information requested on the form may be subject to criminal sanctions (including fines and imprisonment) and/or civil sanctions (including civil penalties).

PS Form 3526, September 2007 (Page 2 of 3)

Moving?

Make sure your subscription moves with you!

To notify us of your new address, find your **Clinics Account Number** (located on your mailing label above your name), and contact customer service at:

Email: journalscustomerservice-usa@elsevier.com

800-654-2452 (subscribers in the U.S. & Canada)
314-447-8871 (subscribers outside of the U.S. & Canada)

Fax number: 314-447-8029

Elsevier Health Sciences Division
Subscription Customer Service
3251 Riverport Lane
Maryland Heights, MO 63043

*To ensure uninterrupted delivery of your subscription, please notify us at least 4 weeks in advance of move.

ELSEVIER

Printed and bound by CPI Group (UK) Ltd, Croydon, CR0 4YY

14/10/2024

01773879-0001